AF669523

Symptom Oriented Otolaryngology Head and Neck Surgery

Rhinology and Facial Plastics

Symptom Oriented Otolaryngology Head and Neck Surgery

Vol. 2

Rhinology and Facial Plastics

Chief Editors

Zahoor Ahmad MBBS MS FRACS
Consultant Otolaryngologist—Head and Neck Surgeon
Counties-Manukau Health, Auckland University Hospitals
Vice-Chairman
Department of Otolaryngology—Head and Neck Surgery
Counties-Manukau Health
Auckland University Hospitals
Auckland, New Zealand

Randall P Morton MBBS MSc FRACS
Consultant Otolaryngologist—Head and Neck Surgeon
Counties-Manukau Health
Professor of Otolaryngology, University of Auckland
Deputy Clinical Director of Surgery in Counties-Manukau Health
Auckland, New Zealand

Malcolm Giles MBChB FRACS
Otolaryngologist, Otolaryngology Clinic
Waikato Hospital
Hamilton, New Zealand

Foreword

Eugene N Myers MD

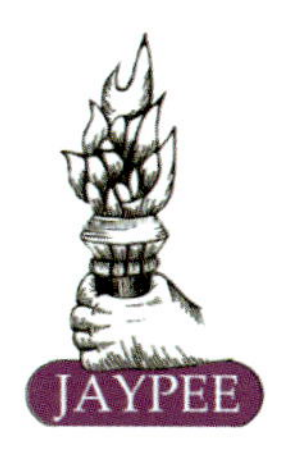

The Health Sciences Publisher
New Delhi | London | Panama

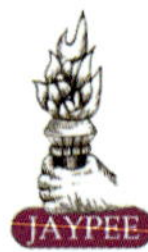

Jaypee Brothers Medical Publishers (P) Ltd

Headquarters

Jaypee Brothers Medical Publishers (P) Ltd.
4838/24, Ansari Road, Daryaganj
New Delhi 110 002, India
Phone: +91-11-43574357
Fax: +91-11-43574314
Email: jaypee@jaypeebrothers.com

Overseas Offices

J.P. Medical Ltd.
83, Victoria Street, London
SW1H 0HW (UK)
Phone: +44-20 3170 8910
Fax: +44 (0)20 3008 6180
Email: info@jpmedpub.com

Jaypee-Highlights Medical Publishers Inc.
City of Knowledge, Bld. 235, 2nd Floor, Clayton
Panama City, Panama
Phone: +1 507-301-0496
Fax: +1 507-301-0499
Email: cservice@jphmedical.com

Jaypee Brothers Medical Publishers (P) Ltd.
17/1-B Babar Road, Block-B, Shaymali
Mohammadpur, Dhaka-1207
Bangladesh
Mobile: +08801912003485
Email: jaypeedhaka@gmail.com

Jaypee Brothers Medical Publishers (P) Ltd.
Bhotahity, Kathmandu, Nepal
Phone +977-9741283608
Email: kathmandu@jaypeebrothers.com

Website: www.jaypeebrothers.com
Website: www.jaypeedigital.com

Inquiries for bulk sales may be solicited at: jaypee@jaypeebrothers.com

Symptom Oriented Otolaryngology—Head and Neck Surgery: (Vol. 2) Rhinology and Facial Plastics

First Edition: **2017**

ISBN 978-93-85891-84-7

Printed at Replika Press Pvt. Ltd.

Dedication

We dedicate this work to our wives and children, whose unconditional love and support have been the source of our inspiration and energy.

Zahoor Ahmad
Randall P Morton
Malcolm Giles

Chief Editors

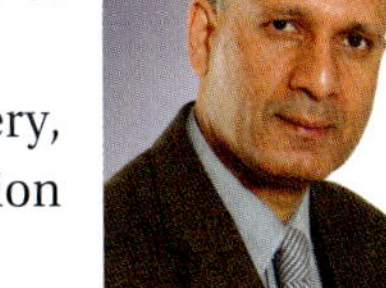

Zahoor Ahmad is Consultant Otolaryngologist—Head and Neck Surgeon, Counties-Manukau Health, Auckland University Hospitals, Auckland, New Zealand. He is the Vice-Chairman, Department of Otolaryngology—Head and Neck Surgery, Counties-Manukau Health, Auckland, New Zealand.

He is a member of the New Zealand Society of Otolaryngology—Head and Neck Surgery, American Academy of Otolaryngology—Head and Neck Surgery and a life member of the Association of Otolaryngologists of India.

He previously served as President of the Northern Regional Society of Otolaryngology—Head and Neck Surgery, New Zealand.

Dr Ahmad has clinical interests in head and neck, salivary, thyroid, nasal, and sinus diseases. His thesis for MS (Masters in Surgery) was on adenoids and middle ear disease in children.

He has lectured in a number of scientific meetings and has been a keynote Lecturer in several International meetings. He participates and instructs in International workshops focusing on salivary diseases and sinus problems. He has about 75 publications in peer-reviewed International journals and has also written chapters in books. He is actively involved in teaching and examining undergraduate and postgraduate medical students.

Dr Ahmad was born in Kashmir, India and after postgraduation has traveled widely before falling in love with New Zealand and made it his home.

He is supported by his wife, two sons, and two granddaughters and has passion for golf and enjoys playing the game. He enjoys listening to classical music. He loves to watch rugby and cricket.

Zahoor Ahmad MBBS MS FRACS

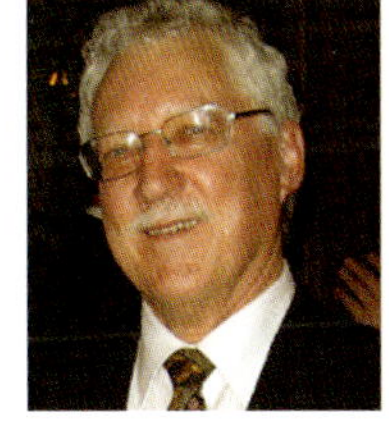

Randall P Morton is Consultant Otolaryngologist—Head and Neck Surgeon, Counties-Manukau Health, Auckland University Hospitals, Auckland, New Zealand. He is Professor of Otolaryngology at Auckland University Medical School and Deputy Clinical Director of Surgery in Counties-Manukau Health, Auckland, New Zealand.

He is currently the Chairman of the Royal Australasian College of Surgeons (RACS), New Zealand National Board. He was previously RACS Councillor, RACS Examiner in Otolaryngology—Head and Neck Surgery, and Chairman of the RACS Head and Neck Section and also served on RACS Board of Otolaryngology-Head and Neck Surgery (O-HNS).

He was the 1999 RACS/RCSI Visiting Professor to Ireland, and the 2005 RACS Foundation Lecturer in Head and Neck Surgery and was awarded the RACS Colin McRae Medal in 2004. He was member of the Board of Studies for the Auckland University Master of Audiology (MAud) Program, and the Medical Advisory Committee of the Auckland Division of the New Zealand Cancer Society, Auckland, New Zealand. He previously served as President of The New Zealand Society of Otolaryngology—Head and Neck Surgery (NZSOHNS), Wellington, New Zealand, Australia & New Zealand Head and Neck Cancer Society, and Asia-Oceania Association of Otolaryngology Societies.

His clinical interest is principally head and neck surgery, with a focus on surgical oncology and non-neoplastic parotid and thyroid diseases. His MSc thesis was on the epidemiology of sinonasal cancer and Triologic Society (USA) thesis was based on research into quality-of-life outcomes in head and neck cancer patients.

He received Presidential Citations from American Head and Neck Society and NZSOHNS. Keynote Lectures in several International meetings, including Eponymous Lectures in the UK, USA, and New Zealand.

He is supported by his wife, two daughters, and two granddaughters. He plays the bagpipes in a Pipe & Drum band and—if at all possible—avoids invitations to play golf. He also loves Australian rules football, soccer and cricket.

Randall P Morton MBBS MSc FRACS

Malcolm Giles is a specialist Otolaryngologist at Waikato Hospital, Hamilton, New Zealand. He qualified from Auckland University School of Medicine, Auckland, New Zealand in 1979, and became a fellow of Royal Australasian College of Surgeons, Melbourne, Australia in 1986. He became a fellow at the Royal Infirmary in Glasglow, UK from 1988 to 89, studying the relationship between hearing loss and disability as well as the management of severe hearing loss.

On completing this Fellowship in late 1989, Dr Giles became a full-time consultant otolaryngologist at Waikato Hospital, Hamilton, New Zealand, where he has worked since then. His main areas of practice are otology, congenital deafness, and otoneurology. He is also heavily involved in teaching medical students, and registrars training in otolaryngology as well as general otolaryngology. He also attends special clinics in otoneurology, congenital hearing loss, and combined clinics caring for children with cleft lip and palate.

Malcolm Giles MBChB FRACS

Associate Editors

Salil B Nair graduated from medical school at University of Dundee, UK in 1991. He obtained his surgical fellowships from both the Royal Colleges of London and Edinburgh. In 1999, he was awarded a prestigious Wellcome Trust Fellowship to pursue basic sciences research. He was awarded his MD in 2002.

Having completed an advanced Rhinology and Skull Base fellowship under the tutelage of Professor Wormald, he was appointed as Consultant Surgeon at Winchester and Southampton Hospitals, UK in 2003. He was elected as a council member under the Rhinology and Laryngology section for the Royal Society of Medicine in 2007, where he served for 4 years.

He was co-founder of the comprehensive endoscopic anterior skull base surgical services for Southampton University hospitals and clinical lead for otolaryngology at Winchester Hospitals for 4 years.

He established the first Advanced Endoscopic Sinus Surgery and Skull Base course in the UK and continues to be an invited faculty member at numerous international courses. He has contributed to a number of book chapters and published widely in Rhinology.

In 2011, he moved to Auckland, where he was appointed as a Senior Rhinologist and Anterior Skull Base Surgeon to Auckland City Hospitals and Counties-Manukau Hospitals. He holds an honorary senior lecturer's post at Auckland University, Auckland, New Zealand.

Salil B Nair MD FRCS (ORL-HNS)

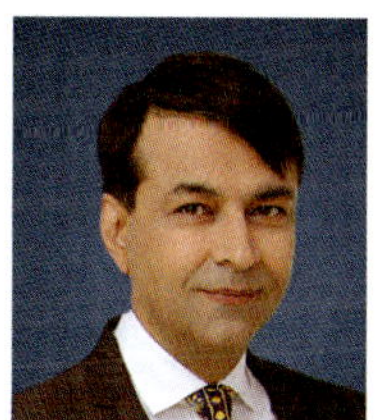

Sandeep Uppal graduated from University of Delhi, India in 1990. He completed his residency in Otolaryngology and Head and Neck Surgery from University of Delhi, India in 1995. Subsequently, he trained and qualified as a Specialist in Otolaryngology and Head and Neck Surgery in UK. He is a Fellow of both the Royal College of Surgeons of England and Royal College of Surgeons in Ireland.

Dr Uppal served a one-year fellowship in Facial Plastic and Reconstructive Surgery conducted by the European Academy of Facial Plastic Surgery. He then completed the certification process of the International and European Boards of Facial Plastic and Reconstructive Surgery. He was awarded the Claus D Walter Award for Academic Excellence by the International Board of Facial Plastic and Reconstructive Surgery in 2012. He has also served a one-year fellowship in Advanced Rhinology and Endoscopic Anterior Skull Base Surgery conducted by the Royal College of Surgeons of England.

Dr Uppal's research and clinical interests have resulted in numerous publications in peer-reviewed international journals as well as presentations at various international courses, workshops, and conferences. He was awarded a PhD by the University of Leeds, UK in 2012. He is actively involved in teaching and examining undergraduate and postgraduate medical students. He conducts three annual courses covering a broad range of topics in Facial Plastic Surgery. He serves as a Director on the Governing Council of Pan-Asia Academy of Facial Plastic and Reconstructive Surgery

Sandeep Uppal PhD MBBS MS FRCSI (Otolaryngology) FRCS (England) FRCS (ORL-HNS)
IBCFPRS EBCFPRS BTEC FAMS (Otorhinolaryngology, Singapore)

Contributors

Zahoor Ahmad MBBS MS FRACS
Consultant
Otolaryngologist—Head and Neck Surgeon
Counties-Manukau Health Auckland
University Hospitals
Vice-Chairman
Department of Otolaryngology—
Head and Neck Surgery
Counties-Manukau Health
Auckland University Hospitals
Auckland, New Zealand

Ashlin J Alexander MD FRCSC
Lecturer
Division of Facial Plastic and
Reconstructive Surgery
Department of Otolaryngology—
Head and Neck Surgery
University of Toronto, Mount Sinai Hospital
Toronto, Ontario, Canada

Robert Almeyda MD FACS
Associate Professor and
Director of Oculofacial Plastic and
Reconstructive Surgery
Albert Einstein College of Medicine
New York, USA
Associate Professor
Montefiore Medical Center
New York, USA

Jamil Asaria MD FRCSC
Clinical Lecturer
Division of Facial Plastic and
Reconstructive Surgery
Department of Otolaryngology—
Head and Neck Surgery
University of Toronto
Humber River Hospital
Toronto, Ontario, Canada

Nadia Ashraf BMedSci (Hon) BMBS (Hon) DA DOHNS FRCS (ORL-HNS)
Specialist Registrar
Department of Otolaryngology
Head and Neck and Facial
Plastic Surgery
Doncaster Royal Infirmary
Thorne Road, Doncaster
South Yorkshire, UK

Yogesh Bajaj MBBS MRCS DLO (RCS) MD MS (ENT) DNB (ENT) FRCS (ORL-HNS)
Consultant Pediatric Otolaryngologist
Department of Otolaryngology—
Head and Neck Surgery
St Bartholomew's Hospital
W Smithfield, London, UK
Royal London Hospital, Whitechapel Road
London, UK

Shan R Baker BA MD MS ABOto ABFPRS ABMS FACS
Division of Facial Plastic and
Reconstructive Surgery
Department of Otolaryngology—
Head and Neck Surgery
Center for Specialty Care
University of Michigan Health System
Livonia, Michigan, USA

Nikhil J Bhatt MD
Clinical Professor of Otolaryngology
Head and Neck Surgery
The University of Illinois Chicago
Consultant for Development, AAO-HNSF
Consultant, International Otolarungology
Committee, AAO-HNSF
Chicago, Illinois, USA

Amit D Bhrany MD ABOto ABFPRS
Associate Professor
Department of Otolaryngology—
Head and Neck Surgery
University of Washington
Medical Center
Seattle, Washington, USA

Lai Juen Bin BDS MDS FRACDS FAMS
Consultant, Department of Oral
and Maxillofacial Surgery
National Dental Center, Singapore
Consultant and Head
Department of Oral and
Maxillofacial Surgery
Co-Director, Integrated Sleep Service
Changi General Hospital, Singapore
Clinical Lecturer, Department of
Oral and Maxillofacial Surgery
National University of Singapore
Adjunct Professor, Department of
Oral and Maxillofacial Surgery
University of Alabama, Birmingham, USA

Michael G Brandt BSc (Hons) MD FRCSC
Clinical Lecturer, Division of Facial
Plastic and Reconstructive Surgery
Department of Otolaryngology—
Head and Neck Surgery
Faculty of Medicine, University of Toronto
Toronto, Ontario, Canada

Claudio Callejas MD
Assistant Professor
Department of Otolaryngology
Pontifical Catholic University of Chile
Santiago, Chile

Raewyn G Campbell FRACS BMed (Hons) BAppSc (Physio) Grad Dip (Ex Sport Sc)
Visiting Medical Officer
Royal Prince Alfred Hospital
Sydney and Macquarie University Hospital
Sydney, Australia

Simon Carney BSc (Hons) MBChB FRCS FRACS MD
Professor of Otolaryngology—
Head and Neck Surgery
Flinders University
Director, Adelaide Sinus Centre
Adelaide, Australia

Sean Carrie MB BCh FRCS (ORL)
Honorary Senior Clinical Lecturer
Newcastle University
Newcastle Upon Tyne
Consultant Rhinologist and
ENT Surgeon, Newcastle upon
Tyne Hospitals NHS Foundation Trust, UK

PP Cheang MD
Maidstone and Tunbridge Wells
NHS Trust
Kent, UK

Yip Chee Chew MBBS (Singapore) MMed (Ophthalmology) (Singapore) FRCS (Edin) FAMS (Singapore)
Head and Senior Consultant
Ophthalmology and Visual Sciences
Department, Khoo Teck
Puat Hospital, Singapore
Head, Oculoplastics
NHG Eye Institute, National
Healthcare Group, Senior Consultant
Department of Ophthalmology
Tan Tock Seng Hospital, Singapore

Humera Babar Craig BSc MRCS DOHNS FRCS (ORL-HNS)
Consultant Otolaryngologist
Department of Otolaryngology—Head and Neck Surgery
East Surrey Hospital
Canada Avenue
Redhill, UK

Richard G Douglas MD FRACS FRACP MRCP
Associate Professor
Department of Surgery
The University of Auckland
Auckland, New Zealand

A D'Souza MBBS FRCS (Otolaryngology) FRCS (ORL-HNS) IBCFPRS EBCFPRS
Consultant Otolaryngologist
Department of Otolaryngology—Head and Neck Surgery
University Hospital Lewisham
Lewisham, UK

Jung Dong Hak MD
Director
Shimmian Clinic, Seocho-Gu, Seocho-Dong, Seoul, South Korea
Clinical Professor
Inha University College of Medicine
Seoul, South Korea

Laura Harrison BMedSci BMBS MRCS DOHNS
ENT SpR Thames Valley Deanery
London, UK

N van Heerbeek MD PhD
Otorhinolaryngologist/IFFPSS-certified Facial Plastic Surgeon:
Radboud University Nijmegan Medical Centre, Nijmegen
The Netherlands

W Heppt MD
Professor and Director
Department of Otorhinolaryngology—Head and Neck Surgery
Facial Plastic Surgery
Klinikum Karlsruhe, Germany
Skin and Face Clinic
Germany

T Hildebrandt MD
Private Practice
Otorhinolaryngology in Association with the Limmat Klink
Zurich, Switzerland

Claire Hopkins DM FRCS (ORL-HNS)
Reader in ENT
King's College London
London, UK

Ilia Ianovski MBChB FRACS (OHNS)
Consultant Otolaryngologist
North Shore Hospital
Waitemata District Health Board
Auckland, New Zealand

Koen JAO Ingels MD PhD
Otorhinolaryngologist/IFFPSS-certified Facial Plastic Surgeon, Radboud University Nijmegen Medical Centre, Nijmegen
The Netherlands

Iman Khodaei MD
Consultant ENT and Facial Plastic Surgeon, Mehregan Hospital
Karaj, Iran

M Kicken MD DDS
Maxillofacial Surgeon
Rijnstate Hospital, Arnhem
The Netherlands

Jennifer Kim MD ABOto ABFPRS
Associate Professor
Facial Plastic and Reconstructive Surgery
Department of Otolaryngology—Head and Neck Surgery
University of Michigan Health System
Center for Specialty Care
Livonia, Michigan, USA

Brett Kotlus MD MS
Allure Medical Spa
Michigan, USA

GAM Krekels MD PhD MBA
Professor
Consultant Dermatologist and Mohs Surgeon
MohsA, Expert Center for Skin Cancer and Mohs Surgery in Eindhoven and Venray
Department of Dermatology and Venereology
The Netherlands

Stephen Lo MD MBA BMedSc FRCS Edin (ORL-HNS)
Consultant Otolaryngologist and Facial Plastic Surgeon
Tan Tock Seng Hospital
Singapore

Ian Loh MRCS MMed FAMS (Singapore)
Consultant Otolaryngologist and Facial Plastic Surgeon, Service Director
Facial Plastic and Reconstructive Surgery
Department of Otolaryngology—Head and Neck Surgery
Changi General Hospital
Singapore

Stuart MacKay BSc (Med) MBBS (Hons) FRACS
Illawarra ENT Head and Neck Clinic
Woolcock Institute
Associate Professor
Graduate School of Medicine
University of Wollongong
Honorary Fellow
University of Western Australia
Sydney, Australia

Emma McNeill MBBS MSc FRCS (ORL-HNS)
Consultant Otolaryngologist
Sunderland Royal Hospital
Kayll Road, Sunderland, UK

Corey C Moore MD MSc FRCSC
Associate Professor
Division of Facial Plastic and Reconstructive Surgery
Department of Otolaryngology—Head and Neck Surgery
Schulich School of Medicine & Dentistry, Western University
London, Ontario, Canada

Craig S Murakami MD ABOto ABFPRS
Clinical Associate Professor
University of Washington
Virginia Mason Medical Center
Seattle, Washington, USA

Salil B Nair MD FRCS (ORL-HNS)
Consultant Rhinologist and Skull Base Surgeon
Honorary Senior Lecturer
Auckland and Counties–Manukau Hospitals
Auckland, New Zealand

Ravinder Natt BSc FRCS (ORL-HNS)
Consultant
ENT Surgeon, Royal Free London NHS Foundation Trust
Pond Street, London, UK

Sarah J Novis MD
Department of Otolaryngology—Head and Neck Surgery
Division of Facial Plastic Surgery
University of Michigan
Ann Arbor, Michigan, USA

Pietro Palma MD
Clinical Professor
Department of Otorhinolaryngology Head and Neck Surgery
University Hospital
Varese, Italy Private Practice
Milan, Italy

Lucio Pereira MD
Otolaryngology—Head and Neck Surgery
Washington Hospital Center
Washington, DC, USA

Ullas Raghavan MS DLO FRCS (Glasgow) FRCS (Edinburgh) FRCS (ORL-HNS)
Consultant Otolaryngologist and
Facial Plastic Surgeon
Doncaster Royal Infirmary
Doncaster, South Yorkshire, UK

Hemal Raja FRCS (ORL-HNS)
Consultant Otorhinolaryngologist
Department of Otolaryngology—
Head and Neck Surgery
Warrington and Halton Hospital
NHS Trust, Lovely Lane, Warrington
Cheshire, Warrington, UK

Julian M Rowe-Jones FRCS (ORL)
The Nose Clinic, Guildford, UK
Consultant Otorhinolaryngologist
Department of Otolaryngology—
Head and Neck Surgery
Royal Surrey County Hospital NHS Trust
Guildford, UK

Anshul Sama BMedSci BMBSc FRCS (Genr Surg) FRCS (Otol)
Consultant Rhinologist
Nottingham University Hospital
Visiting Professor
Loughborough University
Loughborough, UK

Robert Schwarcz MD FACS
Associate Professor and Director of
Oculofacial Plastic and
Reconstructive Surgery
Albert Einstein College of Medicine
New York, USA
Associate Professor
Montefiore Medical Center
New York, USA

Neeraj Sethi MRCS DOHNS ENT
Registrar
Yorkshire and Humber Deanery
Yorkshire, UK

Mahdi Shkoukani MD ABOto ABFPRS
Chief of Craniofacial Surgery
Department of Otolaryngology—
Head and Neck Surgery
Division of Facial Plastic and
Reconstructive Surgery
Wayne State University
Detroit, Michigan, USA

Don Julian De Silva MBBS MD FRCO BSc PGc DIC
Consultant in Oculofacial
Plastic Surgery
Director of the Centre for London Facial
Cosmetic and Plastic Surgery
London, UK

Gordon Soo MBBS (London) FRCS (Glasgow) FCSHK FHKCORL FHKAM (Otorhinolaryngology)
Clinical Associate Professor (Honorary)
Department of Otorhinolaryngology—
Head and Neck Surgery
The Chinese University of Hong Kong
Prince of Wales Hospital
Shatin, New Territories, Hong Kong

Rishi Talwar BSc (Hons) MBBS (Lond) MRCS (Eng) DOHNS (RCS Eng) MFMLM FRCS (ORL-HNS)
Locum Consultant Otolaryngologist
Department of Otolaryngology—
Head and Neck Surgery
Evelina London Children's Hospital
Guy's & St Thomas' Hospital
London, UK

Sandeep Uppal PhD MBBS MS FRCSI (Otolaryngology) FRCS (England) FRCS (ORL-HNS) IBCFPRS EBCFPRS BTEC FAMS (Otorhinolaryngology, Singapore)
Adjunct Assistant Professor
Yong Loo Lin School of Medicine
National University of Singapore, Singapore
Senior Consultant Otolaryngologist
and Facial Plastic Surgeon
Department of Otolaryngology—
Head and Neck Surgery
Khoo Teck Puat Hospital, Singapore

Taher Valika MD
Senior Resident
Eye and Ear Infirmary
University of Illinois
Chicago, Illinois, USA

Irina Vasilenko MD PhD FACS
The Federal Clinical Research
Center for Otorhinolaryngology
Moscow, Russia

M Veenstra MD
Consultant Dermatologist
Department of Dermatology
Radboud University Medical Center
Nijmegen, The Netherlands

Julia Vent MD PhD (USA)
University of Heidelberg
Medical Center at Mannheim
Department of Otorhinolaryngology—
Head and Neck Surgery
Mannheim, Germany

KV Vishwas MBBS MS (ENT) DOHNS (England)
Consultant Otolaryngologist and
Facial Plastic Surgeon
Chord Road Hospital
Bengaluru, Karnataka
Assistant Professor
Department of Otorhinolaryngology—
Head and Neck Surgery
Rajarajeshwari Medical
College and Hospital
Bengaluru, Karnataka, India

Hade Vuyk MD PhD
Consultant Otolaryngologist and
Facial Plastic Surgeon
Department of Otorhinolaryngology—
Head and Neck Surgery
Free University Hospital Amsterdam
The Netherlands

Huib van Waegeningh MD
Resident ENT—Head and Neck surgery
Academic Medical Center
The Netherlands

Victoria Ward FRCSI FRCS (ORL-HNS)
Consultant Otorhinolaryngologist
Mid Yorkshire Hospitals
NHS Trust
Leeds, West Yorkshire, UK

Frederick Wong MBChB (CUHK) MRCS (Ed) FRCSEd (ORL) FHKCORL FHKAM (Otorhinolaryngology)
Clinical Associate Professor (Honorary)
Department of Otorhinolaryngology—
Head and Neck Surgery
The Chinese University of Hong Kong
Prince of Wales Hospital
Shatin, New Territories, Hong Kong

Tim J Woolford MD FRCS (ORL-HNS)
Consultant Otolaryngologist
Manchester Royal Infirmary
Manchester, UK

Chin Chean Yong MB ChB
Manchester Royal Infirmary
Manchester, UK

Foreword

Otolaryngology is a surgical specialty which treats patients of all ages and both sexes, both medically and surgically. As we all learned in our physical diagnosis course early in medical school that when we take a history, we start by asking about specific presenting symptoms and direct the rest of the examination accordingly. *Symptom Oriented Otolaryngology—Head and Neck Surgery* is based on this premise and is designed to provide the reader with the information necessary to proceed with a diagnostic evaluation and plan of management. The reader will benefit from the algorithms presented at the beginning of each chapter, which are supplemented with easy-to-read, well-illustrated text, which will be helpful in the management of their patients. The book is divided into three volumes: Head & Neck and Laryngology, Rhinology and Facial Plastics, and Otology and Pediatrics. There is ample information presented. However, the book is not designed to be a source of information for detailed surgical procedures or as a reference text.

Professor Randall P Morton and his colleagues, Zahoor Ahmad and Malcolm Giles and their associate editors: Patrick J Bradley, Kenneth MacKenzie, Michael J Rutter, Alan TL Cheng, Patrick J Dawes, Salil B Nair, and Sandeep Uppal are all highly qualified, experienced individuals, skilled in teaching and writing for the beginners in our specialty. The contributing authors have been recruited from around the world. Professor Morton has contributed extensively to the scientific literature including articles in high-impact journals as well as numerous book chapters. He has dedicated his entire career to the management of patients with cancer of the head and neck and is recognized as one of the world's leaders in studies of outcome and quality of life in this group. He has held leadership roles in the New Zealand Society of Head and Neck Surgery and the Royal Australasian College of Surgeons, and holds full membership in academic societies worldwide. The high quality of his active pursuit of clinical research and clinical epidemiology has also resulted in invitations to present highly coveted eponymous lectures.

I first met Professor Morton in 1999 in London when Professor Patrick J Bradley, who was the President of the Section of Laryngology of the Royal Society of Medicine, invited both of us to be guest lecturers. Since then, we have met many times across the world. While listening to his lecturers I, recognized that the dominant theme is his dedication to a process of continuous quality improvement in the management of patients with cancer of the head and neck. He spoke eloquently as he shared his thoughts on this topic when he presented the Eugene N Myers Lecture—Quality of Life Assessment in Head and Neck Cancer at the Annual Meeting of the American Academy of Otolaryngology—Head and Neck Surgery in Boston in 2010.

I am honored to have been invited by Professor Morton to write the foreword to this excellent book.

Eugene N Myers MD
Distinguished Professor and Emeritus Chair
Department of Otolaryngology
Pittsburgh, Pennsylvania, USA

Preface

Most textbooks of otolaryngology categorize the field by anatomy or by disease process. However, this bears little relation to the approach needed when facing a patient in the clinic for the first time. With a few exceptions—such as the patient in intensive care presenting with a complication of chronic otitis media or sinusitis, where the diagnosis and presentation are already known—the patient is asking for the Otolaryngologist to manage a problem (presentation), and not a diagnosis.

These volumes attempt to break down all the possible presentations of patients to an Otolaryngologist into manageable and (almost) exclusive categories, and present a diagnostic and management strategy for each of these. Categorizing all possible presentations turned out to be more difficult a task than originally thought, but we believe the chapters cover the vast majority of those likely to be encountered in Otolaryngology.

These texts are designed to demonstrate how a specific presentation can be approached logically, a diagnosis reached where possible, and how common causes of that specific presentation may be treated. Each chapter has a 'Pearls and Pitfalls' section, and flowcharts have been used in the clinical chapters to depict a logical approach to a given presentation.

There have certainly been moments of frustration, but overall, this has been a very stimulating and enjoyable project. We have found the collegial contact between editors to be most satisfying and we have been privileged to have such high-quality associate editors join us in this project. We are also blessed to have had universally high-quality collaboration and support from the contributors and for this, we are most thankful.

We sincerely hope that readers of this book find it a useful guide for the initial care of patients that bring symptoms needing a diagnoses and efficacious management.

Zahoor Ahmad MBBS MS FRACS
Randall P Morton MBBS MSc FRACS
Malcolm Giles MBChB FRACS

Acknowledgments

I think we have succeeded in completing this high-standard book that could be very useful to its readers. However, to produce any high-standard work, one needs help from friends, colleagues, and family.

I have been very fortunate to have some wonderful people around me, who have always made my tasks easy and enjoyable. This book would not have been completed without their help and contribution. My co-authors, Prof Randall P Morton and Dr Malcom Giles have not only been great friends, but a great support for me to complete this book. Their contributions have been enormous and completing this work was only possible with their support. They have spent a number of their valuable days and a lot of their energy in discussions and giving constructive criticism to take this book to its present shape. Their scientific contributions have been of very high quality. I express my gratitude to both of them.

My Associate Editors, Dr Salil B Nair and Dr Sandeep Uppal have been the cornerstones of this volume. It was through them that we could reach to our colleagues and friends to engage them to help us by contributing the individual chapters of this volume. They have spent a number of days of their valuable time to complete this volume. I know this volume would not have reached this high standard without their help and contribution. My sincere thanks to both Dr Salil B Nair and Dr Sandeep Uppal.

I also want to express my appreciation to the individual authors, who have produced a text that is different than most textbooks as it focuses mainly on a symptom-oriented approach and I am glad that this has been done very professionally and scientifically.

My sincere thanks to Eugene N Myers for writing the foreword.

I would also like to thank Mr Jitendar P Vij (Group Chairman), Mr Ankit Vij (Group President), Ms Chetna Malhotra Vohra (Associate Director), Ms Angima Shree (Senior Development Editor), and Production Team of Jaypee Brothers Medical Publishers (P) Ltd., New Delhi, India for being reliable and supportive throughout, providing good guidance and advice for all of us. They have been excellent partners.

Last but not least, I must express my thanks to my wife and family, who have supported me and allowed me to spend a lot of family time completing this project. They have been understanding and supportive throughout the journey of this book.

Zahoor Ahmad MBBS MS FRACS

Contents

Section 1: Rhinology

Section 2: Facial Plastics

Rhinology

Section 1

Chapters Outline

1. Clinical Anatomy of the Nose and Sinuses
2. Acute General Nasal Symptoms
3. Nasal Congestion and Nasal Obstruction
4. Nasal Discharge
5. Postnasal Drip
6. Facial Pain
7. Sneezing
8. Disorders of Smell
9. Bleeding Nose (Epistaxis)
10. Sleep-Disordered Breathing
11. Functional and Aesthetic Analysis of the Nose
12. Trauma to Nose
13. Crooked Nose
14. Saddle Nose
15. The Patient Wanting to Alter Asian Nose
16. Prominent Nose
17. Nasal Valve Collapse
18. Septoplasty
19. Septal Perforation

1 Clinical Anatomy of the Nose and Sinuses

Ilia Ianovski, Laura Harrison, Anshul Sama, Salil B Nair, Zahoor Ahmad

Chapter Overview

Pearls and Pitfalls

Pearls

- Keratinizing squamous epithelium is always abnormal in nose or nasopharynx.
- Nose is supplied by branches of both external carotid artery (ECA) and internal carotid artery (ICA).
- Little's area or Kisselbach's plexus is found on the anterior septum. It is formed by an anastomosis of vessels branching from the ECA and ICA.
- Anatomic relation of sinuses is important to understand to avoid complications in sinus surgery.
- Osteomeatal complex is a unit lateral to middle turbinate that comprises uncinate process, infundibulum, and anterior ethmoidal cells.
- Computerized tomography (CT) scan is a gold standard for radiologic anatomy of sinuses and all views are complementary to each other.
- Variations of Onodi cells should be considered in all cases while operating on sinuses as optic nerve could be in close relation to it.
- Supraorbital ethmoid cells are associated with the anterior ethmoid artery lying in the mesentery and are at greater risk of injury during surgery.
- Agger nasi and uncinate process are key structures in understanding the anatomy of frontal recess.
- The optic nerve and ICA may be dehiscent within sphenoid sinus.

Pitfalls

- Thicker CT slices may miss some important anatomic landmarks.
- Computerized tomography scans are not a substitute for anatomic dissections to learn anatomy.
- Anatomic variations are commonly found and should always be considered.

1.1 OVERVIEW

The nose is a central facial feature, which provides both a cosmetic focus for the complex interplay between light and shadow and serves several important functions: breathing, olfaction, humidification, warming, and filtering of air.

The external nose—the nasal pyramid—is formed by bones, cartilages, and soft tissue. The superior third of the pyramid is boney, being made up of the paired nasal bones, which articulate medially with their counterpart and laterally with the frontal process of maxilla. Superiorly, the boney pyramid is attached to the frontal

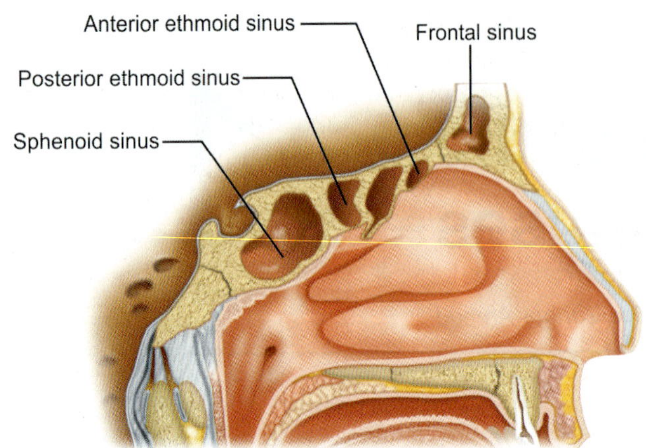

Fig. 1.1: Nasal cavity and paranasal sinuses.

bone. The middle third is made up of the paired *upper lateral cartilages* articulate with the nasal bones superiorly (Keystone area) and with the paired *lower lateral cartilages* inferiorly (the Scroll area)—lower third. Laterally, fibro-fatty tissue and accessory cartilages complete the nasal pyramid. The nose is lined by skin of various thickness: thick skin overlying the boney vault, thinner skin over the middle dorsum, and thick skin with multiple sweat and sebaceous glands overlying the nasal tip and lateral alar region.

The nasal cavity extends from the nostrils to the choanae, which communicate with the nasopharynx, and is bound superiorly by the cribriform plate of the ethmoid bone and inferiorly by the hard palate (maxillary and palatine bones) (Fig. 1.1). The nasal septum splits the nasal cavity in two and provides integral structural support to the nasal pyramid. The four pairs of paranasal sinuses all drain into the nasal cavity at various locations, with all mucus eventually draining into the nasopharynx.

1.2 DEVELOPMENT

The nose begins its development as part of the face in the 4th week of gestation. Five primordial processes begin to grow toward each other around the primitive mouth—the stomodeum. The processes are:

- *Frontonasal process*: A single midline structure that develops the forehead, the nasal dorsum, and the central upper lip, and primary palate
- *Maxillary processes*: Paired and form the upper cheek, the maxilla, and lateral upper lip
- *Mandibular processes*: Paired and form the lower cheek, the lower lip, and chin.

The frontonasal process develops a pair of ectodermal thickenings called nasal placodes, which invaginate to form the nasal pits surrounded by the lateral and medial nasal processes. The lateral nasal process fuses with the *maxillary* process to form the nasolacrimal duct. The medial nasal process fuses with the maxillary process to form the central upper lip—the philtrum and the premaxilla (primary palate). The nasal pits deepen to become nasal sacs, and the epithelial plug (nasobuccal membrane) that fills the nasal cavity becomes resorbed around the 24th week allowing communication between the nose and the nasopharynx.

There is a membrane that separates the nasal pits from the primitive mouth—the oronasal membrane that breaks down between 5th and 6th week of gestation, as the palate develops from the maxilla and forms the floor of the nose.

The structural components of the lateral nasal wall are key to understanding nasal and paranasal sinus anatomy. While the inferior turbinate develops as a separate bone, other lateral nasal wall structures develop from the ethmoid bone. Growths from the ethmoid bone—the ethmoturbinals—are 5 in number.

- 1st ethmoturbinal gives rise to the uncinate bone.
- 2nd ethmoturbinal forms the anterior face of the ethmoidal bulla.
- 3rd ethmoturbinal forms the ground lamella of the middle turbinate (MT).
- 4th ethmoturbinal forms the superior turbinate.
- 5th ethmoturbinal (often absent) gives rise to the supreme turbinate.

The sinuses develop as diverticulae from the walls of the nasal cavity and are rudimentary at birth, apart from the *frontal* sinus, which appears around the age of 2 years. Maxillary, ethmoidal, sphenoid sinuses enlarge throughout early life, but undergo a rapid spurt around the age of 6 years, which coincides with the eruption of secondary dentition, and then again after puberty. The *frontal* sinus develops as the most anterior ethmoidal air cells grow into the frontal bone, and become apparent on X-ray and computerized tomography (CT) imaging around the age of 7 years.

1.3 HISTOLOGY OF THE NASAL CAVITY AND SINUSES

The nasal cavity and paranasal sinuses are lined by respiratory-type epithelium: ciliated pseudo-stratified columnar epithelium with goblet cells as well as mucous and serous glands. Anterior nose—the vestibule and anterior tip of the inferior turbinate are lined by stratified squamous epithelium, with transitional or Schneiderian epithelium. Stratified squamous epithelium is also found in the nasopharynx. This nonkeratinizing stratified squamous epithelium increases in amount with age.

Throughout the mucosa, inflammatory cells can be found that will elicit a rapid release of inflammatory mediators from mast cells, basophils, and other leukocytes in response to microbial or chemical insult. Keratinizing squamous epithelium is always abnormal.

The mucous blanket created by the secreting glands and goblet cells is made up of a thick Gel layer superficially, and a thin Sol layer inferiorly in contact with ciliated cells. The cilia are continually beating, thus providing a constant motion to the mucus blanket within the nose and sinuses. The Gel layer of mucus acts as a filtering and cleaning system for the upper respiratory tract as well as helps to maintain the moisture content within the nose and sinuses.

1.4 ANATOMY

The nasal cavity has a pyriform shape, with a wide base of the hard palate that gradually narrows superiorly to reach the cribriform plate and superior (and occasionally supreme) turbinates.

Lateral Nasal Wall

The lateral nasal wall is made up of six bones: anteriorly the frontal process of the maxilla forms the piriform aperture, and articulates with the ethmoid bone superiorly, lacrimal bone below that, and the inferior turbinate bone inferiorly. Posterior lateral nasal wall is completed by the palatine and the sphenoid (pterygoid process) bones.

The *lateral* nasal wall has its surface area enlarged by the presence of the inferior, middle, superior, and occasionally the supreme turbinates. The space inferior to the turbinate is called the meatus, and is labeled according to the turbinate it is inferior to: inferior meatus lies inferior to the inferior turbinate. The turbinates are lined by mucoperiosteum with a unique submucosal vascular arrangement. The turbinates have capacitance vessels—the sinusoids—connecting capillaries to venules. This arrangement allows congestion and engorgement of the turbinates to take place in one nostril, while the other side is decongested. The sides alternate every 3–6 hours and this process is called the *nasal cycle.*

The inferior turbinate is a separate bone attached to the frontal process of maxilla anteriorly, the ethmoid bone, and the palatine bone posteriorly. The *nasolacrimal* duct drains the nasolacrimal sac into the inferior meatus via the Hasner's valve.

The middle, superior, and supreme turbinates arise from the ethmoid bone. The MT anatomy is key to the understanding of normal sinus drainage pathways. The MT has a complex three-dimensional attachment, which is in the sagittal/vertical plane anteriorly—attaching to the base of skull, coronal/vertical attachment to the lateral wall (the paper-thin *lamina papyracea*) in its middle segment, and horizontal in its posterior attachment to the lateral wall. Anterior to the coronal/vertical part (the ground lamella of the MT)—the remnant of the 2nd ethmoturbinal—lie the anterior ethmoidal air cells. Posterior to this structure lie the posterior ethmoidal air cells. The anterior ethmoidal air cells, thus, drain into the middle meatus, while the posterior ethmoidal cells drain postero-superior to the MT, into the superior meatus.

Nasal Septum

The septum, a median but rarely a perfectly midline structure, divides the cavity into two nostrils. The septum is composed of bones, cartilage, and soft tissue. Anteriorly, the septum is made up of the *quadrangular* cartilage (as it is approximately quadrilateral in shape) and soft tissue of the columella and skin. The quadrangular cartilage articulates postero-inferior with the *vomer* bone, and postero-superior with the perpendicular plate of the ethmoid bone. Superiorly, the septum extends to provide key structural support to the nasal vault anteriorly, and articulates with the cribriform plate of the ethmoid posteriorly. Inferiorly, the cartilaginous septum sits in a groove created by the maxillary bone—the maxillary crest, while posteriorly the vomer articulates with both the maxillary and palatine bones at its base. Posterosuperior vomer also articulates with the rostrum of the sphenoid bone. Partly due to the various components that make up the septum, this structure is seldom perfectly straight, but this does not lead to any discussion in the majority of the population.

Sinonasal Blood Supply and Drainage

The sinonasal blood supply originates from both the internal (ICA) and external carotid arteries (ECAs). The named branches that supply the nasal septum are as follows:

- Anterior and posterior ethmoidal arteries—branches of the *ophthalmic* artery—ICA
- Sphenopalatine artery—terminal branch of the *maxillary* artery—ECA
- Septal branches from *superior labial* artery—branch of the *facial* artery—ECA
- Ascending branch of *greater palatine* artery—subbranch of *maxillary* artery—ECA.

Arteries: The nose is supplied by branches of the ICAs and ECAs. The external nasal pyramid is supplied by the *dorsal* nasal artery (terminal branch of ophthalmic artery, ICA) at the base, and lower by the *external* nasal artery (branch of anterior ethmoidal, ICA) and by the lateral nasal and septal branches of the facial and its superior branch, respectively (ECA). The nasal cavity is supplied superiorly by the anterior and posterior ethmoidal arteries (branches of ophthalmic, ICA). The lateral nasal wall is supplied by conchal branches of the sphenopalatine artery (terminal branch of *maxillary* artery, ECA). The septum is supplied posteriorly by the posterior septal artery (branch of the Sphenopalatine artery), the palatine artery anteriorly (branch of *maxillary*, ECA), and the nasal septal branch of superior labial artery (branch of facial artery, ECA). On the anterior septum, a rich plexus—the Kiesselbach's plexus (also known as Little's area)—thus forms (greater palatine artery, nasal septal artery, ant ethmoidal artery, posterior septal artery). A second—Woodruff's plexus—forms on the posterior-inferior lateral wall (SPA branches, posterior nasal artery, pharyngeal and ascending pharyngeal arteries).

Veins: Veins accompany the arteries and drain in various directions. The pterygoid venous plexus is reached by the sphenopalatine foramen vessels, the internal jugular vein is reached by the facial vein, and the cavernous sinus is reached via the ethmoidal veins draining into the inferior ophthalmic vein.

Lymphatics: Lymphatics run with veins and drain into the submandibular, superior deep cervical, and retropharyngeal nodes.

Neural Innervation

The nose is supplied by special sensory fibers (*olfactory* nerve), sensory fibers [*ophthalmic* (V1) and *maxillary* (V2) branches of the *trigeminal* nerve], parasympathetic fibers (branches from the *pterygopalatine ganglion*), and sympathetic fibers (branches from the internal carotid plexus).

The *olfactory* filaments (approximately 20 in number) pierce the cribriform plate to supply the vault of the nasal cavity, the superior turbinate, and the corresponding part of the septum. The fibers are bipolar cells with cell bodies in the mucosa and synapse with mitral cells in the olfactory bulb located in the anterior cranial fossa (ACF).

The *general sensory* supply includes the branches of the infraorbital nerve in the anterior vestibule, the anterior and posterior ethmoidal nerves (branches of nasociliary nerve, V1) superiorly, posterior superior lateral and posterior inferior lateral nasal nerves (V2) supplying the posterior lateral wall, branch of superior anterior alveolar nerve (V2) supplying anterior lateral wall, and nasopalatine nerve (V2) supplying the septum in combination with greater palatine nerve (V2) via the incisor foramen.

The *parasympathetic* innervation controls the volume, consistency, and viscosity of nasal secretions as well as causes vasodilatation. The innervation arises from the *superior salivary* nucleus in the pons, and initially travels via nervus intermedius that subsequently joins the facial nerve. At the *geniculate ganglion*, the parasympathetic fibers separate as the *greater superficial petrosal nerve* (GSPN), join the *deep petrosal* nerve (*sympathetic* fibers) at the foramen lacerum, and enter the *pterygopalatine fossa* via the *vidian* canal as the *vidian* nerve. Here the parasympathetic fibers synapse at the *pterygopalatine ganglion*. The fibers then follow the branches of maxillary division of trigeminal nerve (V2) into the nose and paranasal sinuses (Fig. 1.2).

The *sympathetic* innervation causes vasoconstriction and also alters the nature of nasal secretions. The fibers arise from the thoracic spinal cord, and after synapsing at the superior cervical ganglion, join the *internal carotid* and follow it as the *internal carotid* sympathetic plexus intracranially. The fibers separate as the deep petrosal nerve and join the GSPN to form the vidian nerve at the foramen lacerum. The sympathetic fibers follow the arteries out of the pterygopalatine fossa into the nose and paranasal sinuses.

Sinus Anatomy (Figs. 1.3 and 1.4)

The paranasal sinuses—frontal, maxillary, ethmoidal, sphenoid—are paired air-filled cavities within the skull that surround the nasal cavity. Their exact function is unknown, but they contribute to lightning of the weight of the skull, protection for the eye and orbit, increasing the surface area of the mucosa providing humidification

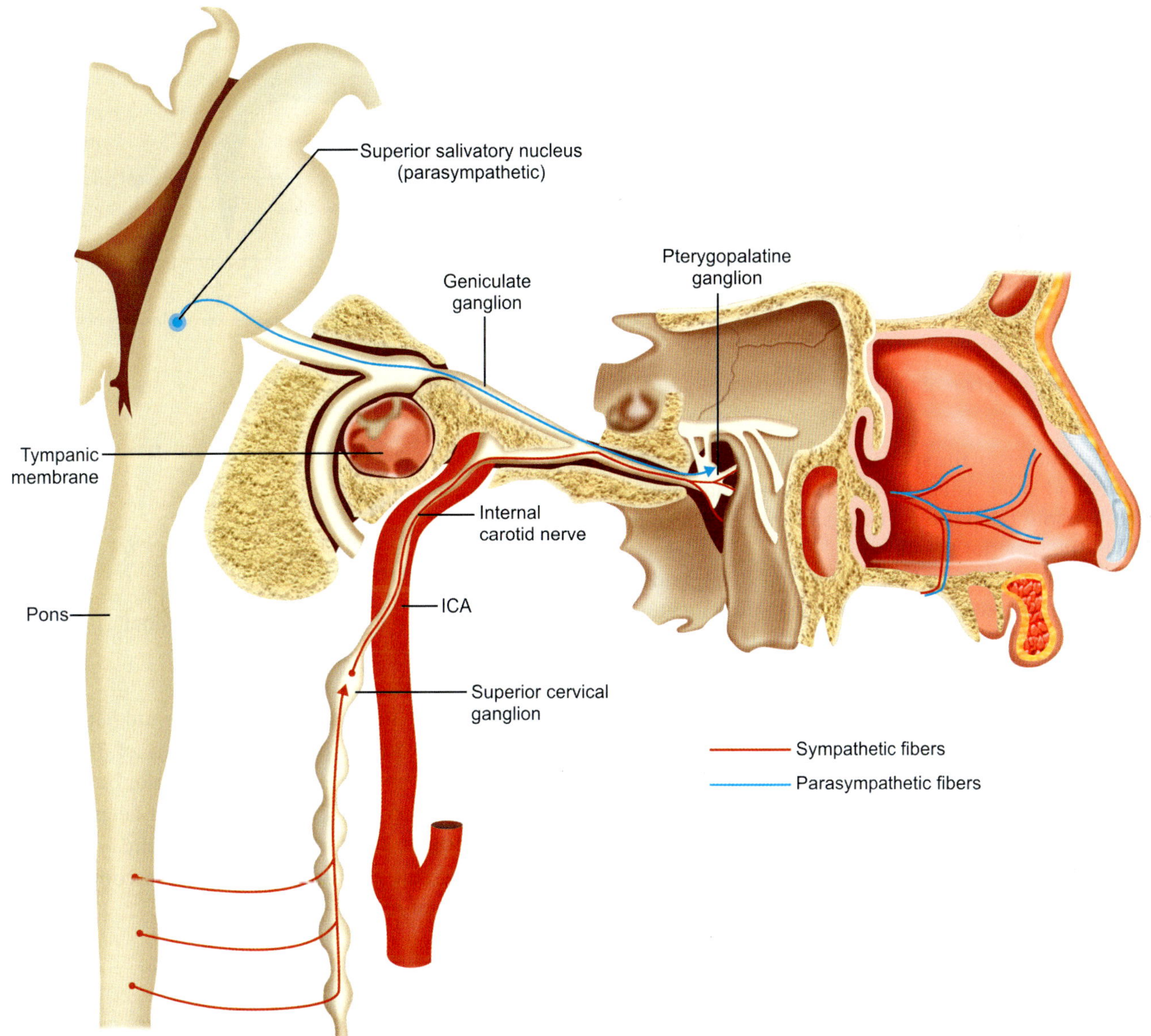

Fig. 1.2: Autonomic nerve supply of nasal cavity. (ICA: Internal carotid artery).

to the inspired air, and altering of the resonance of voice. Anatomically, the relation of each sinus to its surrounding structures is of vital importance. The maxillary sinus roof is the floor of the orbit, while the floor is the maxillary alveolus with dental roots occasionally protruding into the sinus. The ethmoidal air cells are bound laterally by the paper-thin bony plate called lamina papyracea, which is the lateral wall of the orbit. The roof of the ethmoidal air cells is the base of skull, with areas of bone thickness as little as 0.05 mm in certain areas. The sphenoid sinus has the pituitary gland above it, the brainstem posterior to it, and the optic nerve and ICA within its lateral wall. These relationships are important, as they can serve as routes for infection to spread, inadvertent disastrous complications during sinus surgery, as well as provide a surgical approach to otherwise difficult to reach areas.

The drainage pathway of the frontal sinus—the frontal recess—drains anterior to the anterior ethmoidal air cells, and thus also empties into the middle meatus.

The opening of the maxillary sinus—maxillary sinus ostium—is overlapped by a hook-like process of the ethmoid bone called the uncinate process. Thus, on direct examination of the nose, one cannot see inside the maxillary sinus, but the contents of the sinus drain into the middle meatus.

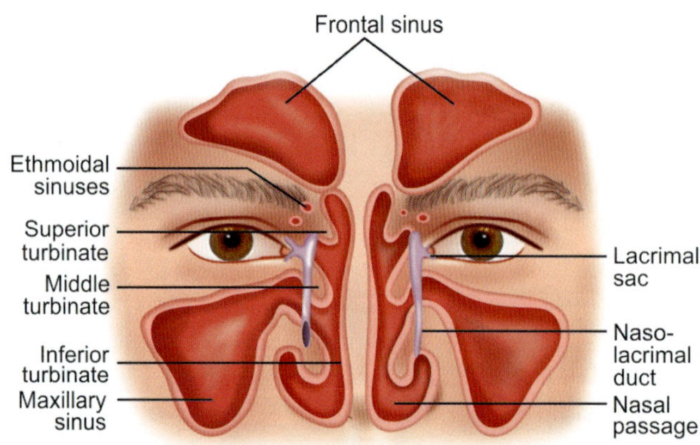

Fig. 1.3: Anterior group of sinuses.

The contents of the sphenoid sinuses drain directly via a sphenoid sinus ostia into the sphenoethmoidal recess, and then join the posterior ethmoid sinus drainage pathway in the superior meatus.

Thus, the contents of the frontal, maxillary, and anterior ethmoidal sinuses empty into the middle meatus and flow posteriorly into the nasopharynx anteroinferiorly to the opening of the Eustachian tube.

This common drainage space within the middle meatus is referred to as the osteomeatal complex.

- Collectively this comprises
  - Uncinate process
  - Infundibulum
  - Anterior ethmoid cells.

Hence, the osteomeatal complex is a three-dimensional space lateral to the MT.

The contents of the posterior ethmoid and sphenoid sinuses empty into the superior meatus and flow posteriorly into the nasopharynx supero-posterior to the Eustachian tube opening. Sphenoid sinuses drain medial to the superior or supreme turbinate via an independent ostia, which in turn communicates with the sphenoethmoid recess.

Hiatus Semilunaris

The *sagittal* cleft between the posterior border of the uncinate process and anterior surface of the ethmoid bulla is called hiatus semilunaris inferior. The cleft between the posterior aspect of the ethmoidal bulla and the basal lamella is the hiatus semilunaris superior.

Hiatus semilunaris inferior opens into a three-dimensional space—ethmoidal infundibulum.

Infundibulum continues superiorly into frontal recess in about 14% cases.

Other 86% infundibulum ends in recess terminalis.

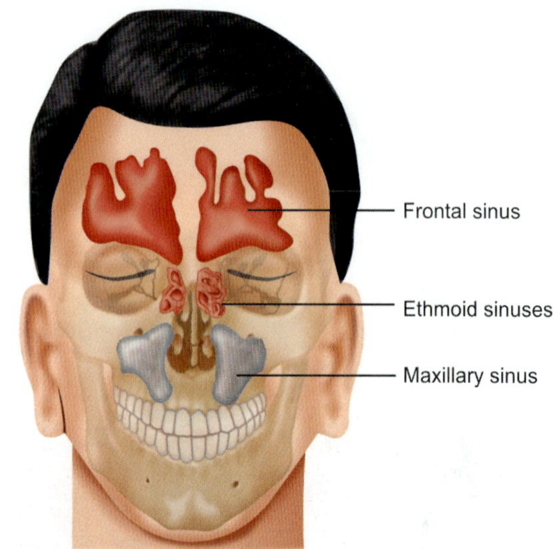

Fig. 1.4: Nasal and sinus anatomy.

Ethmoid Infundibulum

This is a funnel-shaped three-dimensional space. It is V-shaped on CT imaging.

It is bounded:

Medially by the uncinate process, and laterally by the lamina papyracea. The frontal process of the maxilla and lacrimal bone form its anterior-superior boundary. It measures 4 cm in length and is 5–12 mm deep.

Superiorly by the frontal recess (depends on attachment of uncinate process)—14% of them communicate with the frontal recess.

Nasolacrimal Duct

- The duct lies very close to the maxillary ostium. It is approximately 12 mm in length and lies 4–9 mm anterior to the maxillary sinus ostium.
- Bounded by:
  - Maxilla
  - Lacrimal bone
  - Inferior turbinate.

1.5 RADIOLOGIC ANATOMY OF THE SINUSES

- Computerized tomography scans are still the gold standard for radiologic anatomy of the paranasal sinuses.
- The following views are helpful and are complementary to each other:

- Coronal
- Axial
- Sagittal

Following modes are generally viewed: (Figs. 1.5 to 1.7)

- Bone algorithms
- Soft tissue algorithms
- Three-dimensional reconstructions.

Maxillary Sinus

- First to develop

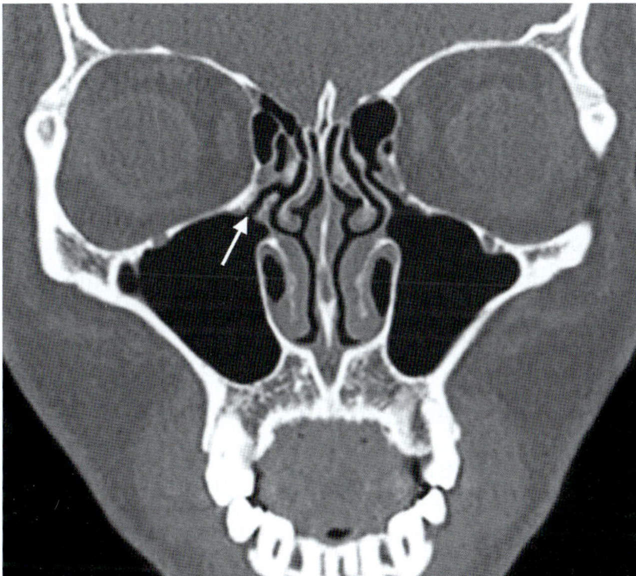

Fig. 1.5: Bone algorithm.

- Fluid filled at birth
- Biphasic growth (0–3 years and 7–12 years)
- Adult sinus is pyramidal, 25 × 34 × 33 mm, 15 mL
- Floor is usually 4–5 mm below the floor of nose
- Infraorbital nerve runs on roof, exits at midsuperior portion (14% dehiscent)
- Thinnest anterior wall—canine fossa
- *Boundaries of maxillary sinus*:
  - Superiorly—orbital floor
  - Inferiorly—hard palate, alveolus, dental part of maxilla
  - Laterally—zygomatic process
  - Medially—uncinate process and inferior turbinate
  - Posteriorly—plate of bone separating from infratemporal fossa and pterygomaxillary fossa
- *Pterygomaxillary fossa contents*:
  - Internal maxillary artery, sphenopalatine ganglion, the vidian canal, the greater palatine nerve, and the foramen rotundum
- *Ostium of maxillary sinus*:
  - The natural maxillary ostium—located at the superior aspect of the medial wall of the sinus—drains into hiatus semilunaris
  - Elliptical, 2.4 mm (1–20 mm in size)
  - 88% times hidden behind uncinate process
  - Accessory ostium is found in 20–50% of cases
  - Accessory ostium is usually in anterior or posterior fontanelle (posterior more common than anterior).

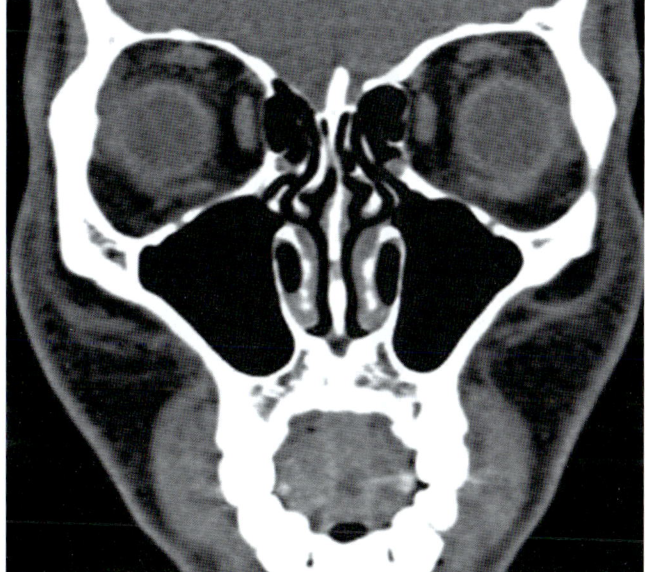

Fig. 1.6: Soft tissue algorithm.

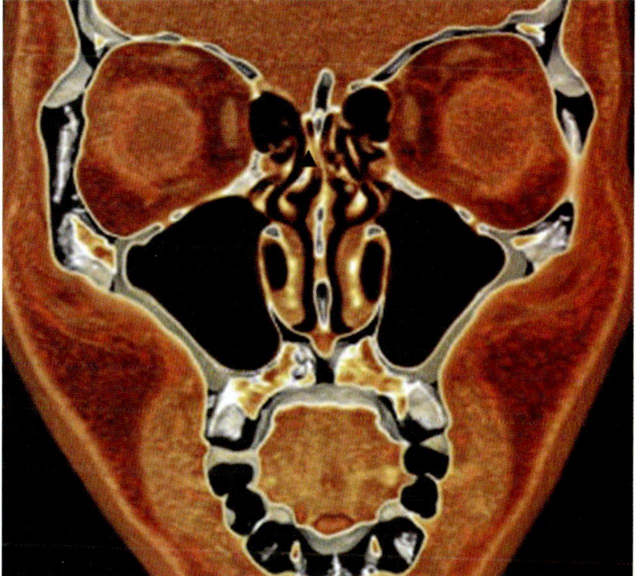

Fig. 1.7: Three-dimensional reconstruction.

Sinus Lateralis

The sinus lateralis may be mistaken as the frontal sinus during sinus surgery. It is not a constant space. When present, it is located posterior and superior to the ethmoid bulla and is also called the suprabullar and retrobullar recess (Fig. 1.8).

- *Boundaries*:
  - Ethmoid roof—superiorly
  - Lamina papyracea—laterally
  - Ethmoid bulla forms roof, posterior, and anterior wall
  - Ground lamella posteriorly.

Ethmoid Sinuses

- Adult size by age 12
- The ethmoid air cells are a paired variable labyrinth of air spaces held together within the ethmoid bone by the lamina cribrosa. Its roof is open superiorly.
- Each lamina cribrosa is separated in the midline by the crista galli
- Laterally separated from orbit by lamina papyracea
- Medially bounded by middle, superior, and supreme turbinates
- Anterior roof is bounded by frontal bones
- *Complex labyrinth is divided into following lamellae* (Fig. 1.9):
  - Uncinate process
  - Bulla ethmoidalis
  - Lamella of superior turbinate
  - Sometimes lamella of supreme turbinate
  - Ground lamella of MT.

Ground lamella is well developed. It divides ethmoid into anterior and posterior parts.

Posterior Ethmoid Sinuses

It is a collection of one to five cells, which drain into the superior/supreme meati.

- *Boundaries*:
  - Anteriorly—ground lamella
  - Posteriorly—anterior wall of sphenoid
  - Laterally—lamina papyracea
  - Medially—superior and supreme turbinates
  - Superiorly—ethmoid roof
- The posterior ethmoids may pneumatize over the sphenoid sinus (sphenoethmoidal or Onodi cells). It is important to be aware of this variation as the optic nerve would be present in the roof of this posterior ethmoid cell rather than the sphenoid.

Other Ethmoid Cells

Ethmoid cells may:

- Pneumatize the orbital plate of the frontal bone. These supraorbital ethmoid (SOE) cells are present in up

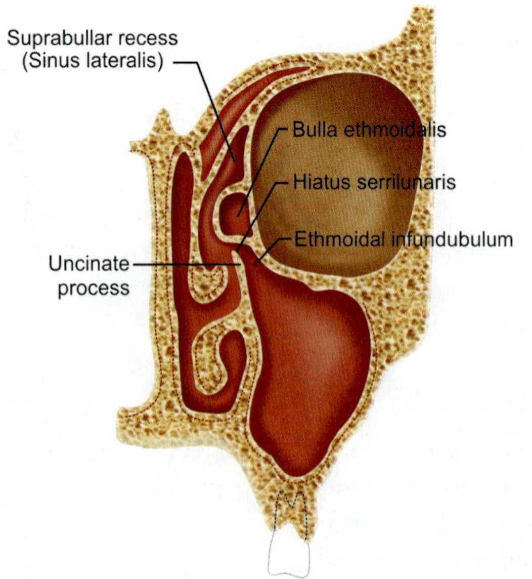

Fig. 1.8: Schematic coronal view of the paranasal sinuses at the level of the osteomeatal complex.

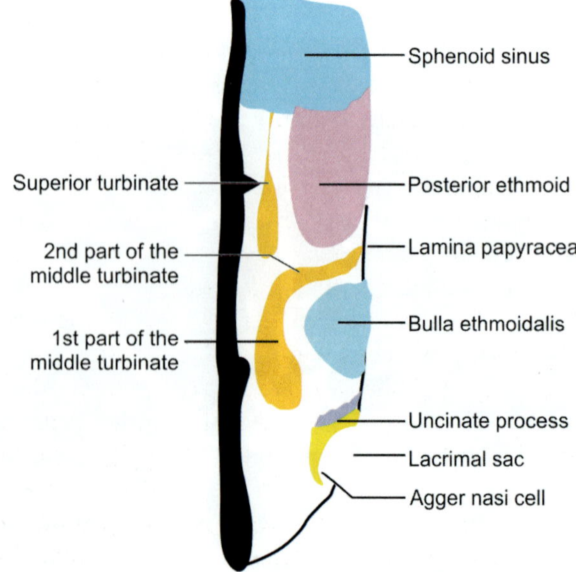

Fig. 1.9: Axial schematic view of the paranasal sinuses.

to 15% of the population. They drain posterior and lateral to the frontal sinus ostium. When extensively pneumatized, SOEs are associated with the anterior ethmoid artery (AEA) being in a mesentery. Arteries in a mesentery are at greater risk of injury during surgery.

- Pneumatize below the orbit. Known as infraorbital or Haller cells, they are present in up to 10% of patients. Haller cells arise from the anterior ethmoid in 88% cases and from the posterior ethmoid in 12% cases. They can obstruct the maxillary ostia, and narrow the infundibulum.
- Pneumatize into the MT—concha bullosa.

Frontal Sinus

The frontal sinus is arguably the most complex of the paranasal sinuses. It demonstrates great variability in size and septation and is rarely symmetrical. In up to 5% of the population, this sinus is absent or rudimentary. The frontal sinus ostium drains into an hourglass-shaped space termed the frontal recess. The frontal recess is a three-dimensional space, which communicates with the ethmoidal infundibulum within the middle meatus. In essence, the ventilation and drainage of both the maxillary and frontal sinuses pass through narrow complex clefts and spaces before they reach the middle meatus.

The Frontal Recess

The frontal recess is bound anteriorly by the agger nasi and the frontal process of the maxilla, the frontal beak. The thickness of the frontal beak depends on the pneumatization of the agger nasi and the presence of frontoethmoidal cells. The medial border of the frontal recess is the superior attachment of the MT, the lateral lamella of the cribriform plate, the height and angle of which can vary considerably. The lateral and posterior boundaries are formed by the lamina papyracea and the upward continuation of the anterior face of the bulla, respectively. If the bulla lamella is absent superiorly, a suprabullar space will communicate directly with the frontal recess. In this situation, the anterior ethmoidal artery is not protected by the bulla lamella and may be at risk during dissection of the frontal recess. The anterior ethmoidal artery, traversing the skull base from laterally posteriorly to medially anteriorly, is more likely to lie in a mesentery when the olfactory fossa depth is >4 mm. Superiorly, the frontal recess communicates with the frontal sinus but posterior to this, the roof is formed by the fovea ethmoidalis.

- Both the agger nasi and uncinate process are key structures in understanding the frontal recess. The agger nasi cell is present in over 90% of patients. The crescent-shaped uncinate process attaches inferiorly to the inferior turbinate, but superiorly it can attach to the lamina papyracea (33%), skull base (10%) or MT, and a combination of these (57%). When present, the medial, posterior, and even superior walls of the agger nasi cell are often attached or intimately related to the superior aspect of the uncinate process.
- There are many complex anatomic variations within the frontal recess. The simplest configuration within the frontal recess is the presence of an agger nasi cell only. In this instance, the uncinate process, curving around the agger cell, would most likely attach directly to the lamina papyracea.

Accessory Cells in the Frontal Recess

- The array of cells within the frontal recess can be complex and confusing. In an attempt to provide clarity, Bent and Kuhn proposed a classification of these cells.
- Frontal ethmoidal cells are frequently present and classified 1–4 (Table 1.1). These are anterior ethmoidal cells that are in contact with the frontal process of the maxilla, the anterior limit of the frontal recess. They sit above the agger nasi cell and are described by their number and degree of extension into the frontal sinus. When multiple or large, they can obstruct ventilation of the frontal sinus.
- Cells can pneumatize forward from the bulla itself (frontal bulla cells) or above the bulla (suprabullar cells).
- The classification has recently been modified in an attempt to simplify the description. The aim is to describe the cells in relation to the position they occupy within the frontal recess: anterior (frontoethmoidal/intersinus), posterior (frontal or suprabullar), medial (intersinus septal), or lateral (frontoethmoidal) (Lund, et al., 2014).

Sphenoid Sinuses

- The sphenoid sinuses are unique in that they do not arise from an outpouching of the nasal cavity.
- These sinuses arise from within the nasal capsule of the embryonic nose.
- Adult size of a sphenoid sinus is 20 × 23 × 17 mm and has a volume of 7.5 mL.

Table 1.1: Frontoethmoid cells (also known as Kuhn cells).

Kuhn type I	Single cell above agger nasi cell
Kuhn type II	Tier of cells in frontal recess above agger nasi cell—not above frontal beak
Kuhn type III	Single massive cell pneumatizing cephalad into frontal sinus (not extending beyond 50% of the vertical height of the frontal sinus (FS) on the CT scan slice that its is evaluated)
Kuhn type IV	Frontoethmoid cell extending >50% of vertical height on a CT scan

(CT: Computerized tomogrpahy).

- Pneumatization can extend as far as the clivus, the sphenoid wings, or foramen magnum.
- The sphenoid sinuses are separated by an intersinus septum.
- The intersinus septum originates in the midline from the vomer anteriorly, but invariably deviates to attach to a bony prominence over ICA.
- The optic nerve and ICA are often dehiscent within the sphenoid.

Types

Conchal: 3% pneumatization does not reach the body of sphenoid bone (Fig. 1.10).
Presella: 21% within the anterior sphenoid bone and does not go beyond tuberculum sella (Fig. 1.11).
Postsella: 76% well pneumatized and causes bulging of sellar floor into the sinus (Fig. 1.12).

- The most posterior position can place the sinus adjacent to the carotid arteries, optic nerves, maxillary branch of the trigeminal N, vidian N, pons, sella turcica, and cavernous sinus.
- These structures are often identified as indentations on the roof and walls of the sinus. A small percentage will have dehiscence of bone over such vital structures (optic nerve and carotid artery).
- The sphenoid sinus ostium drains into the sphenoethmoidal recess.
- The ostium (0.5–4 mm) may appear slit like and is approximately 12–14 mm above the posterior bony choanae. It lies medial to the lower third of the superior turbinate in the same horizontal plane as the roof of the maxillary sinus. Alternatively, it can be identified as being located about 10 mm above the sinus floor, 7 cm from anterior nasal spine.

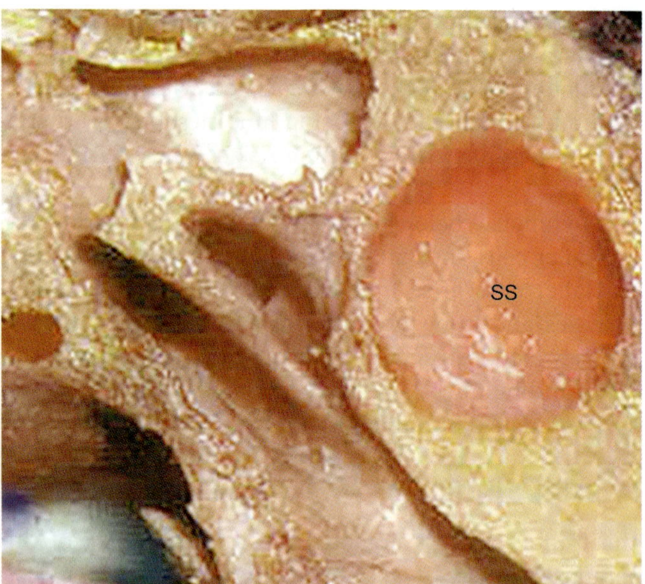

Fig. 1.10: Cadaveric parasagittal section demonstrating conchal pneumatization.

Fovea Ethmoidalis

Fovea ethmoidalis forms the ethmoid roof and frontal bone and is thicker than the adjacent bone. Medially, the region is bound by the lateral lamella of the cribriform plate—lamina cribrosa. This area is one of the weakest areas of the anterior skull base measuring only 0.2–0.5 mm in thickness. The AEA leaves the orbit to enter skull at this point. Here the groove in the lamina cribrosa containing the AEA may be only 0.05 mm in thickness. Point of entry into ACF offers least resistance to probing instruments.

In radiologic evaluation of the sinus scans, the common variability of these cells makes preoperative imaging essential to clarify a patient's individual anatomy.

Skull base evaluation is important in preoperative evaluation of the patients undergoing sinus surgery.

Skull Base Conformations

There are three types of cribriform plate configurations (Keros classification) (Fig. 1.13).
Type I: Olfactory sulcus is 1–3 mm deep (generally safe type).
Type II: Olfactory sulcus is >3–7 mm deep.
Type III: Olfactory sulcus is >7–16 mm deep (hazardous and one should be careful while operating in these cases).

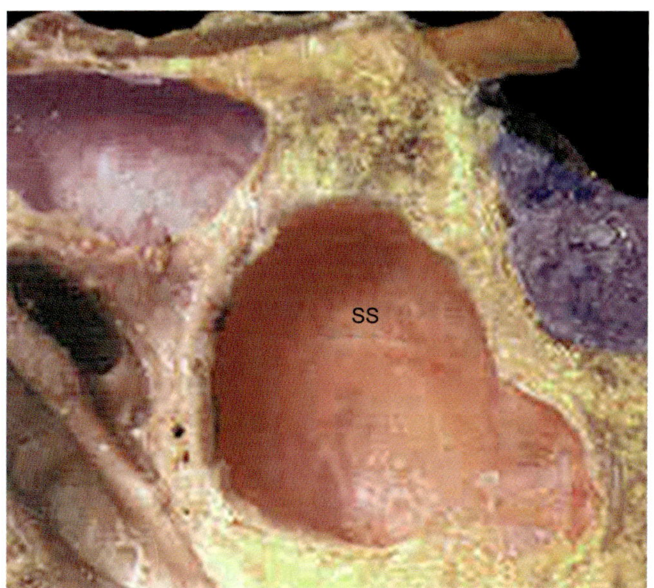

Fig. 1.11: Cadaveric parasagittal section demonstrating presellar pneumatization.

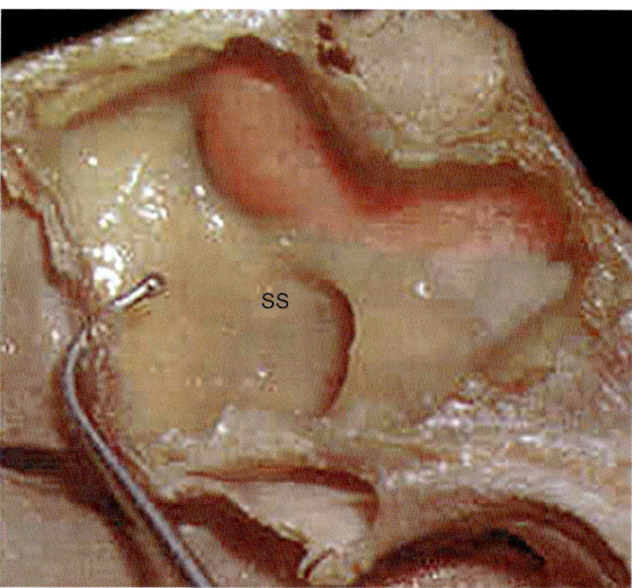

Fig. 1.12: Cadaveric parasagittal section demonstrating sellar pneumatization.

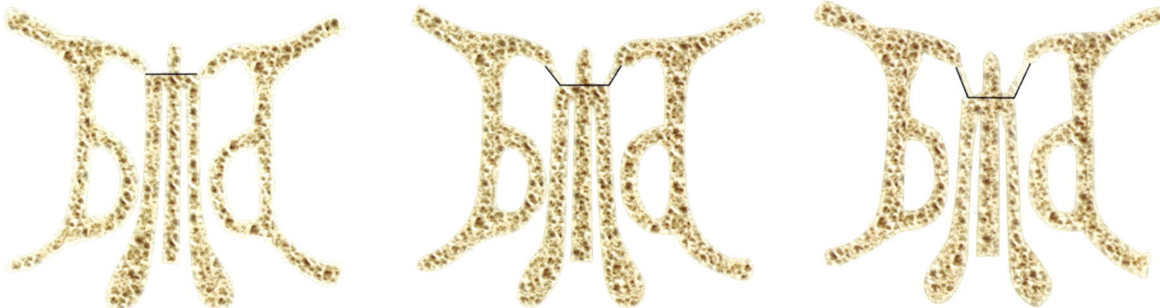

Fig. 1.13: Keros classification of the skull base.

Ethmoid Bulla

It is the largest and most consistent anterior ethmoid cell.

- Created by pneumatization of the bulla lamella (60–70%).
- Located within the middle meatus, behind the uncinate process, anterior to the ground lamella.
- Superiorly, may extend to the skull base to form the posterior limit of the frontal recess. The AEA usually courses across the roof of this cell and would be posterior to the bulla lamella.

Agger Nasi

The agger nasi is the key to the frontal recess.

- It is an ethmoturbinal remnant.
- The cell is in the lacrimal bone anterior and superior to the junction of the MT.
- The uncinate process often makes up the posterior medial wall of the agger nasi cell.
- Drains into hiatus semilunaris.
- Posterior wall of the cell forms the anterior wall of frontal recess.
- The roof is floor of the frontal sinus and it is an important landmark for frontal sinus surgery.

Uncinate Process

It is a sickle-shaped curved structure 3–4 mm wide, 1.5–2 cm in length. It rarely could be pneumatized.

- Attachments:
  Inferiorly: Ethmoid process of inferior turbinate
  Superiorly: Three major variations
- Attaches to lamina papyracea or ethmoid bulla. (Frontal recess opens directly into middle meatus)

- Medially, attaches to lateral surface of MT. (Frontal recess opens into infundibulum)
- Medially and superiorly, attaches to skull base. (Frontal recess opens into infundibulum)

1.6 IMAGING

Plain sinus X-rays are inadequate for the routine diagnosis and management of sinus disease. Scintigraphy is useful in diagnosing osteomyelitis of the frontal bone.

Computer-Assisted Tomography

Computerized tomography is the first choice of radiologic imaging for sinus disease and is essential for planning surgery. In preoperative planning, coronal sinus images are most frequently used due to better correlation of radiologic and clinical findings during surgery. Parasagittal views are very helpful in identifying the drainage pathways. Ideally, CT images should be available in coronal, axial, and parasagittal planes. Advantages of axial scanning include improved patient comfort during scanning and avoidance of dental artifacts. Excellent detail can be achieved with contiguous axial cuts of 0.625 mm thickness. The standard bone window/level settings range between 1500 and 2000/300 Hounsfield units (HU) and 450/50 HU for soft tissue windows.

The following acronym is useful when evaluation CT images of the paranasal sinuses.

CLOSE:

C Cribriform plate
L Lamina payracea
O Optic nerve and Onodi cell
S Sphenoid and skull base
E Ethmoid artery

Magnetic Resonance Imaging

Magnetic resonance imaging (MRI) offers excellent soft tissue detail, but no bony definition. It is very useful in differentiating tumor from retained secretions. Tumors tend to enhance with T1-weighted gadolinium-enhanced scans, while fluids do not. Mucus and secretions tend to avidly enhance on T2-weighted images. Magnetic resonance imaging is very helpful in assessing the dual interfaces between the nasal cavity, and the orbit and the intracranial cavity. It is recommended that in cases of unilateral sinus disease, both CT and MRI are routinely performed. The two imaging modalities are complementary in diagnosing tumors such as inverted papilloma and fungal disease.

Endoscopy

Although anterior rhinoscopy is routinely performed, the accepted gold standard is nasal endoscopy. Traditionally, 4-mm rigid endoscopes have been used to examine the nose. However, smaller 3-mm endoscopes provide very similar optics and tend to be better tolerated by most patients. Narrower 2.7-mm and 1.9-mm endoscopes are available, but compromise image quality and are less robust. Despite the use of narrow endoscopes, access to the middle meatus may be difficult. In patients who have had previous surgery, an angled endoscope (30° or 45°) is useful in examining the frontal recess. In addition, a flexible nasendoscope can be navigated into the frontal sinus for inspection purposes.

REFERENCE

Lund, V.J., Stammberger, S.H., Fokkens, W.J., Beale, T., Bernal-Sprekelsen, M., Eloy, P., Georgalas, C., Gerstenberger, C., Hellings, P., Herman, P., Hosemann, W.G., Jankowski, R., Jones, N., Jorissen, M., Leunig, A., Onerci, M., Rimmer, J., Rombaux, P., Simmen, D., Tomazic, P.V., Tschabitscherr, M. and Welge-Luessen, A., 2014. European position paper on the anatomical terminology of the internal nose and paranasal sinuses. *Rhinology Supplement*, 24, pp. 1-34.

Acute General Nasal Symptoms

2

Ravinder Natt, Claire Hopkins

Chapter Overview

Pearls and Pitfalls

Pearls

- Acute rhinosinusitis most common cause of acute nose related symptoms.
- Most cases are self-limiting and antibiotics are not required.
- Urgent ENT specialist referral in presence of warning signs of actual or impending complications, altered vision, severe headache or other neurological symptoms.

Pitfalls

- Missing acute complications of rhinosinusitis may lead to permanent morbidity.

DIAGNOSTIC SUMMARY OF SYMPTOMS

- Nasal discharge
- Facial pain
- Nasal obstruction
- Facial swelling
- Eye swelling

ACUTE NASAL DISCHARGE

2.1 NASAL FOREIGN BODY

Epidemiology and Pathogenesis

- Common in pediatric population.
- Can be in seen in adult patients with psychiatric problems.
- Organic materials include food and rubber.
- Inorganic materials include metal and plastic.

Clinical Features

Features in Clinical History

- Progressive nasal obstruction.
- Unilateral mucopurulent discharge.
- Painful FBs are highly suspicion of a corrosive agent such as battery.

Flowchart 2.1: Diagnostic tree for acute nasal discharge.

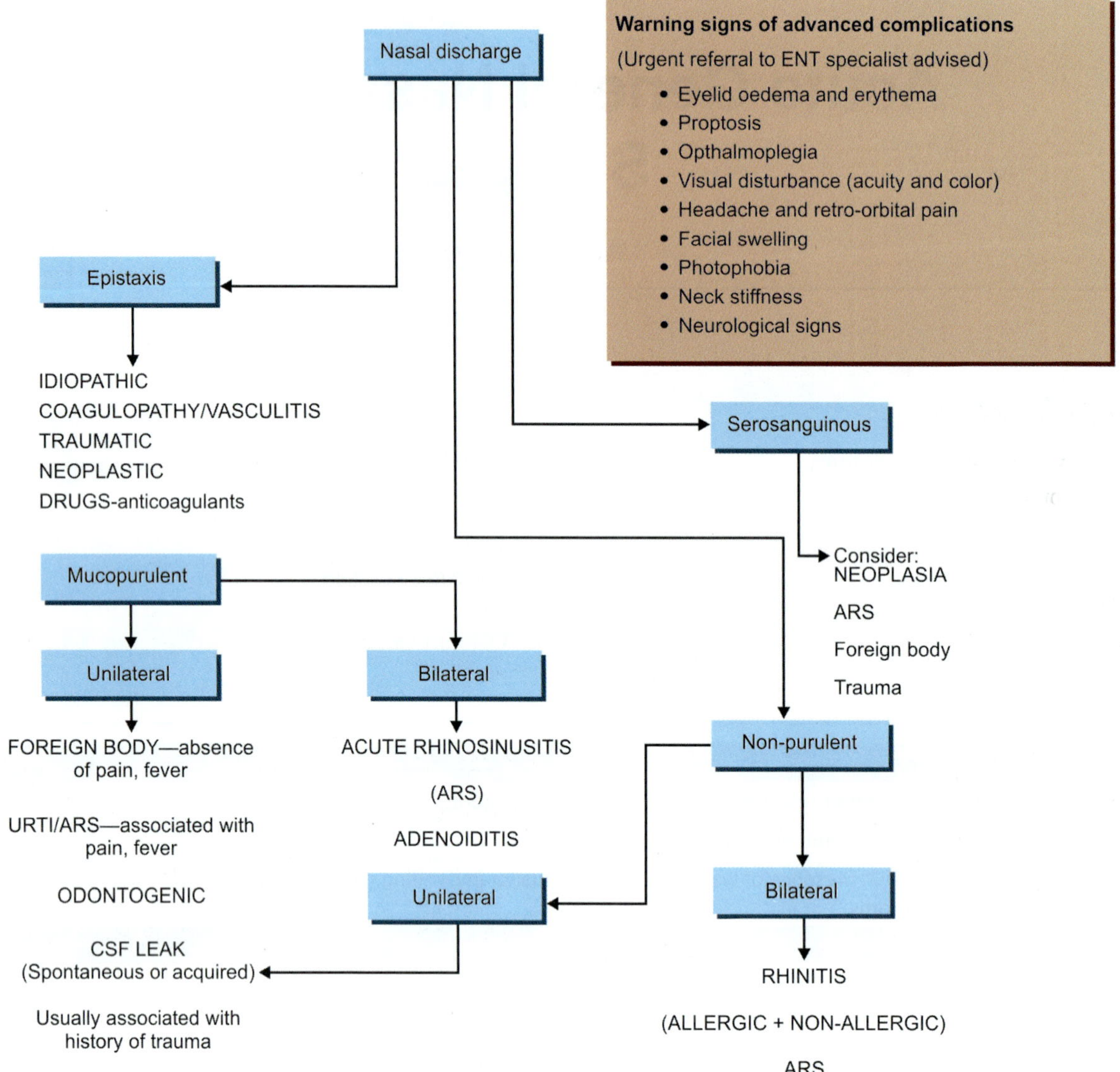

Diagnostic Summary: Nasal Discharge (Flowchart 2.1)

- Serosanguinous:
  - Consider neoplasia—Chapter 4
  - Acute rhinosinusitis (ARS)
  - Foreign body (FB)
- Mucopurulent:
  - Acute rhinosinusitis
  - FB
  - Odontogenic
- Non-mucopurulent:
  - Acute rhinosinusitis
  - Allergic rhinitis (AR)
  - Non-AR (NAR)
  - Cerebrospinal fluid (CSF) rhinorrhea
- Epistaxis—Chapter 9

Typical Findings on Examination

- FBs usually anterior to middle turbinate or below inferior turbinate.
- Must examine both nostrils to exclude occult foreign bodies.

Investigations

Radiograph: To exclude corrosive FB (battery) if history inconclusive and child not cooperating with examination.

Preferred Treatment

- Direct instrumentation and removal under general anesthesia if child is not cooperating.

- Corrosive FB to be removed urgently to avoid complications.
- Positive pressure technique including the Parent's Kiss by the parent delivering air into child's mouth and occluding the unaffected nostril (Alleemudder, Sonsale and Ali, 2007).

Complications of Treatment

- Bleeding if FB very tightly impacted against mucosal surfaces.
- Nasal stenosis and adhesions as a result of mucosal trauma.

Complications of Disease

- Mucosal irritation causing epistaxis.
- Nasal septal perforation/adhesions and stenosis if corrosive FB.
- Posterior dislodgement and tracheal aspiration (rare).
- Rhinolith formation.

2.2 ODONTOGENIC

Epidemiology and Pathogenesis

- Most commonly, the maxillary sinuses are affected because of the anatomical proximity.
- Dental periapical or periodontal abscess secondary to caries.
- Iatrogenic causes of bony sinus wall perforation following dental treatment.
- Benign and malignant odontogenic neoplasia invading into the paranasal sinuses.

Clinical Features

Features in Clinical History

- Facial swelling and pain
- Pyrexia
- Trismus
- Can progress to ARS and cause mucopurulent discharge and nasal obstruction.

Typical Findings on Examination

- Usually, unilateral mucopurulent discharge in the nasal cavity.
- Intraoral examination confirming dental abscess with localized edema of affected teeth.

Investigations

- Orthopantomogram radiograph: to determine site of abscess.
- Computed tomography (CT) scan of paranasal sinuses: if surgical treatment to sinuses considered or diagnostic uncertainty.

Preferred Treatment

- Antibiotic treatment to cover anaerobe organisms, which are the commonest causes of dental abscesses.
- Removal of infected tooth if infection persisting or recurrent.
- Persistent sinus disease may need treatment after dental cause has been treated, or prior to extractions to reduce risk of oroantral fistula.

Complications of Disease

- Development of ARS.
- Formation of dental cyst at site of infected tooth causing recurrent sinus infections.
- Oroantral fistula after dental extraction.
- Osteomyelitis (Longhini, Branstetter and Ferguson, 2012).

2.3 ACUTE RHINOSINUSITIS

Epidemiology and Pathogenesis

- Acute rhinosinusitis can be defined as the sudden onset of two or more symptoms, one of which should be either nasal obstruction of rhinorrhea (anterior or post nasal drip) with the presence or absence of facial pain and hyposmia.
- The symptoms persist by definition for <12 weeks.
- Acute rhinosinusitis is highly prevalent affecting 6–15% of the population (Fokkens, et al., 2012).
- Recurrent ARS is rare.
- Acute viral rhinosinusitis (common cold—rhinovirus) is defined as duration of symptoms of <10 days.
- Acute bacterial rhinosinusitis is usually preceded by an acute viral rhinosinusitis with a phase of further deterioration of symptoms after an initial episode of recovery during the same period of illness (double sickening).
- Bacterial infection thought to occur in 2% cases.
- Usually self-limiting; however, antibiotics often are expected by the patient and subsequently prescribed—92% consultation in primary care result in antibiotic prescription.
- Systematic reviews demonstrate very small clinical benefit from antibiotic use, but number needed to treat is 15, whereas number needed to harm is 7.

Therefore, antibiotics should only be considered in severe cases, or in the presence of complications.
- Analgesia and decongestants may provide symptomatic relief.
- Intranasal corticosteroids are beneficial and associated with low incidence of adverse events.

Clinical Features

Features in Clinical History

- Facial pain may be throbbing, dull, or severe and extends to the frontal, vertex, retro-orbital, and malar regions.
- Facial swelling—suggestive of advanced disease over eyes and frontal region.
- Pyrexia (>39°C), elevated erythrocyte sedimentation rate, purulence on anterior rhinoscopy, purulence in postnasal space, suggested of a bacterial etiology.
- Hyposmia
- Nasal discharge—anterior and/or posterior nasal drip. Purulence alone has positive predictive value of 50% for bacterial infection.
- Children often present with cough—can be difficult to differentiate from acute adenoiditis.
- Exclude warning signs suggestive of complications of ARS—*see* below.

Typical Findings on Examination

- Mucopurulent discharge in the nasal cavity.
- Facial swelling and tenderness.
- Nasal mucosal edema.

Investigations

- *Bacteriology*: Gold standard for diagnosis of bacterial infection is sinus puncture; however, endoscopically guided middle meatal swabs are an alternative.
- *Streptococcus pneumoniae*, *Moraxella catarrhalis*, and *Haemophilus influenzae* are the most common organisms.
- *CT scan of paranasal sinuses*: Indicated only in suspected complications of ARS, as does not differentiate between common cold and ARS, or if surgical intervention considered.
- Contrast CT recommended if suspected orbital or intracranial abscess.
- *Magnetic resonance imaging (MRI) scan*: To determine any intracranial complication.

Preferred Treatment (Flowchart 2.2)

- Complete resolution of symptoms suggests cure. Persistence should lead to re-evaluation of diagnosis and treatment for chronic rhinosinusitis if appropriate.

Complications of Treatment

- Complications of antibiotics usage include severe allergic reactions leading to anaphylactic shock. Gastrointestinal, renal, and neurological disturbance may develop leading to pseudomembranous colitis, convulsions, and renal impairment.
- Antibiotic resistance is a major global health-care problem and the emergence of multidrug resistant pathogens (including methicillin-resistant *Staphylococcus aureus*). The genetic mutations resulting in resistant genes is a consequence of excessive and inappropriate use of antibiotics including indication and duration.
- Antibiotics may also mask sign and symptoms indicating complications of ARS.
- Complications of surgery if required for complicated ARS (endoscopic or external drainage of sinus) are rare but may include epiphora, development of postoperative nasal adhesions, diplopia, visual disturbance, CSF leak, arterial hemorrhage including retrobulbar and cerebral injury with meningitis.

Complications of Disease

- The incidence of complications has been reported as 3 per million populations per year (Hansen, et al., 2012).
- Complications can be categorized with decreasing frequency into orbital (60–75%), intracranial (15–20%), and osseous (5–10%) (Pearlman and Conley, 2008).

Orbital: The close anatomically proximity of the orbit to the paranasal sinuses in particular the ethmoid sinuses makes the orbital region the most commonly involved site of complication. Orbital complications of acute sinusitis have been classified into five categories by Chandler, Langenbrunner and Stevens (1970) as follows:

- *Preseptal cellulitis*:
  - Inflammation of the eyelid and tissue anterior to the orbital septum.
  - Eyelid edema, orbital pain, eyelid erythema.
  - Without reduced or painful eye movements, proptosis, or visual disturbance.
  - Medical therapy for treatment.

Flowchart 2.2: Management of acute rhinosinusitis.

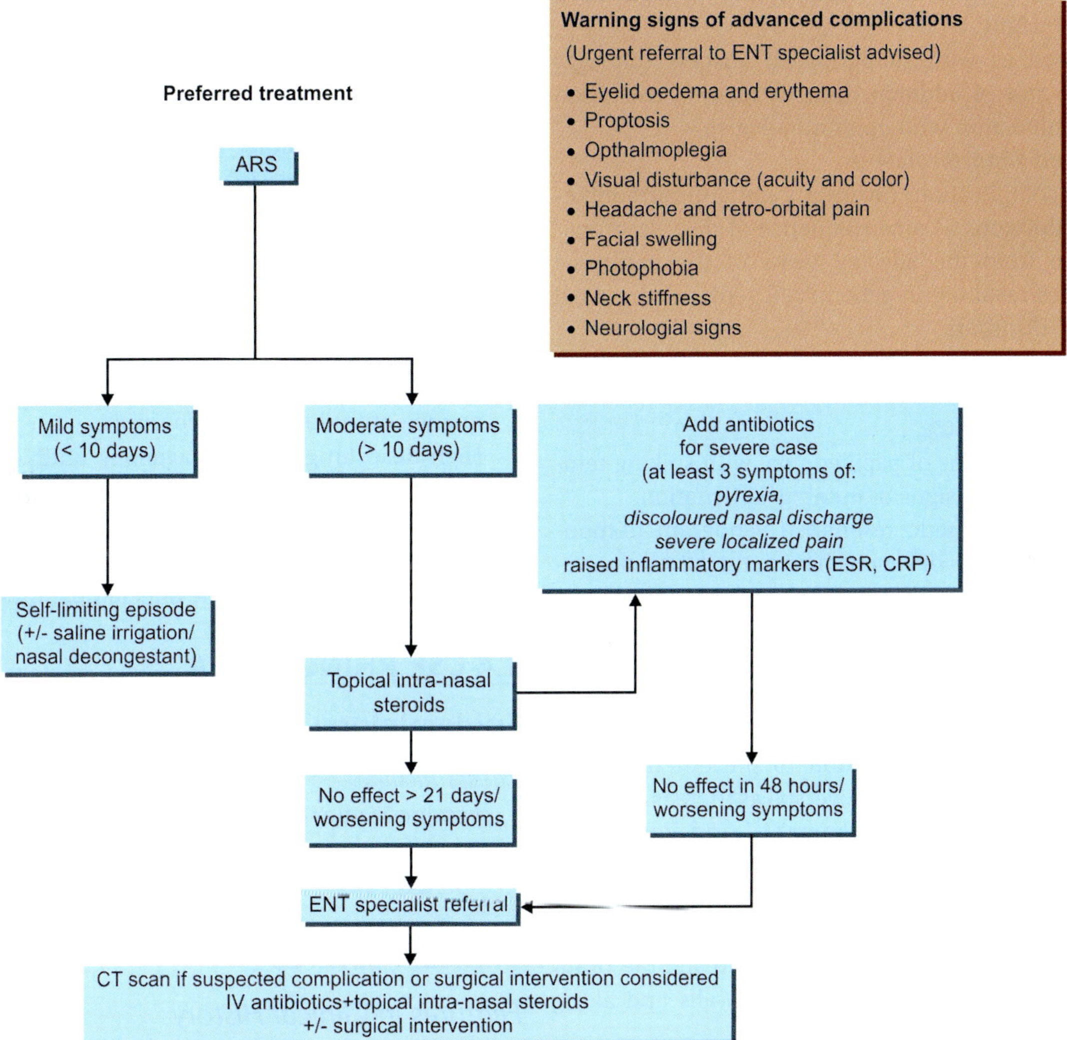

- *Orbital cellulitis*:
  - Inflammation of tissue posterior to the orbital septum.
  - Periorbital cellulitis symptoms with reduced or painful eye movements, proptosis, and chemosis in the presence of NORMAL vision.
  - Medical therapy for treatment.
  - Consider CT if failure to resolve within 24–48 hours, or progressive signs.
- *Subperiosteal abscess*:
  - An extraconal abscess between the periorbita area and lamina papyracea.
  - Orbital cellulitis symptoms with fever and reduced visual acuity with diplopia.
  - Loss of red color vision occurs as early sign—Ishihara charts very useful for assessment (available on smart phones).
  - CT scan reveals edema of the medial rectus muscle with lateralization of the periosteum of the bony orbital margin and displacement of the globe.
  - Surgically drainage of affected paranasal sinus and of abscess through an endoscopic approach involving an ethmoidectomy and opening of lamina papyracea or direct drainage via an external approach.
- *Orbital abscess*:
  - An intraconal abscess within the orbital tissue with significant threat to the optic nerve and irreversible visual loss.

    - Additional symptoms of profound proptosis and opthalmoplegia and significantly deteriorating visual acuity.
    - Proceed as with subperiosteal abscess management and in addition drain intraconal collection in conjunction with ophthalmologist.
- *Cavernous sinus thrombosis*:
    - Rare complication, cavernous sinus thrombophlebitis develops as a consequence of disease propagation from the affected veins of the paranasal sinuses resulting in generalized sepsis and cranial nerve disorders.
    - Symptoms in contralateral eye.
    - There is significant mortality rate of 30% and a morbidity rate of 60%.
    - Additional signs of papilledema, with spiking temperatures and signs of meningeal irritation.
    - Cerebral magnetic resonance venogram demonstrates absence of venous flow in the affected cavernous sinus and filling defects of the ophthalmic veins.
    - Intravenous antibiotics with steroids.
    - Surgical drainage of affected sinus (commonly sphenoid sinus).
    - The use of anticoagulation to prevent thrombus migration remains controversial as there is a potential increased risk of intracranial and intraorbital bleeding (Desa and Green, 2012).

Intracranial: Infections can proceed from the paranasal cavities to the endocranial structures through hematological spread along the diploic veins to reach the brain or via direct bony erosion of the sinus walls and along traumatic fracture lines.

- Most commonly associated with disease involving the frontal, ethmoid, or sphenoid sinuses.
- Specific symptoms and signs include nausea and vomiting, neck stiffness, lethargy and altered conscious levels, focal neurological signs, including cranial nerve palsies and signs of increase intracranial pressure including papilledema.
- Nonspecific symptoms include high pyrexia and severe progressive headache.
- Complications in reducing order of frequency include meningitis, epidural abscess, subdural abscess, intracerebral abscess, and venous sinus thrombosis including sagittal sinus.
- Treatment includes high-dose intravenous antibiotic therapy and steroids with drainage of appropriate sinuses at the same time as neurosurgical drainage of intracranial collection.

Osseus: Sinus infections can involve bony margins causing osteomyelitis and result in thrombophlebitis of the diploic veins leading to intracranial complications.

The frontal sinus bone is most commonly involved.

- Specific symptoms and signs include periorbital and frontal swelling, nasal congestion, rhinorrhea, focal neurological signs, diplopia, photophobia, and meningeal irritation.
- Nonspecific symptoms include high pyrexia and severe progressive headache.
- A Pott's puffy Tumor may develop with features of fluctuant edema over the anterior wall of the frontal bone with subperiosteal pus collection as a consequence of underlying osteomyelitis.
- High-dose long-term intravenous antibiotic therapy and steroids with surgical drainage of subperiosteal abscess and surgical debridement of bone affected by osteomyelitis (Akiyama, Karaki and Mori, 2012).
- Combined drainage of the affected paranasal sinuses.

2.4 CSF RHINORRHEA

Epidemiology and Pathogenesis

Causes include:

- Iatrogenic after surgery
- Head trauma
- Spontaneous

Clinical Features

Features in Clinical History

- Unilateral clear watery nasal discharge
- Increased on tilting head forward or straining
- Salty taste of secretions

Typical Findings on Examination

- May identify on nasal endoscopic examination skull-base defect with active CSF rhinorrhea.

Investigations

- *Immunoelectrophoresis*: β2 transferrin protein detected in nasal secretions, which is highly specific for CSF.
- *CT scan*: May demonstrate skull base defect.
- *MRI scan*: Can demonstrate meningoencephalocele in particular involving sphenoid sinus.

- *Intrathecal fluorescein*: Injection of fluorescein into subarachnoid space prior to surgical repair can reveal fluorescein passing from skull-base fistula into nasal cavity, indicating the site of an occult CSF leak.

Preferred Treatment

- Conservative approach with bed rest and head elevation and stool softeners post-trauma.
- Prophylactic antibiotics remain controversial as they may mask signs of cerebral infections and encourage drug resistance organisms.
- Endoscopic approach for repair now preferred in majority of cases, using abdominal fat, fascia lata, or temporalis fascia graft to repair the defect and secured by nasal mucosal flaps or grafts with fibrin glue (Daele, Goffart and Machiels, 2011).

Complications of Disease

- Risk of meningitis.

Complications of Treatment

- External approaches for repair (including bicoronal and eyebrow incisions) may cause forehead paresthesia following disruption to the supraorbital and supratrochlear nerves.

2.5 RHINITIS

Epidemiology and Pathogenesis

Allergic rhinitis: Inflammation of nasal mucosa primarily but may involve other structures including eyes, middle ear, and pharynx involving inflammatory mediators mediated by immunoglobulin E (IgE).

- Intermittent form of disease is characterized by symptoms < 4 days per week or < 4 weeks per episode.
- Persistent disease of form disease is by symptoms > 4 days per week or > 4 weeks per episode (Bousquet, et al., 2012).

Non-allergic rhinitis: Inflammation of nasal mucosa in the absence of any allergy-based component and can be characterized further into subgroups:

- Infectious rhinitis—commonly viral, of which common cold caused by rhinovirus is the most prevalent with duration of symptoms < 10 days.
- Atrophic rhinitis—impaired mucociliary clearance causing nasal crusting.
- Rhinitis medicamentosa—excess self-use of topical nasal decongestants causing rebound congestion.
- Vasomotor rhinitis—increased vascular tone and permeability triggered by the environment.
- Non-allergic rhinitis with eosinophilia syndrome—presence of nasal eosinophilia without an allergy component.
- Hormonal rhinitis—hormonal imbalance triggers rhinitis (pregnancy, hypothyroidism, and puberty).
- Drug-induced rhinitis—use of certain medications can precipitate rhinitis symptoms including aspirin, oral contraceptives, and beta-blockers.

Clinical Features

Features in Clinical History

- Nasal congestion—bilateral
- Nasal discharge (discoloration suggest and infective cause)
- Ocular symptoms—itchy and watery eyes in AR
- Frequent sneezing—in AR
- Hyposmia

Typical Findings on Examination

- Inflamed nasal mucosa and congested turbinates, clear rhinorrhea
- Conjunctivitis—AR

Investigations

- *Skin-prick test*: Intradermal inoculation of allergens. A positive response results in a wheal and flare appearance when compared to a control solution.
- *Radioallergosorbent test*: In vitro serological analysis of IgE responses to allergens avoiding complication of anaphylaxis with skin-prick testing.
- *CT scan*: Not usually indicated. Consider if no response to medical treatment with suspicion of chronic rhinosinusitis requiring surgical management.

Preferred Treatment (Flowchart 2.3)

- Symptomatic treatment of symptoms with simple analgesics and antipyretics for viral rhinitis.
- Avoidance of allergen, medication, occupational triggers, and correct hormonal imbalances.
- For mainly obstructive symptoms, consider surgical reduction of inferior turbinates.

Flowchart 2.3: Management of rhinitis.

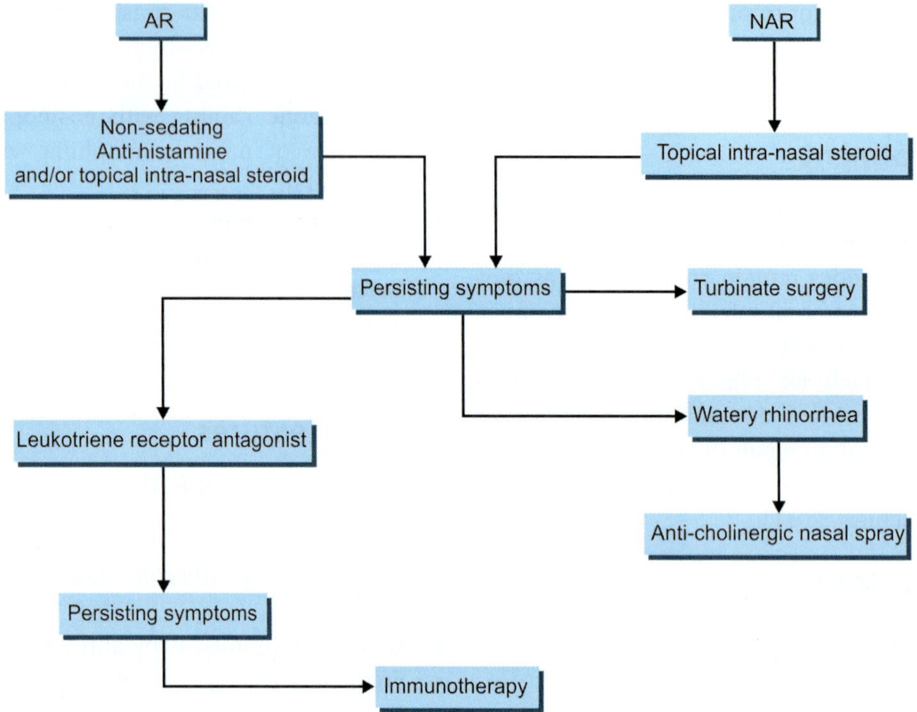

Immunotherapy: Desensitization through controlled application of allergen (Redulovic, et al., 2010).

Complications of Disease

- AR associated with ARS
- Impact on quality of life, reduced performance in school examinations, work.

Complications of Treatment

- Topical nasal sprays can cause localized irritation and epistaxis.
- Allergen immunotherapy carries the risk of anaphylaxis and appropriate management schemes, and clinical environment must be implemented to combat this.
- Hemorrhage and crusting secondary to turbinate reduction.

2.6 ADENOIDITIS

Epidemiology and Pathogenesis

Causes include:

- Inflammation of adenoidal lymphoid tissue.
- Infective cause either viral or bacterial.
- Incidence decreases with age-peak between 3 and 8 years, rare in adolescence, and beyond.

Clinical Features

Features in Clinical History

- Nasal obstruction.
- Mucopurulent discharge.
- Snoring and features suggestive of obstructive sleep apnea (Chapter 10).
- Associated with tonsillitis.
- Associated with otitis media and otitis media with effusion.

Typical Findings on Examination

- Endoscopic nasal examination in cooperative child may demonstrate adenoidal hypertrophy and mucopurulent discharge.

Preferred Treatment

- Usually self-limiting, may require antibiotics in severe infection.
- Prophylactic antibiotics may be considered if recurrent otitis media or adenoiditis.
- Adenoidectomy

Flowchart 2.4: Diagnostic tree for facial pain.

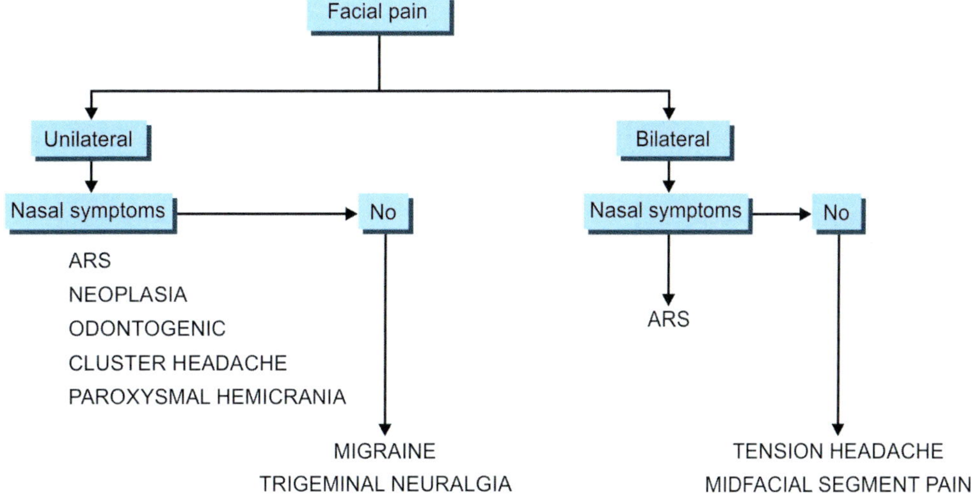

Complications of Treatment

- Infection and hemorrhage.

Complications of Disease

- Extension of infection to surrounding structures causing potential airway obstruction.

Diagnostic Summary: Facial Pain (Flowchart 2.4)

- Unilateral:
  - Neoplasia (*see* section Nasal Discharge)
- Acute rhinosinusitis (*see* section Nasal Discharge):
  - Odontogenic (*see* section Nasal Discharge)
  - Cluster headache
  - Paroxysmal hemicrania
  - Trigeminal neuralgia
- Bilateral:
  - Acute rhinosinusitis (*see* section Nasal Discharge)
  - Migraine
  - Tension headache
  - Midfacial segment pain

Diagnostic Summary: Nasal Obstruction (Flowchart 2.5)

- Unilateral:
  - Neoplasia (*see* section Nasal Discharge)
  - Foreign body (*see* section Nasal Discharge)
  - Odontogenic (*see* section Nasal Discharge)
  - Trauma—(*see* Chapter 12 on Nasal Trauma)
  - Septal abscess
- Bilateral
  - Acute rhinosinusitis (*see* section Nasal Discharge)
  - Allergic rhinitis (*see* section Nasal Discharge)
  - Non-allergic rhinitis (*see* section Nasal Discharge)
  - Adenoiditis (*see* section Nasal Discharge)
  - Trauma (*see* Chapter 12 on Nasal Trauma)

2.7 SEPTAL ABSCESS

Epidemiology and Pathogenesis

- Presence of pus between the cartilaginous septum and overlying layer of mucoperichondrium.
- Associated with nasal trauma or surgery resulting in septal hematoma, which progresses into an abscess and disrupts the blood supply to the septal cartilage.

Clinical Features

Features in Clinical History

- Nasal obstruction
- Pyrexia
- Nasal discharge

Typical Findings on Examination

- Erythema and pain on palpation of nasal tip and dorsum.
- Edema of septum obstructing nasal passage.

Preferred Treatment

- Surgical incision and drainage of abscess with antibiotics.

Flowchart 2.5: Diagnostic tree for nasal obstruction.

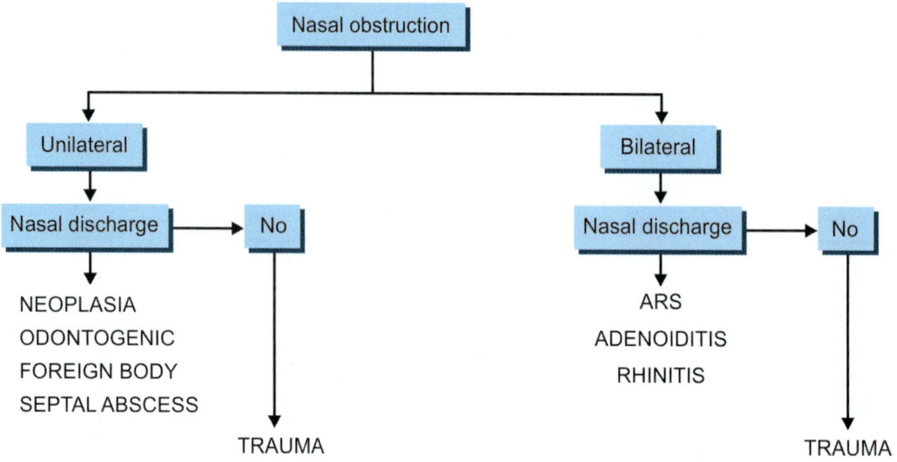

Complications of Disease

- Cosmetic deformity of nose as a consequence of avascular necrosis of septal cartilage.

Diagnostic Summary: Facial Swelling (Flowchart 2.6)

- With fever
  - Acute rhinosinusitis (*see* section Nasal Discharge)
  - Odontogenic (*see* section Nasal Discharge)
  - Cellulitus
- Without fever
  - Trauma (*see* section Facial Trauma)
  - Neoplasia (*see* section Nasal Discharge)

2.8 FACIAL CELLULITIS

Epidemiology and Pathogenesis

- Non-necrotizing inflammation of the skin and subcutaneous tissues secondary to bacterial infection (*Streptococcus* and *Staphylococcal* species) involving the face.
- Danger triangle of face involves the nasal bridge (roof of triangle) and extend to the corners of the mouth (base of triangle) occupying the nose and maxilla.

Clinical Features

Features in Clinical History

- Edema including face, eyes, and lips
- Erythema
- Pain over affected site
- Warmth sensation over inflamed skin
- Pyrexia

Typical Findings on Examination

- Warmth sensation over inflamed skin
- Exclude odontogenic cause of underlying infection

Preferred Treatment

- Use marker pen to demarcate affected area on face to determine further spreading infection.
- Intravenous antibiotics.

Complications of Disease

- Spread of infection along facial veins, which communicate with the cavernous sinus via ophthalmic veins resulting in cavernous sinus thrombosis and associated complications (*see* section Intracranial Complications of ARS).

Diagnostic Summary: Eye Swelling (Flowchart 2.7)

- Unilateral
  - Acute rhinosinusitis (*see* section Nasal Discharge)
  - Trauma
- Bilateral
  - Allergic reaction including AR.

2.9 ALLERGIC REACTION

Epidemiology and Pathogenesis

- Inflammatory reaction following exposure to an allergen.

Flowchart 2.6: Diagnostic tree for facial swelling.

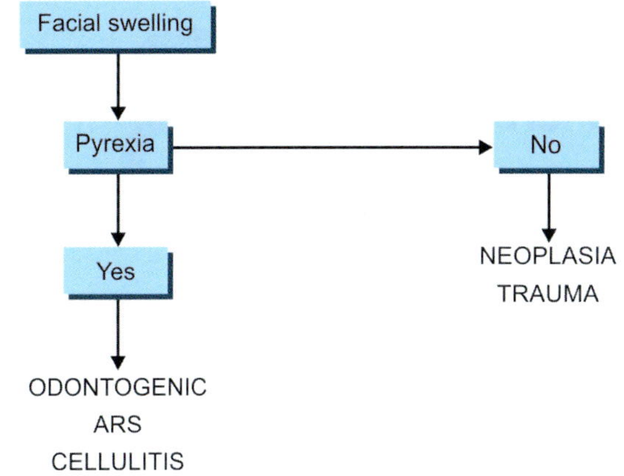

Flowchart 2.7: Diagnostic tree for eye swelling.

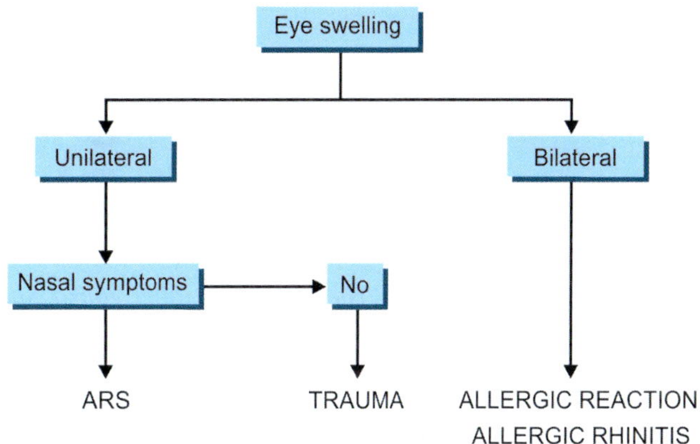

Clinical Features

Features in Clinical History

- Edema including face, eyes, and lips
- Urticaria
- Cough and wheeze
- Sneezing
- Watery eye
- Increased nasal secretions

Typical Findings on Examination

- Look for signs of severe and progress allergic reaction including respiratory and cardiovascular compromise.

Investigations

- Serology: measure baseline mast cell tryptase (Rutkowski, Dua and Nasser, 2012).

Preferred Treatment

- Avoid allergen exposure.
- Combination of antihistamines, bronchodilators, topical nasal steroid sprays, and eye drops depending on severity of reaction.
- Immunotherapy for repeated attacks.
- Progression to anaphylaxis reaction, which is potentially life threatening.

REFERENCES

Akiyama, K., Karaki, M. and Mori, N., 2012. Evaluation of adult Pott's puffy tumor: our five cases and 27 literature cases. *Laryngoscope*, 122(11), pp. 2382-8.

Alleemudder, D., Sonsale, A. and Ali, S., 2007. Positive pressure technique for removal of nasal foreign bodies. *International Journal of Pediatric Otorhinolaryngology*, 71(11), pp. 1809-11.

Bousquet, J., Schünemann, H.J., Samolinski, B., et al., 2012. Allergic Rhinitis and Its Impact on Asthma (ARIA): achievements in 10 years and future needs. *Journal of Allergy and Clinical Immunology*, 130(5), pp. 1049-62.

Chandler, J.R., Langenbrunner, D.J. and Stevens, E.R., 1970. The pathogenesis of orbital complications in acute sinusitis. *Laryngoscope*, 80(9), pp. 1414-28.

Daele, J.J., Goffart, Y. and Machiels, S., 2011. Traumatic, iatrogenic, and spontaneous cerebrospinal fluid (CSF) leak: endoscopic repair. *B-ENT*, 7(Suppl 17), pp. 47-60.

Desa, V. and Green, R., 2012. Cavernous sinus thrombosis: Current therapy. *Journal of Oral and Maxillofacial Surgery*, 70(9), pp. 2085-91.

Fokkens, W.J., Lund, V.J., Mullol, J., et al., 2012. European position paper on rhinosinusitis and nasal polyps 2012. *Rhinology Supplement*, 23:3p preceding table of contents, pp. 1-298.

Hansen, F.S., Hoffmans, R., Georgalas, C. and Fokkens, W.J., 2012. Complications of acute rhinosinusitis in the Netherlands. *Family Practice*, 29(2), pp. 147-53.

Longhini, A.B., Branstetter, B.F. and Ferguson, B.J., 2012. Otolaryngologists' perceptions of odontogenic maxillary sinustis. *Laryngoscope*, 122(9), pp. 1910-4.

Pearlman, A.N. and Conley, D.B., 2008. Review of current guidelines related to the diagnosis and treatment of rhinosinusitis. *Current Opinion in Otolaryngology & Head and Neck Surgery*, 16(3), pp. 226-30.

Radulovic, S., Calderon, M.A., Wilson, D. and Durham, S., 2010. Sublingual immunotherapy for allergic rhinitis. *Cochrane Database of Systematic Reviews*, (12).

Rutkowski, K., Dua, S. and Nasser, S., 2012. Anaphylaxis: current state of knowledge for the modern physician. *Postgraduate Medical Journal*, 88(1042), pp. 458-64.

Nasal Congestion and Nasal Obstruction

3

Nikhil J Bhatt, Taher Valika, Salil B Nair, Zahoor Ahmad

Chapter Overview

Pearls and Pitfalls

Pearls

- Nasal congestion could be due to physical causes of obstruction in nose or due to environmental factors—ranging from allergy/infection to systemic factors affecting nasal physiology.
- Medications causing change in nasal blood flow or affecting nasal secretions should always be kept in mind while managing these patients.

Pitfalls

- Majority of the times, the symptoms are multifactorial and addressing only one factor may not resolve the symptoms.

3.1 INTRODUCTION

The nose has two main functions, the olfaction and the respiration; the latter involves filtration, heating, and humidification of inhaled air. Nasal obstruction can lead to a variety of disorders including, but not limited to, a decreased sense of smell or taste and speech and hearing disorders. Swelling of the nasal mucosa and nasal deformity (both internal and external) are primary causes of nasal obstruction. The nasal airflow cycle changes every 90–180 minutes. Many factors play a role in this including environment, temperature, humidity, body activity, and resting position. The resistance to nasal airflow depends upon the condition of the nasal mucosa, which, in turn, is regulated by our surroundings.

Anatomical abnormalities resulting in obstruction include the following:

- Deviated nasal septum, which can obstruct in various ways. Anterior deflections can cause flaring of the columella. "S"-shaped deflections may result in bilateral obstruction.
- Nasal valve obstruction caused by the protrusion of the caudal end of the upper lateral cartilage and enlarged anterior aspect of the inferior turbinate in relation to the floor of the nose at the nasal vestibule.
- Traumatic causes with injuries to septum and external framework.
- Nasopharyngeal obstruction by enlarged adenoids.
- Other conditions include Wegener's granulomatosis, sarcoidosis, Sjögren's syndrome and tuberculosis. Leprosy or other granulomatous conditions are rarer causes.
- Neoplastic lesions, either benign or malignant, may also produce nasal obstruction.

- Less common are developmental causes leading to nasal obstruction such as cysts, choanal atresia, fibrous dysplasia, and craniofacial abnormalities.

Mucosal congestion and nasal obstruction may occur as a result of the following:

- Inflammatory reactions secondary to viruses, bacteria, pollutants, pollens, chemical irritants, and noxious gases.
- A more common factor producing nasal obstruction is a neurovascular imbalance known as vasomotor rhinitis, which can be difficult to manage.
- Vascular congestion is quite common in patients who are taking antiadrenergic drugs, including, but not limited to, antihypertensive and prostate medications or birth control pills.
- Vascular congestion can occur as a result of metabolic and/or endocrine disorders such as pregnancy and hypothyroidism.
- Lastly, one should not forget the condition known as "empty nose syndrome". This may be iatrogenic or secondary to atrophic rhinitis. In such conditions, though the nasal passages are widely patent, the patient continues to complain of nasal obstruction. This is a result of altered nasal airflow.

Now, let us review the characteristics of common conditions causing nasal congestion or nasal obstruction.

3.2 ALLERGIC RHINITIS

Epidemiology/Pathogenesis

- The second leading cause of chronic disease in the United States.
- Affects nearly 25% of adults and 40% of children.
- Due to immunoglobulin E (IgE)-mediated inflammation of the nasal mucosa by an allergen.
- Commonly associated with other atopic conditions.
- Due to a combination of both genetic and environmental variables.
- Decreased prevalence in third-world countries.
- May be seasonal or perennial.

Clinical History

Most patients present with itchy nose, sneezing, rhinorrhea, and nasal congestion. Other symptoms may include eye and ear itching as well as watery eyes. Pediatric patients commonly present with fatigue as a primary symptom. Symptoms may occur at a specific time of the year or may be present throughout the year and at specific locations, which may change with travel. Other atopic conditions including asthma may be associated with allergic rhinitis.

Clinical Examination

- The presence of a nasal crease can occur due to repetitive rubbing of the nose.
- Abundant clear mucus stranding can be seen along the nasal mucosa.
- The turbinates may be hypertrophied and boggy. The turbinate mucosa may have a purplish hue.
- There can be edema of the lower eyelids, erythema of the conjunctival vessels, and increased secretions from the eye.
- Oral examination may show posterior pharyngeal wall mucosa cobblestoning, erythema, or edema noted due to postnasal drip.
- Otoscopic examination may reveal retracted tympanic membrane or middle ear effusion.
- Nasal endoscopy should be performed to rule out any structural or other obstructive lesions.

Investigations

History alone can be the key to diagnosis! Imaging is usually not necessary unless symptoms of chronic sinusitis are suspected. Allergy testing can help isolate a specific set of antigens to guide therapy.

Allergen skin-prick testing may show positive results in the form of wheal and flare reaction. The risk of anaphylaxis should always be considered when ordering for skin prick tests.

- In vitro specific IgE (immunoglobulin-E) testing or other blood specific testing however does not carry any anaphylaxis risks.

Treatment Options

Treatment involves a combination of environmental control, pharmacotherapy, and immunotherapy.

Allergy testing can be completed to further guide therapy. Environmental changes to reduce allergen exposure include: high efficiency particulate air filter use, low humidity, hard surface flooring, hot water laundry, and pet-free areas. A combination of using the above is the most effective preventive measure.

Allergen avoidance is commonly recommended but not always possible. Pharmacotherapy is the mainstay of treatment and includes the following:

- Antihistamines
  - Oral
  - Topical—nasal and ocular
- Steroids
  - Oral
  - Topical—intranasal corticosteroid (INCS) sprays and ocular steroids.
- Leukotriene modifiers
- Mast cell stabilizers
- Nasal decongestants
- Nasal hygiene (saline rinsing of nose)

Intranasal corticosteroids are the most effective class of medications. These are well tolerated with minimal risk of hypothalamic/pituitary axis suppression. Common side effects include blood spotting from the nose. Stopping the spray or changing to another preparation usually solves this issue. Serious complications such as bone fractures are extremely rare.

Saline nasal irrigations help to improve nasal hygiene and used in combination with other topical therapies, are effective in maintaining symptom control.

Immunotherapy is effective, but not available in many centers. The aim is to desensitize a patient to specific allergens. Therapy can be administered either subcutaneously or sublingually but in either case the treatment protocol may be at least for 2 years.

Surgery may be an option if the inferior turbinate remains hypertrophic while on pharmacotherapy. This can help improve the airway, but in addition, facilitate more effective delivery of the topical medication.

Treatment Outcomes and Prognosis

The most important advice is to ensure patients continue with their topical therapy. Combination therapy monitoring can be performed at follow-up visits with the addition of alternative medications as required.

Long-term studies have demonstrated that nearly 50% of population report an improvement in symptoms with combination therapy.

Possible Complications and Side Effects

Most common issues are associated with side effects from medications. This can include sedation (first-generation antihistamines), nasal irritation and epistaxis (intranasal steroids), hypertension, and sleep disturbances (oral decongestants), and nasal congestion and sneezing (topical anticholinergics).

3.3 NONALLERGIC RHINITIS (CHAPTER 7)

Epidemiology/Pathogenesis

1. Nasal symptoms are present in the absence of allergic triggers.
2. Likely a chronic inflammatory state and a gross imbalance of neuropeptides affect the nasal mucosa.
3. Must exclude allergic, infectious, and obstructive causes of rhinitis first.
4. Some patients may have a mixed rhinitis, which includes allergic and nonallergic triggers.
5. A wide gamut of possible etiologies falls under this diagnosis and include the following:
   a. Idiopathic rhinitis
      i. Imbalance of inflammation and neuromodulators in the nasal mucosa
   b. Occupational rhinitis
      i. Exposure to stimulus at workplace, and not elsewhere
   c. Medication-induced rhinitis
      i. Most commonly seen with antihypertensive medications, antidepressants, antipsychotics, and anti-inflammatory medications.

There is a long list of medicines that cause nasal congestion; however, some commonly used drugs having this side effect are as follows:

1. Nifedipines (e.g. Adalat)
2. Dopaminergic antihypertensives like Aldomet/m-Dopa
3. Baclofen
4. Bromocriptine
5. Beta blockers (e.g. Atenolol)
6. Buspirone
7. Calcitonin
8. Antihistamines-Cetirizine
9. Angiotensin-converting-enzyme inhibitors
10. Cromolyn
11. DDAVP (1-deamino-8-D-arginine vasopressin)
12. Prazosin
13. Risperidone
14. Sildenafil/Viagra
15. Tacrolimus
16. Ventolin
17. Antivirals
18. Progesterones and estrogens

   d. Nonallergic rhinitis with eosinophilia syndrome (NARES)
      i. Allergic symptoms, but with no allergen trigger identifiable

   ii. Likely due to eosinophil-mediated toxicity resulting in decreased mucociliary clearance
e. Rhinitis medicamentosa
   i. From overuse of topical nasal decongestants resulting in tachyphylaxis and thus severe rebound nasal congestion, e.g. xylometazoline (Otrivin) overuse.
f. Hormone-induced rhinitis
   i. Occur during states of increased progesterone and estrogen levels, or decreased thyroid hormone levels
g. Vasomotor rhinitis
   i. Due to autonomic nervous system dysfunction
h. Atrophic rhinitis
   i. Paradoxical nasal congestion; unclear etiology
   ii. Seen in patients with prior nasal surgery and widely patent nasal airways.

Clinical History

- History is important to make the diagnosis. Patients may present with nasal congestion, postnasal drip, rhinorrhea, pressure on the face, sneezing, and occasional sore throat.
- Symptoms occurred after certain medications were started.
- Symptoms occur at work and dissipate when not in that environment.
- Symptoms occur after prolonged nasal decongestant use or use of eye drops.
- Symptoms occur during a period of hormonal imbalance.
- Symptoms occur in response to physical or emotional stimuli.
- Symptoms began after a sinonasal surgical procedure.

Typical Examination Findings

Nasal examination may show dry pale mucosa. The turbinates may be hypertrophic. The nasal cavity may be widely patent as demonstrated by (spatula test) misting of a cold mirror or tongue depressor (like in atrophic rhinitis or empty nose syndrome).

Oral cavity may show posterior pharyngeal wall cobblestone appearance of mucosa.

Nasal endoscopy is indicated to rule out structural or other lesions resulting in the symptoms.

Investigations

A thorough history of the patient's symptoms and general health can help pinpoint the nature of the rhinitis. When symptoms are longstanding, causes of perennial allergy need to be investigated. Specific testing may be necessary.

Treatment Options

Treatment options differ depending on the etiology of the nonallergic rhinitis:

Idiopathic Rhinitis

- Intranasal antihistamines and intranasal steroids may help.
- Daily nasal saline sprays and irrigations in addition to the above.
- Inferior turbinate reduction.

Occupational Rhinitis

- Immunologic testing can be done.
- Intranasal antihistamines and intranasal steroids are helpful.
- Daily nasal saline sprays and irrigations in addition to the above.

Medication-induced Rhinitis

- Substitution of the offending agents.

Nonallergic Rhinitis with Eosinophilia Syndrome

- Allergy testing is usually negative.
- Intranasal steroids and intranasal antihistamines may be helpful.

Rhinitis Medicamentosa

- Discontinuation of the offending agent (nasal decongestants).
- Rule out other causes for the presenting rhinitis complaints (above causes).

Hormone-induced Rhinitis

- Nasal saline irrigations are the mainstay during pregnancy.
- Leukotriene inhibitors and mast cell stabilizers can be used as the second-line therapy.

Atrophic Rhinitis

- Nasal saline irrigations are the mainstay.
- Antibiotic irrigations may be used as well.
- Glycerin with glucose has been used with some success in these patients.
- Surgical options to rebuild the nasal airway are last resort, e.g. modified Young's procedure.

3.4 ADENOID HYPERTROPHY (*SEE* PEDIATRIC CHAPTERS ON NASAL OBSTRUCTION AND SNORING)

Epidemiology/Pathogenesis

There is normal lymphoid tissue known as the adenoids in the nasopharynx. The increase in size of the adenoid lymphoid tissue in relation to the size of the nasopharynx can result in nasal congestion. Growth of adenoid tissue is variable and cannot be attributed to a single factor. Adenoid tissue attains its maximum size around the age of 5. The enlarged adenoid tissue can at times harbor bacteria and result in surrounding chronic inflammation as well.

Clinical History

Clinical history is mostly seen in the pediatric population, but can present in adults as well. Patients present with chronic nasal congestion and chronic mouth breathing complaint is very common.

Patients may complain of recurrent ear or sinus infections, or present with a hyponasal voice. Nasal discharge due to adenoid growth is a common symptom in children.

Typical Examination Findings

Observe the patient. They may be mouth breathing during the encounter. Look for flaring of the nostrils as this may be a sign of increased nasal resistance. Using anterior rhinoscopy, visualize the nasal airways and note their patency. Visualization of the nasopharynx with a mirror is possible in some patients. However, nasal endoscopy is required to adequately examine the nasopharynx. This can be done easily in adults and often in compliant children, which can avoid unnecessary imaging.

Otoscopy may show retracted tympanic membranes or middle ear effusion.

Investigations

Imaging with a lateral neck X-ray may be helpful in confirming the presence of adenoidal hypertrophy; however, it is rarely required.

Treatment Options

The use of topical nasal steroids can improve mild-to-moderate adenoidal hypertrophy. However, significant obstruction secondary to adenoidal hypertrophy may require surgical removal (adenoidectomy).

Increasingly suction diathermy or coblation techniques are being favored over curettage for adenoidectomy.

Treatment Outcomes and Prognosis

Studies suggest that up to 87% of patients note improvement in their symptoms after adenoidectomy. Adenoid regrowth may be seen in 3% of the population, but this was noted not to be associated with significant nasal obstruction.

Possible Complications and Side Effects

Chronic adenoid hypertrophy can result in nasal congestion, fatigue, chronic otitis media, and obstructive sleep apnea. This can affect development of children and result in other comorbidities.

3.5 UNILATERAL CHOANAL ATRESIA

Epidemiology/Pathogenesis

Choanal atresia can occur due to the persistence of the bucconasal membrane of Hochstetter or due to medial outgrowths of the palatine bone. Unilateral atresia is twice as common as bilateral choanal atresia. Unilateral atresia occurs more frequently on the right side. The male-to-female incidence is 1:2. About 90% are secondary to bony obstruction and 10% are membranous obstructions, although most are combination of both (Assanasen and Metheetrairut, 2009).

About 50% of patients have associated with syndromic conditions or chromosomal abnormalities. This is composed of coloboma of the eye (second pupil or a black notch at the edge of the pupil), heart defects, atresia of the choanae, retardation in growth and/or development, genital and/or urinary abnormalities, and ear abnormalities and deafness. Bilateral choanal atresia is noted at birth, may be fatal if not managed urgently, and is rarely seen in the clinical setting in adults.

Clinical History

Patients present with unilateral nasal congestion and often a mucoid discharge as their primary complaint.

Typical Examination Findings

Inspect the nose. Using anterior rhinoscopy, a white mucoid discharge is seen on the floor of the affected nasal cavity. Endoscopic examination confirms the absence of a patent posterior choanae.

Inspect the Oral Cavity

A mirror may be utilized to visualize the nasopharynx and the choanae and nasal endoscopy should be performed for the same. The nature of the obstruction may be determined by the use of the endoscope tip (palpation).

Investigations

A paranasal sinus computed tomography (CT) scan is indicated to assess the degree of choanal atresia. This can help the surgeon to determine whether the obstruction is bony or membranous in nature.

Treatment Options

Surgery is the main treatment option. A complete workup to identify any associated syndromic or chromosomal abnormalities must be completed prior to any surgical intervention. The aim is to restore a normal nasal passage while preserving the integrity of the surrounding structures.

Possible options include an endoscopic approach with powered instrumentation including microdebriders and drills. CO_2 and potassium titanyl phosphate lasers have been used, as have more extensive transpalatal approaches.

Treatment Outcomes and Prognosis

Treatment outcomes depend on the approach chosen. Open approaches may provide more exposure, but can result in increased blood loss and disturbances in facial growth. The endoscopic approach is favored as it provides a good view and is less traumatic. The use of the laser has shown to improve patency, decreasing the need for stenting and revision surgery (Assanasen and Metheetrairut, 2009).

3.6 NASAL SEPTAL DEVIATION

Epidemiology/Pathogenesis

The nasal septum is comprised of bone and cartilage. The bony portion is made of the ethmoid bone and vomer, posteriorly. Anteriorly, the septum is cartilaginous in nature.

Deviation is usually a result of trauma, which may have sustained anytime from the neonatal period through to adulthood.

Clinical History

Patients most commonly presents with unilateral fixed nasal obstruction. They may report other sinonasal complaints including rhinitis, sinusitis, and anosmia. Some may also present with signs of obstructive sleep apnea.

Patients should be asked about the following:
- History of trauma to nose
- History of use of nasal steroid sprays with no relief noted
- History of prior nasal surgery.

Typical Examination Findings

Inspect the nose. Assess the columella and the location of the medial crura footplate. Palpate the base of the nose and assess the strength of the cartilage, if present. Using anterior rhinoscopy, visualize the nasal septum for any deviations or spurs. Examination should be done before and after decongestant has been applied. Nasal endoscopy is warranted to assess the posterior septum, the presence of perforations, and allows for better assessment of the severity of the nasal obstruction.

Treatment

For fixed nasal obstruction due to septal deviation, surgery is the main treatment option. Septoplasty indications include the following:
- Deviation with partial or complete obstruction of the nasal airway or osteomeatal complex
- Persistent or recurrent epistaxis
- Obstructive sleep apnea due to septal deviation
- For surgical access
- Cosmetic, as part of a septorhinoplasty.

Treatment Outcomes and Prognosis

A multicenter study suggests that nearly 90% of patients report a subjective improvement in their nasal symptoms following septoplasty (Gasndomi, Bayat and Kazemei, 2010).

Possible Complications of a Septal Deviation

Chronic septal deviation can cause drying of the nasal mucosa and obstructive symptoms, which can inhibit proper clearance of disease during an acute infectious state.

Septal deviation also predisposes to nasal bleeding as a result of stretching of mucosa and crust formation on deviated parts of septum due to excessive drying effect.

Possible Complications from Surgery

Complications from surgery include hematoma, septal perforation, persistent septal deviation, cerebrospinal fluid leak, toxic shock syndrome, epistaxis, injury to eye, anosmia, cosmetic nasal deformity, and persistent nasal obstruction.

3.7 NASAL VALVE COLLAPSE (CHAPTER 17)

Epidemiology/Pathogenesis

The internal nasal valve is the narrowest portion of the nasal airway and encounters the highest degree of resistance. The valve consists of the upper lateral cartilage, cartilaginous septum, nasal floor, and anterior surface of inferior turbinate. Deformities of the internal nasal valve can result in obstruction of the nasal airway. Patients can present with unilateral or bilateral nasal obstruction.

Clinical History

Most patients present with complaints of a fixed nasal obstruction. Sometimes the obstruction is felt in the inspiratory phase only.

Typical Examination Findings

Inspect the nose. Examine the valve area as the patient inspires. Collapse of the lateral nasal wall resulting in diminished nasal airway is the key to diagnosis.

Perform the Cottle's maneuver. Lift the patient's cheek and have them inspire. If the patient notes a subjective improvement in their obstruction, this test is positive. In our clinical practice, we perform this test using a Q-tip and placing it intranasally at the level of the valve and having the patient inspire (Figs. 3.1 to 3.3).

Investigations

Diagnostic imaging is not necessary for the diagnosis and clinical examination is sufficient.

Treatment Options

Medical management involves adhesive strips (breathe right devices), which patients can apply on the nasal dorsum, and help retract the lateral nasal walls by providing an external lifting pressure.

Surgical management is the definitive treatment. This can involve spreader grafts to widen the nasal valve, alar batten grafts to strengthen the lateral nasal walls or M-plasty of upper lateral cartilage or lateral crural J-skin incisions within the nasal vestibules.

3.8 NASAL POLYPS

Epidemiology/Pathogenesis

Most commonly, nasal polyps occur in response to chronic inflammation, whether from chronic infection or chronic allergic responses. Polyps occur due to the swelling of the nasal mucosal lining and consist of the loose connective tissue and edema. The prevalence is approximately 4% of the US population (Ryan M). There are no specific genetic or racial predilections although they are associated with certain genetically inherited conditions such as cystic fibrosis. There is a higher association with other atopic conditions like in Samter's triad.

Clinical History

Patients may present with a prolonged history of worsening nasal congestion. Other nasal symptoms include anosmia, rhinorrhea, facial pressure, postnasal drip, and headache.

A history of aspirin sensitivity, asthma, and other atopic conditions may be noted. The occasional patient will present with a mass emanating from their nares.

Typical Examination Findings

Observe the patient. A patient may have severe nasal obstruction resulting in obligate mouth breathing.

Inspect the nose. Using anterior rhinoscopy, edematous and polypoid tissue may be visualized in the middle meatus or obstructing the nasal airway. Ensure the polyps are not pulsating.

Inspect the oral cavity. There can be posterior pharyngeal cobblestoning noted due to postnasal drip. Mirror examination of the nasopharynx may reveal polyps in the nasopharynx (commonly seen in antrochoanal polyps).

Nasal endoscopy should be performed to visualize the entire nasal cavity and clearly identify the polyps.

Investigations

A CT sinus is performed to visualize the extent of the polypoidal disease. All unilateral polyps should be biopsied to confirm histology. Prior to any, biopsy the imaging should be studied to ensure that the lesion is not vascular lesion or a meningoencephalocele.

Allergy testing may be requested on the basis of history.

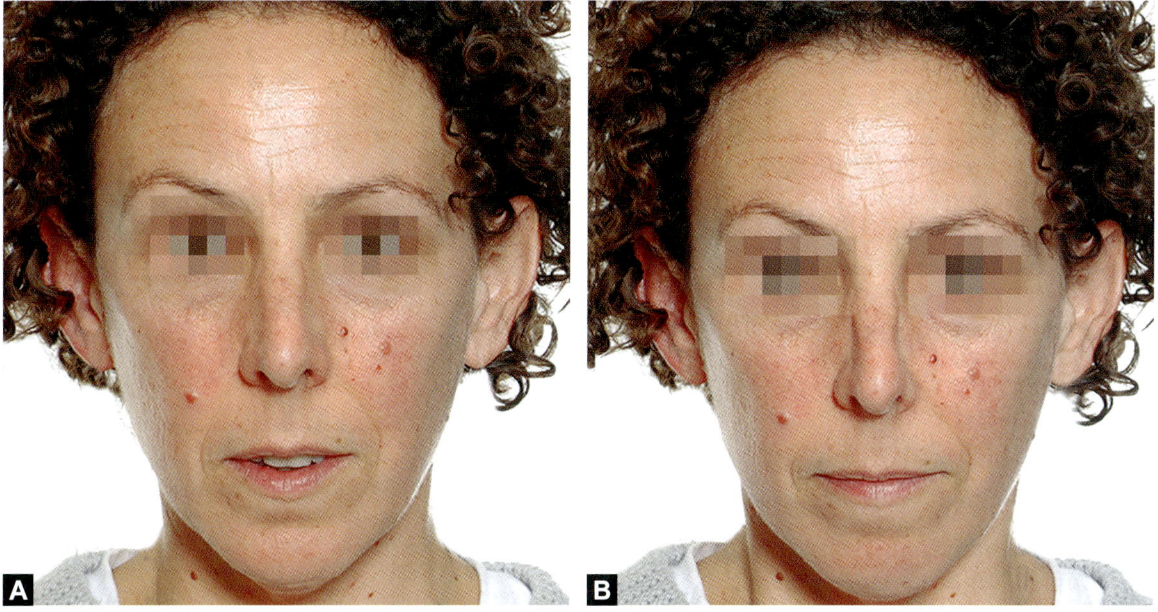

Figs. 3.1A and B: Nasal valve collapse.

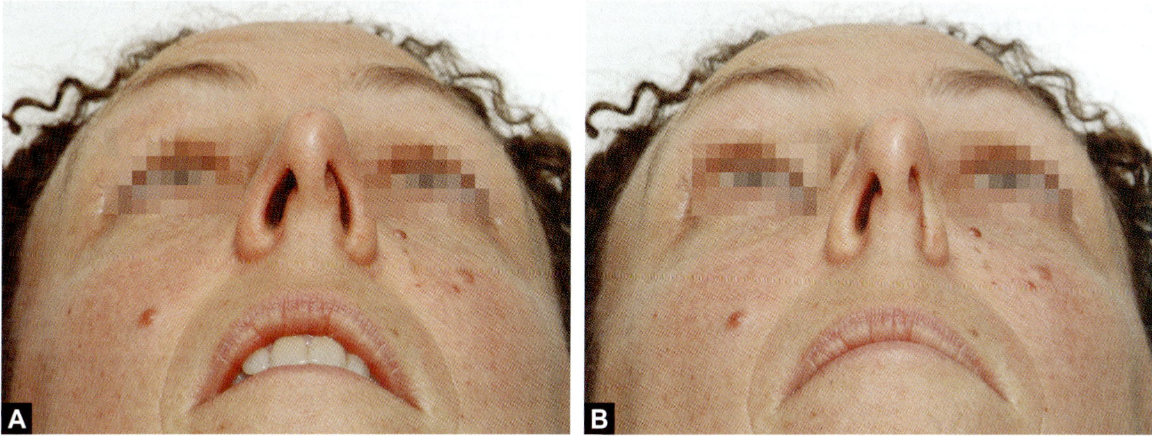

Figs. 3.2A and B: Nasal valve collapse.

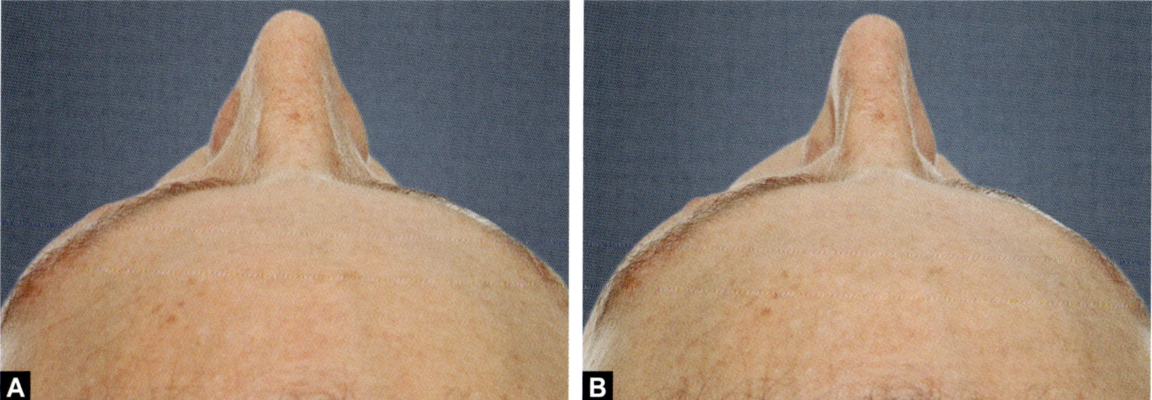

Figs. 3.3A and B: (A) Note the normal alar contour pre-inspiration. (B) Note alar valve collapse post-inspiration.

Treatment Options

Treatment for mild polypoidal disease begins with intranasal corticosteroid use (INCS) use. Nasal saline irrigations are useful in reducing troublesome symptoms.

Symptomatic treatment for acute flare ups could be with a short course of oral steroids.

Surgery may be indicated on the basis of the patients' symptoms and severity of the disease.

Grading of Nasal Polyps

Grade 1. Small size polyps within the middle meatus and not reaching the inferior edge of the middle turbinate.

Grade 2. Polyps within the middle meatus reaching the inferior border of the middle turbinate.

Grade 3. Polyps extending into the nasal cavity below the edge of the middle turbinate but not below the inferior edge of the inferior turbinate.

Grade 4. Polyps filling up the most of the nasal cavity.

Treatment Outcomes and Prognosis

Management involves polyp reduction and symptomatic control.

Possible Complications and Side Effects

Most patients with benign nasal polyps will suffer with nasal obstruction, nasal discharge, hyposmia, and not infrequently facial pressure. Chronic rhinosinusitis with nasal polyps may lead to acute exacerbations of sinusitis and complications related to this.

3.9 FOREIGN BODY

Epidemiology/Pathogenesis

Foreign bodies are most commonly seen in the pediatric population, ages 2–5 years. Most common locations for obstruction include anterior to the middle turbinate and along the inferior meatus. Foreign bodies commonly include food, metal, wood, and batteries.

There is a potential risk of lower airway obstruction with possible nasal dislodgement. If not witnessed and asymptomatic, patients may be carriers for years before a diagnosis is made (Fig. 3.4).

Clinical History

Most cases of nasal foreign bodies are witnessed and reported. Painful foreign bodies suggest a locally irritating object such as a "button" battery, which would require urgent removal.

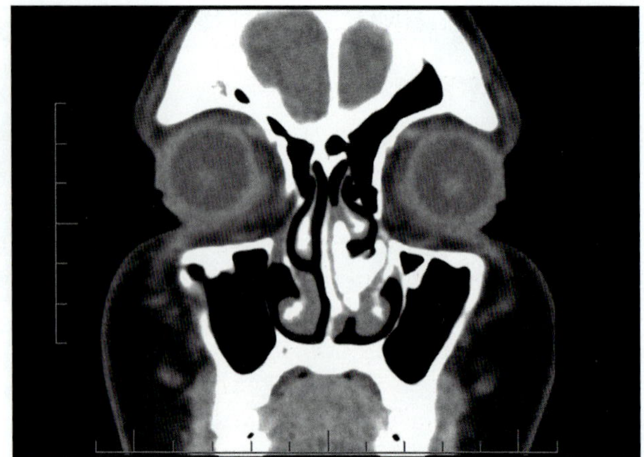

Fig. 3.4: Computed tomographic scan showing a foreign body in nose history of foul odor for many years. The patient recently is in a permanent relationship and forced to see a specialist—had symptoms for 10 years—thought it was normal and was due to sinus infections. Left nasal cavity foreign body. Calcification indicates that this is likely to be long standing. Tumors and fungal debris are differential diagnoses.

Patients present with a unilateral nasal discharge, foul odor, epistaxis, nasal irritation, and pain.

Typical Examination Findings

Inspect the nose. Patient may have purulence, epistaxis, and a foul odor. Identify any areas of excoriation or inflammation as this may lead the way to the foreign body. Nasal endoscopy is imperative.

Investigations

An X-ray or CT scan may be indicated depending on the clinical picture (Fig. 3.4).

Treatment Options

Foreign body needs to be removed. Batteries in the nose, is an emergency and, if left for a longer time, may lead to necrosis of the cartilage and surrounding tissues. Some pediatric patients may tolerate removal at bedside. An examination under anesthesia or with mild sedation is recommended for a thorough bilateral nasal airway examination. The use of balloon catheters and direct instrumentation can facilitate removal.

Alternative techniques involving the "mother's kiss" allows an increase in intranasal positive pressure to remove the object (McMaster, 1970; Botma, Bader and Kubba, 2000; Brown, et al., 2004).

Possible Complications and Side Effects

Epistaxis, sinusitis, otitis media, septal perforation, and cellulitis may occur.

3.10 ACUTE RHINOSINUSITIS

Epidemiology/Pathogenesis

The most common cause of acute sinusitis is a viral infection. Most common virus is the rhinovirus.

Up to 2% of cases can be complicated by the progression to acute bacterial sinusitis. Most common organisms are *Streptococcus pneumonia, Haemophilus influenzae,* and *Moraxella catarrhalis.* An acute viral infection can cause edema and inflammation of the nasal mucosa. This can impair sinus drainage. Decreased mucociliary clearance and mucus stasis thus predispose to secondary bacterial infections. Acute sinusitis is generally classified as symptoms lasting <4 weeks.

Clinical History

The history of upper respiratory tract infection precedes nasal symptoms. Most patients will complain about facial pressure, rhinorrhea, nasal congestion, postnasal drip, dental pain, anosmia, halitosis, otalgia, sinus tenderness, and, possibly, fever. The key to determining the difference between is the duration of the symptoms and their current state. Symptoms that persist >7 days and are getting worse typically tend to favor a bacterial etiology (Hoddeson and Wise, 2013).

Typical Examination Findings

Inspect the face and head. Although it is generally not a reliable sign in the acute setting, palpation over the frontal and maxillary sinuses may reveal point tenderness. Inspect the facial skin for any erythema and soft tissue edema.

Inspect the eyes. Note any deficit in ocular movement. Assess for any proptosis, purulence, or erythema of the globe.

Inspect the nose. The nasal mucosa will be inflamed; edematous and frank purulence may be seen. Mucus stranding will likely be present as well.

Inspect the oral cavity. Thickened postnasal drip or purulent postnasal drip may indicate acute bacterial rhinosinusitis.

Nasal endoscopy is performed after applying a decongestant. Visualization of the sphenoethmoid recess and middle meatus will show inflamed and edematous mucosa with purulence, from which a microbiology swab can be taken.

Investigations

Diagnosis is based on the clinical history and physical examination. Middle meatus culture is done to help direct antimicrobial therapy. A CT sinus in unresponsive/complicated case may be requested.

Treatment Options

Medical management of acute viral rhinosinusitis involves symptomatic treatment of pain and fever. Nasal saline sprays/irrigation and/or mist inhalations will help with mucociliary clearance and hydrate the nasal mucosa. Nasal decongestants may be used on their own (7–10 days) or in combination with a topical nasal steroid.

Medical management of acute bacterial rhinosinusitis involves oral antibiotics in addition to the above. Studies have shown spontaneous resolution of acute bacterial rhinosinusitis in 19–39% by day 14 with mild symptoms (Rosenfeld, Singer and Jones, 2004; Sharp, Dneman and Pumala, 2007).

Antibiotics are necessary in the presence of pain and fever.

Hence, their selection is based on patient's tolerance and general health, and the selection is made between Augmentin and β-lactamase antibiotic. They could be directed after the results of microbiology with sensitivity are available.

Surgical management of acute sinusitis is beyond the scope of this chapter and will not be addressed as it is covered elsewhere in this book.

Treatment Outcomes and Prognosis

Most sinusitis improve with the use of proper antibiotics.

Possible Complications and Side Effects

Extracranial

Orbital complications: Well classified by Chandler, et al.

Preseptal Cellulitis

- Edema and erythema of eyelids, external ocular muscle movements (EOM) normal
- Treated with medical therapy.

Orbital Cellulitis

- Orbital edema, normal EOM
- Treated with medical therapy.

Subperiosteal Abscess

- Orbital edema, proptosis, impaired EOM.
- Medical and surgical management is required.

Orbital Abscess

- Orbital purulence, vision changes, chemosis
- Medical and surgical management is required.

Cavernous Sinus Thrombosis

- Orbital pain, ophthalmoplegia
- Deficits in cranial nerves III, IV, V1, V2, V3, and V1
- Medical and surgical management is required
- Some cases may need anticoagulation.

Intracranial

- Epidural abscess
- Subdural abscess
- Intracerebral abscess
- Meningitis.

3.11 COMMON COLD

Epidemiology/Pathogenesis

- An acute inflammation of the upper respiratory airway.
- Self-limited in its nature course.
- Viral in nature.
- Up to 25 different virus strains can be responsible.

Clinical History

Patient will present with an acute onset of rhinitis, sore throat, malaise, fever, cough, postnasal drip, myalgia, and nasal congestion. The acute onset is the key to diagnosis.

Typical Examination Findings

Inspect the nose. Using anterior rhinoscopy, abundant clear mucus stranding can be seen along the nasal mucosa. The turbinates can be erythematous and/or edematous. There can be posterior pharyngeal wall cobblestoning noted due to postnasal drip. Erythema and edema of the posterior pharyngeal wall can be noted as well. The tonsils can be hypertrophic and erythematous. Nasal endoscopy is indicated only if symptoms persist beyond 7 days.

Investigations

No diagnostic tests are necessary in the first 7–10 days and by that time most of the symptoms are resolved in most of the patients.

Treatment Options

Mainstay is rest, fluids, nasal decongestant, and antihistamines. There is no role of antibiotics in the uncomplicated illness sate.

3.12 NASAL MASSES

Epidemiology/Pathogenesis

Various etiologies form a broad differential diagnosis of nasal masses and some of these are as follows:

Congenital Masses

Congenital lesions include gliomas, dermoid cysts, and encephaloceles.

Inflammatory Masses

Common inflammatory lesion is the nasal polyp, seen in 4% of the population.

Neoplastic Masses

Neoplastic masses include hemangiomas, mucoceles, inverted papillomas, esthesioneuroblastoma, angiofibroma, squamous cell carcinoma, and adenocarcinoma. Over 50% of patients will present with bilateral nasal masses.

Clinical History

Most common presenting symptom is nasal obstruction. Other symptoms can include rhinorrhea, hyposmia, anosmia, epistaxis, headache, orbital complications, and external nasal deformity.

Typical Examination Findings

Anterior rhinoscopy may visualize nasal mass/polyp. Nasal endoscopy is indicated to visualize the entire nasal cavity.

Investigations

Computed tomography of the sinuses delineate the extent of the disease. Magnetic resonance imaging brain with contrast is necessary when the skull base is violated. Biopsy of the nasal mass will add in the diagnosis except when a meningoencephalocele and/or vascular tumors are suspected—it should be avoided in latter cases.

Treatment Options

Treatment varies according to the characteristic of the mass. Some may require surgery, chemotherapy, radiation therapy, embolization, observation, or a combination of all.

3.13 THIS IS HOW WE DO IT (NICK BHAT (USA) APPROACH)

Our diagnostic process begins with a detailed history, generally taken by our clinically oriented nurse. In my opinion, patients are more at ease with and more receptive to our clinical staff. Documentation of the problem in the patient's words is very important. Then, I like to review the history with the patient requesting him/her to correct my understanding of his/her symptoms. By this time, quite often the patient is relaxed and provides valuable history. This becomes a foundation of our relationship. As a rule, I do not like to offer a surgical solution to the problem on the first visit, even though it may be the obvious solution. In our practice, we often come across patients with more than one cause of nasal obstruction. Patients with chronic nasal obstruction with a deviated nasal septum have also been found to have chronic perennial allergy or rhinitis medicamentosa. Hence, it is important to identify associated causes and manage them prior to surgery and/or make the patient understand the limitation of proposed surgery.

At times, it may take the physician two or three office visits and several discussions before confirming the diagnosis and finalizing a plan. Educating the patient and preparing him/her is the art of medicine that we all strive toward perfection.

One of the common causes of nasal congestion that we come across in our clinical practice is allergic rhinitis. Examination does not always reveal a classic picture. While a trial of steroid sprays may help alleviate the symptoms and confirm the diagnosis, it is prudent to offer the patient an allergy workup to help find the specific triggers so to avoid can also be an option. Options in terms of allergy workup include skin testing and/or RAST (radioallergosorbent test) and RIST (radioimmunosorbent test). If the patient does not respond to immunotherapy within a reasonable period of time, a secondary test may be of value in reassessing the allergy.

Another diagnosis that we routinely encounter is nasal valve collapse. The physical examination gives us a clear picture of the problem. Our surgical approach to this condition begins with an analysis of the entire nose. A narrow nasal valve will benefit from spreader grafts. Collapse of the lateral lower cartilages can be strengthened from alar batten grafts. An M-plasty can help modify the lower lateral cartilages to open up nasal valve area.

"Septal surgery" to relieve nasal obstruction, in my opinion, is not as simple as it seems. The surgical procedure is a series of steps, which may include, apart from major septal reconstruction, partial turbinotomy, sculpturing the middle turbinate, and/or reducing the protruding upper lateral cartilage by M-plasty. Since most septal surgeries are a combination of one or more of these steps, I prefer to call the procedure "nasal airway reconstruction".

REFERENCES

Albalawi, Z.H., Othman, S.S. and Alfaleh, K., 2011. Intranasal ipratropium bromide for the common cold. *Cochrane Database of Systematic Reviews*, 7, p. CD008231.

Alobid, I., Benitez, P., Valero, A., Munoz, R. Langdon, C., Mullol, J., 2012. Oral and intranasal steroid treatments improve nasal patency and paradoxically increase nasal nitric oxide in patients with severe nasal polyposis. *Rhinology*, 50, pp. 171-7.

Assanasen, P. and Metheetrairut, C., 2009. Choanal atresia. *Journal of the Medical Association of Thailand*, 92(5), pp. 699-706.

Blaiss, M.S., 2008. Evolving paradigm in the management of allergic rhinitis-associated ocular symptoms: role of intranasal corticosteroids. *Current Medical Research and Opinion*, 24, pp. 821-36.

Botma, M., Bader, R. and Kubba, H., 2000. 'A parent's kiss': evaluating an unusual method for removing nasal foreign bodies in children. *The Journal of Laryngology and Otology*, 114(8), pp. 598-600.

Brook, I., Shah, K. and Jackson, W., 2000. Microbiology of healthy and diseased adenoids. *The Laryngoscope*, 110(6), pp. 994-9.

Brown, L., Denmark, T.K., Wittlake, W.A., Vargas, E.J., Watson, T. and Crabb, J.W., 2004. Procedural sedation use in the ED: management of pediatric ear and nose foreign bodies. *The American Journal of Emergency Medicine*, 22(4), pp. 310-4.

Cengel, S., 2006. The role of topical nasal steroids in the treatment of children with otitis media with effusion and/or adenoid hypertrophy. *International Journal of Pediatric Otorhinolaryngology*, 70(4), pp. 639-45.

Chan, T., 2013. Nonallergic rhinitis. In: J.T. Johnson and C.A. Rosen, eds. *Bailey's head and neck surgery: otolaryngology*. 5th ed. Philadelphia, PA: Lippincott Williams and Wilkins.

Chandler, J.R., Langenbrunner, D.J., Stevens, E.R., 1970. The pathogenesis of orbital complications in acute sinusitis. *Laryngoscope*. 80(9):1414-28.

Chien, C., Chen, A.M., Hwang, C.F., Su, C.Y., et al., 2005. The clinical significance of adenoid-choanae area ratio in children with adenoid hypertrophy. *International Journal of Pediatric Otorhinolaryngology*, 69(2), pp. 235-9.

Courtiss, E.H., 1988. Diagnosis and treatment of nasal airway obstruction due to inferior turbinate hypertrophy. *Clinics in Plastic Surgery*, 15(1), pp. 11-3.

De Sutter, A.I., van Driel, M.L., Kumar, A.A., Lesslar, O., Skrt, A., 2012. Oral antihistamine-decongestant-analgesic combinations for the common cold. *Cochrane Database of Systematic Reviews*, 2, p. CD004976.

Diamantopoulos, I.I., Jones, N.S. and Lowe, J., 2000. All nasal polyps need histological examination: an audit-based appraisal of clinical practice. *The Journal of Laryngology and Otology*, 114, pp. 755-9.

Gasndomi, B., Bayat, A. and Kazemei, T., 2010. Outcomes of septoplasty in young adults, the Nasal Obstruction Septoplasty Effective study. *American Journal of Otolaryngology*, 31(3), pp. 189-92.

Gehani, M. and Houser, S., 2013. Septoplasty, turbinate reduction, and correction of nasal obstruction. In: J.T. Johnson and C.A. Rosen, eds. *Bailey's head and neck surgery: otolaryngology*. 5th ed. Philadelphia, PA: Lippincott Williams and Wilkins.

Giannoni, C., 2013. Complications of rhinosinusitis. In: J.T. Johnson and C.A. Rosen, eds. *Bailey's head and neck surgery: otolaryngology*. 5th ed. Philadelphia, PA: Lippincott Williams and Wilkins.

Hackman, T.G. and Ferguson, B.J., 2005. Powered instrumentation and tissue effects in the nose and paranasal sinuses. *Current Opinion in Otolaryngology and Head and Neck Surgery.*, 13(1), pp. 22-6.

Hassan, M., AboEl-Ezz, T. and Youssef, T., 2011. Combined transoral-transnasal approach in the repair of congenital posterior choanal atresia: clinical experience. *Journal of Otolaryngology and Head and Neck Surgery*, 40(3), pp. 271-6.

Hoddeson, E. and Wise, S., 2013. Acute rhinosinusitis. In: J.T. Johnson and C.A. Rosen, eds. *Bailey's head and neck surgery: otolaryngology*. 5th ed. Philadelphia, PA: Lippincott Williams and Wilkins.

Huang, S. and Giannoni, C., 2001. The risk of adenoid hypertrophy in children with allergic rhinitis. *Annals of Allergy, Asthma and Immunology*, 87(4), pp. 350-5.

Hwang, P.H., McLaughlin, R.B., Lanza, D.C. and Kennedy, D.W., 1999. Endoscopic septoplasty: indications, technique, and results. *Otolaryngology and Head and Neck Surgery*, 120(5), pp. 678-82.

Kaliner, M.A., 2007. A novel and effective approach to treating rhinitis with nasal antihistamines. *Annals of Allergy, Asthma and Immunology*, 99, pp. 383-90.

Kalish, L., Snidvongs, K., Sivasubramaniam, R., et al., 2012. Topical steroids for nasal polyps. *Cochrane Database of Systematic Reviews*, 12, p. CD006549.

Khosh, M.M., Honrado, C. and Pearlman, S.J., 2004. Nasal valve reconstruction. *Archives of Facial Plastic Surgery*, 6, pp. 167-71.

Kiger, J.R., Brenkert, T.E. and Losek, J.D., 2008. Nasal foreign body removal in children. *Pediatric Emergency Care*, 24(11), pp. 785-92.

Kubba, H. and Bingham, B., 2001. Endoscopy in the assessment of children with nasal obstruction. *Journal of Laryngology and Otology*, 115(5), pp. 380-4.

Lathi, A., Syed, M.M.A., Kalakoti, P., Qutub, D., Kishve, S.P., 2011. Clinico-pathological profile of sinonasal masses: a study from a tertiary care hospital of India. *ACTA Otorhinolaryngologica Ita Lica*, 31, pp. 372-7.

Li, J.T., 2000. Immunotherapy for allergic rhinitis. *Immunology and Allergy Clinics of North America*, 20, pp. 381-400.

McMaster, W.C., 1970. Removal of foreign body from the nose. *JAMA: the Journal of the American Medical Association*, 213(11), p. 1905.

Meltzer, E.O., Hamilos, D.L., Hadley, J.A., Lanza, D.C., Marple, B.F., Nicklas, R.A., Bachert, C., Baraniuk, J., Baroody, F.M., Benninger, M.S., Brook, I., Chowdhury, B.A., Druce, H.M., Durham, S., Ferguson, B., Gwaltney, J.M., Kaliner, M., Kennedy, D.W., Lund, V., Naclerio, R., Pawankar, R., Piccirillo, J.F., Rohane, P., Simon, R., Slavin, R.G., Togias, A., Wald, E.R., Zinreich, S.J., 2004. Rhinosinusitis: establishing definitions for clinical research and patient care. *The Journal of Allergy and Clinical Immunology*, 114, pp. 155-212.

Meltzer, E.O., Nathan, R.A., Derebery, J., Dalal, A.A., Stanford, R.H., Corrao, M.A., McMorris, B.J., 2009. Physician perceptions of the treatment and management of allergic and nonallergic rhinitis. *Allergy and Asthma Proceedings*, 30, pp. 75-83.

Mims, J. Allergy testing. In: J.T. Johnson and C.A. Rosen, eds. 2013. *Bailey's head and neck surgery: otolaryngology*, 5th ed. Philadelphia, PA: Lippincott Williams and Wilkins.

Naclerio, R., 2008. Intranasal corticosteroids reduce ocular symptoms associated with allergic rhinitis. *Otolaryngology and Head and Neck Surgery*, 138, pp. 129-39.

Nassef, M., Shapiro, G. and Casale, T.B., 2006. Identifying and managing rhinitis and its subtypes: allergic and non-allergic components—a consensus report and materials from the Respiratory Allergic Disease Foundation. *Current Medical Research and Opinion*, 22, pp. 2541-8.

O'Neil, J. and Mims, J., 2013. Allergic rhinitis. In: J.T. Johnson and C.A. Rosen, eds. 2013. *Bailey's head and neck surgery: otolaryngology*, 5th ed. Philadelphia, PA: Lippincott Williams and Wilkins.

Panwar, S.S. and Martin, F.W., 1996. Trans-nasal endoscopic holmium: YAG laser correction of choanal atresia. *The Journal of Laryngology and Otology*, 110(5), pp. 429-31.

Piccirillo, J.F., 2004. Clinical practice. Acute bacterial sinusitis. *The New England Journal of Medicine*, 351, pp. 902-10.

Radulovic, S., Calderon, M.A., Wilson, D., et al., 2010. Sublingual immunotherapy for allergic rhinitis. *Cochrane Database of Systematic Reviews*, 12, p. CD002893.

Riedler, J., Braun-Fahrlander, C., Eder, W., Schreuer, M., Waser, M., Maisch, S., Carr, D., Schierl, R., Nowak, D., von Mutius, E.; ALEX Study Team. 2001. Exposure to farming in early life and development of asthma and allergy: a cross-sectional survey. *Lancet*, 358, pp. 1129-33.

Rosenfeld, R.M., Andes, D., Bhattacharyya, N., Cheung, D., Eisenberg, S., Ganiats, T.G., Gelzer, A., Hamilos, D., Haydon, R.C. 3rd, Hudgins, P.A., Jones, S., Krouse, H.J., Lee, L.H., Mahoney, M.C., Marple, B.F., Mitchell, C.J., Nathan, R., Shiffman, R.N., Smith, T.L., Witsell, D.L., 2007. Clinical practice guideline: adult sinusitis. *Otolaryngology and Head and Neck Surgery*, 137(Suppl 3), pp. S1-31.

Rosenfeld, R.M., Singer, M. and Jones, S., 2004. Systematic review of antimicrobial therapy in patients with acute rhinosinusitis. *Otolaryngology and Head and Neck Surgery*, 130, pp. 1-45.

Rudmik, L.1., Schlosser, R.J., Smith, T.L., Soler, Z.M., 2012. Impact of topical nasal steroid therapy on symptoms of nasal polyposis: a meta-analysis. *The Laryngoscope*, 122, pp. 1431-7.

Ryan, M., 2013. Chronic rhinosinusitis with nasal polyposis. In: J.T. Johnson and C.A. Rosen, eds. *Bailey's head and neck surgery: otolaryngology*, 5th ed. Philadelphia, PA: Lippincott Williams and Wilkins.

Schoem, S.R., 2004. Transnasal endoscopic repair of choanal atresia: why stent? *Otolaryngology and Head and Neck Surgery*, 131(4), pp. 362-6.

Sharp, H.J., Denman, D., Puumala, S., Leopold, D.A., 2007. Treatment of acute and chronic rhinosinusitis in the United States 1999-2002. *Archives of Otolaryngology and Head and Neck Surgery*, 133, pp. 260-5.

Sheen, J.H.,1984. Spreader graft: a method of reconstructing the roof of the middle nasal vault following rhinoplasty. *Plastic and Reconstructive Surgery*, 73(2), pp. 230-9.

Siegel, N.S., Gliklich, R.E., Taghizadeh, F., and Chang, Y., 2000. Outcomes of septoplasty. *Otolaryngology and Head and Neck Surgery*, 122(2), pp. 228-32.

Skoner, D.P., 2001. Allergic rhinitis: definition, epidemiology, pathophysiology, detection, and diagnosis. *The Journal of Allergy and Clinical Immunology*, 108, pp. S2-8.

Staevska, M. and Baraniuk, J.N., 2005. Persistent nonallergic rhinosinusitis. *Current Allergy and Asthma Reports,* 5, pp. 233-42.

Stevenson, M.D., Sellins, S., Grube, E., Schroer, K., Gupta, J., Wang, N., Khurana, Hershey, G.K., 2007. Aeroallergen sensitization in healthy children: racial and socioeconomic correlates. *The Journal of Pediatrics,* 151, pp. 187-91.

Swierczyńska, M., Strek, P., Składzień, J., Nizankowska-Mogilnicka, E., Szczeklik, A., 2003. Nonallergic rhinitis with eosinophilia syndrome: state of knowledge. *Otolaryngologia polska. The Polish otolaryngology,* 57, pp. 81-4.

Toriumi, D.M., Josen, J., Weinberger, M., and Tardy, M.E., Jr, 1997. Use of alar batten grafts for correction of nasal valve collapse. *Arch Otolaryngology and Head and Neck Surgery,* 123(8), pp. 802-8.

Walker, S.M., Durham, S.R., Till, S.J., Roberts, G., Corrigan, C.J., Leech, S.C., Krishna, M.T., Rajakulasingham, R.K., Williams, A., Chantrell, J., Dixon, L., Frew, A.J., Nasser, S.M., 2011. Immunotherapy for allergic rhinitis. *Clinical and Experimental Allergy,* 41, pp. 1177-200.

Wallace, D.V., Dykewicz, M.S., Bernstein, D.I., Blessing-Moore, J., Cox, L., Khan, D.A., Lang, D.M., Nicklas, R.A., Oppenheimer, J., Portnoy, J.M., Randolph, C.C., Schuller, D., Spector, S.L., Tilles, S.A., 2008. The diagnosis and management of rhinitis: an updated practice parameter. *The Journal of Allergy and Clinical Immunology,* 122(Suppl 2), pp. S1-84.

Wood, R.A., Johnson, E.F., Van, Natta, M.L., Chen, P.H., Eggleston, P.A., 1998. A placebo-controlled trial of a HEPA air cleaner in the treatment of cat allergy. *American Journal of Respiratory and Critical Care Medicine,* 158, pp. 115-20.

Yaniv, E., Hadar, T., Shvero, J., Stern, Y. and Raveh, E., 2007. Endoscopic transnasal repair of choanal atresia. *International Journal of Pediatric Otorhinolaryngology,* 71(3), pp. 457-62.

Nasal Discharge

4

Laura Harrison, Anshul Sama, Salil B Nair

Chapter Overview

Pearls and Pitfalls

Pearls

- Skin tests and radioallergosorbent test are negative in nonallergic rhinitis.
- Chronic cerebrospinal fluid (CSF) leak carries a risk for bacterial meningitis.
- All suspected CSF leaks should be tested for b-2 transferrin to confirm CSF.
- The most common bacteria causing acute rhinosinusitis are *Streptococcus pneumoniae, Haemophilus influenzae, Moraxella catarrhalis*, and *Staphylococcus aureus.*
- Button battery (foreign body) in the nose is an emergency and should be taken out as soon as possible.
- Bilateral choanal atresia is an emergency at birth and presents with cyanosis, which is reversed on crying.

Pitfalls

- Unilateral nasal polyps in adults may prove inverted papillomas on histology.

4.1 DEFINITION OF RHINORRHEA

Rhinorrhea is characterized as an excess anterior discharge of fluid from the nasal cavity. It can be clear (serous), gray and cloudy (mucoid), thick and green (purulent) or bloody or serosanguinous and could be unilateral or bilateral (Flowcharts 4.1 and 4.2).

What to Elicit in the History?

There are important history-taking questions, which can be used to differentiate between the different diagnostic categories in rhinorrhea. These are as follows:

- Patient's age
- Unilateral or bilateral rhinorrhea
- Character of the discharge—blood stained, purulent, or clear and watery
- Acute or chronic onset
- Personal or family history of atopy
- *Associated nasal symptoms*: Hyposmia, reduced taste, nasal blockage, trauma, nasal congestion, and facial pain.

Examination

The following examinations should be performed in patients with rhinorrhea.

Examination	*Findings*
Anterior rhinoscopy	Can visualize turbinate hypertrophy and occasionally nasal polyposis, vestibular lesions, nasal septal perforations
Oral cavity examination	Evidence of postnasal drip or postnasal lesion
Endoscopy (flexible/rigid)	To visualize the turbinates, osteomeatal complex, sphenoethmoid recess and superior meatus if possible, posterior choanae, Eustachian tubes, and associated tubal ridges

Diagnostic Flowcharts

Flowchart 4.1: Acute rhinorrhea (duration < 4 weeks).

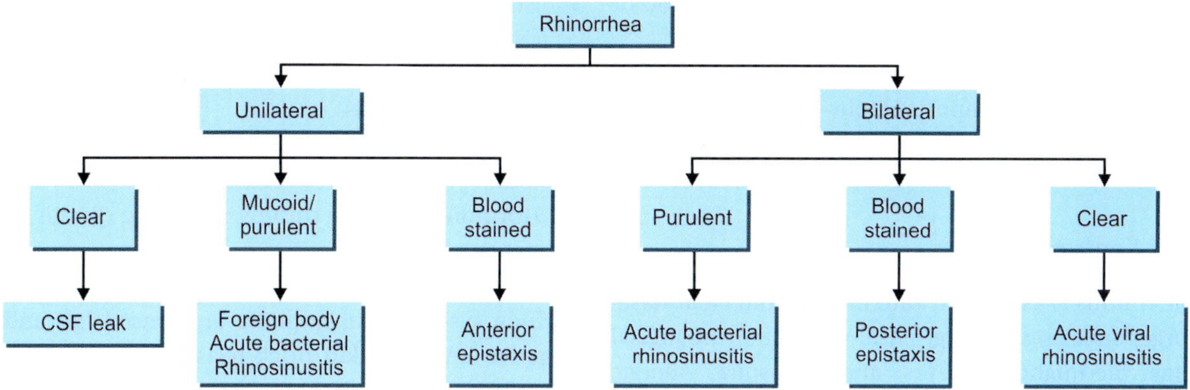

Flowchart 4.2: Chronic rhinorrhea.

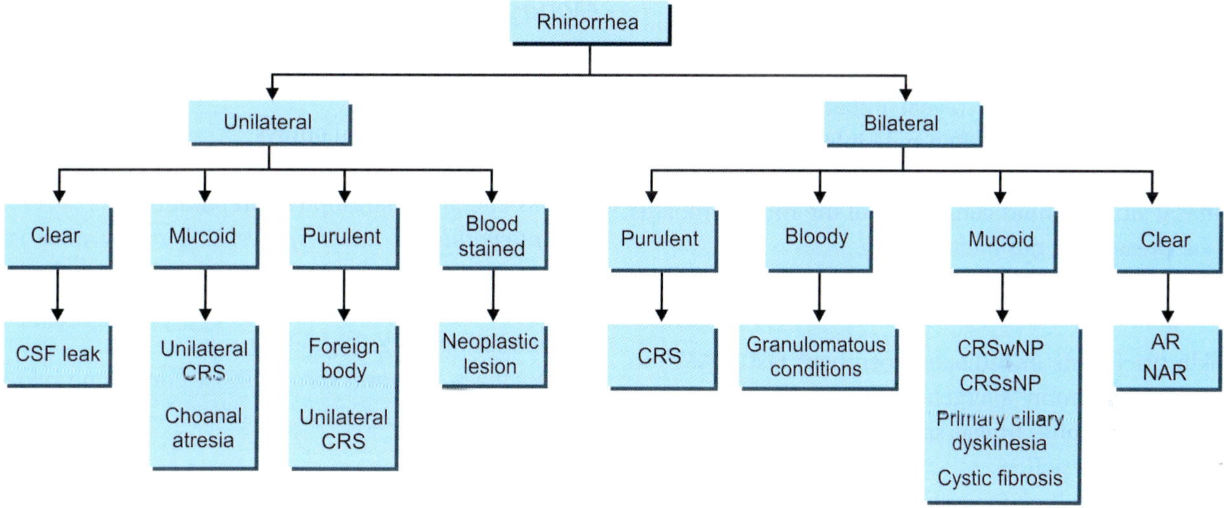

4.2 CLEAR RHINORRHEA

Diagnostic Synopsis

Allergic rhinitis (seasonal, perennial)
Nonallergic rhinitis
Cerebrospinal rhinorrhea

There are two main types of rhinitis: allergic rhinitis and nonallergic rhinitis (NAR).

Allergic Rhinitis

Allergic rhinitis (AR) is defined as inflammation of the membranous lining of the nasal cavity in response to allergens leading to one of the following: clear or mucoid rhinorrhea, congestion, sneezing, nasal itching, and nasal obstruction.

Allergic rhinitis affects 10–20% of the adult population and is sustained by an immunoglobulin-E (IgE)-triggered type-1 hypersensitivity reaction, classically following exposure to an allergen. This results in histamine release, followed by an inflammatory response, which involves cells, mediators, cytokines, and adhesion molecules. The inflammatory response propagates increased vascular permeability and edema, which is the cause of the clear rhinorrhea.

Symptoms of AR can be either intermittent or seasonal, which manifest in the presence of seasonal allergens such as pollen and grass or perennial where symptoms persist all year round. Nonseasonal allergens include house dust mite, animal dander, and mold.

Historically, personal or family history of atopy (asthma, eczema, and Hay fever) is a strong risk factor for the development of rhinitis symptoms. This is irrespective of the varying prevalence and environmental risk factors in different societies and environments. Atopy has a strong familial tendency, usually starting in childhood or adolescence.

Environmental factors (air pollution and bacterial/viral infection) play an important role in the development of AR. Environmental endotoxin may also affect the balance of the Th1/Th2 cytokine level.

Clinical Features

Allergic rhinitis is associated with mucoid and clear nasal discharge, sneezing, itching, nasal congestion postnasal drainage, lacrimation of eyes, and hyposmia. Allergic rhinitis may be associated with asthma and eczema. It is important to enquire about pets, hobbies, feather-pillows, and smoking in the history.

Examination

Anterior rhinoscopy may reveal inflamed mucosa with enlarged, engorged, and often pale inferior turbinates.

As the nasal mucosa is continuous with that of the paranasal sinuses, mild congestion of the middle meatus may be present on nasal endoscopy.

Investigation

- Skin prick tests or radioallergosorbent test (RAST) to identify common allergen sensitivity (grass, pollen, house dust mite, fungal spores, cat and dog dander, feathers, tree pollen
- Blood tests to look for systemic IgE levels and eosinophilia
- In exceptional cases, nasal provocation tests may be indicated.

Management

- Allergen avoidance can assist in control of symptoms
- Topical or systemic histamine receptor antagonists
- Topical steroid sprays
- Allergen immunotherapy.

Nonallergic Rhinitis

Nonallergic rhinitis is characterized by a perennial rhinitis in relation to nonallergic, noninfectious triggers.

These patients have negative skin prick or RAST test for relevant allergens and symptoms and clinical findings consistent with rhinitis.

Nonallergic rhinitis subtypes are as follows:

- Idiopathic NAR
- Nonallergic rhinitis with eosinophilia syndrome (NARES)
- Atrophic rhinitis
- Gustatory rhinitis
- Drug-induced rhinitis, including rhinitis medicamentosa
- Hormonal induced rhinitis, including rhinitis of pregnancy.

Investigations are same as AR. It is important to exclude systemic eosinophilia and raised IgE and have negative RAST or skin prick tests. Nasal smears can be submitted for analysis and >25% eosinophilia is diagnostic of NARES.

Management

Treatments depend on severity and effect on quality of life

- Saline nasal sprays
- Corticosteroid nasal sprays
- *Antihistamine nasal sprays*: Oral antihistamines appear less effective than topical preparations.
- *Anticholinergic nasal sprays*: If a runny nose is the main complaint (Ipratropium bromide).
- *Oral decongestants*: These include pseudoephedrine-containing drugs (Sudafed)
- *Decongestant nasal sprays*: Those containing xylo/oxymetazoline.

Cerebrospinal Fluid Rhinorrhea

Cerebrospinal fluid (CSF) rhinorrhea is the drainage of CSF into the nasal cavity or paranasal sinuses, caused by a breach in the dural and pia-arachnoid layer, through a skull base defect.

Traumatic head injuries resulting in fractures of the anterior skull base can breach the dural and pia-arachnoid layer leading to a CSF leak. Eighty percent of CSF leaks occur following nonsurgical trauma and complicate 2% of all head traumas. Cerebrospinal fluid leak is a documented complication of nasal or sinus surgery. Occasionally, CSF leak can occur spontaneously or secondary to intracranial hypertension.

Clinical Features

Unilateral clear watery rhinorrhea from the nasal cavity, accentuated by leaning forward.

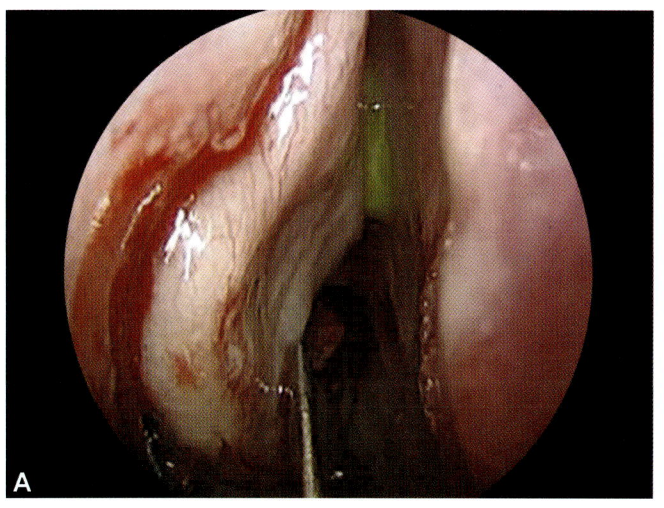

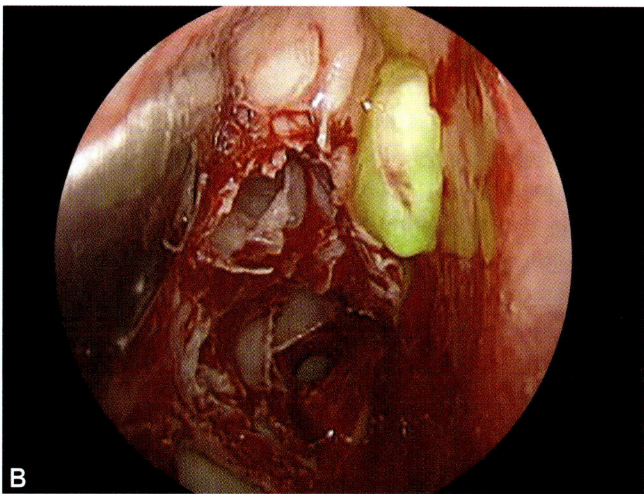

Figs. 4.1A and B: (A) Endoscopic view of fluorescein medial to the middle turbinate in the olfactory niche (B) an encephalocoele is seen after administration of intrathecal fluorescein.

Investigation

- A sample of the nasal discharge should be sent for b-2 transferrin analysis.
- High-definition computed tomography (CT) imaging may show small defects in the anterior skull base or sphenoid sinus.
- Magnetic resonance imaging (MRI) is useful to define the site of the leak if none or multiple areas of inflammation are evident on CT. Magnetic resonance imaging is helpful in identifying meningocele and meningoencephaloceles (Figs. 4.1A and B).

Management

Most post-traumatic CSF leaks close spontaneously within 7–10 days with conservative management.

Conservative management includes strict bed rest, head elevation, avoidance of straining, retching, or nose blowing.

Chronic CSF leaks carry a risk of bacterial meningitis at a rate of 10% per year. Prophylactic antibiotics have not been shown to reduce the risk of meningitis and can lead to more virulent organisms.

Endoscopic endonasal approaches are the preferred standard of repair with a success rate of >90%. However, in a small minority of cases, open transcranial approaches may be indicated.

4.3 MUCOPURULENT RHINORRHEA

Diagnostic Synopsis
Acute rhinosinusitis (viral, post-viral, and bacterial)
Chronic rhinosinusitis (CRS with nasal polyps and without nasal polyps, allergic fungal rhinosinusitis)
Foreign body nasal cavity
Choanal atresia

Rhinosinusitis

Clinical definition of rhinosinusitis in adults form is defined in European Paper on Sinusitis (EPOS) papers as: (Ref EPOS 2012):

Acute rhinosinusitis (ARS) includes the following symptoms for up to 4 weeks.

Chronic rhinosinusitis (CRS) includes the following symptoms for >12 weeks.

- Inflammation of the nose and the paranasal sinuses characterized by two or more symptoms, one of which should be either nasal blockage, obstruction, congestion, or nasal discharge (anterior/posterior nasal drip)
- +/– Facial pain/pressure
- +/– Reduction or loss of smell
- And either endoscopic signs of:
- Nasal polyps and/or
- Mucopurulent discharge primarily from middle meatus and/or
- Computed tomography showing mucosal changes within the osteomeatal complex and/or sinuses.

Acute Rhinosinusitis

Acute rhinosinusitis is highly prevalent affecting 6–15% of the population. It can be induced by viral, postviral, and bacterial infections. The most common viruses isolated in adult viral rhinitis and rhinosinusitis are rhinoviruses and coronaviruses. Bacterial ARS is generally preceded by a virus and can be described as postviral phenomenon. The viral infection induces epithelium disruption increasing the number of goblet cells and decreasing the number of ciliated cells, which reduces the efficacy to which mucous containing microorganisms can be cleared and can result in a bacterial superinfection. The most common bacteria are *Streptococcus pneumoniae, Haemophilus influenzae, Moraxella catarrhalis,* and *Staphylococcus aureus.* Other causes are *Klebsiella, Pseudomonas aeruginosa,* and *Escherichia coli.*

Environmental factors and anatomic factors such as septal deviation, nasal polyps, and choanal obstruction by benign adenoid tissue or odontogenic sources of infections, may be predictive of the development of ARS. Studies have also shown a link between allergy and frequency of ARS.

Investigation

- Imaging studies are not required for a diagnosis of ARS.
- Inflammatory markers such as white cell count and C-reactive protein can be used to monitor more severe infections.
- CT is reserved for patients developing complications secondary to ARS.

Management

A recent Cochrane review concluded that there was no place for antibiotics in uncomplicated ARS in adults. The benefits of antibiotics need to be reviewed in the context of the possibility of developing complications. Management entails symptomatic support. Bed rest, analgesia, and the use of a decongestant (topical or systemic) can be helpful, but do not change the course or time frame of the episode. Decongestants should only be used for a limited period (5 days) due to the risk of developing rhinitis medicamentosa. Topical steroid sprays have been shown to reduce the length of ARS. Antibiotics should be reserved for prolonged symptoms (>10 days) and where there are concerns regarding complications. A suitable broad spectrum antibiotic to use would be co-amoxiclav. In those with penicillin-resistant pneumococci, a second generation cephalosporin should be considered.

Surgical management is only indicated in those with extra sinus extension of pus or to obtain fluid for microbiology. Surgery is tailored to drain the extra sinus sepsis and can be approached endoscopically or externally.

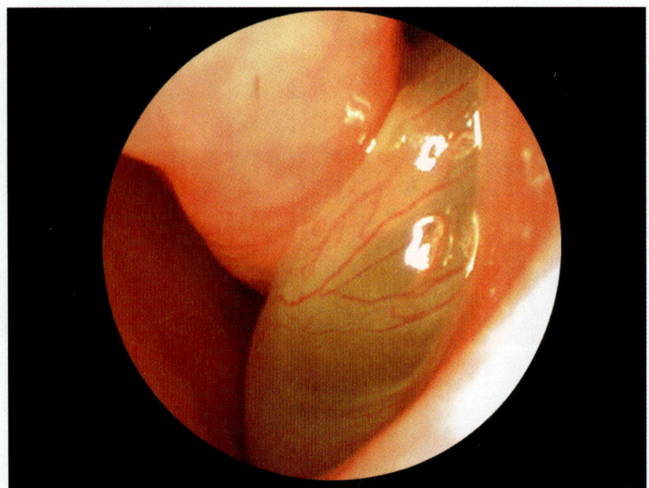

Fig. 4.2: Nasal polyps.

Complications of ARS
Orbital cellulitis
Orbital abscess (subperiosteal or intraconal)
Intracranial sepsis (meningitis, subdural, extradural or intracerebral abscess)
Cavernous sinus thrombosis

Chronic Rhinosinusitis

There are two main subtypes of CRS. This can be diagnosed on nasal endoscopy.

- CRS with nasal polyps (CRSwNP) (Fig. 4.2)
- CRS without nasal polyps (CRSsNP)

Many hypotheses exist for the pathophysiology of CRS. The current consensus is that the deranged interaction between immunological and host factors leads to chronic inflammation and remodeling in the airway. Additionally several medical conditions predispose patients to this disease process such as primary ciliary dyskinesia, cystic fibrosis, and immunodeficiency.

Nasal polyps cause direct obstruction within the airway. Several theories exist for the development of nasal polyposis, but the exact cause remains unknown. It is thought that activated epithelial cells may mediate the influx of inflammatory cells such as eosinophils and fibroblasts leading to nasal polyp formation. Cytokines, chemokines, and growth factors play an important role in the persistence of mucosal inflammation associated with nasal polyps. Infectious agents may be responsible for the initial activation of these mediators. In those with aspirin-exacerbated respiratory disease (AERD), suffering with nasal polyposis, asthma, and aspirin hypersensitivity, it is thought that the arachidonic acid metabolites are responsible for the development of nasal polyps. Inhibition of cyclooxygenase-1 induces attacks of upper and lower airway reactions, including rhinorrhea and varying degrees of bronchospasm and laryngospasm.

Clinical Features

Symptoms are as listed in the definition above. Examination findings may show inflamed mucosa, edematous middle meatus with or without mucopurulent discharge, postnasal discharge, and nasal polyps.

Investigations

- Routine blood tests are not necessary, but if one suspects a granulomatous disease, erythrocyte sedimentation rate (ESR), anti-neutrophil cytoplasmic antibody (ANCA), and acetylcholinesterase levels are helpful.
- Skin prick and RAST testing to exclude an allergic component
- *Endoscopy*: Significant polyps are a feature of AERD
- CT scan of paranasal sinuses to assess the disease extent and assist with surgical planning if medical treatment fails.

Management

Algorithm in Flowchart 4.3.

Management strategy for chronic rhinosinusitis without nasal polyps	*Level of evidence*
Steroid—topical	Ia
Nasal saline irrigation	Ib
Oral antibiotic therapy <4 weeks	II
Oral antibiotic therapy >12 weeks	Ib
Oral steroids	IV

Management strategy for chronic rhinosinusitis with nasal polyps	*Level of evidence*
Topical steroids	Ia
Oral steroids	Ia
Oral antibiotics <4 weeks	Ia/Ib
Oral antibiotics >12 weeks	III
Nasal saline irrigation	No data in single use

Foreign Body in the Nasal Cavity

Foreign body in the nose is a common presentation in any pediatric ENT department. It is typically seen in children aged 2–3 years, but may present in adults with learning difficulties. Rarely, in adults they present as a rhinolith. Foreign bodies are usually inorganic—beads, sponge, plastic, and buttons—but can be organic matter including nuts, peas, etc.

Clinical features: One may witness insertion of a foreign body. Most commonly however this is not the case and the main clinical feature is the presence of a unilateral, foul smelling nasal discharge. This can be purulent or in the first instance or a unilateral foul smelling discharge, which can be purulent or sanguineous if the foreign body has been present for longer than a week.

If there is pain, one should be suspicious of a button battery. These are very corrosive and unless removed promptly can cause significant nasal damage including septal perforation.

It is important to enquire about coughing, choking, and blue episodes, as a nasal foreign body does pose a potential airway risk if aspirated.

On examination, the foreign body may be visualized in the anterior nasal cavity.

Investigation: Using an auroscope with illumination should reveal the foreign body. The use of a topical nasal decongestant can improve the view. If the history is convincing and there is a high index of suspicion that a nasal foreign body exists, a general anesthetic may be required for examination and for its removal.

Chest X-ray should be performed if there is a suspicion of aspiration. Collapse or hyperinflation may be seen on the chest radiograph.

Management: Management includes removal of the foreign body. Batteries and organic matter, which cause a severe inflammatory reaction or impacted foreign bodies, may require a general anesthetic for removal and to allow the nasal cavity to be irrigated.

Choanal Atresia

Choanal atresia is a congenital condition that is a result of failure of the primitive bucconasal membrane to rupture before birth. The choana is blocked by either bone or soft tissue. It occurs in one in 7,000 births, is twice as prevalent in females as in males, and there is a familial tendency. Choanal atresia can be associated with CHARGE

Flowchart 4.3: Management of chronic rhinosinusitis.

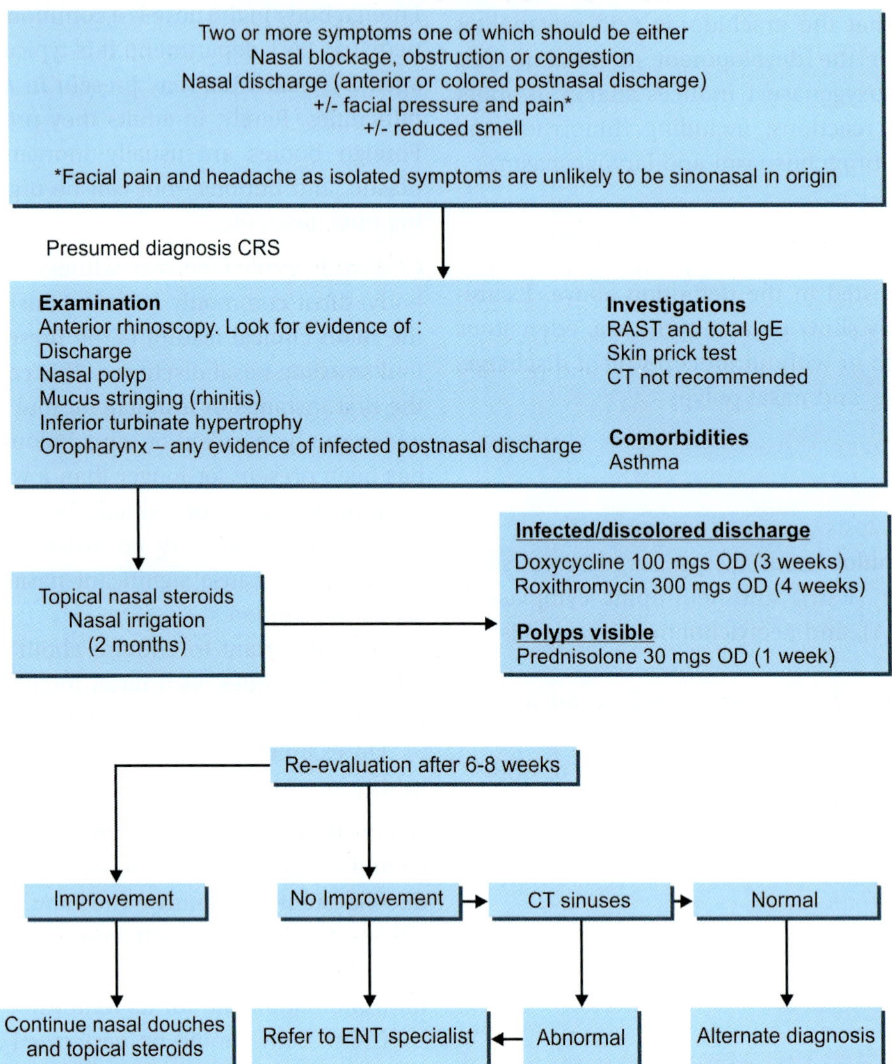

(coloboma, heart defects, atresia of nasal choanae, retardation of growth, genital abnormalities, ear abnormalities) syndrome.

Clinical features: A unilateral choanal atresia can present with a thick gelatinous secretion on the affected side. It may be asymptomatic at birth and is often detected later in life.

Bilateral choanal atresia is a serious life-threatening condition as neonates are obligate nasal breathers. Neonates with bilateral choanal atresia will present with cyanosis at birth, which is reversed on crying.

Investigation: Inability to insert a nasal catheter should raise suspicion for choanal atresia. Computed tomography scan confirms diagnosis.

Management: For bilateral choanal atresia, an oral airway will alleviate cyanosis in the first instance. The neonate will require intubation before definitive surgery is performed.

Surgical procedures aim to provide adequate functional choanal patency and a low rate of restenosis. These are generally performed endoscopically.

4.4 BLOODY RHINORRHEA

Diagnostic Synopsis
Granulamatous disease of nasal cavity
Sinonasal tumors (benign and malignant)
Epistaxis

Granulomatous Diseases of the Nose

Wegener's Granulomatosis

Wegener's granulomatosis (WG) is a chronic, relapsing, systemic necrotizing vasculitis with typical pathologic findings of granulomatous inflammation and autoimmune vasculitis. It affects small and medium sized vessels in the kidneys, lungs, brain, larynx, ears, and nose. The nose is the most commonly affected organ. Antineutrophil cytoplasmic antibodies (ANCAs) have a key role in the pathogenesis of the disease. It is uncertain how ANCAs develop, but it is thought to be associated with B-cells, which are precursors of ANCA-producing plasma cells and possibly antigen-presenting and cytokine-producing cells.

Clinical features: Granulomatosis with polyangiitis presents with a blood-stained rhinorrhea, marked crusting, nasal obstruction, and widespread friable inflammation on examination. This can progress to nasal septum perforation and in advanced cases a saddle-nose deformity.

Although many other organs are affected by WG, nasal symptoms and involvement is often the first sign. Glomerulonephritis resulting in chronic renal failure may present as hematuria. Pulmonary nodules known as coin lesions may cause hemoptysis and dyspnea. Associated otologic symptoms include both sensorineural and conductive hearing loss.

Investigations
- c-ANCA (cytoplasmic ANCA)
- Chest X-ray
- Urinalysis
- Renal biopsy (if indicated)
- Nasal biopsy of an area where the disease is active on examination.

Management: Immunosuppression is the mainstay of treatment. Initially, cyclophosphamide and corticosteroids are administered to achieve remission. Following this, azathioprine and methotrexate are used for long-term immunosuppression. B-cell depletion using rituximab is replacing the use of cyclophosphamide as recent studies have supported its use.

Sarcoidosis

Sarcoidosis is an idiopathic granulomatous disease that can affect any part of the body. Most frequently, the condition affects the lymph nodes, skin, lungs, eyes, liver, spleen, and small bones of hand and feet. The nose, when involved, can present with external and internal nasal changes.

Clinical features: Intranasal involvement is commonest and can present with yellow or grayish slightly raised nodules affecting the nasal septum or inferior turbinate. The patients complain of nasal obstruction, crusting, mucopurulent or often blood-stained mucus. Saddling of the nose, synechiae, and stenosis are late sequelae.

Investigations
- ESR
- Chest X-ray
- Serum angiotensin-converting enzyme
- Nasal biopsy if the above tests are equivocal. Histology shows noncaseating epithelioid cell tubercles or granuloma.

Management: Corticosteroids are the mainstay of therapy. Nonsteroid medication are increasingly used. These include Methotrexate, Azathioprine and antimalarial drugs with immunomodulating properties.

Sinonasal Tumors

Benign neoplasms include epithelial and nonepithelial tumors.

Inverted Papilloma

Inverted papilloma (IP) is the commonest primary nasal tumor. It is associated with a high propensity to recur, local aggressiveness, and 4–14% risk of malignant conversion. It is commonly found in Caucasian males in the sixth to seventh decades of life. Inverted papilloma comprises between 0.5% and 4% of all nasal tumors (2–3% of all nasal polyps); they are most commonly found in the lateral wall of the nasal cavity and often involve ethmoid and maxillary sinuses (Fig. 4.3).

Inverted papilloma has an endophytic growth pattern with downgrowth of epithelium into underlying stroma. The epithelial basement membrane is preserved. Human papillomavirus family of type 6,11 and 16,18 DNA has been observed in IP and associated with severe dysplasia and development of squamous cell carcinoma.

Clinical features
- IP commonly presents as a unilateral polyp, which should raise suspicion. A polyp(s) can be visualized on endoscopy.
- Symptoms include nasal obstruction, blood-stained rhinorrhea or epistaxis, facial pain, headaches, and visual disturbances.

Investigation
- Biopsy of the polyp

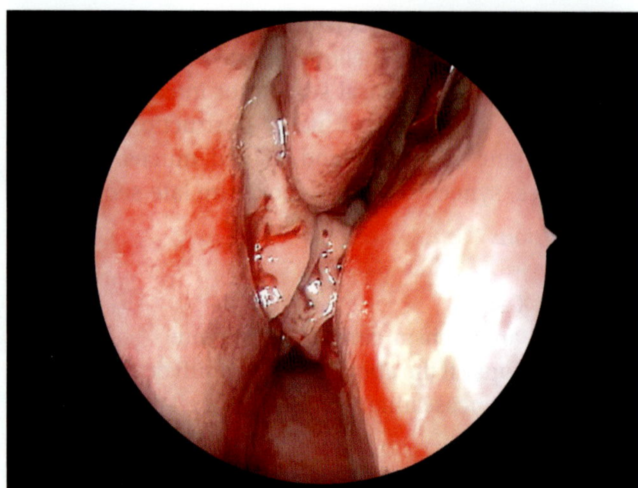

Fig. 4.3: Inverted papilloma.

- High-definition CT will often identify the extent of the tumor, erosion, and expansion of the surrounding structures. MRI is useful in differentiating between tumor and mucosal disease and for evaluating the extra sinus involvement and for operative planning.

Management

- Recommended treatment of IP is complete surgical excision.
- Endoscopic resection is the preferred approach. Lateral rhinotomy and midfacial degloving are alternative approaches.

Sinonasal Malignancies

Sinonasal malignancies are rare accounting for approximately 3% of all head and neck malignancies. They are more common in Asia, particularly in Japan and have a well-known association with exposure to nickel dust, mustard gas, wood dust, isopropyl oil, chromium, or dichlorodiethyl. Wood dust has classically been associated with adenocarcinoma.

Sinonasal Malignancy Includes
Squamous cell carcinoma
Adenocarcinoma
Adenoid cystic carcinoma
Malignant melanoma
Esthesioneuroblastomas
Undifferentiated sinonasal carcinoma

Clinical features

- Clinical features are comparable to IP.
- Sinonasal malignancies can grow to a considerable size before presentation.
- Extra sinus spread results in signs and symptoms that relate to expansion and invasion of adjacent structures, i.e. proptosis, facial paresthesia, visual symptoms, and headaches.

Investigations

- Staging requires a clinical and endoscopic examination with histologic diagnosis and imaging. As per head and neck malignancy, imaging of the primary site, neck, chest, and abdomen in the form of CT is necessary for staging. MRI is useful in assessing the extent of spread and involvement of adjacent critical structures such as the orbit and dura.

Management

- Best prognosis lies with surgical excision followed by radiotherapy if appropriate. Success of surgical resection is dependent on extent and location of the lesion.
- As with any oncologic disease, treatment consists of a multidisciplinary approach.

Epistaxis

The vast majority of bleeds occur in the anterior nasal cavity from Kiesselbach's plexus; in comparison, posterior bleeds are less common and more difficult to control. For a more detailed description, please refer to Chapter 9 on Epistaxis.

Local factors associated with epistaxis include nasal fracture or injuries, septal perforations, inflammatory reactions secondary to granulomatous diseases, foreign bodies, and tumors. Epistaxis can be secondary to prolonged use of nasal sprays, nasal cannula oxygen, and inhalation drugs such as cocaine. Iatrogenic causes such as sinonasal surgery are not uncommon, e.g. septoplasty and functional endoscopic sinus surgery.

Clinical Features

- Fresh blood from the nasal cavity, which can be intermittent, constant, unilateral or bilateral, and anterior or posterior. In the history, it is important to ask about anticoagulation, hypertension, and clotting disorders to ascertain the cause of the epistaxis.

- Recurrent epistaxis may be related to hereditary hemorrhagic telangiectasia.
- On examination, epistaxis patients should be assessed for signs of shock.

Investigation

- Rigid nasendoscopy can be used to visualize and cauterize bleeding points.
- Investigations should include a full blood count, renal profile, clotting, group and save.

Management

Safety equipment such as eye protection, gloves, and an apron should always be worn to manage these patients. Specific management techniques include:

- Packing
- Cautery
- Nasopore, tranexamic acid
- *Floseal*: Hemostatic matrix
- *Surgery*: Sphenopalatine or anterior ethmoidal artery ligation
- Embolization.

Postnasal Drip

5

Raewyn G Campbell, Richard G Douglas

Chapter Overview

Pearls and Pitfalls

Pearls

- Postnasal drip (PND) is a symptom and may be only a sensation (globus).
- The most common causes of PND are sinonasal in origin or reflux related.
- The treatment of PND should be directed to its cause.

Pitfalls

- Chronic cough could be due to PND.
- Most of the times there is no postnasal discharge on examination in patients with history of PND.

5.1 INTRODUCTION

Postnasal drip (PND) is the increased awareness of mucus in the nasopharynx passing to the pharynx and was first described by Johann Peter Frank, a German physician and hygienist, in 1794 (Frank, 1974). Whether PND is a syndrome or merely a symptom is a matter of debate (Morice, 2004). Further, patient descriptions of PND vary widely, from excess nasal mucus that can be sniffed back into the throat, to the sensation of mucus moving down the back of the throat, the inability to expectorate mucus, a sensation of fullness in the nasopharynx or a sensation of a lump in the throat (globus pharyngeus).

Postnasal drip has been described as one of the 3 most common causes of chronic cough (41%), the other two causes being asthma (24%) and gastroesophageal reflux disease (GORD – 21%) (Morice, et al., 2012; Irwin, et al., 1990). Since 2006, cough associated with upper airway conditions, including PND, has been termed upper airway cough syndrome (UACS) in North America due to the uncertain aetiology of a cough associated with PND (Pratter, et al., 2006). The localization of sensation by the mucosa of the upper airway is not very accurate and the symptom of PND may have anatomically and physiologically diverse origins from laryngopharyngeal reflux (LPR) to rhinosinusitis (Morice, 2004). Surprisingly, a perception

Flowchart 5.1: Management of postnasal drip.

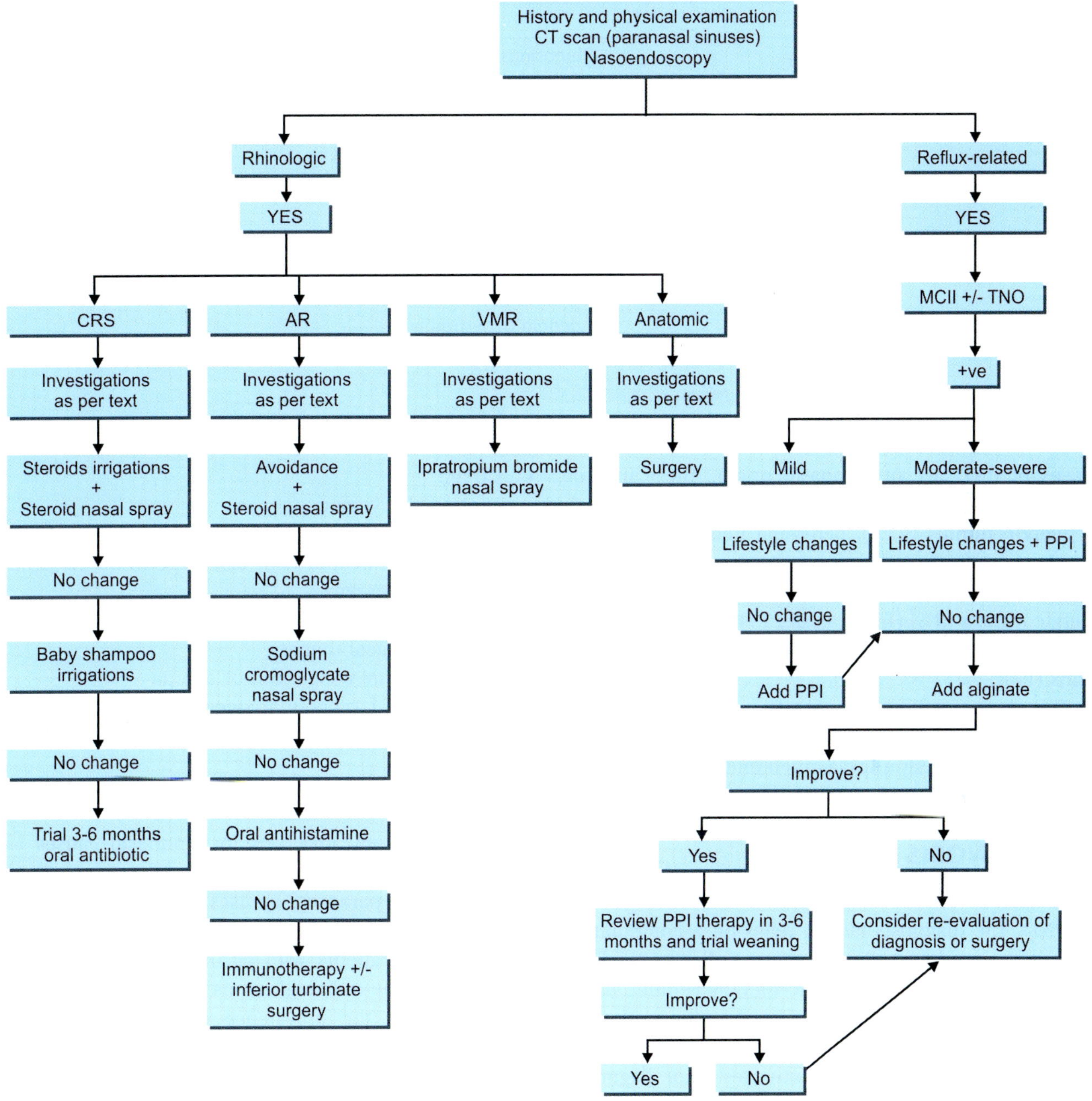

(CRS: Chronic rhinosinusitis; AR: Allergic rhinitis; VMR: Vasomotor rhinitis; PPI: Proton pump inhibitor; TNO: Transnasal esophagoscopy; MCII: Multichannel intraluminal impedance).

of PND can be triggered by anesthetizing the nasopharynx (Ryan, 2010). Postnasal drip can also be present in the absence of any evidence of postnasal drainage of mucus (O'Hara and Jones, 2006). In the United Kingdom, the term rhinosinusitis is preferred (Morice, 2004) over UACS as most patients with purulent rhinosinusitis and symptoms of PND do not complain of cough (O'Hara and Jones, 2006; Irwin and Madison, 2002). In fact, only 20% of patients with chronic cough due to rhinosinusitis experience PND (Tatar, 2009).

The incidence of PND varies geographically and this variation is probably due to differences in the definition of PND and "societal differences in the appreciation of symptomatology" (Morice, 2004). The most common

Table 5.1: Etiology of postnasal drip (PND).

Etiology of PND			
Rhinologic	Inflammatory	Rhinosinusitis	Chronic rhinosinusitis (CRS)
		Rhinitis	
	Anatomic abnormalities	Septal deviation	
		Accessory maxillary sinus ostia	
		Complications of Surgery	Mucosal stripping
			Bone chips
			Residual disease
	Other	Antrochoanal polyps	
		Adenoid hypertrophy	
		Thornwaldt cyst	
Reflux related	Laryngopharyngeal reflux		

causes of PND are of sinonasal origin. These include rhinosinusitis (39%) and varying forms of rhinitis such as allergic rhinitis (23%), perennial nonallergic rhinitis (17%), postinfectious rhinitis (6%), vasomotor rhinitis (2%), drug-induced rhinitis (2%) and environmental non-allergic rhinitis (2%) (Irwin, et al., 1990). The most common non-rhinologic cause of PND is laryngopharyngeal reflux (LPR).

This chapter will use the term "postnasal drip" rather than UACS and will focus on chronic causes of PND. These can be most simply classified under rhinologic and reflux-related causes.

5.2 DIAGNOSIS

No diagnostic criteria or pathognomonic findings exist for PND. The diagnosis largely relies on a combination of patient symptoms, clinical signs, radiographic findings and/or response to specific therapy (Pratter, et al., 2006). PND can be difficult to diagnose due to the differing patient perceptions and descriptions of PND. Unfortunately, there are no objective tests, nor diagnostic methods, to quantify PND.

5.3 CLINICAL FEATURES

Features in clinical history:

- Can often be non-specific and insensitive
- Sensation of fluid in the back of the nose then throat
- Nasal congestion
- Rhinorrhea
- Throat clearing
- Halitosis
- Cough
- Globus pharyngeus

Typical findings on examination:

- Mucoid or mucopurulent discharge in the nasopharynx or oropharynx
- A cobblestone appearance of the oropharyngeal or nasopharyngeal mucosa
- Nasal mucosal congestion or edema
- Evidence of laryngopharyngeal reflux on nasoendoscopy (*see* below).

5.4 INVESTIGATIONS

- Nasoendoscopy to assess for sinonasal causes and LPR
- CT scan of paranasal sinuses where there is a suspicion of sinusitis
    - Among patients with chronic cough, up to 38% have some radiologic sinus abnormality.
    - However, the prevalence of incidental mucosal changes in an asymptomatic population is approximately 30%.
- For further investigations, *see* individual conditions.

5.5 DIAGNOSTIC SUMMARY

The etiology of PND can be classified according to conditions that either:

- Increase sinonasal mucous production
- Alter mucous viscoelasticity/rheologic properties
- Impaired mucociliary clearance (MCC)

The conditions causing these alterations are categorized as in Table 5.1.

5.6 RHINOLOGIC

Inflammatory

Inflammation results in mucous hypersecretion, ciliary dysfunction and alterations to the rheologic properties and composition of mucus (Rubin, 2002; Rogers and Barnes, 2006). Metaplastic epithelial alterations have been noted in chronically inflamed sinus tissue, including cilial loss and squamous metaplasia (Pacini, et al., 1993). Squamous metaplasia results in an epithelium with a reduced MCC (Naclerio, et al., 2007). Chronic inflammation can also result in goblet cell and submucosal gland hypertrophy and hyperplasia (Rubin, 2002). In fact, a mucous hypersecretory phenotype has been described as developing secondary to chronic respiratory tract exposure to particulate matter, allergens, irritants and/or pathogens (Jackson, 2001). Two mucin genes, *MUC5AC* and *MUC5B*, are responsible for the production of excess mucus. These gene products have been found to be the major mucin species in secretions from patients with COPD, asthma, and cystic fibrosis (Rogers, 2007).

As most acute rhinologic conditions generally resolve and do not warrant review by an otorhinolaryngologist, only chronic conditions will be discussed in this chapter.

5.7 CHRONIC RHINOSINUSITIS

Epidemiology and Pathogenesis

Chronic rhinosinusitis (CRS) affects between 5 and 16% of the population (Melen, 1994; Adams, et al., 1999; Blackwell, et al., 2002) and is the primary diagnosis in approximately 2% of attendances at primary care physicians in the USA (Schappert, 1992). The pathogenesis of CRS is uncertain. It is currently thought to result from an interaction of multiple factors including infection, mucosal inflammation and impaired MCC (Sturgess, et al., 1979; Zacharak and Krouse, 2003; Timperley, et al., 2010; Takeuchi, et al., 1991).

Postnasal drip is included in the diagnostic criteria for CRS (*see* below). In CRS, mucous volume, viscosity and elasticity are all increased. The composition changes are due to increases in sodium ion content and the volume increase can be attributed to hyperplasia and hypertrophy of nasal acinar cells (Majima, et al., 1997, Boat, et al., 1994). As mucus becomes infected, its viscosity increases and MCC decreases (Luc and Dulfano, 1983). Further, both viruses and bacteria increase vascular permeability, damage cilia, reduce ciliary beat frequency (CBF), increase mucous volume and viscosity and reduce mucous elasticity (Quraishi, et al., 1998; Tegner, et al., 1979; Carson, et al., 1985; Proctor, et al., 1973).

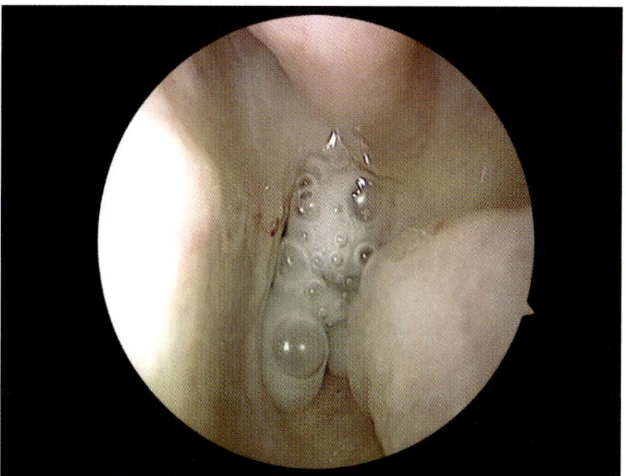

Fig. 5.1: Endoscopic image of mucopurulent discharge in a patient with chronic rhinosinusitis.

Rhinosinusitis and allergic rhinitis have been demonstrated to increase cough sensitivity (Tatar, 2009; Plevkova, et al., 2005). This may explain the cough often associated with these conditions as opposed to cough due to direct aspiration of nasal mucus (often described as PND). Finally, rhinosinusitis often coexists with other conditions that could cause cough such as GORD and eosinophilic airway diseases (e.g. asthma) (Tatar, 2009). Importantly, therefore, cough associated with rhinosinusitis may be unrelated to sinonasal disease.

Clinical Features

Features in history and on examination:

- CRS is classified as an inflammatory disorder of the nose and paranasal sinuses with symptoms of either nasal obstruction or discharge (anterior or PND) plus facial pain or pressure and/or a reduction in sense of smell for a minimum of 12 weeks' duration.
- These symptoms must be accompanied by either endoscopic findings of nasal polyps, mucopurulent discharge (Fig. 5.1) or mucosal edema and/or CT changes within the ostiomeatal complex and/or sinuses (Fokkens, et al., 2012).

Investigations

Hematologic:

- Full blood count with differential (e.g. eosinophil count)
- Immunoglobulins—for CRS refractory to maximal medical and surgical therapy and/or when associated with other conditions such as bronchiectasis

Histopathologic:
- Biopsy of polyps or masses

Radiologic:
- CT scan
- Rarely, magnetic resonance imaging (MRI) (can help diagnose fungal disease).

Symptom Scores

- Visual analog scale (VAS):
  - Correlates well with CT scores (Wabnitz, et al., 2005)
  - Quick and relatively simple
- Sinonasal Outcome Score-22 (SNOT-22):
  - Validated questionnaire (Hopkins, et al., 2009)
  - Correlates with other quality of life outcome measures (e.g. VAS) (Zheng, et al., 2010).

Other:

Cystic fibrosis chloride sweat testing and/or genetic testing.

Ciliary dysmotility studies such as cilial ultrastructure and motility analysis if conditions such as primary ciliary dyskinesia are suspected.

Preferred Treatment

Most clinical trials for the management of CRS have not focused specifically on the management of PND associated with CRS. Generally, studies use global symptom scores that may or may not include PND. The therapies listed below are those specific for PND associated with CRS.

Topical Therapies

Saline irrigation: The mechanism of action of saline irrigations is not precisely understood. Saline irrigations may improve MCC, cleanse the nasal mucosa (Kurtaran, et al., 2003; Homer, et al., 2000), reduce mucosal edema, (Tomooka, et al., 2000), reduce the viscosity of mucus, prevent secondary infection, promote mucosal healing (Homer, et al., 2000; Rabago and Zgierska, 2009), prevent postoperative adhesion formation and ostial stenosis (Talbot, et al., 1997) or remove inflammatory mediators (Georgitis, 1994).

Hypertonic vs isotonic saline: Both hypertonic (3.5%) and normal saline significantly improve PND in adults and children with PND and allergic rhinitis or CRS (Homer, et al., 2000; Tomooka, et al., 2000; Talbot, et al., 1997; Shoseyov, et al., 1998; Ural, et al., 2009). Hypertonic saline has shown superior results over isotonic saline in the symptoms of nasal drainage in postoperative patients, however, hypertonic saline can be painful (Pinto, et al., 2006). Saline concentrations above 3%, have been shown to cause ciliostasis (Boek, et al., 1999), and are therefore not recommended.

Buffered saline solutions: Although buffered solutions may improve absorption (Washington, et al., 2000), no clinically significant difference in PND has been demonstrated between buffered and non-buffered solutions in clinical trials (Homer, et al., 2000; Bachmann, et al., 2000).

Delivery device: Large volume (>200 mL), positive pressure nasal irrigation results in a more uniform intranasal distribution of solution and a greater reduction in overall symptoms (including PND) compared to nasal sprays (low volume, positive pressure) or negative pressure techniques (Miller, et al., 2004; Olson, et al., 2002; Pynnonen, et al., 2007; Khianey and Oppenheimer, 2012).

Rinse devices should be cleaned daily, to avoid cross contamination. The following techniques are useful:
- Rinsing with boiling water
- Rinsing with Milton's solution (Ceuta Healthcare Ltd)
- Microwaving for 1.5 minutes on high (Psaltis, et al., 2012).

Adverse effects:

Adverse effects from saline irrigation are rare and generally mild. These include:
- Aural fullness
- A burning or stinging sensation
- Epistaxis (Tomooka, et al., 2000; Rabago and Zgierska, 2009; Pynnonen, et al., 2007; Khianey and Oppenheimer, 2012)
- Nasal drainage
- Potential recontamination (Keen, et al., 2010; Foreman, et al., 2011; Sowerby and Wright, 2012).

Topical steroids: Studies have shown conflicting results regarding the effect of intranasal steroids on PND (Meltzer, et al., 2000; Meltzer, et al., 2012). On a practical note, twice daily mometasone has been found to be superior to once daily treatment for overall CRS symptoms which included PND (Meltzer, et al., 2012). Patients often express concern regarding the possible systemic effects of intranasal steroids. Multiple studies have demonstrated a lack of systemic steroid absorption and adrenocortical suppression from topical intranasal steroid use (DelGaudio and Wise, 2006; Bhalla, et al., 2008; Welch, et al., 2010).

Adverse effects:
- Epistaxis, headaches, cough.

Other Topical Therapies

Anticholinergics:

- Reduce mucus secretion by inhibiting vagally-mediated serous and seromucous gland secretion.
- Inhaled ipratropium bromide reduces mucus secretion however, does not improve MCC or PND (Ohi, et al., 1984; Houtmeyers, et al., 1999; Macedo, et al., 2009).
- Therefore, anticholinergics cannot be recommended.

Xylitol: Xylitol is a sugar alcohol that behaves as an osmolyte in the airway surface liquid (ASL) coating the airway epithelia. By reducing the bacterial load in the ASL, symptoms of PND may improve with xylitol irrigations. Five percent xylitol in water irrigations resulted in significantly improved SNOT-20 scores in recalcitrant CRS patients (Weissman, et al., 2011). The specific effect on PND was not mentioned. Further study in this area is required.

Topical antibiotics: Multiple studies have demonstrated that there is no clinical benefit from the topical intranasal antibiotics in CRS (Rudmik, et al., 2012). In fact, one study demonstrated increased nasal congestion after nebulized tobramycin (Desrosiers and Salas-Prato, 2001).

Topical antifungals: There is no evidence to support the use of topical antifungals in the treatment of PND or CRS (Rudmik, et al., 2012; Sacks, et al., 2011; Isaacs, et al., 2011).

Surfactants: Surfactants reduce mucus adherence to the epithelium, thereby aiding MCC (Allegra, et al., 1985). Surfactant added to saline irrigation solutions improves the sinus penetration in unoperated sinuses (Rohrer, et al., 2012).

Baby shampoo:

- Irrigations with a 1% solution of baby shampoo improve MCC (Isaacs, et al., 2011; Outzen and Svane-Knudsen, 1993) and reduce symptoms of PND in 53.3% of recalcitrant CRS patients in one prospective, non-randomized study (Chiu, et al., 2008).
- Adverse effects:
  - Nasal burning, headache, reduced sense of smell, epistaxis.

Mucolytics:

N-acetylcysteine (NAC).

NAC reduces mucous viscosity but there are no studies to recommended its use for PND.

Systemic Therapies

Antibiotics: A prolonged course (3 months) of erythromycin, doxycycline or clarithromycin reduces mucous viscosity and PND in patients with recalcitrant CRS (Cervin, et al., 2002; Hashiba and Baba, 1996; Van Zele, et al., 2010) and in patients with milder disease (Kimura, et al., 1997). In fact, a 6 month postoperative course of clarithromycin (200 mg/day) has been shown to result in greater improvement in symptoms of PND and rhinorrhea when compared to a 3 month course (Nakamura, et al., 2013).

Adverse effects:

- Gastrointestinal (cramping, diarrhoea)
- Clostridium difficile colitis
- Anaphylaxis
- Bacterial resistance.

5.8 ALLERGIC RHINITIS

Epidemiology and Pathogenesis

Allergic rhinitis (AR) is a rhinologic expression of IgE-mediated, atopic disease in response to allergen exposure. Approximately 8–15% of the western population suffers from AR which also has a strong association with eczema and asthma. Atopy is determined by a combination of genetic and environmental factors and is classified as:

- Intermittent (previously seasonal)
  - Symptoms < 4 days/week or lasting < 4 weeks.
- Persistent (previously perennial)
  - Symptoms > 4 days/week or lasting > 4 weeks.

The pathogenesis of PND in AR can be explained by the following factors: patients with AR have an increased number of submucosal glands when compared to controls (Mygind, et al., 1974; Tos, et al., 1977). Nasal mucus viscoelasticity is less, and volume greater, after an allergen challenge in patients with AR. Mucociliary clearance is reduced in a congested nose (Puchelle, et al., 1981).

Clinical Features

Findings on history and examination:

- Nasal and ocular pruritus
- Rhinorrhea—usually watery
- Sneezing
- Nasal obstruction
- PND
- Epiphora

- Symptoms reversible with or without treatment
- Physical findings are often non-specific
  - Nasal mucosal edema
  - Hypertrophy of lymphoid tissue in Waldeyer's ring.

Risk factors:
  - Family history of atopy
  - First-born, or only, child
  - Cigarette smoke exposure
  - Higher socioeconomic status
  - Total IgE > 100 IU/L before 6 years of age (Skoner, 2001).

Investigations

Hematologic:
- Full blood count (FBC) with differential (e.g. eosinophil count)
  - Eosinophil count is non-specific
  - Eosinophils can be elevated in AR, nonallergic rhinitis with eosinophilia syndrome (NARES) and parasitic infection
- IgE level
  - Total level not as useful as specific IgE testing
  - However, may be used as a screening tool
- Allergy testing
  - Blood antigen-specific IgE (Radioallergosorbent test [RAST])
    - Better clinical correlation than total IgE
    - Less sensitive than skin prick testing
    - Specificity varies when compared to skin prick testing
      - Sensitivity 60–95%
      - Specificity 30–95%
    - Semi-quantitative measure
    - Do not reflect clinical severity of allergy
  - Skin prick testing
    - Gold standard
    - Qualitative measure
    - Grading is subjective
    - High negative predictive value

Nasal Function Tests:
- Peak inspiratory flow
- Acoustic rhinometry
- Rhinomanometry

Symptom scores:

See section in Chronic Rhinosinusitis.

Note: Always exclude CSF rhinorrhea when investigating AR.

Preferred Treatment

Avoidance:

Bedroom-based hygiene programs; mattress, bedding and pillow covers, acaricide sprays and vacuum HEPA filters have been shown to be effective in managing atopic rhinitis. Isolated use of impermeable bedding is unlikely to be effective (Sheikh, et al., 2010).

Topical Therapies:
1. *Intranasal steroids*: Intranasal fluticasone and triamcinolone acetonide have been shown to significantly reduce PND associated with AR in adults (Gawchik and Lim 1997; Parameswaran, et al., 2006) and children (Ngamphaiboon, et al., 1997).
2. *Sodium cromoglycate*: Eight weeks treatment with 4% sodium cromoglycate nasal spray (5.2 mg/nostril 6 times daily) demonstrated a significant reduction in PND associated with allergic rhinitis (ragweed allergy) (Welsh, et al., 1977).

Systemic Therapies:

Anti-histamines: Oral loratadine (10 mg/d) improved PND in patients suffering from seasonal ragweed-induced rhinitis (Gawchik and Lim, 1997). Azelastine, however, did not reduce PND in patients with rhinitis or CRS (Macedo, et al., 2009).

Immunotherapy: Subcutaneous (SCIT) and sublingual immunotherapy (SLIT) are effective in patients who do not respond to medical therapy and whose symptoms significantly impact quality of life (Purkey, et al., 2013). CBF and MCC have been found to increase after 1 year of injection immunotherapy for dust mites/dermatophagoides farina (Ohashi, et al., 1989; Cmejrek, et al., 2005).

Acupuncture: Has been shown to significantly reduce overall symptom scores in allergic rhinitis (Choi, et al., 2013).

Surgery:

Inferior turbinate (IT) surgery: Partial IT reduction surgery was found not to be successful in relieving PND in patients with varying types of rhinitis (Schmelzer, et al., 1999). However, patients with allergic rhinitis achieved the best results (Zagolski, 2010).

5.9 VASOMOTOR RHINITIS

Vasomotor rhinitis (VMR) is an idiopathic, perennial, nonallergic rhinitis (NAR) characterized by non-specific nasal hyperreactivity on exposure to nonimmunologic stimuli. Vasomotor rhinitis is the most common cause of NAR and is responsible for approximately 61% of causes. Vasomotor rhinitis affects approximately 6% of the US population (Shah and McGrath, 2012), is more common in women and the age of onset tends to be after the age of 40 years. Despite its name, no vascular or neurologic dysfunction has been identified in VMR. It is likely related to multiple causes, yet is unrelated to allergy, infection, structural lesions, systemic disease or pharmacologic causes. Links between VMR and LPR have been postulated based on evidence of autonomic dysfunction (Jaradeh, et al., 2000). Vasomotor rhinitis can include sub-categories such as gustatory rhinitis (rhinitis provoked by eating certain foods), pregnancy rhinitis and exercise-induced rhinitis.

Clinical Features

Findings on history and examination:

- Nasal congestion
- Rhinorrhea
- PND
- Sneezing
- Triggers include:
  - Irritants—smoke, perfumes, chemicals
  - Change in weather
  - Cold air

Investigations:

- Skin prick testing
  - Negative in VMR.

Preferred Treatment

- Ipratropium bromide may be effective in treating PND due to VMR (Irwin and Madison, 2002).
- However, Fluticasone did not improve PND in patients with VMR (Jacobs, et al., 2009).
- Vidian neurectomy
  - Whilst effective in alleviating symptoms of rhinorrhea and nasal obstruction, vidian neurectomy is not effective for the treatment of PND associated with VMR (Robinson and Wormald, 2006).

5.10 IRRITANTS/TOXINS/OCCUPATIONAL RHINITIS

Tobacco smoke: Chronic tobacco smoke exposure (both passive and active) causes hypertrophy of submucosal glands, an increase in nasal mucosal goblet cell number, a reduction in CBF and a reduction in cilial number (Goodman, et al 1978; Stanley, et al., 1986; Hadar, et al., 2009; Elwany and Ibrahim, 2012).

5.11 ANATOMICAL ABNORMALITIES

Septal Deviations

Epidemiology and Pathogenesis

Up to 79% of the population have a deviated septum (Gray, 1978). Mucus tends to move around, rather than over, septal deviations. However, occasionally, no movement is noted around a septal deviation (Proctor, 1982; Waguespack, 1995). Septal deviations will reduce nasal airflow, which will therefore, reduce MCC. Septal deviation has been associated with an increased prevalence of rhinosinusitis (Orlandi 2010) and reduced MCC (Ginzel and Illum, 1980; Kamani, et al., 2006; Ulusoy, et al., 2007).

Preferred Treatment

Septoplasty (Ginzel, et al., 1980; Ulusoy, et al., 2007; Polat and Dostbil, 2010).

Accessory Ostia and Mucous Recirculation

Epidemiology and Pathogenesis

Accessory ostia most commonly involve the maxillary sinus. The incidence of maxillary sinus ostia varies between 4% and 41% (Hollinshead, 1982) and has been found in the posterior fontanelle in up to 25% of patients (Stammberger, 1991).

Mucous recirculation most commonly occurs in 4 scenarios:

- Between the natural and accessory ostium (Albu and Tomescu 2004; Kennedy and Shaalan 1989; Yanagisawa and Yanagisawa 1997)
- Between a middle meatal antrostomy and accessory ostium
- Between a natural ostium and middle meatal antrostomy (Kennedy and Shaalan, 1989)
- Between middle and inferior meatal antrostomies (Gutman and Houser 2003).

Although technically, recirculation can occur in any sinus and has been noted in the ethmoid and sphenoid sinuses (Waguespack 1995; Yanagisawa and Weaver, 1996). As mucus recirculates it becomes more viscous and includes a greater concentration of inflammatory and infectious agents (Matthews and Burke, 1997). This recirculation forms a ring visible on CT (Chung, et al., 2002) and predisposes the patient to recurrent infection before it finally makes its way to the nasopharynx.

Missed accessory ostia are a common cause of endoscopic sinus surgery (ESS) failure (Albu and Tomescu, 2004; Kennedy and Zinreich, 1988; Parsons, et al., 1996) and PND has been described as a common symptom of accessory ostia (Yanagisawa and Tanagisawa, 1997; Gutman and Houser, 2003; Chung, et al., 2002).

Preferred Treatment

Surgery to connect the natural ostia with the accessory ostia. Using an angled endoscope following an uncinectomy will ensure that an accessory ostium has not been missed. Natural ostia tend to be oval shaped compared to more circular accessory ostia. Careful review of the CT scan preoperatively will alert the surgeon to the presence of an accessory ostium.

Complications of Surgery

Residual Disease

Most patients with persistent mucosal disease post-ESS will report PND, yet only 50–60% of patients with resolution of mucosal disease post-ESS report PND (Wise, et al., 2006).

Mucosal Stripping

Mucosal stripping results in exposed bone, altered and dysfunctional regenerated mucosa and nonphysiological mucosal healing. Poorly ciliated mucosa will result in a dysfunctional sinus with poor drainage that relies on gravity, mucus stasis, recurrent infection and, ultimately, PND.

Preferred Treatment

Mucosal preservation techniques in sinus surgery will maximise mucosal regeneration and preservation of healthy mucosa. Increasing frequency of postoperative debridement was not found to improve PND in a prospective randomized study (Lee and Byun, 2008).

5.12 OTHER

Thornwaldt Cyst

A Thornwaldt cyst is a persistent notochord remnant presenting as a cystic mass in the nasopharynx. When infected, it can discharge mucus and be a cause of PND (Woodbury and Ferguson, 2011).

Preferred Treatment

These are easily identified via endoscopic examination and may be confirmed by CT imaging. Most are asymptomatic. Inflamed or infected cysts not responding to a course of systemic antibiotics are best managed surgically by marsupialization.

Adenoid Hypertrophy

Adenoid hypertrophy has been noted in 16% of patients with PND (Liu, et al., 2008).

Preferred Treatment

Adenoidectomy: Limited evidence to supports the use of intranasal steroid sprays in the management of adenoid hypertrophy.

Future Directions

Therapies targeting the hypersecretory phenotype are currently under investigation. These therapies aim to reverse this phenotype and reduce airway inflammation, the number of goblet cells and the size of submucosal glands (Rogers, 2007). This may occur via an alteration in the *MUC5B* to *MUC5AC* ratio. Therapies include chemokine receptor antagonists to reduce mucus production and goblet cell hyperplasia (Chapman, et al., 2007).

5.13 REFLUX-RELATED

Gastroesophageal Reflux

Epidemiology and Pathogenesis

Extraesophageal symptoms of reflux occur in approximately one-third of adults with GORD (Jaspersen, et al., 2003). In particular, over 50% of patients with GORD also experience PND (Bucca, et al., 2010; Pawar, et al., 2007). Gastroesophageal reflux disease can be divided into erosive (40%) and nonerosive (60%) disease according to pH studies and endoscopic examination. Gastroesophageal reflux disease affects between 10 and 20% of the Western population (Dent, et al., 2005) and is increasing in prevalence (El-Serag, 2007). There is some evidence supporting a genetic predisposition for GORD (Dent, et al., 2005). It has been reported that patients with CRS have a higher incidence of positive pH tests when compared to non-CRS patients (Flook and Kumar, 2011). In one series 78% of patients with refractory CRS had GORD (DiBiase, et al., 2002). GORD has certainly been shown to be associated with a reduction in MCC (Delehaye, et al., 2009) and has been identified as a predictor of poor outcome in endoscopic sinus surgery (ESS) (Chambers, et al., 1997).

The pathophysiology behind the extraesophageal manifestations of GORD is unknown and a causal link between the two has not been convincingly documented. Many symptoms may be due to the direct effect of gastric fluids on nasal tissue (Delehaye, et al., 2009). More recently, it has been proposed that a vagally-mediated esophageal-nasal reflex, stimulated by acid coming into contact with esophageal mucosa, may be responsible for the association between CRS and GORD (Chambers, et al., 1997; Phua, et al., 2010; Megale, et al., 2006; Vaezi, et al., 2010). However, two recent reviews found no evidence of a causal link between CRS and GORD (Woodbury and Ferguson, 2011; Flook and Kumar, 2011).

Laryngopharyngeal reflex is an extraesophageal manifestation of GORD and the most likely cause of reflux-related PND.

Laryngopharyngeal Reflux

Epidemiology and Pathogenesis

Laryngopharyngeal reflux is the result of retrograde flow of gastric contents to the laryngopharynx (Ford, 2005). Up to 75% of people with LPR experience PND (Irwin, et al., 1990; Issing and Karkos, 2003) and up to 93% complain of PND in conjunction with another symptom such as throat clearing or rhinorrhea (Irwin, et al., 1990). Postnasal drip is included as one of the 9 items in the Reflux Symptom Index, a validated and commonly utilized tool to measure LPR severity (Belafsky, et al., 2002).

Laryngopharyngeal reflux differs from GORD in many ways (Table 5.2). Firstly, the majority of patients with LPR do not have oesophagitis or the associated symptoms of heartburn (Koufman, et al., 2002). Laryngopharyngeal reflux patients predominantly suffer daytime, upright reflux whereas GORD patients reflux at night whilst supine. Finally, most patients with LPR do not have GORD (Koufman, et al., 2002).

The association between LPR and PND has long been debated. However, reflux of gastric acid into the nasal cavity is a rare event in adult patients with GORD and chronic rhinosinusitis (CRS) (Wong, et al., 2010). Alternatively, non-acid reflux may play a role in the cause of PND associated with LPR (Ozmen, et al., 2008; Piper and Fenton, 1965; Panetti, et al., 2001).

Table 5.2: Comparison of LPR with GORD.

	GORD	*LPR*
Symptoms		
• Heartburn/indigestion	++++	+
• Hoarseness, cough, dysphagia, globus, throat clearing, PND	+	++++
Etiology		
• Defective lower esophageal sphincter	++++	+
• Defective upper esophageal sphincter	+	++++
Reflux pattern		
• Nocturnal/supine	++++	+
• Daytime/upright	+	++++
Examination findings		
• Esophagitis	++++	+
Laryngeal findings:		
• Vocal fold granuloma, ulcers, edema, erythema, etc.	+	++++
Effectiveness of treatment		
• Diet and lifestyle modification	++	+
• Antacids	++	+
• PPI daily	+++	+
• PPI bd for >3 months	++++	+++

(GORD: Gastroesopheageal reflux disease; LPR: Laryngopharyngeal reflux; PPI: Proton pump inhibitor; bd: Twice daily).

Laryngopharyngeal reflux damages the laryngeal respiratory epithelium resulting in ciliary dysfunction and a reduction in the MCC (Hanson and Jiang, 2000). The resulting local inflammation also up-regulates laryngeal sensory nerves causing hypersensitivity (Hanson and Jiang, 2000). This may produce a PND sensation and stimulate throat clearing and swallowing.

Autonomic nervous system (ANS) dysfunction may also be involved in the pathogenesis of LPR and PND. Reflux stimulates hyperreactivity of the ANS and subsequently results in upper respiratory tract signs and symptoms such as nasal edema and discharge (Loehrl, et al., 2002).

Whatever the mechanism, it appears that LPR does have a role to play in patients with PND (Wise, et al., 2006).

Features in Clinical History

- Symptoms are protean and intermittent, yet chronic
- Typical symptoms such as heartburn and indigestion are usually absent (Tatar, et al., 2009; Koufman, et al., 2002)

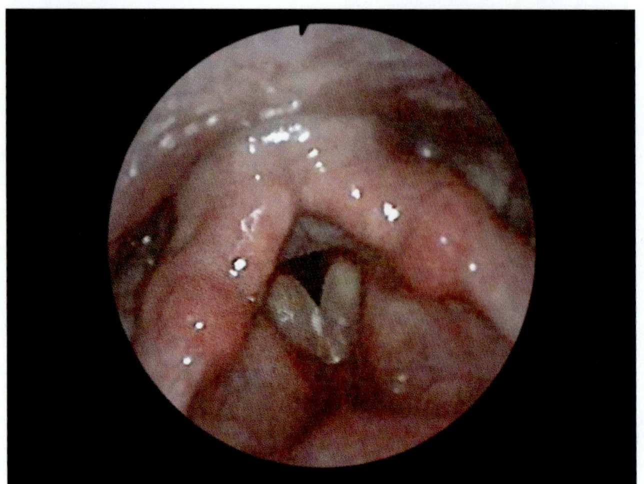

Fig. 5.2: Endoscopic image of the larynx of a patient with postnasal drip due to laryngopharyngeal reflux demonstrating thickening, erythema and edema of posterior larynx.

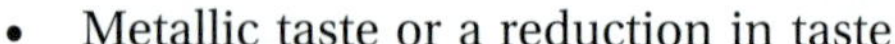

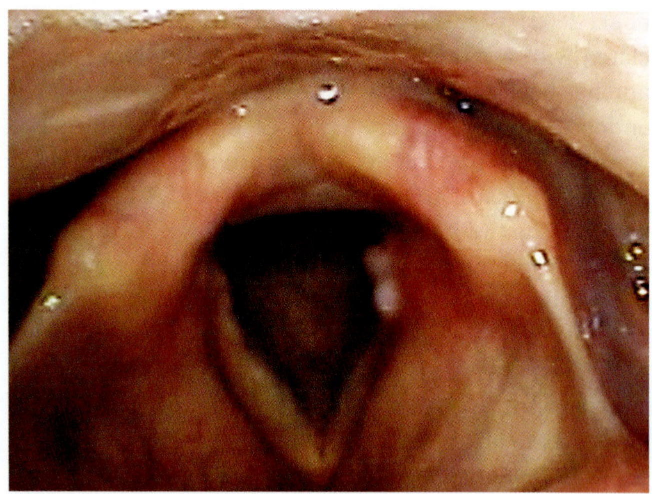

Fig. 5.3: Endscopic image of the larynx of a patient with postnasal drip due to laryngopharyngeal reflux demonstrating a left sided contact granuloma.

- Metallic taste or a reduction in taste
- Hoarseness
- Laryngospasm
- Throat burning/sore throat
- Throat clearing—more common in LPR than in GORD (Koufman, et al., 2002)
- Persistent cough
- Dysphagia
- Globus pharyngeus (GP)
  - PND is included in the Glasgow Edinburgh Throat Scale (GETS), a tool to assess the severity of GP symptoms. Fifty-five percent of patients with GP complain of PND (Ali and Wilson, 2007).
- Also otalgia, cervical pain, burning in buccal and lingual regions (Wise, et al., 2006).

Findings on Clinical Examination

- Nasoendoscopy
  - Thickening, erythema, edema of posterior larynx (Ylitalo, et al., 2001) (Fig. 5.2)
  - Contact granuloma (Ohman, et al., 1983; Ylitalo and Ramel, 2002) (Fig. 5.3)
  - Vocal fold edema (Koufman, et al., 2002)
  - Vocal fold contact ulcers (Koufman, et al., 2002)
  - Vocal fold nodules
  - Subglottic pseudosulcus (Belafsky, et al., 2002; Hickson, et al., 2001)
    - 70% sensitivity and 77% sensitivity of finding pseudosulcus in LPR
  - LPR is associated with:
    - Subglottic stenosis
    - Laryngeal carcinoma
    - Laryngospasm
    - Paradoxical vocal fold movement
  - Sinusitis.

Investigations

- Reflux Symptom Index
  - >13 considered abnormal
- Reflux Finding Score (Belafsky, et al., 2001)
  - >7 indicates a 95% certainty of LPR
- Transnasal esophagoscopy (TNE)
- pH monitoring
  - Gold standard for diagnosis of GORD, not for diagnosis of LPR
  - Does not record non-acid reflux or gaseous reflux
- Multi-channel intraluminal impedance monitoring (MCII)
  - Rather than pH, therefore, records nonacid reflux
  - Invasive
- esophagogastroduodenoscopy
  - Abnormal in < 20% of LPR patients
  - Useful for detecting lesions in GORD patients
- CT scan
  - *Neck*: To investigate suspicious signs or symptoms, thyroid gland, osteophytes, etc.
  - *Sinuses*: To include or exclude sinonasal pathology as an associated factor. Does not exclude rhinitis as a cause of symptoms.

Preferred Treatment

Lifestyle Modification: Suitable for all LPR patients, yet only suitable as the sole therapy in those with mild signs and symptoms.

- Weight loss if overweight
- Smoking cessation (nicotine)
- Alcohol avoidance/reduction
- Dietary restrictions
  - Chocolate, fats, citrus fruit/juices, carbonated drinks, tomato-based foods, spicy foods, alcohol, and caffeine
- Avoid eating within 2–3 hours of going to bed
- Small frequent meals
- Elevate head of bed.

Acid Suppressive Therapy: *Proton pump inhibitors*: The majority of patients with LPR will require proton pump inhibitor (PPI) therapy.

The twice daily use of PPIs has been demonstrated to result in significant improvement in PND severity when compared to placebo in adults and children (Pawar, et al., 2007; Vaezi, et al., 2010; Bothwell, et al., 1999). PPIs for LPR are best taken twice daily (Park, et al., 2005; DelGaudio and Waring, 2003) as PPIs suppress acid for less than 16.8 hours (Pawar, et al., 2007; Koufman, et al., 2002; Chiverton, et al., 1992; Kahrilas, et al., 2000). PPIs should also be taken a minimum of 30 minutes before food for optimum effect (Hatlebakk, et al., 2000). LPR requires more aggressive and prolonged treatment compared to GORD as LPR symptoms take longer to respond (months), and do not respond as strongly, to PPIs as oesophageal symptoms (DelGaudio and Waring, 2003). Therefore, PPIs for an extended period (up to 6 months) are recommended for LPR (Ford, 2005; Koufman, et al., 2002; Park, et al., 2005; DelGaudio and Waring, 2003). Finally, the response of LPR to PPIs is highly variable and may require a prolonged taper or chronic treatment.

Side Effects:

- Uncommon
- Headache, rash, dizziness, somnolence, mental confusion, impotence
- May reduce absorption of vitamin B12 due to hypochlorhydria
- Hypergastrinemia due to prolonged (>12 months) suppression of gastric acid
- Category B3 in pregnancy.

H2-Receptor Antagonists:

- Of limited use in LPR (Fackler, et al., 2002; Kibblewhite and Morrison, 1990)
- Less effective than PPIs and do not benefit if prescribed in addition to a PPI (Park, et al., 2005; Fackler, et al., 2002).

Antacids:

- Liquid alginate suspension has been shown to improve symptoms in patients with LPR (McGlashan, et al., 2009).

Surgery:

- For medically resistant patients
- Laparoscopic fundoplication (either partial or full) for patients with LPR reduces the associated symptom of PND (Iqbal, et al., 2009).

Outcomes of Treatment

Approximately 25% of patients with LPR will experience spontaneous resolution of symptoms and 50% will suffer a relapsing and remitting course (Koufman, et al., 2002). Most patients experience symptomatic improvement after 2 months of lifestyle changes and 3–4 months of PPI therapy (Ford 2005; Park, et al., 2005). Laryngeal changes and other physical findings resolve after 6 months.

SUMMARY

Postnasal drip is a symptom with a variety of causes, however, the most common are sinonasal in origin or reflux-related. Whether it is one of the major causes of chronic cough is controversial. Once the predominant cause is determined, a multitude of therapeutic options exist and outcomes can be very satisfying for both patients and surgeons.

REFERENCES

Adams, P.F., Hendershot, G.E. and Marano, M.A., 1999. Current estimates from the National Health Interview Survey, 1996. *Vital and Health Statistics*, 10(200), pp. 1-203.

Agastya, G., West, B.C. and Callahan, J.M., 2000. Omeprazole inhibits phagocytosis and acidification of phagolysosomes of normal human neutrophils in vitro. *Immunopharmacology and Immunotoxicology*, 22, pp. 357-72.

Albu, S. and Tomescu, E., 2004. Small and large middle meatus antrostomies in the treatment of chronic maxillary sinusitis. *Otolaryngology—Head and Neck Surgery*, 131, pp. 542-7.

Ali, K.H.M. and Wilson, J.A., 2007. What is the severity of globus sensation in individuals who have never sought health care for it? *Journal of Laryngology and Otology*, 121(9), pp. 865-8.

Allegra, L., Bossi, R. and Braga, P. 1985. Influence of surfactant on mucociliary transport. *European Journal of Respiratory Diseases*, 142(Suppl), pp. 71-6.

Bachmann, G., Hommel, G. and Michel, O., 2000. Effect of irrigation of the nose with isotonic salt solution on adult patients with chronic paranasal sinus disease. Hyperlink. http://www.springer.com/medicine/otorhinolaryngology/journal/405. *European Archives of Oto-Rhino-Laryngology*, 257, pp. 537-41.

Bassiouny, A., Atef, A.M., Raouf, M.A., et al., 2003. Ultrastructural ciliary changes of maxillary sinus mucosa following functional endoscopic sinus surgery: an image analysis quantitative study. *Journal of Laryngology and Otology*, 117, pp. 273-9.

Becker, J.C., Grosser, N., Waltke, C., et al., 2006. Beyond gastric acid reduction: proton pump inhibitors induce heme oxygenase-1 in gastric and endothelial cells. *Biochemical and Biophysical Research Communications*, 345, pp. 1014-21.

Belafsky, P.C., Postma, G.N. and Koufman, J.A., 2001. The validity and reliability of the reflux finding score (RFS). *Laryngoscope*, 111, pp. 1313-7.

Belafsky, P.C., Postma, G.N. and Koufman, J.A., 2002. Validity and reliability of the reflux symptom index (RSI). *Journal of Voice*, 16(2), pp. 274-7.

Bhalla, R.K., Payton, K. and Wright, E.D., 2008. Safety of budesonide in saline sinonasal irrigations in the management of chronic rhinosinusitis with polyposis: lack of significant adrenal suppression. *Journal of Otolaryngology—Head and Neck*, 37, pp. 821-5.

Biswas, K., Bandyopadhyay, U., Chattopadhyay, I., Varadaraj, A., Ali, E. and Banerjee, R.K., 2003. A novel antioxidant and antiapoptotic role of omeprazole to block gastric ulcer through scavenging of hydroxyl radical. *Journal of Biological Chemistry*, 278, pp. 10993-1001.

Blackwell, D.L., Collins, J.G. and Coles, R., 2002. Summary health statistics for U.S. adults: National Health Interview Survey, 1997. *Vital and Health Statistics*, 10(205), pp. 1-109.

Boat, T.F., Cheng, P.W. and Leigh, M.W., 1994. Biochemistry of mucus. In: T. Takishima and S. Shimura, eds. *Airway secretion: lung biology in health and disease*. New York: Dekker. pp. 217-82.

Boek, W.M., Keles, N., Graamans, K. and Huizing, E.H., 1999. Physiologic and hypertonic saline solutions impair ciliary activity in vitro. *Laryngoscope*, 109, pp. 396-9.

Bothwell, M.R., Parsons, D.S., Talbot, A., Barbero, G. and Wilder, B., 1999. Outcome of reflux therapy on pediatric chronic sinusitis. *Otolaryngology—Head and Neck Surgery*, 121(3), pp. 255-62.

Brozek, J.L., Bousquet, J., Baena-Cagnani, C.E., Bonini, S., Canonica, G.W., Casale, T.B., van Wijk, R.G., Ohta, K., Zuberbier, T., Schünemann, H.J.; Global Allergy and Asthma European Network; Grading of Recommendations Assessment, Development and Evaluation Working Group, 2010. Allergic Rhinitis and its Impact on Asthma (ARIA) guidelines: 2010 revision. *Journal of Allergy and Clinical Immunology*, 126(3), pp. 466-76.

Bucca, C.B., Bugiani, M., Culla, B., Guida, G., Heffler, E., Mietta, S., Moretto, A., Rolla, G. and Brussino, L., 2010. Chronic cough and irritable larynx. *Journal of Allergy and Clinical Immunology*, 127(2), pp. 412-9.

Carson, J.L., Collier, A.M. and Hu, S.S., 1985. Acquired ciliary defects in nasal epithelium of children with acute viral upper respiratory infections. *The New England Journal of Medicine*, 312, pp. 463-8.

Cervin, A., Kalm, O., Sandkull, P. and Lindberg, S., 2002. One-year low-dose erythromycin treatment of persistent chronic sinusitis after sinus surgery: clinical outcome and effects on mucociliary parameters and nasal nitric oxide. *Otolaryngology—Head & Neck Surgery*, 126(5), pp. 481-9.

Chambers, D.W., Davis, W.E., Cook, P.R., Nishioka, G.J. and Rudman, D.T., 1997. Long-term outcome analysis of functional endoscopic sinus surgery: correlation of symptoms with endoscopic examination findings and potential prognostic variables. *Laryngoscope*, 107(4), pp. 504-10.

Champion, G., Richter, J.E., Vaezi, M.F., et al., 1994. Duodenogastroesophageal reflux: relationship to pH and importance in Barrett's esophagus. *Gastroenterology*, 107, pp. 747-54.

Chapman, R.W., Minnicozzi, M., Celly, C.S., Phillips, J.E., Kung, T.T., Hipkin, R.W., et al., 2007. A novel, orally active, C.X.CR1/2 receptor antagonist, Sch527123, inhibits neutrophil recruitment, mucus production, and goblet cell hyperplasia in animal models of pulmonary inflammation. *Journal of Pharmacology and Experimental Therapeutics*, 322(2), pp. 486-93.

Chiu, A.G., Palmer, J.N., Woodworth, B.A., Doghramji, L., Cohen, M.B., Prince, A. and Cohen, N.A., 2008. Baby shampoo nasal irrigations for the symptomatic post-functional endoscopic sinus surgery patient. *American Journal of Rhinology*, 22(1), pp. 34-7.

Chiverton, S.G., Howden, C.W. and Burget, D.W., 1992. Omeprazole (20 mg) daily given in the morning or evening: a comparison of effects on gastric acidity, and plasma gastrin and omeprazole concentration. *Alimentary Pharmacology & Therapeutics*, 6, pp. 103-11.

Choi, S.M., Park, J.E., Li, S.S., Jung, H., Zi, M., Kim, T.H., Jung, S., Kim, A., Shin, M., Sul, J.U., Hong, Z., Jiping, Z., Lee, S., Liyun, H., Kang, K. and Baoyan, L., 2013. A multicenter, randomised, controlled trial testing the effects of acupuncture on allergic rhinitis. *Allergy*, 68(3), pp. 365-74.

Chung, S.K., Cho, D.Y. and Dhong, H.J., 2002. Computed tomogram findings of mucous recirculation between the natural and accessory ostia of the maxillary sinus. *American Journal of Rhinology*, 16(5), pp. 265-8.

Cmejrek, R.C., Gutman, M.T., Torres, A.J., Keen, K.J. and Houser, S.M., 2005. The effect of injection immunotherapy on mucociliary clearance in allergic patients. *Otolaryngology—Head and Neck Surgery*, 133(1), pp. 9-15.

Contencin, P. and Narcy, P., 1991. Nasopharyngeal pH monitoring in infants and children with chronic rhinopharyngitis. *International Journal of Pediatric Otorhinolaryngology*, 22(3), pp. 249-56.

Cvorovic, L., Brajovic, D., Strbac, M., Milutinovic, Z. and Cvorovic, V., 2008. Detection of Helicobacter pylori in nasal polyps: preliminary report. *Journal of Otolaryngology—Head and Neck Surgery*, 37, pp. 192-5.

Dasgupta, B. and King, M., 1996. Reduction in viscoelasticity in cystic fibrosis sputum in vitro using combined treatment with Nacystelyn and rhDNase. *Pediatric Pulmonology*, 22(3), pp. 161-6.

Delehaye, E., Dore, M.P., Bozzo, C., Mameli, L., Delitala, G. and Meloni, F., 2009. Correlation between nasal mucociliary clearance time and gastroesophageal reflux disease: our experience on 50 patients. *Auris, Nasus, Larynx*, 36(2), pp. 157-61.

DelGaudio, J.M., 2005. Direct nasopharyngeal reflux of gastric acid is a contributing factor in refractory chronic rhinosinusitis. *Laryngoscope*, 115, pp. 946-57.

DelGaudio, J.M. and Waring, J.P., 2003. Empiric esomeprazole in the treatment of laryngopharyngeal reflux. *Laryngoscope*, 113, pp. 598-601.

DelGaudio, J.M. and Wise, S.K., 2006. Topical steroid drops for the treatment of sinus ostia stenosis in the postoperative period. *American Journal of Rhinology*, 20, pp. 563-7.

Dent, J., El-Serag, H.B., Wallander, M.A. and Johansson, S., 2005. Epidemiology of gastro-oesophageal reflux disease: a systematic review. *Gut*, 54(5), pp. 710-17.

De Poortere, D., Kofonow, J.M., Chiu, A.G. and Cohen, N.A., 2011. Polyhydrated ionogen enhances postoperative sinonasal ciliated remucosalization. *International Forum of Allergy & Rhinology*, 1(2), pp. 83-7.

Desrosiers, M.Y. and Salas-Prato, M., 2001. Treatment of chronic rhinosinusitis refractory to other treatments with topical antibiotic therapy delivered by means of a large-particle nebulizer: results of a controlled trial. *Otolaryngology—Head and Neck Surgery*, 125, pp. 265-9.

DiBiase, J.K., Olusola, B.F., Huerter, J.V., et al., 2002. Role of GERD in chronic recalcitrant sinusitis: A prosective, open label, pilot trial. *The American Journal of Gastroenterology*, 97, pp. 843-50.

El-Serag, H.B., 2007. Time trends of gastroesophageal reflux disease: a systematic review. *Clinical Gastroenterology and Hepatology*, 5(1), pp. 17-26.

Elwany, S., Ibrahim, A.A., Mandour, Z. and Talaat, I., 2012. Effect of passive smoking on the ultrastructure of the nasal mucosa in children. *Laryngoscope*, 122(5), pp. 965-9.

Fackler, W.K., Ours, T.M., Vaezi, M.F. and Richter, J.E., 2002. Long-term effect of H2RA therapy on nocturnal gastric acid breakthrough. *Gastroenterology*, 122, pp. 625-32.

Flook, E.P. and Kumar, B.N., 2011. Is there evidence to link acid reflux with chronic sinusitis or nasal symptoms? A review of the evidence. *Rhinology*, 49(1), pp. 11-16.

Fokkens, W.J., Lund, V.J., Mullol, J., Bachert, C., Alobid, I., Baroody, F., Cohen, N., Cervin, A., Douglas, R., Gevaert, P., Georgalas, C., Goossens, H., Harvey, R., Hellings, P., Hopkins, C., Jones, N., Joos, G., Kalogjera, L., Kern, B., Kowalski, M., Price, D., Riechelmann, H., Schlosser, R., Senior, B., Thomas, M., Toskala, E., Voegels, R., Wang, D.Y. and Wormald, P.J., 2012. European position paper on rhinosinusitis and nasal polyps 2012. *Rhinology—Supplement*, 23(3), pp. 1-298.

Ford, C.N., 2005. Evaluation and management of laryngopharyngeal reflux. *JAMA*, 294(12), pp. 1534-40.

Foreman, A. and Wormald, P.J., 2011. Can bottle design prevent bacterial contamination of nasal irrigation devices? *International Forum of Allergy & Rhinology*, 1(4), pp. 303-7.

Forsgren, K., Otori, N., Stierna, P., et al., 1999. Microvasculature, blood flow, and vasoreactivity in rabbit sinus mucosa after surgery. *Laryngoscope*, 109(4), pp. 562-8.

Forsgren, K., Stierna, P., Kumlien, J., et al., 1993. Regeneration of maxillary sinus mucosa following surgical removal. Experimental study in rabbits. *Annals of Otology, Rhinology & Laryngology*, 102(6), pp. 459-66.

Frank, J., 1794. De curandis hominum morbis epitome. *Mannhemii*, pp. 124-5.

Gawchik, S.M. and Lim, J., 1997. Comparison of intranasal triamcinolone acetonide with oral loratadine in the treatment of seasonal ragweed-induced allergic rhinitis. *American Journal of Managed Care*, 3(7), pp. 1052-8.

Gaynor, E.B., 1991. Otolaryngologic manifestations of gastroesophageal reflux. *The American Journal of Gastroenterology*, 86(7), pp. 801-8.

Georgalas, C., Thomas, K., Owens, C., Abramovich, S. and Lack, G., 2005. Medical treatment for rhinosinusitis associated with adenoidal hypertrophy in children: an evaluation of clinical response and changes on magnetic resonance imaging. *Annals of Otology, Rhinology & Laryngology*, 114(8), pp. 638-44.

Georgitis, J.W., 1994. Nasal hyperthermia and simple irrigation for perennial rhinitis. Changes in inflammatory mediators. *Chest*, 106, pp. 1487-92.

Gilljam, H., Ellin, A. and Strandvik, B., 1989. Increased bronchial chloride concentration in cystic fibrosis. *Scandinavian Journal of Clinical and Laboratory*, 49, pp. 121-4.

Ginzel, A. and Illum, P., 1980. Nasal mucociliary clearance in patients with septal deviation. *Rhinology*, 18, pp. 177-81.

Goel, H., Jindal, N.K., Wig, U., Chawla, R.K. and Yadav, S.P.S., 1989. Effect of bromhexine on nasal mucus clearance in chronic maxillary sinusitis. *The Indian Journal of Chest Diseases & Allied Sciences*, 31(1), pp. 33-6.

Goodman, R.M., Yergin, B.M., Landa, J.F., Golivanux, M.H. and Sackner, M.A., 1978. Relationship of smoking history and pulmonary function tests to tracheal mucous velocity in nonsmokers, young smokers, ex-smokers, and patients with chronic bronchitis. *American Review of Respiratory Disease*, 117(2), pp. 205-14.

Gray, L.P., 1978. Deviated nasal septum. Incidence and etiology. *Annals of Otology, Rhinology, and Laryngology Supplement*, 87(3 Pt 3 Suppl 50), pp. 3-20.

Guercio, J.P., Birch, S., Fernandez, R.J., et al., 1980. Deposition of Ragweed pollen and extract on nasal mucosa of patients with allergic rhinitis: effect on nasal airflow resistance and nasal mucus velocity. *Journal of Allergy and Clinical Immunology*, 66, pp. 61-9.

Guo, Y., Majima, Y., Hattori, M., Seki, S. and Sakakura, Y., 1997. Effects of functional endoscopic sinus surgery on maxillary sinus mucosa. *Archives of Otolaryngology—Head and Neck Surgery*, 123, pp. 1097-100.

Gutman, M. and Houser, S., 2003. Iatrogenic maxillary sinus recirculation and beyond. *Ear, Nose and Throat Journal*, 82(1), pp. 61-3.

Hadar, T., Yaniv, E., Shvili, Y., Koren, R. and Shvero, J., 2009. Histopathological changes of the nasal mucosa induced by smoking. *Inhalation Toxicology*, 21(13), pp. 1119 22.

Handa, O., Yoshida, N., Fujita, N., et al., 2006. Molecular mechanisms involved in anti-inflammatory effects of proton pump inhibitors. *Inflammation Research*, 55, pp. 476-80.

Hanson, D.G. and Jiang, J.J., 2000. Diagnosis and management of chronic laryngitis associated with reflux. *American Journal of Medicine*, 108(Suppl 4a), pp. 112S-9S.

Harvey, R.J., Goddard, J.C., Wise, S.K. and Schlosser, R.J., 2008. Effects of endoscopic sinus surgery and delivery device on cadaver sinus irrigation. *Otolaryngology—Head and Neck Surgery*, 139, pp. 137-42.

Hashiba, M. and Baba, S., 1996. Efficacy of long-term administration of clarithromycin in the treatment of intractable chronic sinusitis. *Acta Otolaryngologica Supplementum*, 525, pp. 73-8.

Hatlebakk, J.G., Katz, P.O., Camacho-Lobato, L. and Castell, D.O., 2000. Proton pump inhibitors: better acid suppression when taken before a meal than without a meal. *Alimentary Pharmacology & Therapeutics*, 14(10), pp. 1267-72.

Hattori, M., Majima, Y., Ukai, K. and Sakakura, Y., 1993. Effects of nasal allergen challenge on dynamic viscoelasticity of nasal mucus. *Annals of Otology, Rhinology & Laryngology*, 102(4 Pt 1), pp. 314-7.

Hickson, C., Simpson, C.B. and Falcon, R. Laryngeal pseudosulcus as a predictor of laryngopharyngeal reflux. *Laryngoscope*, 111(10), pp. 1742-5.

Hollinshead, W.H., 1982. The head and neck. In: *Anatomy for surgeons, Vol. 1*, 3rd ed. Philadelphia, PA: Harper & Row. pp. 223-67.

Homer, J.J., Dowley, A.C., Condon, L., El-Jassar, P. and Sood, S., 2000. The effect of hypertonicity on nasal mucociliary clearance. *Clinical Otolaryngology and Allied Sciences*, 25(6), pp. 558-60.

Hopkins, C., Gillett, S., Slack, R., Lund, V.J. and Browne, J.P., 2009. Psychometric validity of the 22-item sinonasal outcome test. *Clinical Otolaryngology*, 34(5), pp. 447-54.

Houtmeyers, E., Gosselink, R., Gayan-Ramirez, G. and Decramer, M., 1999. Effects of drugs on mucus clearance. *European Respiratory Journal*, 14(2), pp. 452-67.

Hwang, P.H. and Chan, J.M., 2006. Retinoic acid improves ciliogenesis after surgery of the maxillary sinus in rabbits. *Laryngoscope*, 116(7), pp. 1080-85.

Iqbal, M., Batch, A.J., Moorthy, K., Cooper, B.T. and Spychal, R.T., 2009. Outcome of surgical fundoplication for extra-oesophageal symptoms of reflux. *Surgical Endoscopy*, 23(3), pp. 557-67.

Irwin, R.S., Curley, F.J. and French, C.L., 1990. Chronic cough: the spectrum and frequency of causes, key components of the diagnostic evaluation, and outcome of specific therapy. *American Review of Respiratory Disease*, 141(3), pp. 640-47.

Irwin, R.S. and Madison, J.M., 2002. Diagnosis and treatment of chronic cough due to gastro-esophageal reflux disease and postnasal drip syndrome. *Pulmonary Pharmacology and Therapeutics*, 15(3), pp. 261-6.

Isaacs, S., Fakhri, S., Luong, A. and Citardi, M.J., 2011. A meta-analysis of topical amphotericin B for the treatment of chronic rhinosinusitis. *International Forum of Allergy & Rhinology*, 1, pp. 250-54.

Issing, W.J. and Karkos, P.D., 2003. Atypical manifestations of gastro-oesophageal reflux. *The Journal of the Royal Society of Medicine*, 96, pp. 477-80.

Jackson, A.D., 2001. Airway goblet cell mucus secretion. *Trends in Pharmacological Sciences*, 22(1), pp. 39-45.

Jacobs, R., Lieberman, P., Kent, E., Silvey, M., Locantore, N. and Philpot, E.E., 2009. Weather/temperature-sensitive vasomotor rhinitis may be refractory to intranasal corticosteroid treatment. *Allergy & Asthma Proceedings*, 30(2), pp. 120-27.

Jaradeh, S.S., Smith, T.L., Torrico, L., Prieto, T.E., Loehrl, T.A., Darling, R.J. and Toohill, R.J., 2000. Autonomic nervous system evaluation of patients with vasomotor rhinitis. *Laryngoscope*, 110(11), pp. 1828-31.

Jaspersen, D., Kulig, M., Labenz, J., Leodolter, A., Lind, T., Meyer-Sabellek, W., et al., 2003. Prevalence of extra-oesophageal manifestations in gastro-oesophageal reflux disease: an analysis based on the ProGERD Study. *Alimentary Pharmacology & Therapeutics*, 17(12), pp. 1515-20.

Johnston, N., Bulmer, D., Gill, G.A., Panetti, M., Ross, P.E., Pearson, J.P., Pignatelli, M., Axford, S.E., Dettmar, P.W. and Koufman, J.A., 2003. Cell biology of laryngeal epithelial defenses in health and disease: further studies. *Annals of Otology, Rhinology & Laryngology*, 112(6), pp. 481-91.

Joris, L., Dab, I. and Quinton, P.M. Elemental composition of human airway surface fluid in healthy and diseased airways. *American Review of Respiratory Disease*, 148(6 pt 1), pp. 1633-7.

Kahrilas, P.J., Falk, G.W., Johnson, D.A., et al., 2000. Esomeprazole improves healing and symptom resolution as compared with omeprazole in reflux esophagitis patients: a randomized controlled trial. *Alimentary Pharmacology & Therapeutics*, 14, pp. 1249-58.

Kamani, T., Yilmaz, T., Surucu, S., Turan, E. and Brent, K.A., 2006. Scanning electron microscopy of ciliae and saccharine test for ciliary function in septal deviations. *Laryngoscope*, 116(4), pp. 586-90.

Kapanci, Y. and Elemer, G., 1983. Ambroxol and surfactant secretion. Experimental studies on the incorporation of 3H-palmitate into pulmonary surfactant. *Symposia Giovanni Lorenzini Foundation*, 16, pp. 263-72.

Kedika, R.R., Souza, R.F. and Spechler, S.J., 2009. Potential anti-inflammatory effects of proton pump inhibitors: a review and discussion of the clinical implication. *Digestive Diseases and Sciences*, 54, pp. 2312-7.

Keen, M., Foreman, A. and Wormald, P.J., 2010. The clinical significance of nasal irrigation bottle contamination. *Laryngoscope*, 120, pp. 2110-14.

Kennedy, D.W. and Shaalan, H., 1989. Reevaluation of maxillary sinus surgery: experimental study in rabbits. *Annals of Otology, Rhinology & Laryngology*, 98(11), pp. 901-6.

Kennedy, D.W. and Zinreich, S.J., 1982. The functional endoscopic approach to inflammatory sinus disease: current perspectives and technique modifications. *American Journal of Rhinology*, 2(3), pp. 89-96.

Khianey, R. and Oppenheimer, J., 2012. Is nasal saline irrigation all it is cracked up to be? *Annals of Allergy, Asthma & Immunology*, 109(1), pp. 20-8.

Kibblewhite, D.J. and Morrison, M.D., 1990. A double-blind controlled study of the efficacy of cimetidine in the treatment of the cervical symptoms of gastroesophageal reflux. *Journal of Otolaryngology*, 19, pp. 103-9.

Kimura, N., Nishioka, K., Nishizaki, K., Ogawa, T., Naitou, Y. and Masuda, Y., 1997. Clinical effect of low-dose, long-term roxithromycin chemotherapy in patients with chronic sinusitis. *Acta Medica Okayama*, 51(1), pp. 33-7.

King, E., 1935. A clinical study of the functioning of the maxillary sinus mucosa. *Annals of Otology, Rhinology & Laryngology*, 44, pp. 480-82.

Koch, T.R., Petro, A., Darrabie, M. and Opara, E.C., 2004. Effect of the, H, K-ATPase inhibitor, esomeprazole magnesium, on gut total antioxidant capacity in mice. *The Journal of Nutritional Biochemistry*, 15, pp. 522-6.

Koufman, J.A., Aviv, J.E., Casiano, R.R., et al., 2002. Laryngopharyngeal reflux: position statement of the Committee on Speech, Voice, and Swallowing disorders of the American Academy of Otolaryngology—Head and Neck Surgery. *Otolaryngology—Head and Neck Surgery*, 127, pp. 32-5.

Koyuncu, M., Yilmaz, M., Yalcin, S., Metin, N., Gunduz, S. and Karatas, E., 1989. The existence of sinusitis in rabbits and the use of bromhexine as a mucolytic nose drop in the treatment of sinusitis. *Mikrobiyoloji Bulteni*, 23(2), pp. 133-44.

Kuroda, M., Yoshida, N., Ichikawa, H., et al., 2006. Lansoprazole, a proton pump inhibitor, reduces the severity of indomethacin-induced rat enteritis. *International Journal of Molecular Medicine*, 17, pp. 89-93.

Kurtaran, H., Karadag, A., Catal, F. and Avci, Z., 2003. A reappraisal of nasal saline solution use in chronic sinusitis. *Chest*, 124(5), pp. 2036-7; author reply 7-8.

Lapenna, D., de Gioia, S., Ciofani, G., Festi, D. and Cuccurullo, F., 1996. Antioxidant properties of omeprazole. *FEBS Letter*, 382, pp. 189-92.

Lee, J.Y. and Byun, J.Y., 2008. Relationship between the frequency of postoperative debridement and patient discomfort, healing period, surgical outcomes, and compliance after endoscopic sinus surgery. *Laryngoscope*, 118(10), pp. 1868-72.

Leung, M.K. and Hwang, P.H., 2007. Rehabilitation of surgically traumatized paranasal sinus mucosa using retinoic acid. *American Journal of Rhinology*, 21(3), pp. 271-5.

Little, F.B., Koufman, J.A., Kohut, R.I., et al., 1985. Effect of gastric acid on the pathogenesis of subglottic stenosis. *Annals of Otology, Rhinology & Laryngology*, 94, pp. 516-9.

Liu, H., Sun, C., Han, Y. and Shang, G., 2008. Analysis of the causes and treatment of postnasal drip syndrome. *Journal of Clinical Otorhinolaryngology, Head, & Neck Surgery (Chinese)*, 22(2), pp. 68-9.

Loehrl, T.A., Smith, T.L., Darling, R.J., Torrico, L., Prieto, T.E., Shaker, R., Toohill, R.J. and Jaradeh, S.S., 2002. Autonomic dysfunction, vasomotor rhinitis, and extraesophageal manifestations of gastroesophageal reflux. *Otolaryngology—Head and Neck Surgery*, 126(4), pp. 382-7.

Luc, C.K. and Dulfano, M.J., 1983. Effect of pH, viscosity and ionic strength changes on the ciliary beat frequency of human bronchial explants. *Clinical Science*, 64, pp. 449-51.

Macedo, P., Saleh, H., Torrego, A., Arbery, J., MacKay, I., et al., 2009. Postnasal drip and chronic cough: an open interventional study. *Respiratory Medicine*, 103(11), pp. 1700-5.

Majima, Y., Masuda, S. and Sakakura, Y., 1997. Quantitative study of nasal secretory cells in normal subjects and patients with chronic sinusitis. *Laryngoscope*, 107(11), pp. 1515-8.

Martinez, S.D., Malagon, I.B., Garewal, H.S., Cui, H. and Fass, R., 2003. Non-erosive reflux disease (NERD)—acid reflux and symptom patterns. *Alimentary Pharmacology & Therapeutics*, 17(4), pp. 537-45.

Matthews, B.L. and Burke, A.J., 1997. Recirculation of mucus via accessory ostia causing chronic maxillary sinus disease. *Otolaryngology—Head and Neck Surgery*, 117, pp. 422-3.

McGlashan, J.A., Johnstone, L.M., Sykes, J., Strugala, V. and Dettmar, P.W., 2009. The value of a liquid alginate suspension (Gaviscon Advance) in the management of laryngopharyngeal reflux. *European Archives of Otorhinolaryngology*, 266 (2), pp. 243-51.

Megale, S.R., Scanavini, A.B., Andrade, E.C., Fernandes, M.I. and Anselmo-Lima, W.T., 2006. Gastroesophageal reflux disease: its importance in ear, nose, and throat practice. *International Journal of Pediatric Otorhinolaryngology*, 70(1), pp. 81-8.

Melen, I., 1994. Chronic sinusitis: clinical and pathophysiological aspects. *Acta Oto-Laryngologica Supplementum*, 515, pp. 45-8.

Meltzer, E.O., Charous, B.L., Busse, W.W., Zinreich, S.J., Lorber, R.R. and Danzig, M.R., 2000. Added relief in the treatment of acute recurrent sinusitis with adjunctive mometasone fumarate nasal spray. *Journal of Allergy and Clinical Immunology*, 106(4), pp. 630-37.

Meltzer, E.O., Gates, D. and Bachert, C., 2012. Mometasone furoate nasal spray increases the number of minimal-symptom days in patients with acute rhinosinusitis. *Annals of Allergy, Asthma & Immunology*, 108(4), pp. 275-9.

Merker, V.H.J., Bublitz, G., Kruger, U. and Zimmermann, B., 1969. Morphologic examinations in the respiratory epithelium using Bisolvon. *Deutsches Medizinisches Journal*, 20(9), pp. 288-90.

Miller, T.R., Muntz, H.R., Gilbert, M.E. and Orlandi, R.R., 2004. Comparison of topical medication delivery systems after sinus surgery. *Laryngoscope*, 114, pp. 201-4.

Monk, B.C., Mason, A.B., Abramochkin, G., Haber, J.E., Seto-Young, D. and Perlin, D.S., 1995. The yeast plasma membrane proton pumping ATPase is a viable antifungal target. I. Effects of the cysteine-modifying reagent omeprazole. *Biochimica et Biophysica Acta*, 1239, pp. 81-90.

Morice, A.H., 2004. Post-nasal drip syndrome—a symptom to be sniffed at? *Pulmonary Pharmacology and Therapeutics*, 17(6), pp. 343-5.

Morice, A.H., McGarvey, L.P.A. and Dicpinigaitis, P.V., 2012. Cough hypersensitivity syndrome is an important clinical concept: a pro/con debate. *Lung*, 190(1), pp. 3-9.

Moriyama, H., Yanagi, K., Ohtori, N., Asai, K. and Fukami, M., 1996. Healing process of sinus mucosa after endoscopic sinus surgery. *American Journal of Rhinology*, 10(2), pp. 61-6.

Mygind, N., Viner, A.S. and Jackman, N., 1974. Histology of nasal mucosa in normals and in patients with perennial rhinitis: a blind study of plastic embedded specimens. *Rhinology*, 12, pp. 131-6.

Naclerio, R., Pinto, J., Assanasen, P. and Baroody, F.M., 2007. Observations on the ability of the nose to warm and humidify inspired air. *Rhinology*, 45(2), pp. 102-11.

Nakamura, Y., Suzuki, M., Yokota, M., Ozaki, S., Ohno, N., Hamajima, Y., Nakayama, M., Hashiba, M. and Murakami, S., 2013. Optimal duration of macrolide treatment for chronic sinusitis after endoscopic sinus surgery. *Auris Nasus Larynx*, 40, pp. 366-72.

Nakao, M. and Malfertheiner, P., 1998. Growth inhibitory and bactericidal activities of lansoprazole compared with those of omeprazole and pantoprazole against Helicobacter pylori. *Helicobacter*, 3, pp. 21-7.

Ngamphaiboon, J., Thepchatri, A., Chatchatee, P. and Chumdermpadetsuk, S., 1997. Fluticasone propionate aqueous nasal spray treatment for perennial allergic rhinitis in children. *Annals of Allergy, Asthma, & Immunology*, 78(5), pp. 479-84.

Ngo, P., Furuta, G.T., Antonioli, D.A. and Fox, V.L., 2006. Eosinophils in the esophagus—peptic or allergic eosinophilic esophagitis? Case series of three patients with esophageal eosinophilia. *The American Journal of Gastroenterology*, 101, pp. 1666-70.

Ohashi, Y., Nakai, Y., Ikeoka, H., et al., 1989. Increased ciliary beating frequency of nasal mucosa following immunotherapy for allergy. *Annals of Otology, Rhinology & Laryngology*, 98, pp. 350-4.

Ohi, M., Sakakura, Y., Murai, S. and Miyoshi, Y., 1984, Effect of ipratropium bromide on nasal mucociliary transport. *Rhinology*, 22(4), pp. 241-6.

Ohman, L., Olofsson, H., Tibbling, L. and Ericsson, G., 1983. Esophageal dysfunction in patients with contact ulcer of the larynx. *Annals of Otology, Rhinology & Laryngology*, 92(3 Pt 1), pp. 228-30.

Olson, D.E., Rasgon, B.M. and Hilsinger, R.L., Jr., 2002. Radiographic comparison of three methods for nasal saline irrigation. *Laryngoscope*, 112, pp. 1394-8.

Orlandi, R.R, 2010. A systematic analysis of septal deviation associated with rhinosinusitis. *Laryngoscope*, 120(8), pp. 1687-95.

Outzen, K.E. and Svane-Knudsen, V., 1993. Effect of surface-active substance on nasal mucociliary clearance time: a comparison of saccharin clearance time before and after the use of surface-active substance. *Rhinology*, 31(4), pp. 155-7.

Ozdek, A., Cirak, M.Y., Samim, E., Bayiz, U., Safak, M.A. and Turet, S., 2003. A possible role of Helicobacter pylori in chronic rhinosinusitis: a preliminary report. *Laryngoscope*, 113, pp. 679-82.

Ozmen, S., Yucel, O.T., Sinici, I., Ozmen, O.A., Suslu, A., Ogretmenoglu, O. and Onerci, M., 2008. Nasal pepsin assay and pH monitoring in chronic rhinosinusitis. *Laryngoscope*, 118(5), pp. 890-94.

O'Hara, J. and Jones, N.S., 2006. Post-nasal drip syndrome: most patients with purulent nasal secretions do not complain of chronic cough. *Rhinology*, 44(4), pp. 270-73.

Pacini, P., Gulisano, M., Dallai, S., et al., 1993. The human nasal mucous membrane during chronic inflammation, before and after muco-active therapy: a study using scanning electron microscopy. *The Italian Journal of Anatomy and Embryology*, 98, pp. 231-41.

Panetti, M., Pearson, J.P., Dettmar, P.W., et al., 2001. Active pepsin in airway secretions: Possible evidence for new supraesophageal pH criteria. *Gastroenterology*, 120, pp. A118-19.

Parameswaran, K., Fanat, A. and O'Byrne, P.M., 2006. Effects of intranasal fluticasone and salmeterol on allergen-induced nasal responses. *Allergy*, 61, pp. 731-6.

Park, W., Hicks, D.M., Khandwala, F., Richter, J.E. Abelson, T.I. Milstein, C. and Vaezi, M.F., 2005. Laryngopharyngeal reflux: prospective cohort study evaluating optimal dose of proton-pump inhibitor therapy and pretherapy predictors of response. *Laryngoscope*, 115(7), pp. 1230-38.

Parsons, D.S., Stivers, F.E. and Talbot, A.R., 1996. The missed ostium sequence and the surgical approach to revision functional endoscopic sinus surgery. *Otolaryngologic Clinics of North America*, 29(1), pp. 169-83.

Pawar, S., Lim, H.J., Gill, M., et al., 2007. Treatment of postnasal drip with proton pump inhibitors: a prospective randomised, placebo-controlled study. *American Journal of Rhinology*, 21(6), pp. 695-701.

Phipps, C.D., Wood, E., Gibson, W.S. and Cochran, W.J., 2000. Gastroesophageal reflux contributing to chronic sinus disease in children: a prospective analysis. *Archives of Otolaryngology—Head and Neck Surgery*, 126(7), pp. 831-6.

Phua, S.Y., McGarvey, L., Ngu, M. and Ing, A., 2010. The differential effect of gastroesophageal reflux disease on mechanostimulation and chemostimulation of the laryngopharynx. *Chest*, 138(5), pp. 1180-85.

Pinto, J.M., Elwany, S., Baroody, F.M. and Naclerio, R.M., 2006. Effects of saline sprays on symptoms after endoscopic sinus surgery. *American Journal of Rhinology*, 20(2), pp. 191-6.

Piper, D.W. and Fenton, B.H., 1965. PH stability and activity curves of pepsin with special reference to their clinical importance. *Gut*, 6, 506-8.

Plevkova, J., Brozmanova, M., Pecova, R. and Tatar, M., 2005. Effects of intranasal histamine on the cough reflex in subjects with allergic rhinitis. *Journal of Physiology and Pharmacology*, 56(Suppl 4), pp. 185-95.

Polat, C. and Dostbil, Z., 2010. Evaluation of the nasal mucociliary transport rate by rhinoscintigraphy before and after surgery in patients with deviated nasal septum. *European Archives of Otorhinolaryngology*, 267(4), pp. 529-35.

Postma, G.N., 2000. Ambulatory pH monitoring methodology. *Annals of Otology, Rhinology & Laryngology Supplement*, 184, pp. 10-14.

Pratter, M.R., et al., 2006. Chronic upper airway cough syndrome secondary to rhinosinus disease (Previously Referred to as Postnasal Drip Syndrome) ACCP Evidence-Based Clinical Practice Guidelines. *Chest*, 129(1 Suppl), pp. 63S-71S.

Proctor, D.F., 1982. The mucociliary system. In: D.F. Proctor and I. Andersen, eds. *The nose: upper airway physiology and the atmospheric environment* (Ch 10). Amsterdam: Elsevier Biomedical Press. pp. 245-78.

Proctor, D.F., Andersen, I. and Lundqvist, G., 1973. Clearance of Inhaled Particles from the human nose. *Archives of Internal Medicine*, 131, pp. 132-9.

Psaltis, A.J., Foreman, A. and Wormald, P.J., et al., 2012. Contamination of sinus irrigation devices: a review of the evidence and clinical relevance. *American Journal of Rhinology & Allergy*, 26(3), pp. 201-3.

Puchelle, E., Aug, F., Pham, Q.T., et al., 1981. Comparison of Three Methods for Measuring Nasal Mucociliary Clearance in Man. *Acta Otolaryngologica* (Stockh), 91, pp. 297-303.

Purkey, M.R., Smith, T.L., Ferguson, B.J., Luong, A., Reisacher, W.R., Pillsbury, H.C. 3rd and Toskala, E., 2013. Subcutaneous immunotherapy for allergic rhinitis: an evidence based review of the recent literature with recommendations. *International Forum of Allergy & Rhinology*, 3(7), pp. 519-31.

Pynnonen, M.A., Mukerji, S.S., Kim, H.M., Adams, M.E. and Terrell, J.E., 2007. Nasal saline for chronic sinonasal symptoms: a randomized controlled trial. *Archives of Otolaryngology—Head and Neck Surgery*, 133, pp. 1115-20.

Quraishi, M.S., Jones, N.S. and Mason, J., 1998. The rheology of mucus: a review. *Clinical Otolaryngology*, 23, pp. 403-13.

Rabago, D. and Zgierska, A., 2009. Saline nasal irrigation for upper respiratory conditions. *American Family Physician*, 80, pp. 1117-9.

Reavis, K.M., Morris, C.D., Gopal, D.V., Hunter, J.G. and Jobe, B.A., 2004. Laryngopharyngeal reflux symptoms better predict the presence of esophageal adenocarcinoma than typical gastroesophageal reflux symptoms. *Annals of Surgery*, 239, pp. 849-56.

Riise, G.C., Qvarfordt, I., Larsson, S., Eliasson, V. and Andersson, B.A., 2000. Inhibitory effect of N-acetylcysteine on adherence of Streptococcus pneumoniae and Haemophilus influenzae to human oropharyngeal epithelial cells in vitro. *Respiration*, 67(5), pp. 552-8.

Ritter, M., Schratzberger, P., Rossmann, H., et al., 1998. Effect of inhibitors of Na+/H+-exchange and gastric H+/K+ ATPase on cell volume, intracellular pH and migration of human polymorphonuclear leucocytes. *The British Journal of Pharmacology*, 124, pp. 627-38.

Robinson, S.R. and Wormald, P.J., 2006. Endoscopic vidian neurectomy. *American Journal of Rhinology*, 20(2), pp. 197-202.

Rochat, T., Lacroix, J.S. and Jornot, L., 2004. N-acetylcysteine inhibits Na+ absorption across human nasal epithelial cells. *Journal of Cellular Physiology*, 201(1), pp. 106-16.

Rogers, D.F., 2007. Mucoactive agents for airway mucus hypersecretory diseases. *Respiratory Care*, 52(9), pp. 1176-97.

Rogers, D.F., Godfrey, R.W., Majumdar, S. and Jeffery, P.K., 1988. Oral N-acetylcysteine speeds reversal of cigarette smoke-induced mucous cell hyperplasia in the rat. *Experimental Lung Research*, 14(1), pp. 19-35.

Rogers, D.F. and Barnes, P.J., 2006. Treatment of airway mucous hypersecretion. *Annals of Medicines*, 38(2), pp. 116-25.

Rogers, D.F. and Jeffery, P.K., 1986. Inhibition by oral N-acetylcysteine of cigarette smoke-induced "bronchitis" in the rat. *Experimental Lung Research*, 10(3), pp. 285-98.

Rohrer, J.W., Dion, G.R., Brenner, P.S., Abadi, W.M., McMains, K.C., Thomas, R.F. and Weitzel, E.K., 2012. Surfactant improves irrigant penetration into unoperated sinuses. *American Journal of Rhinology & Allergy*, 26(3), pp. 197-200.

Rubin, B.K., 2002. Physiology of airway mucus clearance. *Respiratory Care*, 47(7), pp. 761-8.

Rudmik, L., Hoy, M., Schlosser, R.J., Harvey, R.J., Welch, K.C., Lund, V. and Smith, T., 2012. Topical therapies in the management of chronic rhinosinusitis: an evidence-based review with recommendations. *International Forum of Allergy & Rhinology*, 3(4), pp. 281-98.

Ryan, M.W., 2010. The patient with "postnasal drip". *Medical Clinics of North America*, 94(5), pp. 913-21.

Sacks, P.L., Harvey, R.J., Rimmer, J., Gallagher, R.M. and Sacks, R., 2011. Topical and systemic antifungal therapy for the symptomatic treatment of chronic rhinosinusitis. *The Cochrane Database of Systematic Reviews*, CD008263.

Sasaki, T., Yamaya, M., Yasuda, H., et al., 2005. The proton pump inhibitor lansoprazole inhibits rhinovirus infection in cultured human tracheal epithelial cells. *European Journal of Pharmacology*, 509(2-3), pp. 201-10.

Schappert, S.M., 1992. National Ambulatory Medical Care Survey: 1990 summary. Advance Data from *Vital and Health Statistics*, Vol. 213. Hyattsville, MD: National Center for Health Statistics. pp. 1-11.

Schmelzer, B., Katz, S. and Vidts, G., 1999. Long-term efficacy of our surgical approach to turbinate hypertrophy. *American Journal of Rhinology*, 13(5), pp. 357-61.

Seagrave, J.C., Albrecht, H., Park, Y.S., Rubin, B., Solomon, G. and Kim, K.C., 2010. Effect of guaifenesin on mucin production, rheology, and mucociliary transport in differentiated human airway epithelial cells. *Experimental Lung Research*, 37(10), pp. 606-14.

Shah, R. and McGrath, K., 2012. Nonallergic rhinitis. *Allergy and Asthma Proceedings*, 33(Suppl 1), pp. S19-21.

Sheikh, A., Hurwitz, B., Nurmatov, U. and van Schayck, C.P., 2010. House dust mite avoidance measures for perennial allergic rhinitis (review). *The Cochrane Database of Systematic Reviews*, Issue 7. Art. No.: CD001563. DOI: 10.1002/14651858.CD001563.pub3.

Shoseyov, D., Bibi, H., Shoseyov, N., Shazberg, G. and Hurvitz, H., 1998. Treatment with hypertonic saline versus normal saline nasal wash of pediatric chronic sinusitis. *Journal of Allergy and Clinical Immunology*, 101(5), pp. 602-5.

Simon, W.A., Sturm, E., Hartmann, H.J. and Weser, U., 2006. Hydroxyl radical scavenging reactivity of proton pump inhibitors. *Biochemical Pharmacology*, 71, pp. 1337-41.

Sisson, J.H., Yonkers, A.J. and Waldman, R.H., 1995. Effects of guaifenesin on nasal mucociliary clearance and ciliary beat frequency in healthy volunteers. *Chest*, 107(3), pp. 747-51.

Skoner, D., 2001. Allergic rhinitis: definition, epidemiology, pathophysiology, detection, and diagnosis. *Journal of Allergy and Clinical Immunology*, 108, pp. S2-8.

Smith, J.J., Travis, S.M., Greenberg, E.P. and Welsh, M.J., 1996. Cystic fibrosis airway epithelia fail to kill bacteria because of abnormal airway surface fluid. *Cell*, 85, pp. 229-36.

Sowerby, L.J. and Wright, E.D., 2012. Tap water or "sterile" water for sinus irrigations: what are our patients using? *International Forum of Allergy & Rhinology*, 2(4), pp. 300-302.

Stammberger, H., 1991. Secretion transportation. In: *Functional endoscopic sinus surgery*, Chap. 2. Philadelphia, PA: B.C. Decker. pp. 17-47.

Stanley, P.J., Wilson, R., Greenstone, M.A., MacWilliam, L. and Cole, P.J., 1986. Effect of cigarette smoking on nasal mucociliary clearance and ciliary beat frequency. *Thorax*, 41(7), pp. 519-23.

Sturgess, J.M., Chao, J., Wong, J., Aspin, N. and Turner, J.A., 1979. Cilia with defective radial spokes: a cause of human respiratory disease. *New England Journal of Medicine*, 300(2), pp. 53-6.

Sun, F., Tai, S., Lim, T., Baumann, U. and King, M., 2002. Additive effect of dornase alfa and Nacystelyn on transportability and viscoelasticity of cystic fibrosis sputum. *Canadian Respiratory Journal*, 9(6), pp. 401-6.

Suzuki, M., Mori, M., Miura, S., et al., 1996. Omeprazole attenuates oxygen-derived free radical production from human neutrophils. *Free Radical Biology and Medicine*, 21, pp. 727-31.

Suzuki, M., Nakamura, M., Mori, M., Miura, S., Tsuchiya, M. and Ishil, H., 1995. Lansoprazole inhibits oxygen-derived free radical production from neutrophils activated by Helicobacter pylori. *Journal of Clinical Gastroenterology*, 20(Suppl 2), pp. S93-6.

Suzumura, E. and Takeuchi, K., 1992. Antigen reduces nasal transport epithelial electric potential differences and alters ion transport in allergic rhinitis in vivo. *Acta Otolaryngologica* (Stockh), 112(3), pp. 552-8.

Takeuchi, K., Suzumura, E., Hirata, K., Majima, Y. and Sakakura, Y., 1991. Role of transepithelial ion transport as a determinant of mucus viscoelasticity in chronic/inflammation of the maxillary sinus. *Acta Otolarygology* (Stockh), 111(6), pp. 1133-8.

Takeyama, K., Jung, B., Shim, J.J., Burgel, P.R., Dao-Pick, T., Ueki, I.F., Protin, U., Kroschel, P. and Nadel, J.A., 2001. Activation of epidermal growth factor receptors is responsible for mucin synthesis induced by cigarette smoke. *American Journal of Physiology—Lung Cellular and Molecular Physiology*, 280(1), pp. L165-72.

Talbot, A.R., Herr, T.M. and Parsons, D.S., 1997. Mucociliary clearance and buffered hypertonic saline solution. *Laryngoscope*, 107(4), pp. 500-503.

Tatar, M., Plevkova, J., Brozmanova, M., Pecova, R. and Kollarik, M., 2009. Mechanisms of the cough associated with rhinosinusitis. Pulmonary *Pharmacology and Therapeutics*, 22(2), pp. 121-6.

Tegner, H., Ohlsson, K., Toremalm, N.G., et al., 1979. Effect of human leucocyte enzymes on tracheal mucosa and its mucociliary activity. *Rhinology*, 17, pp. 199-206.

Therapeutic Guidelines November 2012—Gastrointestinal. www.etg.hcn.com.au.

Timperley, D., Schlosser, R.J. and Harvey, R.J., 2010. Chronic rhinosinusitis: an education and treatment model. *Otolaryngology—Head and Neck Surgery*, 143(5(Suppl 3)), pp. S3–8.

Todisco, T., Polidori, R., Rossi, F., Iannacci, L., Bruni, B., Fedeli, L. and Palumbo, R., 1985. Effect of N-acetylcysteine in subjects with slow pulmonary mucociliary clearance. *European Journal of Respiratory Diseases (Supplementary)*, 139, pp. 136-41.

Tomooka, L.T., Murphy, C. and Davidson, T.M., 2000. Clinical study and literature review of nasal irrigation. *Laryngoscope*, 110(7), pp. 1189-93.

Tos, M. and Mogensen, C., 1977. Nasal glands in nasal allergy. *Acta Otolaryngologica*, 83(5-6), pp. 498-504.

Ulusoy, B., Arbag, H., Sari, O. and Yondemli, F., 2007. Evaluation of the effects of nasal septal deviation and its surgery on nasal mucociliary clearance in both nasal cavities. *American Journal of Rhinology*, 21(2), pp. 180-83.

Ural, A., Kocak Oktemer, T.K., Kizil, Y., Ileri, F. and Uslu, S., 2009. Impact of isotonic and hypertonic saline solutions on mucociliary activity in various nasal pathologies: clinical study. *Journal of Laryngology and Otology*, 123(5), pp. 517-21.

Vaezi, M.F., Hagaman, D.D., Slaughter, J.C., et al., 2010. Proton pump inhibitor therapy improves symptoms in postnasal drainage. *Gastroenterology*, 139(6), pp. 1887-93.

Van Zele, T., Gevaert, P., Holtappels, G., Buele, A., Wormald, P.J., Mayr, S., Hens, G., Hellings, P., Ebbens, F.A., Fokkens, W., Van Cauwenberge, P. and Bachert, C., 2010. Oral steroids and doxycycline: two different approaches to treat nasal polyps. *Journal of Allergy and Clinical Immunology*, 125(5), pp. 1069-1076e4.

Vela, M.F., Camacho-Lobato, L., Srinivasan, R., et al., 2001. Simultaneous intraesophageal impedance and pH measurement of acid and nonacid gastroesophageal reflux: effect of omeprazole. *Gastroenterology*, 120, pp. 1599-606.

Vesper, B.J., Jawdi, A., Altman, K.W., Haines G.K. 3rd, Tao, L. and Radosevich, J.A., 2009. The effect of proton pump inhibitors on the human microbiota. *Current Drug Metabolism*, 10, pp. 84-9.

Vincent, D.A., Garrett, J.D., Radionoff, S.L., et al., 2000. The proximal probe in esophageal pH monitoring: development of a normative database. *Journal of Voice*, 14, pp. 247-54.

Wabnitz, D.A., Nair, S. and Wormald, P.J., 2005. Correlation between preoperative symptom scores, quality-of-life questionnaires, and staging with computed tomography in patients with chronic rhinosinusitis. *American Journal of Rhinology*, 19(1), pp. 91-6.

Waguespack, R., 1995. Mucociliary clearance patterns following endoscopic sinus surgery. *Laryngoscope*, 105(7 Pt 2 Suppl 71), pp. 1-40.

Wandall, J.H., 1992. Effects of omeprazole on neutrophil chemotaxis, super oxide production, degranulation, and translocation of cytochrome b-245. *Gut*, 33, pp. 617-21.

Washington, N., Steele, R.J., Jackson, S.J., et al., 2000. Determination of baseline human nasal pH and the effect of intranasally administered buffers. *International Journal of Pharmaceutics*, 198, pp. 139-46.

Weissman, J.D., Fernandez, F. and Hwang, P.H., 2011. Xylitol nasal irrigation in the management of chronic rhinosinusitis: a pilot study. *Laryngoscope*, 121(11), pp. 2468-72.

Welch, K.C., Thaler, E.R., Doghramji, L.L., Palmer, J.N. and Chiu, A.G., 2010. The effects of serum and urinary cortisol levels of topical intranasal irrigations with budesonide added to saline in patients with recurrent polyposis after endoscopic sinus surgery. *American Journal of Rhinology & Allergy*, 24, pp. 26-8.

Welsh, P.W., Yunginger, J.W., Kern, E.B. and Gleich, G.J., 1977. Preseasonal IgE ragweed antibody level as a predictor of response to therapy of ragweed hay fever with intranasal cromolyn sodium solution. *Journal of Allergy and Clinical Immunology*, 60(2), pp. 104-9.

Wise, S.K., Wise, J.C. and DelGaudio, J.M., 2006. Association of nasopharyngeal and laryngopharyngeal reflux with postnasal drip symptomatology in patients with and without rhinosinusitis. *American Journal of Rhinology*, 20(3), pp. 283-9.

Wong, I.W., Rees, G., Greiff, L., Myers, J.C., Jamieson, G.G. and Wormald, P.J., 2010. Gastroesophageal reflux disease and chronic sinusitis: In search of an esophageal-nasal reflex. *American Journal of Rhinology & Allergy*, 24(4), pp. 255-9.

Woodbury, K. and Ferguson, B.J., 2011. Recalcitrant chronic rhinosinusitis: investigation and management. *Current Opinion in Otolaryngology & Head and Neck Surgery*, 19(1), pp. 1-5.

Yanagisawa, E. and Weaver, E.M., 1996. Endoscopic view of the recirculation phenomenon of sphenoid sinus drainage. *Ear, Nose, and Throat Journal*, 75, pp. 68-70.

Yanagisawa, E. and Yanagisawa, K., 1997. Endoscopic view of recirculation phenomenon of the maxillary sinus. *Ear, Nose, and Throat Journal*, 76(4), pp. 196-8.

Ylitalo, R., Linstead, P.A. and Ramel, S., 2011. Symptoms, laryngeal findings, and 24-hour pH monitoring in patients with suspected gastroesopho-pharyngeal reflux. *Laryngoscope*, 111(10), pp. 1735-41.

Ylitalo, R. and Ramel, S., 2002. Esophageal reflux in patients with contact granuloma: a prospective controlled study. *Annals of Otology, Rhinology & Laryngology*, 111(5 Pt 1), pp. 441-6.

Zacharek, M.A. and Krouse, J.H., 2003. The role of allergy in chronic rhinosinusitis. *Current Opinion in Otolaryngology and Head and Neck Surgery*, 11(3), pp. 196-200.

Zagolski, O., 2010. Factors affecting outcome of inferior turbinate mucotomy in treatment of postnasal drip syndrome. *American Journal of Rhinology & Allergy*, 24(6), pp. 459-63.

Zedtwitz-Liebenstein, K., Wenisch, C., Patruta, S., Parschalk, B., Daxbock, F. and Graninger, W., 2002. Omeprazole treatment diminishes intra- and extracellular neutrophil reactive oxygen production and bactericidal activity. *Critical Care Medicine*, 30, pp. 1118-22.

Zhang, L., Mendoza-Sassi, R.A., Cesar, J.A. and Chadha, N.K., 2008. Intranasal corticosteroids for nasal airway obstruction in children with moderate to severe adenoidal hypertrophy. *The Cochrane Database of Systematic Reviews*, 3, CD006286.

Zheng, Y., Zhao, Y., Lv, D., Liu, Y., Qiao, X., An, P. and Wang, D., 2010. Correlation between computed tomography staging and quality of life instruments in patients with chronic rhinosinusitis. *American Journal of Rhinology & Allergy*, 24(1), pp. e41-5.

Ziment, I., 1986. Acetylcysteine: a drug with an interesting past and a fascinating future. *Respiration*, 50(Suppl 1), pp. 26-30.

6 Facial Pain

Chin Chean Yong, Tim J Woolford

Chapter Overview

Pearls and Pitfalls

Pearls

- A thorough history is essential to obtain the correct diagnosis.
- Employ a systematic approach to provide clarity in history taking.
- Nasendoscopy is mandatory in all patients presenting with facial pain to exclude sinusitis.
- Sinusitis is a rare cause of chronic facial pain.
- Sinogenic pain is typified by episodes of pain brought on by an upper respiratory tract infection, associated with nasal symptoms and responds to a course of antibiotics.
- Midfacial segment pain is common and frequently misdiagnosed as sinusitis.
- Patients with trigeminal neuralgia require magnetic resonance imaging to exclude causative pathology.
- Atypical facial pain is diagnosed by exclusion. Referral to a pain clinic for comprehensive management is often beneficial.

Pitfalls

- When diagnosing sinusitis, do not fall into the trap of relying solely on the combination of nasal symptoms and facial pain or computed tomographic findings showing thickened sinonasal mucosa.
- Migraine can also be accompanied by nasal symptoms, causing misdiagnosis of sinusitis.

6.1 INTRODUCTION

Patients with facial pain are frequently referred to otorhinolaryngologists, and most have a provisional diagnosis of sinusitis. The fact is that only a minority of these patients actually have sinogenic pain. It is therefore the duty of the specialist to make an accurate diagnosis, offer appropriate treatment, and avoid unnecessary surgery.

Chronic facial pain is a complex symptom with numerous possible etiologies. It is helpful to employ a systematic approach when trying to obtain a diagnosis of facial pain and this chapter will describe a practical approach related to patient symptoms and examination findings. A brief guide to the outpatient management of these various conditions is outlined, although a detailed description is of course beyond the scope of this chapter.

6.2 HISTORY

A thorough history is essential to make the right diagnosis. Sometimes, it may require more than one consultation to achieve this and on occasion, asking patients to

Flowchart 6.1: Diagnosis of Facial Pain (*see* individual pages for management).

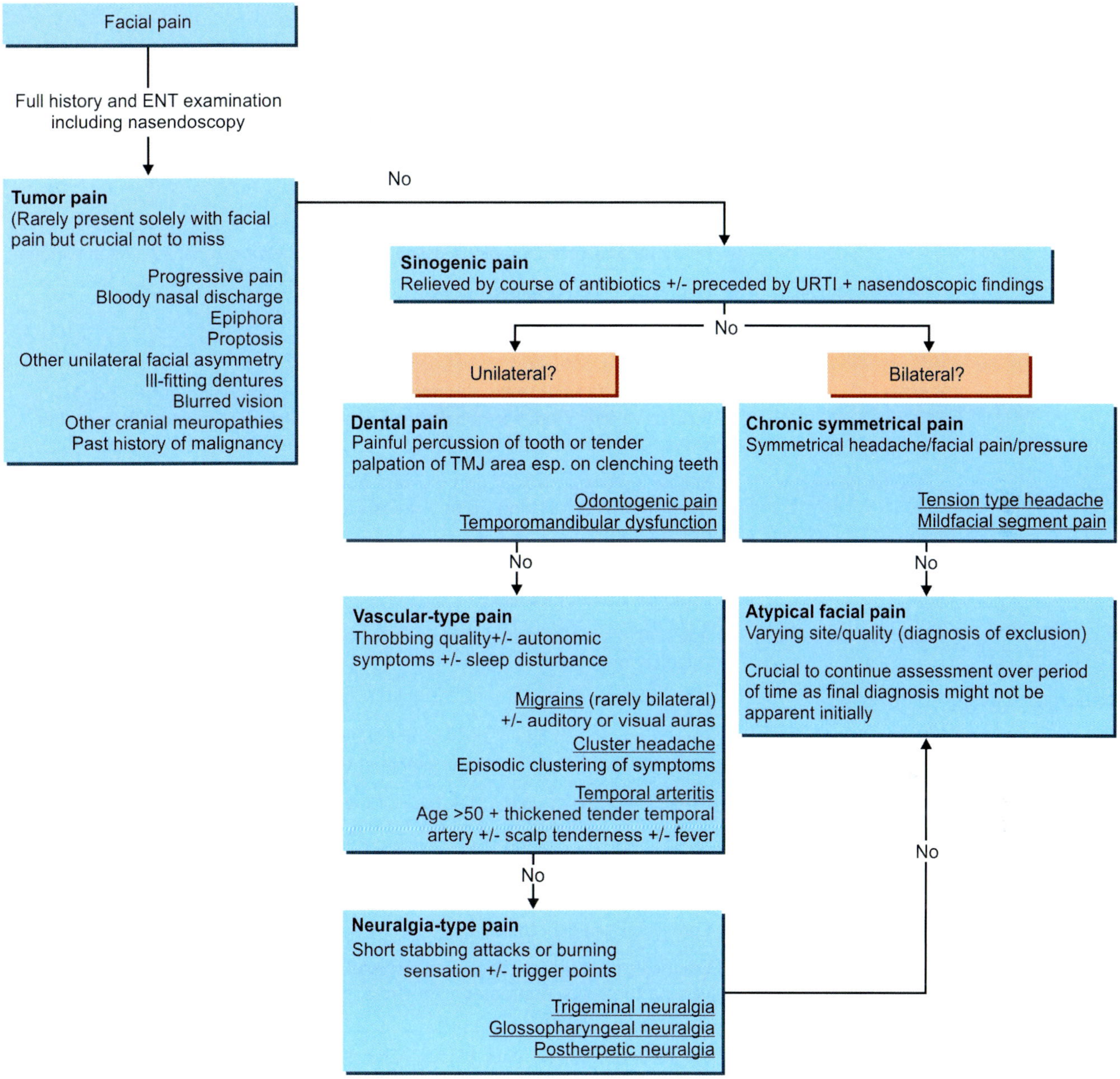

Facial pain

Full history and ENT examination including nasendoscopy

Tumor pain
(Rarely present solely with facial pain but crucial not to miss

Progressive pain
Bloody nasal discharge
Epiphora
Proptosis
Other unilateral facial asymmetry
Ill-fitting dentures
Blurred vision
Other cranial meuropathies
Past history of malignancy

No

Sinogenic pain
Relieved by course of antibiotics +/- preceded by URTI + nasendoscopic findings

No

Unilateral?

Dental pain
Painful percussion of tooth or tender palpation of TMJ area esp. on clenching teeth

Odontogenic pain
Temporomandibular dysfunction

No

Vascular-type pain
Throbbing quality+/- autonomic symptoms +/- sleep disturbance

Migrains (rarely bilateral)
+/- auditory or visual auras
Cluster headache
Episodic clustering of symptoms
Temporal arteritis
Age >50 + thickened tender temporal artery +/- scalp tenderness +/- fever

No

Neuralgia-type pain
Short stabbing attacks or burning sensation +/- trigger points

Trigeminal neuralgia
Glossopharyngeal neuralgia
Postherpetic neuralgia

Bilateral?

Chronic symmetrical pain
Symmetrical headache/facial pain/pressure

Tension type headache
Mildfacial segment pain

No

Atypical facial pain
Varying site/quality (diagnosis of exclusion)

Crucial to continue assessment over period of time as final diagnosis might not be apparent initially

No

keep a diary of their symptoms is helpful. It is beneficial to have a "diagnostic map" when taking the history and to ask a number of key questions. The classification of facial pain and specific findings for each condition are summarized in Table 6.1. Furthermore, the detailed description of each condition can be found under its own subheading.

Useful questions are: Where do you feel the pain and where does it spread to? This can, particularly, help identify temporomandibular joint (TMJ) disorders, dental pain, temporal arteritis, and referred pain from the cervical spine.

Is It Only on One Side or Both?

Migraines and TMJ dysfunction are often unilateral while midfacial segment pain is usually bilateral. Sinogenic pain can either be unilateral or bilateral. Pain related to malignancy is usually, although not always, unilateral.

Table 6.1: Classification of facial pain with summary of key clinical findings.

Condition findings		*Classical history/examination*
Sinogenic pain		Episodic pain with nasal congestion and infected rhinorrhea. Triggered by URTIs and responds to antibiotics. Mucopus on nasendoscopy
Dental pain	"Dull ache localized to a dental cause"	
	Painful teeth	Localized to culprit tooth. Tender percussion
	TMJ disorder	Unilateral pain localized to a tender TMJ. Can radiate to middle ear, periauricular, temporal and cervical regions. Made worse by chewing or lateral jaw movement
	Myofascial pain	Pain akin to TMJ disorder but less localized
Vascular pain	Unilateral "throbbing" or "pulsing" pain	
	Migraine	Lasts up to 72 hours with autonomic dysfunction. Preceding auras. Triggers include various food, hormonal changes, sleep disturbance and withdrawal of stress. Pain can be bilateral
	Cluster headache	Middle-aged man woken up by severe frontal and/or temporal pain. Clustering of episodes, each lasting up to 2 hours accompanied by ipsilateral autonomic dysfunction
	Paroxysmal hemicrania	Akin to cluster headaches except commoner in women. Differentiated by good response to indomethacin
	Temporal arteritis	Age >50 years old. Tender thickened temporal artery. Scalp tenderness and jaw claudication. Fever, malaise
Neuralgia "stabbing" "burning" pain		
	Trigeminal neuralgia	Paroxysms of pain along affected divisions of trigeminal nerve territories. Associated with specific trigger points in the face.
	Glossopharyngeal neuralgia	Rare. Paroxysms of pain at the back of the throat, tongue base, tonsils and middle ear. Triggered by chewing, talking, swallowing, or yawning
	Postherpetic neuralgia	Persistent/recurrent pain at site of shingles. Hyperesthesia
Midfacial segment pain		Similar profile to tension-type headaches but affects midface/periorbital areas. Commonest in ENT clinics
Atypical facial pain		Diagnosis of exclusion. Vague, widespread pain that is constant or daily, with varying locations. Associated with stress, depression and other significant psychological factors
Tumors		Constant progressive pain. Bloody nasal discharge, epiphora, and proptosis. History of past malignancy

(TMJ: Temporomandibular joint; URTI: Upper respiratory tract infection; ENT: Ear–nose–throat).

Please Describe to Me What the Pain Feels Like

A "burning" quality or sudden pangs of pain that "shoots" or "stabs" hint toward a neuralgic type pain. Vascular-type pain is often described as having a "throbbing" or "pulsatile" quality. A "tension" or "pressure" pain points toward midfacial segment pain.

How Often Does It Occur?

Midfacial segment pain or atypical facial pain is likely to be described as a continuous or daily feature. Sinogenic pain is typically episodic corresponding to bouts of upper respiratory tract infection (URTI).

As the name suggests, cluster headaches are recurrent in high frequency during an active cluster period that can last for weeks. Each acute episode lasts up to 2 hours, and each cluster period is separated by weeks to months of remission. Migraines can have a cyclical presentation when associated with the premenstrual period. If pain is constant and progressive, be wary of possible malignancy.

Have You Noticed Anything Else that Accompanies the Pain?

Sinogenic pain is invariably associated with rhinological symptoms such as nasal obstruction and infected catarrh. However, migraines and cluster headaches can also present with congestion and rhinorrhea due to autonomic dysfunction. Other autonomic dysfunctions include nausea and lacrimation. Preceding auras, photophobia, and phonophobia are typical of migraines.

Have You Noticed Anything that Might Trigger the Pain or Make It Worse?

Although described in numerous textbooks, facial pain made worse by bending forward is actually a rather nonspecific sign and not indicative of sinogenic pain. Migraines can have specific triggers such as certain foods withdrawal of stress or sleep disruption. Alcohol is known to trigger episodes in cluster headaches. For TMJ disorders, chewing can trigger or worsen the pain, while clicking is a nonspecific finding.

What Makes the Pain Better? Or What Do You Do to Lessen the Pain?

An episode of sinogenic pain usually responds to antibiotics. With midfacial segment pain or atypical facial pain, patients might describe how analgesics were helpful initially, but become less effective with time. Those who find a dark and quiet environment particularly helpful during an episode of pain are frequently suffering from migraines.

6.3 CLINICAL EXAMINATION

Inspection should begin with the face, noticing any swelling, skin changes, or asymmetry. Palpation can yield specific signs. Look for tenderness associated with the TMJ and associated muscles. A specific tender point linked to TMJ disorders is at the insertion of the lateral pterygoid muscle at the superoposterior end of the buccal sulcus. Lateral jaw movement will also trigger pain. Examine the eye for protosis, chemosis, or epiphora.

In temporal arteritis, expect scalp (temporal areas) tenderness and a visibly thickened and tender temporal artery. Do not forget to feel for neck lumps, tenderness, or crepitus during neck movements. Inspect the oral cavity for any dental caries or gum swelling. Other findings might include malocclusion with a cross-bite or ill-fitting dentures, which can give rise to TMJ pain.

Nasendoscopy is mandatory if a diagnosis of sinusitis is being considered. Inspection of the middle meatus and nasal cavity can reveal mucopus or inflammatory changes on the afflicted side. Be aware of any suspicious masses or bloody discharge indicating possible malignancy.

6.4 SPECIFIC CONDITIONS CAUSING FACIAL PAIN

Sinogenic Pain

Acute sinusitis can cause severe facial pain, and the diagnosis is usually straightforward. Chronic sinusitis can also cause facial pain especially during acute exacerbations; however, sinogenic pain tends to be overdiagnosed by patients and clinicians alike. Daily or constant pain over a number of weeks is rarely due to sinusitis. Sinogenic pain is commonly described as a unilateral dull ache near the medial canthus of the eye and surrounding areas. The episode is associated with nasal symptoms and responds well to antibiotics. Nasendoscopic findings of mucopus during an acute episode add further diagnostic confidence. Note, however, that these nasendoscopic findings should never be used solely to guide diagnosis. Rhinosinusitis is common and only a small proportion of these patients have facial pain. Very few patients with nasal polyps have facial pain. The absence of nasendoscopic findings of infection during an active or recent episode of facial pain makes sinogenic pain most unlikely (Jones and Cooney, 2003).

Imaging should generally be considered as part of preoperative planning, or to exclude more serious pathology. Plain sinus X-rays have been shown to be a poor diagnostic tool for chronic sinusitis due to poor sensitivity and specificity and are largely redundant. Computed tomographic (CT) scans are excellent for viewing anatomy and inflammatory changes. However, correlation to clinical symptoms with a high sensitivity is reduced by a low specificity to clinically significant disease. As many as 30% of asymptomatic patients will demonstrate mucosal thickening in one or more sinuses in their CT scans (Jones, et al., 1997). Therefore, these findings have to be treated with caution as they do not confirm a sinogenic origin of pain.

Medical treatment of sinogenic pain requires intranasal corticosteroids, nasal saline douches, and appropriate antibiotics, with a long course of a macrolide, such as clarithromycin, often proving effective. Surgical treatment should only be reserved for those with sinogenic pain who have failed medical treatment.

Dental Pain

Patients with a dental origin for facial pain are rarely seen in ear-nose-throat (ENT) clinics. With a painful tooth, most patients will be able to identify the source themselves. Those seen at otorhinolaryngology clinics often have poorly localized pain. This pain radiates to the maxilla or mandible on the same side, confusing the patient. Painful percussion of the offending tooth will lead to the diagnosis.

Temporomandibular Joint Dysfunction

This is a spectrum of disorders relating to the TMJ. The facial pain described is usually unilateral, localized; TMJ is tender to palpation; and pain can radiate to the periauricular, temporoparietal, and/or cervical regions. Shared innervation gives rise to referred otalgia. This condition is generally managed by a maxillofacial surgeon including the use of occlusal devices or surgical correction of causative factors.

Myofascial Pain

This clinical entity presents similarly to TMJ dysfunction but with a less defined area of dull aching pain in the neck, mandible and/or ear. Poor dental occlusion or neck posture can contribute to tender points found in the sternomastoid and trapezoid muscles. It is found to be strongly linked to stress and five times more common in postmenopausal women.

Vascular Pain

Migraine

Migraines are common, and reported to have a prevalence of 18% in women and 6% in men. Only 25% of patients have "classical" migraine with preceding auras, which include visual disturbances, hallucinatory smells or taste, and tinnitus. A unilateral headache of "pulsating" or "throbbing" quality then ensues. Photophobia is highly suggestive of migraine. Other autonomic symptoms, such as nausea and phonophobia, can accompany the episode. Common migraines can be identified by having no associated visual aura or other neurological symptoms. An episode of migraine can last up to 72 hours and can be related to various dietary factors, sleep disturbance, withdrawal of stress, or hormonal changes during menstruation.

Basic advice would be to identify and avoid trigger factors. During an acute episode, aspirin and antiemetics are used for symptomatic relief. Sumatriptan or rizatriptan, which are serotonin agonists are also effective (Derry, et al., 2012). Consider starting prophylaxis if the patient experiences >3 episodes of migraine per month. First-line prophylaxis includes pizotifen or propranolol. If migraine is refractory to treatment, a referral to a neurologist is appropriate.

Cluster Headache

Cluster headaches are estimated to have a prevalence of 1 in 1,000. Although termed as a headache, the pain is actually a unilateral facial pain that is frontal and/or temporal, and can radiate over the maxilla or teeth. Patients experience a clustering of episodes, each lasting 15 minutes to 2 hours. The pain is characterized by particular severity, which can be totally disabling to the patient. Ipsilateral autonomic symptoms are frequently present during an episode (lacrimation, sweating, nasal congestion, and rhinorrhea).

These cluster periods last for weeks and in between there are often months of remission. Alcohol may be linked to these episodes. Drug treatment is similar to migraines, and triptans are effective for an acute episode. In addition, prophylaxis during the active cluster period should be considered, with verapamil. Refractory cases warrant a referral to the neurologist.

Paroxysmal Hemicrania

Paroxysmal hemicranias are rare and have the very similar pain profile as that of cluster headaches. The location and quality of pain is analogous; it occurs in 15–30-minute episodes several times a day, and it is also accompanied by ipsilateral autonomic symptoms. However, paroxysmal hemicranias are classified separately as they are instead found to occur predominantly in women and have an absolute response to treatment with indomethacin.

Sluder's Neuralgia

Sluder's neuralgia has been historically used to describe a syndrome encompassing a range of neuralgic, motor, sensory, and gustatory symptoms thought to be caused by inflammation of the sphenopalatine ganglion. This theory was later extended to include nasal mucosal contact points as a potentiating factor. Treatment modalities were centered around ablation of the ganglion or surgical correction of these contact points.

In recent years, this clinical syndrome, particularly the significance of contact points, has largely been discredited and is no longer recognized. Sluder's neuralgia bears underlying similarities to vascular-type pain, and in particular, cluster headaches, and patients are now classified as such.

Arteritis (Giant Cell Arteritis)

Recognizing temporal arteritis is important as delay of treatment could lead to involvement of the opthalmic artery with permanent visual loss. This condition occurs in adults who are over 50 years old and is more common in women. Nearly two thirds present with headache localized to the temporal region. Useful clues include a thickened and tender temporal artery, scalp tenderness, and jaw claudication. Constitutional symptoms such as fever and malaise can precede the pain. Blood tests would reveal a significantly elevated erythrocyte sedimentation rate. To confirm the diagnosis, an arterial biopsy is required. However, it would be prudent to commence high-dose steroids if clinical suspicion is high.

Neuralgias

Trigeminal Neuralgia

Trigeminal neuralgia is identified by paroxysmal attacks of neuralgia-type pain induced by a trigger point. Pain follows the distribution of the trigeminal nerve branches: one-third of cases involve both maxillary and mandibular divisions; one fifth of cases involve the maxillary division alone and in 3% the ophthalmic division. Specific trigger points can include the lips, nasolabial folds, and gingiva. Patients also report triggering of pain with hot or cold drinks, chewing, or talking. A brief facial spasm or flush may also occur; however, there is no sensory disturbance in primary trigeminal neuralgia.

Primary trigeminal neuralgia is thought to be caused by compression of the nerve roots by vascular structures. Secondary causes of trigeminal neuralgia include neuromas, aneurysmal, or tumor-related compression. Although rare, trigeminal neuralgia may be the presenting feature for multiple sclerosis in younger patients.

Magnetic resonance imaging scanning is mandatory to exclude multiple sclerosis and possible tumors such as posterior fossa meningiomas. Carbamazepine remains the first-line treatment (van Kleef, et al., 2009), and another commonly prescribed drug is gabapentin. Refractory cases require referral to specialist centers for consideration of other drugs' treatment or, in rare cases, surgery.

Glossopharyngeal Neuralgia

Glossopharyngeal neuralgia is very rare and causes short severe stabbing pains in the tongue base, tonsillar fossae, posterior pharynx, and middle ear. Triggers include actions such as coughing, sneezing, swallowing, or yawning. These painful episodes can recur for weeks and then return after a period of remission. Management is along the same lines as trigeminal neuralgia. This includes imaging to exclude secondary causes and exclude any malignancy.

Postherpetic Neuralgia

A history of shingles with persisting or recurrent neuralgic-type pain at the site usually makes this diagnosis clear. Patients can also describe hyperesthesia and itching at the site. Up to 50% of patients aged 50 and above develop postherpetic neuralgia and the condition may be particularly distressing. During acute shingles, administration of antiviral medication within 72 hours of rash onset helps with ongoing pain and reduces the risk of developing persisting neuralgia. For chronic neuralgia, if basic analgesia has been tried, regimes such as low-dose amitriptyline, carbamazepine, pregabalin, or gabapentin can be helpful. Specialist pain clinics provide further guidance to treatment.

6.5 MIDFACIAL SEGMENT PAIN (TENSION-TYPE FACIAL PAIN)

In our experience, midfacial segment pain is the commonest underlying diagnosis in patients with facial pain referred to ENT, although most of these patients believe that they have sinusitis. Midfacial segment pain is a specific syndrome where there is bilateral symmetrical pain involving the midface and periorbital region. The quality of pain described is similar to that of tension-type headache, with a dull or "tension-like" quality and hyperesthesia of the affected areas. There can be further overlap, with many patients having coexisting tension-type headaches.

Psychological factors are seen to have a lesser role in midfacial segment pain compared to atypical facial pain. The pain generally lasts for many hours on a daily basis, but with little disability or consequence to daily activities. It does not interfere with the patient's sleep, and episodes are reduced at times of reduced stress, such as weekends or holidays. Patients reaching the specialist's clinic will also often report how analgesics initially helped them, but have become less effective.

Explanation and reassurance is an important aspect of the treatment. Showing normal nasendoscopic findings to patients can provide much needed reassurance. With appropriate counseling, many patients are happy enough to cope without relying on any medication. Advise on how lifestyle changes can break pain cycles, such as a change to their work routine or taking up regular exercise. Complimentary therapy, such as acupuncture, may be helpful. Drug treatment is similar to tension headaches, and the first-line treatment is with low-dose amitriptyline once daily for 6 weeks, titrate to response and maintain for at least 3 months once responding (Bendtsen and Rigmor, 2009). There is often an overlap with migraine, and other drugs such as propranolol may be helpful.

6.6 ATYPICAL FACIAL PAIN

Atypical facial pain is a diagnosis by exclusion. Caution is required when making this diagnosis even if there is a history of multiple past consultations and investigations. The history and description of the pain are often vague and inconsistent, and the location may be widespread in the face onto other areas of the head and neck. Some patients are convinced that their sinuses are to blame, and describe how they can feel mucous moving in their sinuses.

Other clues might be found in the body language used while describing their pain. Dramatic gestures alongside the association of stressful life events can be apparent. There is commonly a background of other coexisting pain syndromes. Many have had previous "failed" surgery and remain resentful about this. Ongoing depression or other psychological disturbance is strongly associated with perception of the pain. Most patients are pessimistic about any treatment options.

There are some patients who have persistent facial pain after trauma or previous surgery, months after direct effects should have resolved. There may be a history of assault with ongoing psychological stress or particular dissatisfaction with previous surgery. We would categorize such pain as atypical facial pain, and caution is required, especially when considering further surgery.

A thorough history and full head and neck examination including nasendoscopy are required. Management is predictably challenging. It is emphasized that confrontation is counterproductive and acknowledging the patient's pain and remaining empathetic are helpful.

In reality, the role of the surgeon is to exclude significant pathology, and explain that further surgery is not indicated and will actually be counterproductive. Most patients with atypical facial pain are best managed in a specialist pain clinic where a comprehensive approach, including psychological support, can be offered.

6.7 PAIN DUE TO MALIGNANCY

Malignancy may present with facial pain, although rarely as the only symptom. Suspicions should be raised if the patient complains of a constant, progressive pain, associated with other clinical findings such as a past history of malignancy, bloody nasal discharge, epiphora, proptosis, other structural asymmetries, or nerve palsies. Pain itself is commonly a late-presenting feature of malignancy. Be aware as well that neuromas, which take on a slow clinical course, can cause persisting pain for many years. Choice of imaging modality depends on the suspected cause and specific management is outside the limits of this symptom-based chapter.

REFERENCES

Bendtsen, L. and Rigmor, J., 2009. Tension-type headache. *Neurologic Clinics,* 27(2), pp. 525-35.

Derry, C.J., Derry, S. and Moore, R.A., 2012. Sumatriptan (subcutaneous route of administration) for acute migraine attacks in adults. *Cochrane Database of Systematic Reviews*, 2, pp. CD009665.

Jones, N.S. and Cooney, T.R., 2003. Facial pain and sinonasal surgery. *Rhinology*, 41(4), pp. 193-200.

Jones, N.S., Strobi, A. and Holland, I., 1997. A study of the CT findings in 100 patients with rhinosinusitis and 100 controls. *Clinical Otolaryngology*, 22, pp. 47-51.

van Kleef, M., van Genderen, W.E., Narouze, S., et al. 2009. Trigeminal neuralgia. *Pain Practice*, 9(4), pp. 252-9.

Sneezing 7

Neeraj Sethi, Victoria Ward

Chapter Overview

Pearls and Pitfalls

Pearls

- Allergic rhinitis is the most common cause of sneezing—look for other signs of allergy.
- In allergic rhinitis, look for nasal crease on tip of nose and on columella (allergic salute).
- Skin-prick test forms an important part of the investigations.

Pitfalls

- Absence of the reaction to common skin tests does not rule out allergic rhinitis.
- It is important to remember that non-rhinitic causes for sneezing occur and not to fit rhinitis to every case.

7.1 RHINITIS

Allergic Rhinitis

Epidemiology and Pathogenesis

- Very common with highest prevalence in industrialized countries (Bousquet, Van Cauwenberge and Khaltaev, 2001).
- Affects people of all ages with peak in teens (Bousquet, Van Cauwenberge and Khaltaev, 2001).
- Closely linked to other inflammatory diseases affecting respiratory mucous membranes including asthma, allergic conjunctivitis, and rhinosinusitis (Greiner, et al., 2011).
- Specific inhaled allergens precipitate an immunoglobulin E (IgE)-mediated immune response with immediate and late-phase reactions.

Clinical Features

Features in clinical history: two or more of the following symptoms for >1 hour on most days:

- Watery anterior rhinorrhea
- Sneezing (especially paroxysmal)
- Nasal obstruction
- Nasal pruritus
- +/- Conjunctivitis (Bousquet, Van Cauwenberge and Khaltaev, 2001; Bousquet, et al., 2008).

Classified as intermittent or persistent, mild or moderate-to-severe (Chapter 5)

Risk factors include:

- Past history of other atopic disorder
- Family history of atopy
- Occupational factors (e.g. woodworking, farming)
- Ethnic origin other than white European

- High socioeconomic status
- Environmental pollution.

Typical findings on examination are as follows:

- Nasal crease on tip of nose (allergic salute) and along columella (Fig. 7.1).
- Anterior rhinoscopy may reveal classically pale, edematous, wet mucosa, but it may be normal or erythematous (Fig. 7.2). Inferior turbinates may be hypertrophied and have a bluish hue.

Nonallergic Rhinitis

Classification of nonallergic rhinitis:

- Infectious
- Occupational
- Drug-induced
- Hormonal
- Nonallergic rhinitis with eosinophilia syndrome (NARES)
- Idiopathic.

Epidemiology and Pathogenesis

Infectious: Affecting millions of people annually, the most common cause being viral (common cold). The most common viral cause are human rhinoviruses (van Kempen, Bachert and Van Cauwenberge, 1999). The most common bacterial causes are *Streptococcus pneumoniae, Haemophilus influenzae,* and *Moraxella catarrhalis* (Scadding, 2001).

Occupational: It occurs secondary to exposure in the workplace of high-molecular-weight, low-molecular-weight, and irritant substances through immunologic and nonimmunologic pathways. These include cigarette smoke, cold air, air fresheners, formaldehyde, among others (Gautrin, Desrosiers and Castano, 2006; Sublett and Bernstein, 2011). It is diagnosed with an occupational history and the presence of IgE-mediated inflammation in response to the causative agent.

Drug-induced: In addition to the classical aspirin and nonsteroidal anti-inflammatory drug sensitivity, drug-induced rhinitis associated with sneezing can be caused by beta-blockers and other antihypertensives (e.g. guanethidine, hydralazine, and prazosin) (Varghese, Glaum and Lockey, 2010). Rhinitis medicamentosa is a drug-induced rhinitis in response to excessive use of topical decongestants (Varghese, Glaum and Lockey, 2010).

Hormonal: It may occur in the presence of increased levels of estrogen (e.g. pregnancy, menstrual cycle, puberty) (Ellegard, Karlsson and Ellegard, 2007).

NARES: A nasal hypersensitivity in which eosinophils exceed 20% of the total leukocyte count in the absence of IgE-dependent allergy. It is thought to be due to the infiltration of eosinophils into the nasal mucosa due to increased levels of substance P (Mullarkey, Hill and Webb, 1980).

Idiopathic: This is characterized by short episodes of nasal blockage, rhinorrhea, and sneezing of unknown etiology generally associated with triggers such as changes in temperature and inhaled irritants (Saleh and Durham, 2007).

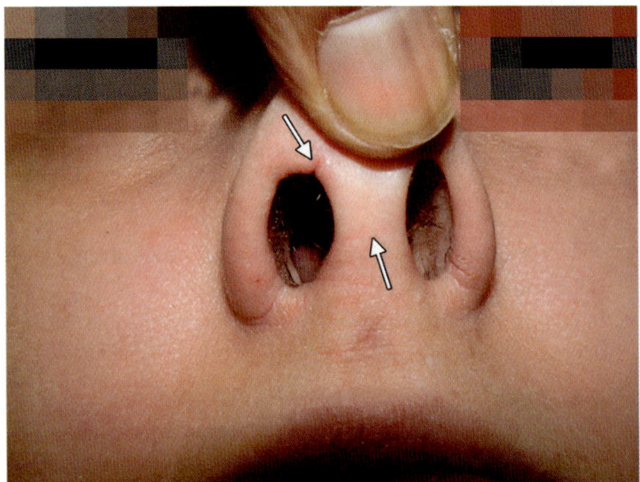

Fig. 7.1: Alar trauma (upper arrow) and columella creases (lower arrow) typical of significant nose rubbing secondary to allergic rhinitis.

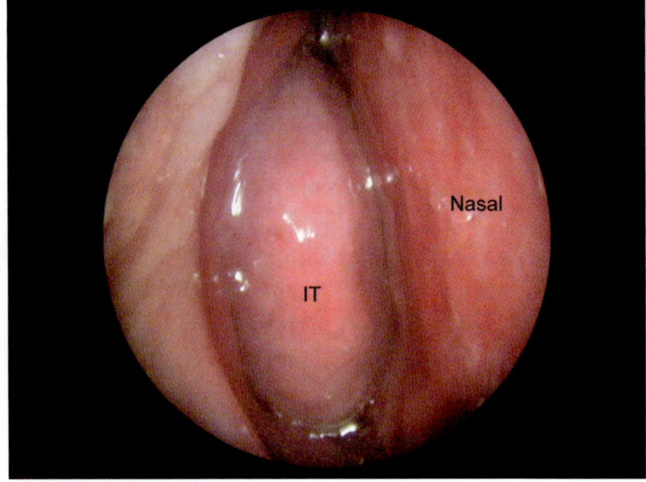

Fig. 7.2: Allergic rhinitis with a pale swollen inferior turbinate (IT) occluding the airway.

Clinical Features

Features in clinical history:

Infectious: Can be accompanied by fevers, fatigue, and malaise. Characterized by nasal blockage/obstruction/congestion, anterior/posterior nasal discharge, facial pain/pressure, sneezing, and hyposmia. Acute viral rhinosinusitis is defined as symptom duration <10 days. Acute nonviral rhinosinusitis is defined as increase of symptoms after 5 days or persistent symptoms after 10 days with <12 weeks' durations (Fokkens, Lund and Mullol, 2012).

Occupational: Watery rhinorrhea, sneezing, nasal congestion, hyposmia chronologically associated with occupation, though symptoms may persist outside the work environment.

Drug-induced: Primarily nasal congestion, watery rhinorrhea, and essential to enquire specifically about any over-the-counter medications being used currently or in the past.

Hormonal: Nasal symptoms are limited to times of increased estrogen; therefore it is imperative to ask about time course as well as relapsing and remitting symptoms. Not associated with asthma or rhinitis prior to pregnancy (Ellegard, Karlsson and Ellegard, 2007).

NARES: Perennial sneezing attacks, watery rhinorrhea, nasal pruritus, nasal congestion, and hyposmia (Saleh and Durham, 2007).

Idiopathic: Episodic watery rhinorrhea, congestion, and paroxysmal sneezing in response to triggers. It is important to ask about change in temperatures, environment, chronology and, if necessary, for the patient to keep a symptom diary to assist with identifying triggers.

Typical findings on examination:

Infectious: Edematous, erythematous nasal mucosa with yellowish (viral) or green (bacterial) discharge. Polyps are often not present, though people with polyps may be predisposed to acute rhinosinusitis.

Occupational: Erythematous, wet mucosa with watery, clear discharge present. However, anterior rhinoscopy may be normal if symptoms are only present at work.

Drug-induced: Erythematous, nasal mucosa with copious secretions, often with hypertrophied inferior turbinates.

Hormonal: Erythematous, edematous mucosa.

NARES: Erythematous, mucosa with hypertrophied inferior turbinates, watery secretions. These patients frequently develop nasal polyps and asthma in later life.

Idiopathic: Erythematous mucosa, though excess secretions may be absent as some patients complain mainly of congestion.

Investigations

Skin prick test: It confirms specific IgE reactivity to airborne allergens within 15 minutes and helps guide treatment. Patients should stop taking any antihistamines 48 hours prior to testing as this can affect the results. These are contraindicated in severe eczema, any history of anaphylaxis, or dermographism (Bousquet, Van Cauwenberge and Khaltaev, 2001).

Serum IgE: Total IgE is not usually helpful as a patient may have a specific allergy with normal overall IgE levels.

Specific IgE levels by radioallergosorbent test (RAST): These can be used when skin pricks tests are contraindicated, unavailable, or produce equivocal results.

Nasal allergen challenge: This is useful if occupational rhinitis is suspected, though difficult to perform as it takes several hours and requires trained staff and resuscitation equipment to be available.

Computed tomography scan: In the absence of clinical evidence of chronic rhinosinusitis and planning surgery, this is of little benefit.

Preferred Treatment

Allergic rhinitis: Allergen avoidance and patient education about environmental control is the first-line treatment. Pharmacotherapy can then be introduced as per the box below (Bousquet, Van Cauwenberge and Khaltaev, 2001; Bousquet, et al., 2008):

Severity	*Treatment options*
Mild, intermittent	Saline douche Oral/intranasal antihistamine (nonsedating) And/or decongestant (<10 days) And/or antileukotriene
Moderate-severe, intermittent Mild, persistent Moderate-severe, persistent	Saline douche Oral/intranasal antihistamine (nonsedating) Intranasal corticosteroids Decongestants (<10 days) Intranasal cromone Specific immunotherapy may be considered if the above is insufficient

Infectious: For acute viral rhinosinusitis, symptomatic relief with decongestants is appropriate. For acute nonviral rhinosinusitis, adding in topical corticosteroids and oral antibiotics if necessary for 7–14 days (Fokkens, Lund and Mullol, 2012). For chronic rhinosinusitis, maximal medical therapy as per the European position paper is preferred with surgical intervention reserved for patients refractory to this (Fokkens, Lund and Mullol, 2012).

Occupational: With an established diagnosis, protective measures in the workplace should be employed (altered duties, masks, gloves, etc). Medical treatment is otherwise similar to allergic rhinitis as above.

Drug-induced: Withdrawal of the responsible medication if possible. If not, then medical treatment as per allergic rhinitis. In the specific case of decongestants, "rebound rhinitis" should be expected on withdrawal and topical corticosteroids introduced.

Hormonal: During pregnancy, some topical corticosteroids may be considered and/or intranasal cromone.

NARES/idiopathic: Medical therapy as per allergic rhinitis may be considered.

Treatment Outcomes

Patient-based: Persistent rhinitis has been shown to have as detrimental an effect on health-related quality of life as asthma and effective treatment has not only been shown to improve quality-of-life measures, but also patient compliance with treatment (Greiner, et al., 2011; Marple, et al., 2007).

Disease-based: Twenty percent of patients are not helped by guideline-directed treatment (Greiner, et al., 2011). There is some degree of trial and error in managing patients, but good education is key to improving outcomes and controlling rhinitic symptoms has been shown to have beneficial effects on comorbid airway disease (e.g. asthma) (Greiner, et al., 2011; Peters, 2007).

Complications of Treatment

Complications of medical therapy for rhinitis are uncommon. It is important to remember topical decongestants can only be used for a maximum of 10 days and repeated users should try and reduce even that. Topical corticosteroids may cause dryness or epistaxis and those taking ethanol-based preparations can complain of discomfort on use. In patients on antiretrovirals, the systemic absorption of fluticasone is increased and adrenal suppression with iatrogenic Cushing's syndrome is a serious risk (Whitlock, et al., 2012).

7.2 PHOTIC SNEEZE REFLEX

Epidemiology and Pathogenesis

Sneezing in response to bright light is called the photic sneeze reflex, also termed the autosomal dominant compelling helio-ophthalmic outburst (ACHOO) syndrome (Collie, et al., 1978).

Reports have suggested it occurs in around one in four of studied populations (Songu and Cingi, 2009).

Theories exist regarding the reflex:

- The optical-trigeminal summation theory suggests intense light stimulation of the optic nerve triggers cross-stimulation of the ophthalmic division of the trigeminal nerve, which generates the nasal stimulation via the maxillary division of the trigeminal nerve.
- Parasympathetic generalization hypothesizes that adjacent parasympathetic branches are stimulated when light of sufficient intensity falls on the retina; it stimulates a nasal tickling sensation.

Clinical Features

Features in clinical history:

- It is characterized by sneezing in response to sudden exposure by a dark-adapted subject to intensive sunlight.
- Traditionally associated with sunlight, but has been reported and demonstrated with artificial light.

Typical findings on examination:

- No physical abnormality is found associated with this.

Investigations

No investigations are clinically useful.

Preferred Treatment

Patient should be educated on avoiding/preparing for potentially dangerous situations, e.g. driving out of a tunnel or piloting an aeroplane (Songu and Cingi, 2009; Benbow, 1991).

Complications of Disease

Numerous case reports describe sneezing as the final precipitant event prior to events such as aortic dissection, orbital emphysema, and retinal hemorrhage (Songu and Cingi, 2009).

7.3 NEUROGENIC SNEEZING

Epidemiology and Pathogenesis

Sneezing can accompany temporal lobe and grand mal epilepsy. It can occur within the aura prior to seizure or as an autonomic manifestation during the seizure.

Paroxysmal sneezing is also known to precede lateral medullary syndrome (Wallenberg's syndrome) and has been blamed as the cause of the vertebral artery dissection/occlusion, though it has been reported in patients with no evidence of vertebral artery pathology (Swenson and Leira, 2007).

Physical stimulation of the trigeminal nerve can trigger sneezing, such as pulling nasal hair, tearing off eyebrows, or orbital injections during local anesthetic procedures (Songu and Cingi, 2009).

7.4 PSYCHOGENIC SNEEZING

Epidemiology and Pathogenesis

Psychogenic (intractable) sneezing is a rare disorder, which occurs mainly in teenage girls and is regarded as a somatic conversion disorder (Gopalan and Browning, 2002).

Clinical Features

Features in clinical history:

- Sneezes occur with an atypical rate or rhythm and are absent when the patient is asleep or alone (Gopalan and Browning, 2002). Previous psychiatric history or somatic symptoms should be asked about as well as any negative life events or stresses. They will have been refractory to any previous treatments (e.g. topical corticosteroids).

Typical findings on examination:

- Physical examination is generally normal.
- Observation of sneezing reveals a short inspiratory phase with minimal expulsion of secretions and the eyes may remain open (Songu and Cingi, 2009). Beware of any primary or secondary gains that occur as a result of the disorder (Gopalan and Browning, 2002). Topical intranasal anesthetic will have no effect on the sneezing (Gopalan and Browning, 2002).

Investigations

Skin prick tests can be useful to exclude allergy (or RAST tests if contraindicated or unavailable).

Preferred Treatment

The mainstay of treatment is counseling and supportive psychotherapy including an explanation of the diagnosis and cognitive behavioral therapy to reduce symptoms (Fochtmann, 1995). Antidepressants or anxiolytics have a role in conjunction with this.

Treatment Outcomes

The condition responds well to the above treatments with often reported complete resolution of symptoms (Songu and Cingi, 2009; Gopalan and Browning, 2002).

Complications of Disease

The condition itself may cause psychosocial complications if untreated. Patients with conversion disorder are at risk of developing other psychiatric problems in later life (Fochtmann, 1995).

7.5 SNATIATION REFLEX

Epidemiology and Pathogenesis

It is a rarely reported condition, wherein a reflex with an autosomal dominant inheritance pattern causes paroxysmal sneezing on a full stomach (Teebi and al-Saleh, 1989). Hall (1990) named this the Sneezing Noncontrollably At a Tune of Indulgence of the Appetite—a Trait Inherited and Ordained to be Named. The mechanism of this reflex is not understood.

Clinical Features

Features in clinical history:

- Paroxysmal sneezing (in the absence of other nasal symptoms) after eating, especially when particularly full is reported (Teebi and al-Saleh, 1989).

Typical findings on examination:

- Examination is normal.

Investigations

Patients may be concerned over food allergy, though nasal symptoms are rare in this situation. Double-blind placebo-controlled food challenge is the gold standard, but needs to be performed by competent staff and is difficult to arrange and perform practically and probably unnecessary (Bruijnzeel-Koomen, et al., 1995).

Preferred Treatment

No treatment is required.

Complications of Disease

None reported.

7.6 SEXUAL IDEATION/ORGASM

The incidence of this sneezing associated with sexual ideation or orgasm is unknown, though has been suggested to be more common than thought (Bhutta and Maxwell, 2008). The mechanism is unknown.

Clinical Features

Features in clinical history:

- Paroxysmal sneezing is described in association with sexual thought or immediately following orgasm (Bhutta and Maxwell, 2008).

Typical findings on examination:

- Examination is normal.

Investigations and Treatment

No investigations are indicated. No treatment is recognized.

Complications of Disease

Patients may find this condition embarrassing.

REFERENCES

Benbow, E.W., 2007. Practical hazards of photic sneezing. *British Journal of Ophthalmology*, 75(7), p. 447.

Bhutta, M.F. and Maxwell, H. Sneezing induced by sexual ideation or orgasm: an under-reported phenomenon. *Journal of the Royal Society of Medicine*, 101(12), pp. 587-91.

Bousquet, J., Khaltaev, N., Cruz A.A., et al., 2008. Allergic Rhinitis and its Impact on Asthma (ARIA) 2008 update (in collaboration with the World Health Organization, GA(2)LEN and AllerGen). *Allergy*, 63(Suppl 86), pp. 8-60.

Bousquet, J., Van Cauwenberge, P. and Khaltaev, N., 2001. Allergic rhinitis and its impact on asthma. *Journal of Allergy and Clinical Immunology*, 108(5 Suppl), pp. S147-334.

Bruijnzeel-Koomen, C., Ortolani, C., Aas, K., Bindslev-Jensen, C., Björkstén, B., Moneret-Vautrin, D. and Wüthrich, B., 1995. Adverse reactions to food. European Academy of Allergology and Clinical Immunology Subcommittee. *Allergy*, 50(8), pp. 623-35.

Collie, W.R., Pagon, R.A., Hall, J.G. and Shokeir, M.H., 1978. ACHOO syndrome (autosomal dominant compelling helio-ophthalmic outburst syndrome). *Birth Defects Original Article Series*, 14(6B), pp. 361-3.

Ellegard, E.K., Karlsson, N.G. and Ellegard, L.H., 2007. Rhinitis in the menstrual cycle, pregnancy, and some endocrine disorders. *Clinical Allergy and Immunology*, 19, pp. 305-21.

Fochtmann, L.J., 1995. Intractable sneezing as a conversion symptom. *Psychosomatics*, 36(2), pp. 103-12.

Fokkens, W.J., Lund, V.J., Mullol, J., et al., 2012. European position paper on rhinosinusitis and nasal polyps 2012. *Rhinology Supplement*, (23), p. 3 (preceding table of contents, 1-298).

Gautrin, D., Desrosiers, M. and Castano, R., 2006. Occupational rhinitis. *Current Opinion in Allergy and Clinical Immunology*, 6(2), pp. 77-84.

Gopalan, P. and Browning, S.T., 2002. Intractable paroxysmal sneezing. *The Journal of Laryngology and Otology*, 116(11), pp. 958-9.

Greiner, A.N., Hellings, P.W., Rotiroti, G. and Scadding, G.K., 2011. Allergic rhinitis. *Lancet*, 378(9809), pp. 2112-22.

Hall, J.G., 1990. The SNATIATION reflex. *Journal of Medical Genetics*, 27(4), p. 275.

Marple, B.F., Fornadley, J.A., Patel, A.A., Fineman, S.M., Fromer, L., Krouse, J.H., Lanier, B.Q. and Penna, P.; American Academy of Otolaryngic Allergy Working Group on Allergic Rhinitis, 2007. Keys to successful management of patients with allergic rhinitis: focus on patient confidence, compliance, and satisfaction. *Otolaryngology—Head and Neck Surgery*, 136(6 Suppl), pp. S107-24.

Mullarkey, M.F., Hill, J.S. and Webb, D.R., 1980. Allergic and nonallergic rhinitis: their characterization with attention to the meaning of nasal eosinophilia. *Journal of Allergy and Clinical Immunology*, 65(2), pp. 122-6.

Peters, S., 2007. The impact of comorbid atopic disease on asthma: clinical expression and treatment. *Journal of Asthma*, 44(3), pp. 149-61.

Saleh, H.A. and Durham, S.R., 2007. Perennial rhinitis. *BMJ*, 335(7618), pp. 502-7.

Scadding, G.K., 2001. Non-allergic rhinitis: diagnosis and management. *Current Opinion in Allergy and Clinical Immunology*, 1(1), pp. 15-20.

Songu, M. and Cingi, C., 2009. Sneeze reflex: facts and fiction. *Therapeutic Advances in Respiratory Disease*, 3(3), pp. 131-41.

Sublett, J.W. and Bernstein, D.I., 2011. Occupational rhinitis. *Immunology and Allergy Clinics of North America*, 31(4), pp. 787-96, vii.

Swenson, A.J. and Leira, E.C., 2007. Paroxysmal sneezing at the onset of lateral medullary syndrome: cause or consequence? *European Journal of Neurology*, 14(4), pp. 461-3.

Teebi, A.S. and al-Saleh, Q.A., 1989. Autosomal dominant sneezing disorder provoked by fullness of stomach. *Journal of Medical Genetics*, 26(8), pp. 539-40.

van Kempen, M., Bachert, C. and Van Cauwenberge, P., 1999. An update on the pathophysiology of rhinovirus upper respiratory tract infections. *Rhinology*, 37(3), pp. 97-103.

Varghese, M., Glaum, M.C. and Lockey, R.F., 2010. Drug-induced rhinitis. *Clinical and Experimental Allergy*, 40(3), pp. 381-4.

Whitlock, G.G., Patel, A., Edwards, S.G., Benn, P.D. and Miller, R.F., 2012. The current system for prescribing antiretroviral therapy puts HIV-infected patients at risk of serious drug-drug interactions: is now the time for a paradigm shift in HIV care delivery? *Clinical Medicine*, 12(3), pp. 300-1.

8 Disorders of Smell

Emma McNeill, Sean Carrie

Chapter Overview

Pearls and Pitfalls

Pearls

- There is limited evidence to recommend any medication other than a trial of corticosteroids in patients with hyposmia.
- Computed tomography imaging is better for the assessment of sinonasal disease, whereas magnetic resonance imaging is preferable for the diagnosis of olfactory apparatus abnormalities and parenchymal disease.
- Patients with olfactory distortions should always be imaged.
- Patients should be advised of risks associated with reduced smell and detection of environmental hazards.

Pitfalls

- It is easy to underestimate the impact that the loss of smell can have on a person's quality of life.

8.1 INTRODUCTION

The importance of an intact sense of smell is underestimated. It plays a significant part in the enjoyment of food and has a strong association with memory and emotion. Some occupations depend on an intact sense of smell, e.g. cooking and fire fighting. A reduced or distorted sense of smell may be the primary manifestation of intracranial pathology. Twenty percent of people describe olfactory dysfunction, 14% with hyposmia and 6% with anosmia. The ability to assess olfactory disorders appropriately is a vital skill for the otolaryngologist.

8.2 DEFINITION OF OLFACTION

Olfaction is the sensation arising from the nasal cavity, following stimulation of the olfactory epithelium by volatile compounds.

Types of olfactory disorders (dysosmia) are as follows:

- Reduced or absent sense of smell—hyposmia or anosmia
- Distorted sense of smell
  - Parosmia/troposmia—distorted quality of perceived odorant
  - Phantosmia—perceived smell in absence of olfactory stimulant
  - Cacosmia—perception of unpleasant smell in absence of olfactory stimulation
  - Hyperosmia—increased olfactory acuity
- Olfactory disorders can be total, partial, or specific to certain smells.

8.3 PHYSIOLOGY OF OLFACTION

- Olfaction is mediated by cranial nerves I and V. The olfactory nerve (I) is responsible for identification of

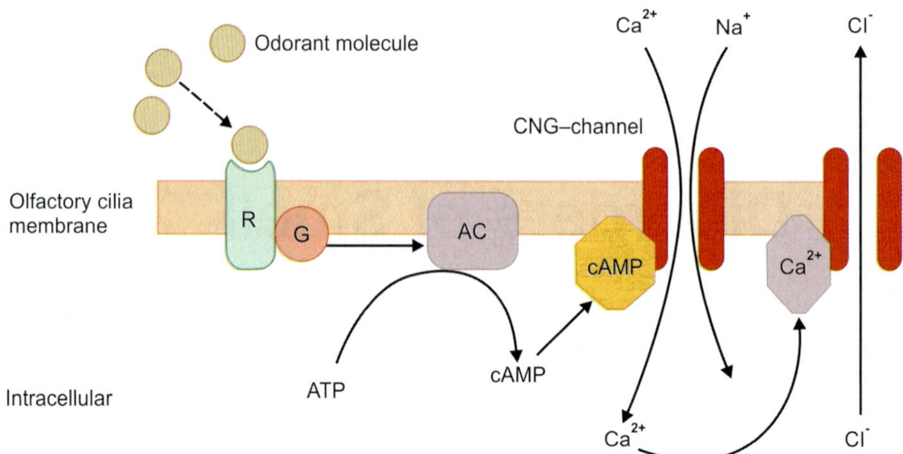

Fig. 8.1: Olfactory transduction—interaction of odorant molecules with olfactory neurons. (cAMP: Cyclic adenosine monophosphate; ATP: Adenosine triphosphate: AC: Adenylate cyclase). *Source*: Reprinted with permission from Harish Viswanathan and ENT News.

odorants via specialized olfactory epithelium. The trigeminal nerve (V) is responsible for the perception of chemical irritants and detection of pungency.

- The olfactory mucosa is an area of 1 mm thickness of specialized neuroepithelium overlying the cribriform plate, within the olfactory cleft. It extends over the superior turbinate, below the anterior middle turbinate and onto the nasal septum (Leopold, et al., 2000). It is accessed by orthonasal (direct inspiration into nasal cavity) and retronasal (via the mouth and postnasal space) airflow.
- Olfactory pathway—mediated by cyclic AMP
  - Odorant molecules interact with olfactory mucus.
  - Molecules bind with olfactory receptor cells (bipolar neurons, with single, cilia-bearing, club-shaped peripheral receptor). Each receptor can combine with a range of odorant molecules (Fig. 8.1).
  - The unmyelinated axons of receptor cells are then ensheathed by Schwann cells and pass through the cribriform plate (via 15-20 foramina) and synapse in the olfactory bulb (Jafek, 1983; Holley, et al., 1974; Mombaerts, et al., 1996).
  - Each odor has an "olfactory code," where the activation of set pattern of receptors and glomeruli is recognized by the olfactory cortex and identified as a specific odor (Vassar, et al., 1994).
  - The primary olfactory cortex (primary odor identification) is the prepyriform and periamygdaloid areas of medial aspect of temporal lobe, while the secondary olfactory cortex (affective aspects of olfaction) is located in the amygdala and entorhinal areas of the pyriform lobe. The associations between odor perception, memory, and emotional stimuli result from projections to thalamus, forebrain, and limbic system.
  - The vomeronasal organ (Jacobson's organ) is an accessory olfactory organ in mammals, with a role in pheromone perception. It is situated in the anterior septum, but its role as an active sensory organ in humans is debatable.

8.4 CLINICAL EVALUATION OF THE PATIENT WITH DYSOSMIA

The clinical evaluation of the patient with dysosmia is summarized in Flowchart 8.1.

History

- Presenting complaint
  - *Duration*: Knowledge of the duration of symptoms may give an indication of the likelihood of recovery.
  - Speed of onset/precipitant, e.g. upper respiratory tract infection (URTI), head injury: Awareness of the potential etiology of the olfactory disorder will guide treatment options and indicate the likelihood of recovery.
  - *Pattern of olfactory disturbance*: An obstructive cause, e.g. rhinitis may present with intermittent or persistent hyposmia. Parosmia and phantosmia are more suggestive of a neurologic cause.
  - Associated nasal symptoms are likely to be present in hyposmia secondary to chronic rhinosinusitis, e.g. obstruction, discharge, facial pain.

Flowchart 8.1: Clinical evaluation of the patient with dysosmia.

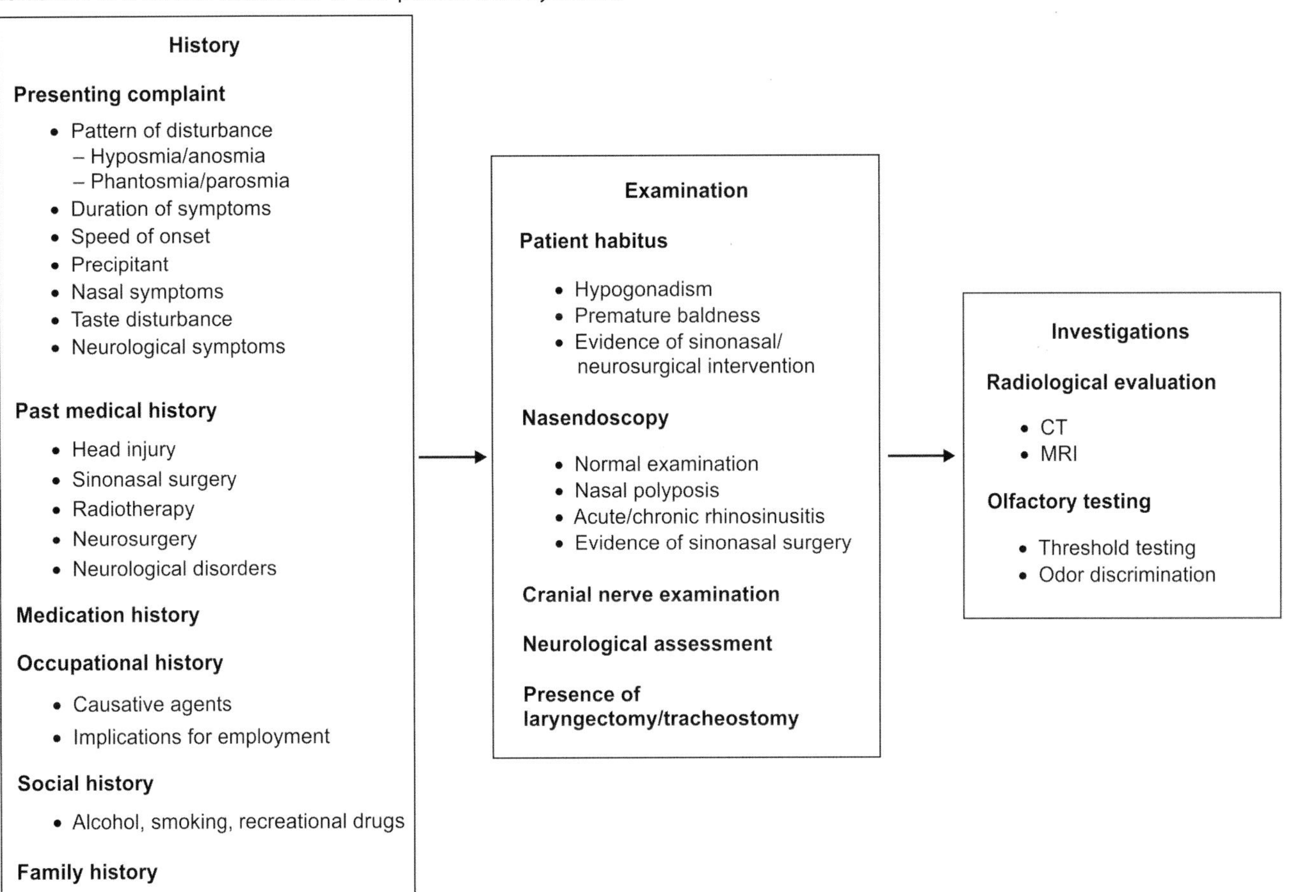

  - Taste disturbance is present in 80% of patients with smell disorders.
  - A neurologic history is an important part of the assessment, e.g. headache, speech disturbance, limb weakness, gait abnormalities.
- Past medical history
  - *Head injury*: Inquiries should be made into the severity of any head injury, including loss of consciousness, direction of impact, and any known radiologic finding as this has implications for recovery (Ogawa et al., 1999; Green et al., 2003; Callahan et al., 2002).
  - A history of sinonasal surgery, radiotherapy, or neurosurgical interventions may indicate the underlying cause of an olfactory disturbance or the consequences of medical intervention on a patient's sense of smell.
  - Olfactory disorders are found in patients with Alzheimer's disease, multiple sclerosis, and Parkinson's disease among others (Jones, et al., 1998).
- Medication history
  - Anosmia has been reported following the use of amiodarone, antidepressants, zinc-based cold products, and anti-inflammatory medication.
- Occupational history
  - This is a very important part of the history with regard to both the cause and the effects of the smell pathology. Exposure to noxious chemicals, such as formaldehyde and benzene, is associated with hyposmia. The smell abnormality can also have a significant impact on a patient's ability to perform their job, e.g. chef, wine taster, cosmetics industry.
- Social history
- Smoking, alcohol, and cocaine use all reduce olfactory sensitivity.
- Family history
  - Congenital conditions with associated olfactory disorders include primary congenital anosmia and Kallmann's syndrome. An association between anosmia, premature baldness and vascular headache

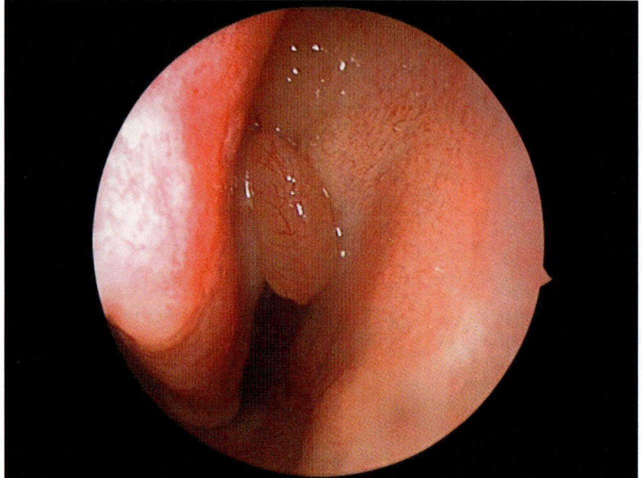

Fig. 8.2: Nasal polyps causing a "conductive" olfactory loss.

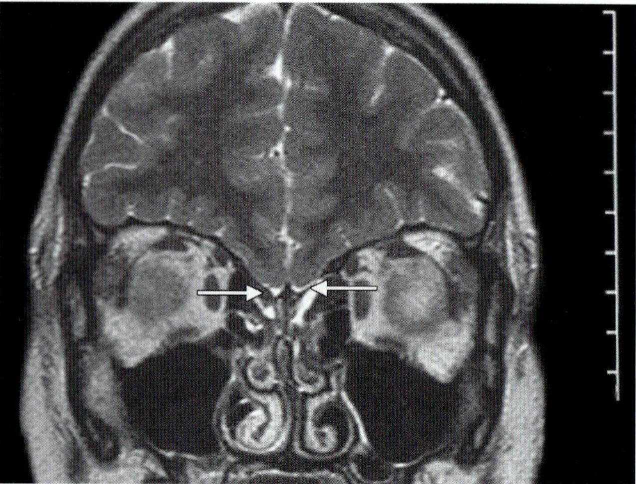

Fig. 8.3: Magnetic resonance imaging scan demonstrating absent olfactory apparatus (white arrow).

with a dominant inheritance pattern has also been described (Singh, et al., 1970).

Clinical Examination

- *Patient habitus*: Assess the patient for evidence of hypogonadism (Kallmann's syndrome), premature baldness.
- The presence of a tracheostomy/laryngectomy.
- Nasendoscopy may show evidence of rhinosinusitis, nasal polyposis, or may be completely normal (Fig. 8.2)
- There may be endoscopic or external evidence of sinonasal or neurosurgical intervention.
- Cranial nerve examination and neurologic assessment, e.g. speech, gait, motor function, should be performed.

Investigations

Radiologic Evaluation of Olfactory Dysfunction

- There are no current guidelines for the radiologic evaluation of olfactory dysfunction. However, computed tomography imaging is better for the assessment of sinonasal disease, particularly when relating to surgical planning. Magnetic resonance imaging is the gold standard for the diagnosis of olfactory apparatus abnormalities and parenchymal disease (Fig. 8.3).
- Phantosmias and olfactory hallucinations should always be imaged (Leopold, 2002).
- Accurate diagnosis of site of skull fracture and associated parenchymal injuries may allow the prediction of likelihood of recovery of smell following head injury.

Olfactory Testing

- Necessary criteria to maximize odor recognition in olfactory testing:
  - Odors must be familiar to patient
  - Requires a longstanding association between the odor and its name.
  - Help should be given to recall the name (Cain, 1979).
- Principles of formal smell testing:
  - Reliability is improved by using threshold testing and odor discrimination.
  - Threshold testing identifies the concentration at which an odorant is reliably perceived. Butanol or phenylethylalcohol are used, due to minimal associated trigeminal nerve stimulation.
  - Varying dilutions of the olfactory stimulant (4% highest concentration) are presented to the patient in random order. The patient chooses between the odorant and two controls, as to which they can smell. The lowest concentration that can be perceived is documented and repeated until the lowest concentration that is reliably perceived.
  - "Forced-choice" testing reduces response bias. Patients scoring less than chance are likely to be malingering, as are those who fail to identify trigeminal nerve stimulants, such as ammonia.
  - Formal olfactory testing allows monitoring of progression or resolution of dysosmia, particularly following therapeutic intervention.
  - There is considerable variation in the reliability of olfactory tests. Results from different testing

Flowchart 8.2: Demonstrating the etiology of olfactory disorders.

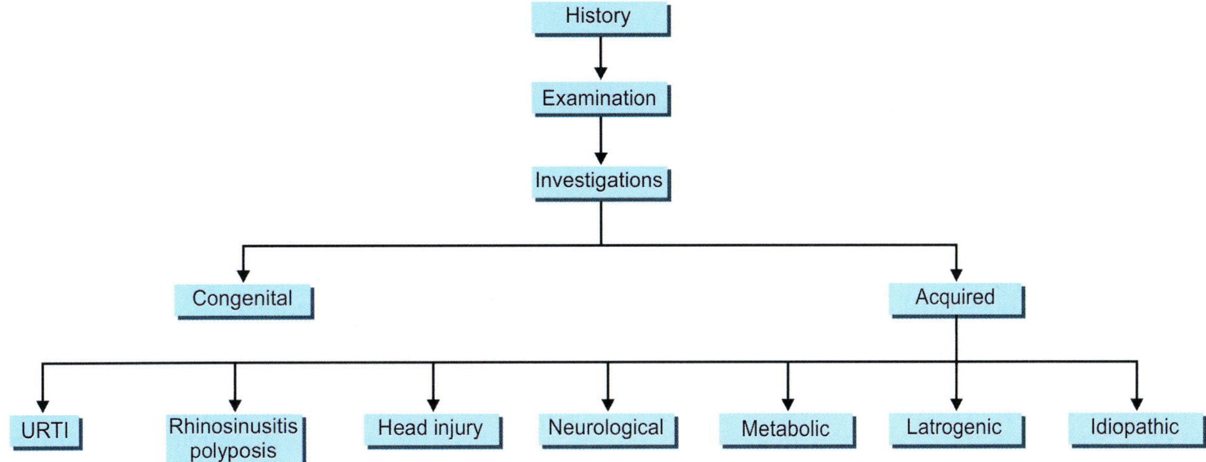

methods should not be compared, as variations may result from differing reliabilities rather than reflecting clinical findings.

- Commonly used olfactory testing kits include:
  - University of Pennsylvania Smell Identification Test (UPSIT)—a forced-choice suprathreshold test with 40 microencapsulated odors, acting as a "scratch and sniff" test. The test indicates a level of smell function, i.e. mild to total anosmia and has score ranking for age and gender (Doty, 1997).
  - Cross-Cultural Smell Identification Test (CCSIT)—a self-administered 12-item test based on UPSIT, which can be carried out in 5 minutes (Doty, et al., 1996).
  - "Sniffin' Sticks"—a test of olfactory function based on felt-tip pens and assesses odor threshold, discrimination, and identification. University of Pennsylvania Smell Identification Test and "Sniffin' Sticks" tests were developed in the United States and Germany, respectively—some odorants may not be familiar to different populations (Koba, et al., 1996).
  - The Combined Olfactory Test is a test designed and validated in the UK and assesses odor discrimination and threshold testing (Robson, et al., 1996).
- Other olfactory tests
  - Electrophysiology testing aims to provide an objective olfactory assessment. It is rarely used beyond specialist olfactory centers as it is expensive and technically demanding with high interindividual response variability. Tests include the electro-olfactogram and olfactory event-related potentials.
  - "Taste powders" are an assessment of retronasal olfactory function. They are placed in the mouth and forced choice questionnaires used to identify the taste. Truly anosmic patients are only able to detect sweet, sour, bitter, salty, and umami.

8.5 CAUSES OF OLFACTORY LOSS

The causes of olfactory disorder are summarized in Flowchart 8.2.

Causes

- Congenital or acquired
- The pathology can be divided into
  - "Conductive losses"—failure of odorant molecules to access olfactory mucosa, e.g. nasal polyps.
  - "Sensory losses"—damage to the olfactory mucosa, e.g. by chemical exposure, viral infection.
  - "Neural losses"—defect in peripheral or central neural pathways, e.g. head injury.
  - Most common causes—trauma, viral infections, nasal pathology.
- Congenital
  - 3% of cases
  - Primary congenital anosmia is the absence of sense of smell from birth and may be associated with the absence/hypoplasia of olfactory bulbs on imaging. Kallmann's syndrome is the genetic condition of anosmia and the failure to start or complete puberty due to hypogonadotropic hypogonadism. This may be apparent on clinical assessment.

- Head injury
  - 17% of cases of olfactory disturbances.
  - Dysosmia may result from damage to nasal mucosa, shearing of olfactory fibers due to cribriform plate fracture, and edema of the olfactory tracts and bulbs. The anterior temporal lobes and orbitofrontal poles are most vulnerable.
  - Damage to peripheral olfactory apparatus results in anosmia, while central olfactory damage results in the inability to discriminate odors.
  - Post-traumatic olfactory impairment is more pronounced with less chance of recovery than in chronic rhinosinusitis or postinfection.
  - Negative predictive factors include a Glasgow Coma Scale score of <13 at presentation, loss of consciousness >1 hour, post-traumatic amnesia, and radiologic abnormalities with occipital, frontal, and skull base fracture (Ogawa, et al., 1999; Green, et al., 2003).
  - Forty percent of patients who suffer a significant head injury will develop an olfactory deficit. This may only manifest on formal testing.
  - Recovery has been noted up to 5 years post-injury (Callahan, et al., 2002; Doty, 1997; Duncan, 1995).
- Upper respiratory tract infections
  - 20–30% of identified olfactory losses are due to viral URTI, which may be temporary or permanent (Seiden, 2004).
  - Temporary anosmia occurs when edema prevents odorant molecules reaching the olfactory cleft. Permanent olfactory impairment is due to the reduction in olfactory receptors with replacement by respiratory epithelium.
  - Stem cells may persist in olfactory mucosa with regenerative potential.
  - Recovery varies in the literature from 6 months to 3 years, although other studies describe minimal recovery.
  - Olfaction may remain permanently distorted, particularly in women (70–80%) and in those aged between 40 and 60, partly due to age-related cumulative degeneration of olfactory apparatus (Cullen, et al., 1999).
- Nasal pathology
  - 20% of cases.
  - Temporary loss of smell occurs when nasal airflow is impaired secondary to edema and inflammatory changes within the olfactory mucosa. Nasal polyposis results in the failure of odorant molecules to reach olfactory mucosa due to obstruction by polyps.
  - Permanent olfactory dysfunction can occur due to a reduction in olfactory epithelium and replacement with normal respiratory mucosa, e.g. chronic rhinosinusitis (Lee, et al., 2000).
  - Recovery of smell in chronic rhinosinusitis/polyposis is time-dependent. The outcome is less satisfactory in prolonged disease (Kern, 2000).
  - Chronic inflammatory conditions such as sarcoidosis and Wegener's granulomatosis can cause dysosmia. Nasal signs may be visible, e.g. crusting, bleeding, nasal deformity.
- Neurologic causes
  - Olfactory acuity deteriorates with age.
  - There is an association with dysosmia and Alzheimer's disease, Huntington's disease, multiple sclerosis, and motor neuron disease. It is found in over 95% patients with Parkinson's syndrome (preceding the development of motor symptoms) (Leopold, 2002).
  - Phantosmia is associated with epilepsy, migraine, schizophrenia, and head injury. There may be other associated neurologic symptoms, including a preceding aura, visual disturbance, headache, altered mood, speech, and motor symptoms. Odors can be pleasant or unpleasant and can last from seconds to hours.
  - Altered smell may be the presenting feature of olfactory neuroblastoma or anterior skull base tumors.
  - A thorough neurologic assessment should be part of the evaluation of a patient with phantosmia/parosmia, with a low threshold for imaging.
- Metabolic/Endocrine
  - Hyposmia is described in chronic liver and renal failure.
  - There are reported associations with endocrine disorders, including diabetes mellitus, hypothyroidism, and hypo/hyperadrenalism.
  - 76% of pregnant females experience significant changes in olfaction and taste perception.
- Iatrogenic
  - Reduced olfactory acuity post-laryngectomy/tracheostomy is due to reduced nasal airflow. Retronasal olfactory function is likely to be preserved.
  - Radiotherapy/surgery to the anterior skull base can cause hyposmia.
  - Sinonasal surgery can cause hyposmia due to the underappreciated extent of olfactory mucosa, highlighting the importance of preserving normal tissue (Lee, et al., 2000).

- Surgery on olfactory areas (resection of olfactory neuroblastoma) would cause postoperative anosmia.
- Medications associated with reduced olfactory acuity include cocaine, immunosuppressants, e.g. methotrexate, antidepressants, e.g. amitriptyline, and topical zinc applications for coryzal symptoms.

- Idiopathic
  - Accounts for 20% of cases of hyposmia.

8.6 MANAGEMENT OF OLFACTORY DISORDERS

- Treatment should ideally be directed toward a specific etiologic cause.
- A trial of oral corticosteroids may be useful in hyposmic patients with allergic rhinitis, chronic rhinosinusitis, and nasal polyposis, e.g. prednisolone 0.5 mg/kg for 7 days. An improvement is likely to be due to a reduction in mucosal edema. Hyposmic patients may not return to normosmia, and truly anosmic patients show minimal improvement in olfactory scores.
- Corticosteroid nasal sprays are less effective in improving olfactory scores and symptoms, but reduce edema in the olfactory cleft in inflammatory nasal conditions. They can maintain the effect of an initial response to oral steroids or following functional endoscopic sinus surgery (FESS).
- There is limited evidence to recommend the use of any medication other than steroids in anosmia or hyposmia (Martinez-Devesa and Patiar, 2011).
- Antidepressants, e.g. venlafaxine, and anticonvulsants are used in the treatment of olfactory distortions. A neurologic or psychiatric disorder needs to be established as part of the patient's investigations and treated accordingly, e.g. Parkinson's disease, complex partial seizures.
- Improvements in subjective and objective measures of olfactory functions following FESS and nasal polypectomy have been demonstrated and may be maintained by continued use of nasal steroids. Ten percent of patients show no improvement and 6% have experienced olfactory deterioration at 5 years post-FESS.
- Risk of damage to normal olfactory mucosa is possible during all nasal surgery.
- "Odor gymnastics" targets the potential for olfactory neural plasticity by the use of olfactory training. Olfactory ability was shown to improve on formal testing, at least in the short term, by structured exposure to intense odors, post-URTI and head trauma. However, spontaneous remission needs to be separated from genuine therapeutic effect (Hummel, 2011).
- Other surgical techniques include bifrontal craniotomy and removal of the olfactory bulbs or excision of the olfactory mucosa via an endonasal approach for olfactory distortions. These result in permanent anosmia and carry a significant risk of morbidity to the patient.

8.7 QUALITY-OF-LIFE ISSUES

- An impaired sense of smell can have a significant impact on a patient's quality of life.
- Almost 75% of dysosmic patients have problems with cooking food and 50% report inadvertently eating spoiled food.
- Some occupations depend heavily on an intact sense of smell, including wine tasting, cosmetic and perfume manufacturing, and the catering industry.
- Altered mood and difficulty in perception of their own body odor can put a significant strain on a patient's daily life. The loss of sentimental smell memory has been associated with depression.
- Patients should be advised of risks associated with reduced smell, particularly regarding detection of environmental hazards, e.g. smoke and gas detection.

REFERENCES

Cain, W.S., 1979. To know with the nose: keys to odor identification. *Science*, 203(4379), pp. 467-70.

Callahan, C.D., and Hinkebein, J.H., 2002. Assessment of anosmia after traumatic brain injury: performance characteristics of the University of Pennsylvania Smell Identification Test. *J Head Trauma Rehab*, 17(3), pp. 251-6.

Cullen, M.M., and Leopold, D.A., 1999. Disorders of smell and taste. *Med Clin North Am*, 83(1), pp. 57-74.

Doty, R.L., Marcus, A. and Lee, W.W., 1996. Development of the 12-item Cross-Cultural Smell Identification Test (CC-SIT). *Laryngoscope*, 106(3, Pt 1), pp. 353-6.

Doty, R.L., 1997. Studies of human olfaction from the University of Pennsylvania Smell and Taste Centre. *Chem Senses*, 22(5), pp. 565-86.

Doty, R.L., Yousem, D.M., Pham, L.T., Kreshak, A.A., Geckle, R., and Lee, W.W., 1997. Olfactory dysfunction in patients with head trauma. *Arch Neurol*, 54(9), pp. 1131-40.

Duncan, H.J. and Seiden, A.M., 1995. Long-term follow-up of olfactory loss secondary to head trauma and upper respiratory tract infection. *Arch Otolaryngo Head Neck Surg*, 121(10), pp. 1183-7.

Green, P., Rohling, M.L., Iverson, G.L., and Gervais, RO., 2003. Relationships between olfactory discrimination and head injury severity. *Brain Inj*, 17(6), pp. 479-96.

Holley, A., Duchamp, A., Reviel, M., and Juge, A., 1974. Qualitative and quantitative discrimination in frog olfactory receptors: analysis from electrophysiological data. *Ann N Y Acad Sci*, 237, pp. 102-14.

Hummel, T., Landis, B.N., and Huttenbrink, K.B., 2011. Smell and taste disorders. GMS current topics in Otorhinolaryngology, Head and Neck Surgery at http://www.egms.de/static/en/journals/cto/2012-10/cto000077.shtml

Jafek, B., 1983. Ultrastructure of human nasal mucosa. *Laryngoscope*, 93, p. 1576.

Jones, N. and Rog, D., 1998. Olfaction: a review. *Journal of Laryngology & Otology*, 112(1), pp. 11-24.

Kern, R.C., 2000. Chronic sinusitis and anosmia: pathologic changes in the olfactory mucosa. *Laryngoscope*, 110(7), pp. 1071-7.

Kobal, G., Hummel, T., Sekinger, B., Barz, S., Rischer, S., and Wolf, S., 1996. "Sniffin" sticks—screening of olfactory performance. Rhinology, 34(4), pp. 222-6.

Lee, S.H., Lim, H.H., Lee, H.M., Park, H.J., and Choi, J.O., 2000. Olfactory mucosal findings in patients with persistent anosmia after endoscopic sinus surgery. *Ann Otol Rhinol Laryngol*, 109(8 Pt 1), pp. 720-5.

Leopold, D.A., Hummel, T., Schwob, J.E., Hong, S.C., Knecht, M. and Kobal, G., 2000. Anterior distribution of human olfactory epithelium. *Laryngoscope*, 110(3 Pt 1), pp. 417-21.

Leopold, D., 2002. Distortion of olfactory perception: Diagnosis and Treatment. *Chem Senses*, 27, pp. 611-5.

Martinez-Devesa, P., and Patiar, S., 2011. Oral steroids for nasal polyps. *Cochrane Database for Systematic Reviews* at http://www.ncbi.nlm.nih.gov/pubmed/21735400

Mombaerts, P., Wang, F., Dulac, C. and Chao, S., et al., 1996. Visualising an olfactory sensory map. *Cell*, 87, pp. 675-86.

Ogawa, T. and Rutka, J., 1999. Olfactory dysfunction in head injured workers. *Acta Otolaryngol Supp*, 540, pp. 50-7.

Robson, A.K., Woollons, A.C., Ryan, J., Horrocks, C., Williams, S. and Dawes, P.J., 1996. Validation of the combined olfactory test. *Clin Otolaryngol Allied Sci*, 21(6), pp. 512-8.

Seiden, A.M., 2004. Postviral olfactory loss. *Otolaryngol Clin North Am*, 37(6), pp. 1159-66.

Singh, N., Grewal, M.S., and Austin, J.H., 1970. Familial anosmia. *Arch Neurol*, 22(1), pp. 40-4.

Vassar, R., Chao, S., Sitcheran, R and Nunez J, et al., 1994. Topographic organisation of sensory projections to the olfactory bulb. *Cell*, 79, pp. 981-91.

Bleeding Nose (Epistaxis)

9

Claudio Callejas, Salil B Nair

Chapter Overview

Pearls and Pitfalls

Pearls

- Epistaxis should be considered a symptom, not a diagnosis. The underlying cause must be identified.
- History taking, examination, and treatment are important and often performed simultaneously.
- Patients with epistaxis often present with elevated blood pressure. Some controversy exists regarding its best management.
- In fit patients with severe bleeding, a small dose of oral diazepam (2 mg) is a useful measure to help reduce anxiety. This can improve both blood pressure and the discomfort associated with examination.
- Associated unilateral or asymmetric sinonasal symptoms should raise the possibility of a neoplasm.

Pitfalls

- Epistaxis in the children under 2 years of life is uncommon and nonaccidental injury should be excluded.
- Caution is required in the cessation of antiaggregant and anticoagulant therapy. Consultation with an hematologist is recommended.

9.1 INTRODUCTION

Epistaxis is the commonest emergency in otorhinolaryngology. Most cases are mild and can be solved with ease; however, a proportion with severe epistaxis can be associated with significant morbidity and sometimes even mortality.

9.2 EPIDEMIOLOGY AND CLASSIFICATION

Most people experience some form of a nosebleed during their lifetime, but only a small proportion seek medical attention. Epistaxis accounts for about 1 in 200 emergency department visits in the United States (Pallin, et al., 2005).

The age-related frequency of epistaxis in patients who seek medical attention has a bimodal distribution. There is a small peak among children younger than 10 years (although unusual in the first 2 years of life) and then the frequency steadily increases from 30 years age onward, with the highest rates in the elderly, reaching a peak in the eighth decade of life.

Epistaxes can be classified as either primary (idiopathic) or secondary. Primary epistaxis occurs without any obvious cause.

From a therapeutic point of view, epistaxes are usefully classified as either anterior or posterior, depending on the region of the nose they arise from. This classification reflects the anatomy of the nasal cavity blood supply, which originates from branches of the internal and external carotid arteries (Fig. 9.2). Posterior epistaxes are characteristically more severe than anterior bleeds and can be life threatening.

Typically, childhood epistaxes are anterior and tend to present as recurrent nonlife-threatening bleeding. They are usually managed by improving nasal hygiene, ointment application, or cauterization. Hospitalization is seldom required. On the other hand, with age, severe episodes of nosebleeds become more usual. In elderly patients, severe bleedings can decompensate pre-existing conditions (e.g. cardiovascular disease). Hospital admissions due to epistaxis steadily increase after 30 years of age (Walker, Macfarlane and McGarry, 2007).

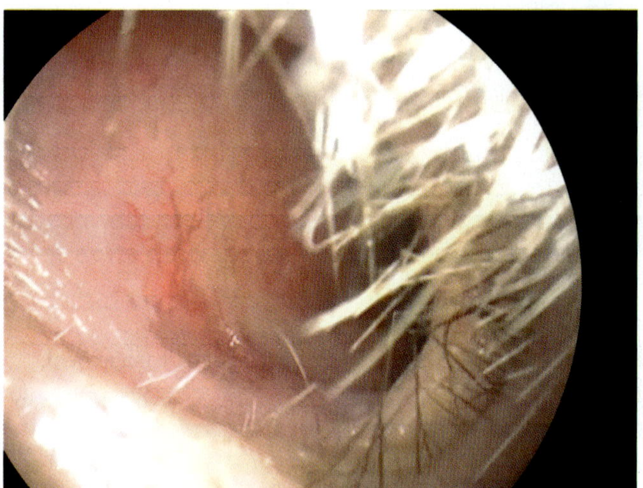

Fig. 9.1: Prominent blood vessels of the Kiesselbach's plexus in the Little's area of the left nasal cavity.

9.3 VASCULAR ANATOMY

Approximately 90% of epistaxes are anterior, and the great majority of these arise from the *Kiesselbach's plexus* (Fig. 9.1) in the anterior region of the nasal septum (*Little's area*). This plexus is a consistent arterial anastomotic crossroad, composed of large, thin-walled vessels supplied by the terminal branches of the *sphenopalatine artery* (SPA), the *superior labial branch of the facial artery*, and the branches of *anterior* and *posterior ethmoidal arteries* (Fig. 9.2).

Posterior bleeds account for approximately 10% of epistaxes and the SPA (main blood supply to the posterior region of the nose) is responsible for most cases. Although relatively uncommon, posterior epistaxes can arise from the anterior and posterior ethmoidal arteries (branches of the ophthalmic artery), which supply the mucosa of the superior lateral wall of the nose. Ethmoidal artery bleeds are mostly secondary to facial trauma and may be associated with skull base fractures. Posterior epistaxis could also be due to bleeding from Woodruff's plexus.

Woodruff's plexus: This area is located over the posterior end of the middle turbinate. The anastomosis here is made up of branches from the internal maxillary artery, namely, its sphenopalatine and ascending pharyngeal branches.

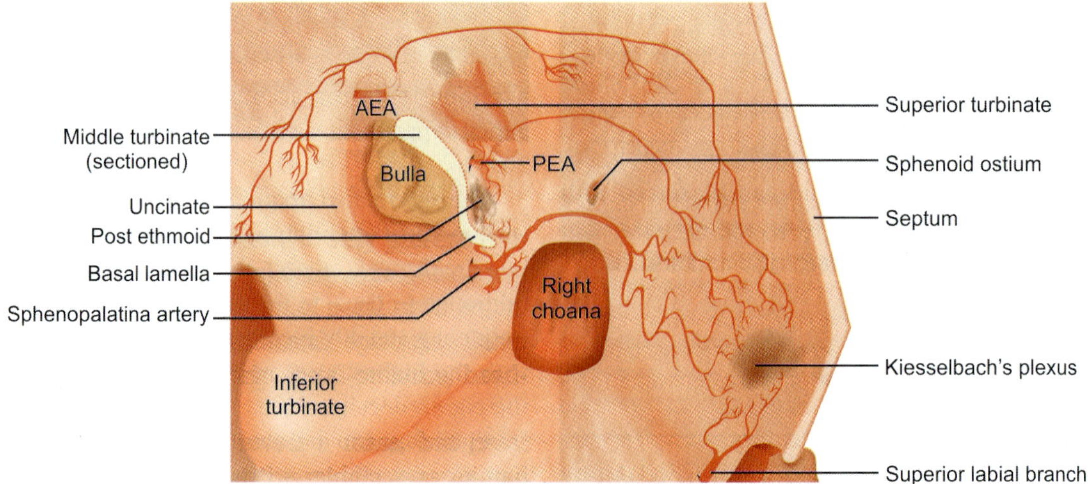

Fig. 9.2: Vascular anatomy of the nose. (AEA: Anterior ethmoidal artery; PEA: Posterior ethmoidal artery).

Table 9.1: Focused medical history.
Present history
• Trigger – Upper respiratory tract infection, nose picking, trauma, other • Side • Magnitude • Anterior vs. posterior • First episode/recurrent (previous treatments) • Chronic unilateral nasal symptoms (tumor?)
Medications
• Anticoagulants • Antiaggregants • Complementary and alternative medicine • Topical nasal drugs (e.g. corticosteroids sprays) • *Others*: Isotretiroin (acne treatment), anti-angiogenic drugs (cancer treatment)
Adverse drug reactions
Past medical history • Diseases associated with hemostasis disorders – Hematological diseases, chronic liver disease, chronic renal failure, other • Diseases whose treatment can affect hemostasis – Cardiovascular (epistaxis my also decompensate it), malignancies, other • Rhinitis • Known septal perforation or vasculitis • Cocaine abuse • Family or known personal history of hereditary hemorrhagic telangiectasia • Severe maxillofacial trauma (Pseudoaneurysm?)

9.4 HISTORY TAKING AND EXAMINATION

History taking is important even in the acute setting. The aim is to determine the circumstances of the event, relevant background information, and any possible cause or associated predisposing conditions (Table 9.1).

Physical examination is continuous, and often simultaneous, with history taking and treatment.

Appropriate protective clothing, face masks, and gloves should be worn when examining patients with epistaxes.

Initial assessment and resuscitation should be performed on all patients. The *Advance Trauma Life Support Guidelines of the American College of Surgeons* (ATLS) is a widely accepted approach.

After life-threatening situations that require immediate actions have been ruled out, a thorough examination of the nose and oropharynx should be performed. Patients should be seated upright and encouraged to lean forward and clear any clots from their pharynx. Appropriate headlight and suction are required. Nasal clots can be removed by gentle suction or by asking the patients to gently blow their own nose. *Anterior rhinoscopy* will identify the site of bleeding in most cases. If the bleeding point cannot be identified, the use of an *endoscope* is useful. The use of topical anesthesia and vasoconstriction (when not contraindicated) will make examination easier and less uncomfortable.

Blood studies should be guided according to history taking. A full blood count is recommended in elderly patients and in cases of severe and/or recurrent bleeding (Flowchart 9.1).

9.5 STOPPING THE BLEEDING

First aid measures are important and rarely conducted effectively. Most anterior bleeds are easily stopped with bilateral digital compression of the nostrils, and leaning forward. A small pledget soaked with local anesthetic and decongestant, placed in the anterior nares is very useful. Once active bleeding stops, cautery with silver nitrate is possible (*see* Little's area bleeding section). Persistent bleeding despite cautery or when a bleeding point cannot be identified requires nasal packing. *Anterior nasal packing* is most commonly performed using nondegradable commercially available dressings (e.g. Merocel®, Medtronic®, Rapid Rhino®, and ArthroCare).

Posterior epistaxis usually requires posterior tamponade if these do not settle with longer anterior nasal tampons. The most used materials are a Foley catheter (French 12–14) combined with anterior packing. There are also commercially available inflatable devices (e.g. Epistat, Medtronic).

Broad spectrum antibiotic cover is recommended as *Staphylococcal Toxic Shock Syndrome*, although very rare, has been reported. The duration of packing varies considerably (24 hours to 7 days) depending on the site, cause, associated morbidity, and the physician's judgment. After packing removal, the use of topical emollients promotes mucosal healing.

Flowchart 9.1: Assessment and treatment of epistaxis.

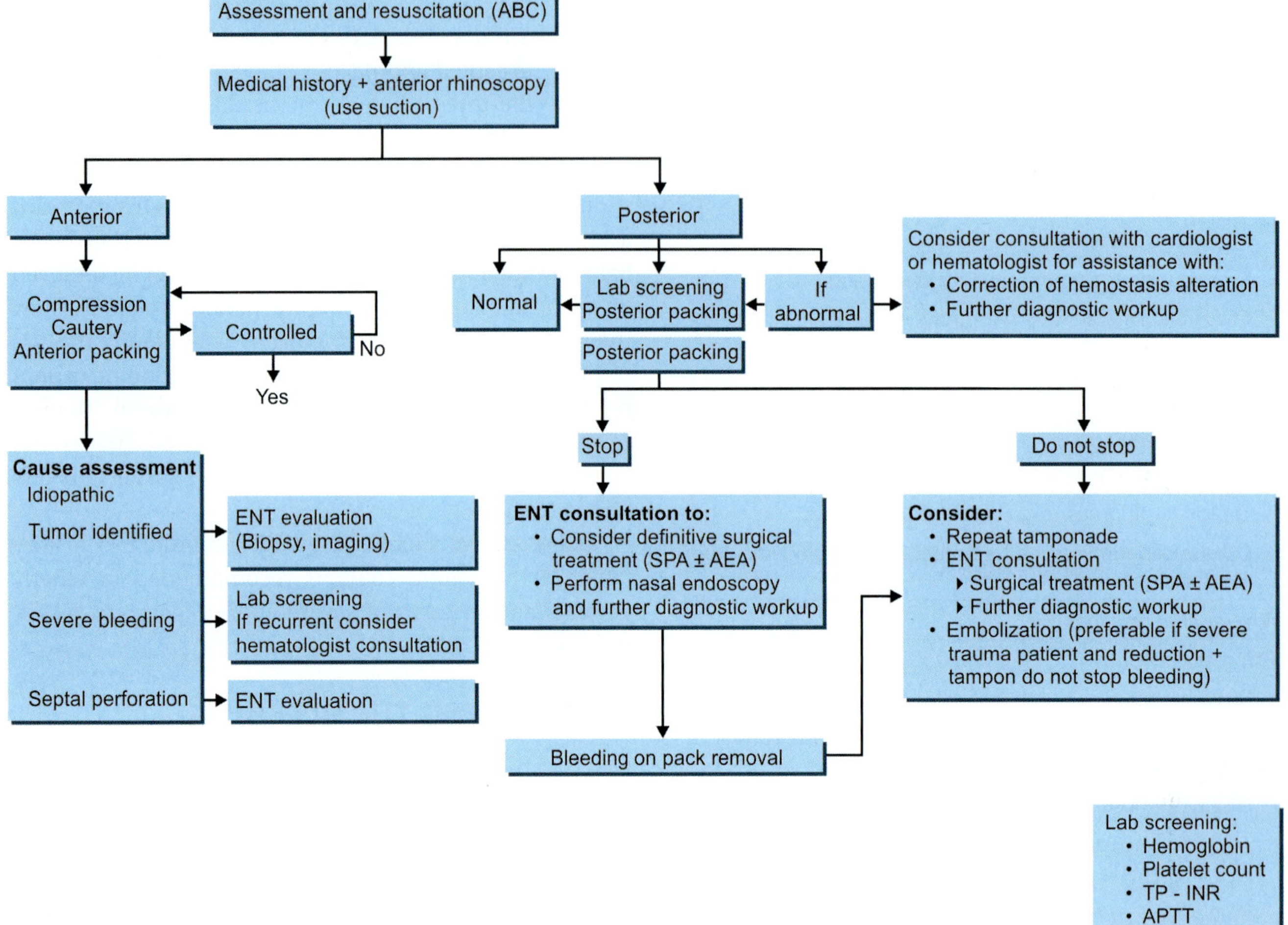

(ABC: Assessment and resuscitation according to ATLS®; ENT: Ear nose throat specialist; SPA: Sphenopalatine artery; AEA: Anterior ethmoidal artery).

When available, *endoscopic ligation of the SPA* should be considered. The use of posterior packing may be considered a transitory measure before definitive surgical treatment is undertaken. Controversy exists in the timing of a SPA ligation as many posterior bleeds will settle with conservative packing measures alone. However, this can be uncomfortable for the patient, requires prolonged hospital stays, and is not without risk (aspiration, alar necrosis, septal perforation).

Life-threatening nose bleeding needs prompt resolution as part of the resuscitation maneuvers, with little time for assessment, in order to secure the airway (e.g. associated swallow disorder) or to assure maintenance of an adequate circulation. Usually nasal packing will allow control of the bleeding in an expeditious manner. Flowchart 9.1 summarizes the assessment and treatment of epistaxis. For a detailed description on epistaxis management, *see* Barnes, Spielmann and White, 2012.

9.6 CAUSES AND ASSOCIATED CONDITIONS ASSESSMENT

While a significant percentage of epistaxes are idiopathic, often the cause or an associated condition predisposing to the bleeding can be identified (Table 9.2).

Their prevalence varies according to the age and the characteristics of the population considered. In general, traumatic and idiopathic causes are frequent across all ages. In children, Little's area bleeding is the most common cause. Tumors tend to affect a slightly older age group and their frequency increases from 50 years of age.

Mucosal Insults

Infection and Inflammation

Nosebleed secondary to infection (viral or bacterial *rhinosinusitis*) or inflammation (e.g. Wegener's granulomatosis)

Table 9.2: Secondary causes and associated conditions.

- Mucosal insults
- Infection/inflammation
- Little's area
- Septal perforation and ulcers
- Foreign body

Vasculitis (Wegener's, etc.) or nonspecific inflammation

Trauma

Hemostasis alterations

- Drugs
- Hematologic diseases
- Other diseases
- Sinonasal tumors

Vascular malformations

- Hereditary hemorrhagic telangiectasia

may manifest as a blood-stained nasal discharge within a constellation of sinonasal symptoms. Bleeding is rarely the leading symptom.

Little's Area

Epidemiology and Pathogenesis

- By far the most common cause of epistaxis, being responsible for approximately 90% of all nosebleeds.
- In children above 2 years of age, nearly all bleeding episodes arise from this area. However, epistaxis is rare under this age and nonaccidental injury should be considered (McIntosh, Mok and Margerison, 2007).
- Vestibulitis, nose picking, and mucosal drying are among the most common forms of trauma to the large, thin-walled vessels that characterize this area.
  - Mucosal drying may be secondary to local factors (e.g. intranasal steroid spray use) or systemic medications (e.g. isotretinoin for acne treatment).

Clinical Features

Little's area bleeding tends to present as recurrent non-life-threatening bleeding. Diagnosis is made by anterior rhinoscopy, which shows the active bleeding point or evidence of recent bleeding (e.g. clot or bloody crust).

Investigations

Pediatric patients with recurrent severe epistaxis who fail medical therapy warrant consideration for a comprehensive hematologic evaluation as a higher prevalence of bleeding disorders has been observed in this select group of patients, most with normal screening studies (Elden, Reinders and Witmer, 2012).

Preferred Treatment

Patient education: Emphasize the importance of avoiding *nose picking*. Advice on the correct use of nasal sprays: Apply nasal sprays pointing away from the septum.

Acute episodes of bleeding can be managed by pinching the region of the nasal vestibule.

Emollients and/or *silver nitrate cautery* are used to avoid recurrence. Petroleum jelly (Vaseline) and creams or ointments with antibiotics are used as moisturizers. Patients should not apply creams with cotton buds, but use either a clean finger under direct vision or preferably just the nozzle of the ointment tube.

Silver nitrate cauterization in children should be preferably done under topical application of lignocaine. Four percent of lignocaine is applied on a cotton wool and placed over the septum for few minutes before application of silver nitrate, which should remain in contact with the septal vessel for at least 30 seconds to achieve good cauterization.

Monopolar or bipolar *diathermy* of the septum under general anesthesia (at least in children) may be required if the above measures fail (Flowchart 9.2).

Treatment Outcomes

Although a recent Cochrane review has found limited evidence for the use of nasal antiseptic creams (Qureishi and Burton, 2012), a number of studies do demonstrate a benefit, which is enhanced when used in conjunction with silver nitrate cautery.

Complications of Treatment

Septal perforation: Bilateral cautery in theory poses a potential risk for septal perforation, although this is not uncommonly performed. In general, it is recommended to defer the cautery of the less compromised side (approximately 4–6 weeks) to provide time for mucosal healing. However, when applied in an appropriate concentration (75%) and at an appropriate duration in a healthy mucosal environment, bilateral cautery appears to have a low rate of complications and allows treatment at a single visit.

Complication of Disease

Septal perforation: In theory, septal perforation may originate as a consequence of recurrent insults to Little's area, although at present this cannot be substantiated by the literature (Lanier, et al., 2007).

Flowchart 9.2: Epistaxis management.

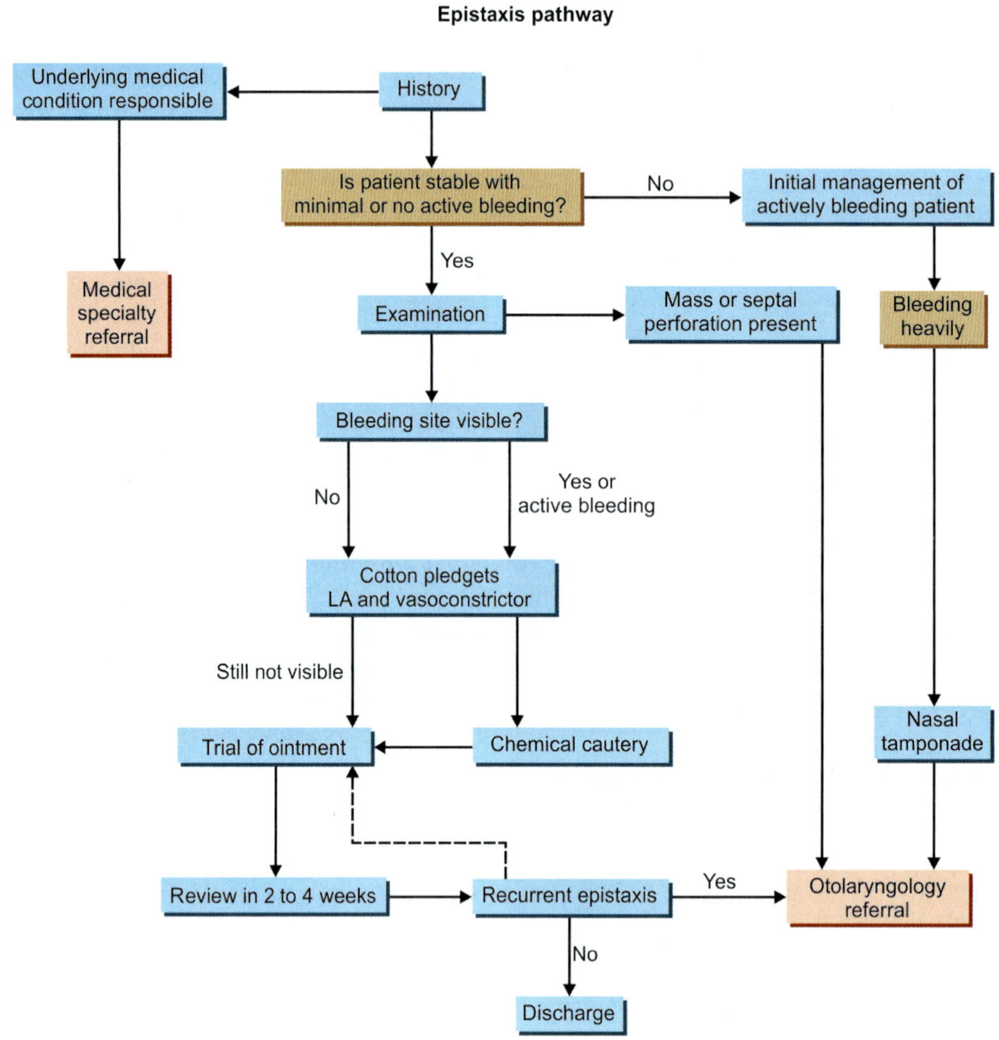

Septal Perforation and Ulcers

Diagnostic Summary

Idiopathic
Traumatic
- Nose picking
- Nasal surgery
- Trauma (e.g. nasal fracture)

Inflammatory
- Wegener's granulomatosis, sarcoidosis, lupus erythematosus, vasculitis

Infectious
- Nonspecific
- Specific: syphilis, leprosy, and tuberculosis

Drugs (e.g. cocaine abuse)
Malignancy
- High-grade lymphomas present with aggressive signs and symptoms including nonhealing ulcer, epistaxis, septal perforation, and bony destruction

Foreign body (button-battery)
Others
- Radiation-induced
- Nasal mucosal occupational irritants

Clinical Features

Most patients are asymptomatic. Common symptoms include recurrent epistaxis, nasal obstruction, crusting, whistling, and discharge.

Symptomatic septal perforations are usually anterior and easily detected by anterior rhinoscopy (Fig. 9.3). The most common finding is a smooth, well-circumscribed septal lesion with an occasional bleeding point. Often the

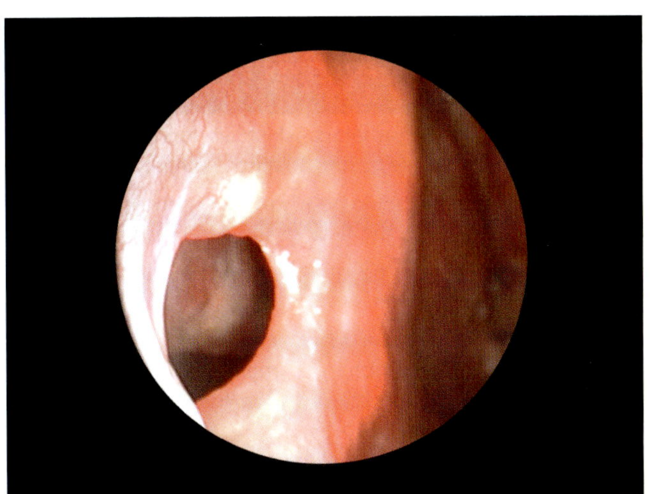

Fig. 9.3: Postsurgical septal perforation in the anterior region of the septum.

posterior edge of the perforation is swollen and inflamed and can contribute to the symptoms of obstruction.

Investigations

Biopsy: nasal septal biopsy should be performed when there is a suspicion of malignancy (e.g. bony erosion). Studies have shown a poor diagnostic yield following a biopsy and furthermore rarely contribute toward clinical management, even when vasculitis is suspected (Murray and McGarry, 2000; Diamantopoulos and Jones, 2001).

Preferred Treatment

Conservative management includes nasal irrigation, lubrication with ointments, and prosthesis (e.g. silastic *septal button*).

Patients with debilitating symptoms in spite of conservative management may benefit from surgical closure of the septal perforation.

Treatment Outcomes

A significant number of patients do well with conservative measures. Most of the perforations with unusual appearance revert to well-circumscribed clean edges and epithelialized margins within a few weeks of local treatment.

The success of surgical closure varies greatly in the literature (50–100%). The size of the perforation is the most significant predictor of successful closure (Kim and Rhee, 2012).

Complications of Treatment

Unsuccessful closure is not uncommon. Other complications include persistent nasal obstruction in spite of successful closure and postoperative synechia.

Foreign Body

Although they may manifest as a blood-stained nasal discharge, rarely is bleeding the leading symptom. Most characteristic symptoms are nasal obstruction, unilateral mucopurulent discharge, and foul odor.

Trauma

Epidemiology and Pathogenesis

- Epistaxis secondary to trauma affects mostly young adults during the third and fourth decade of life and has a male preponderance (Pallin, et al., 2005).
- Depending on the trauma, bleeding can range from relatively minor and self-limiting episodes to severe and life-threatening ones.
- Facial and *nasal fractures* may be associated with bleeding from the anterior ethmoidal artery.
- *Maxillary artery* injury is responsible for most major epistaxis secondary to facial trauma.

Clinical Features

Most bleeds are mild and related to minor trauma (e.g. nasal fracture).

Episodic arterial bleeding following a nasal fracture suggests injury to the anterior ethmoidal artery (AEA).

Serious life-threatening hemorrhage is rare and related to severe maxillofacial trauma.

History and Examination

Where possible, a careful history and examination are essential to ascertain the nature and site of the injury.

Investigations

Imaging: When facial fractures are suspected, computed tomography (CT) imaging is essential. It can help identify injuries to the skull base, orbit, and cervical spine.

Angiography: Where significant vascular injury is suspected, angiography can identify site of injury and enables treatment by means of selective angiographic embolization.

Preferred Treatment

Although epistaxis due to nasal trauma is usually self-limiting, initial assessment and resuscitation is performed on all patients. The ATLS is a widely accepted approach.

Nasal packing is the first choice to stop active bleeding. If attempted, posterior tamponade with a Foley catheter is effective, but should be used with caution in trauma cases as intracranial placement of the catheter has been described Woo, et al. (2008).

Fracture reduction: Temporary reduction may be attempted in the emergency room when nasal packing fails and excessive bleeding or hemodynamic instability precludes formal reduction. Nasal packs should be removed first as packing may actually distract the fractures and promote hemorrhage.

Surgical arterial ligation: It is considered when other measures fail. Direct ligation of the bleeding vessels is preferred. *Endoscopic* approach is the method of choice in case of SPA bleeding. *External ligation* is the preferred method to stop AEA bleeding, as it is a straightforward procedure with low risks in comparison with embolization of these vessels, which carries a risk of blindness. External ligation of the posterior ethmoidal artery (PEA) is associated with significant morbidity due to the close proximity of the orbital apex. Fortunately, severe PEA bleeding is rare. Indirect ligation of the bleeding vessel by means of external carotid artery ligation has met with unpredictable success due to the rich collateral blood flow.

Selective angiographic embolization: It is usually the preferred method to stop severe arterial bleeding secondary to serious trauma when conservative measures fail (except ethmoidal arteries bleeding). Severe maxillofacial fractures may distort the nasal anatomy making endoscopic ligation of the SPA extremely challenging. Furthermore, patients are frequently unstable. Where the imaging suggests stable fractures and preserved anatomic landmarks, an endoscopic ligation is possible.

Treatment Outcomes

Epistaxis due to nasal trauma is usually self-limiting or easily stopped with nasal packing; however, management of massive hemorrhage secondary to severe maxillofacial trauma can be a challenging task.

Complications of Treatment

Posterior tamponade: Intracranial migration of the Foley catheter: recommendations have been made to avoid this complication (Table 9.3).

Table 9.3: Recommendations to avoid intracranial migration of Foley catheter while performing posterior tamponade in trauma setting (Woo, et al, 2008).

- Use large diameter catheters, which are less prone to intracranial penetration (e.g. 12–14 French gauge).
- The Foley catheter should be advanced in a straight direction parallel and close to the floor of the nasal cavity.
- The catheter tip must be identified in the oropharynx before inflation of the balloon.
- An insertion length over 13 cm without visualization of the catheter tip in the oropharynx implies that the catheter is in the wrong position (the distance from the nares to the oropharynx is about 11 to 13 cm).
- A lateral skull X-ray is a useful way to confirm the appropriate position of the tip or balloon after the procedure.

Alar necrosis: It is caused by persistent pressure of the catheter against the ala of the nose. Avoiding direct contact of the catheter with the alar skin with loose cotton wool vestibular pack and routinely rotating the catheter along the nares perimeter are useful preventive measures.

Soft palate necrosis: It is caused by pressure ischemia. To prevent it, avoid overinflating the balloon and long periods with too much pressure.

Synechia: It is not an unusual complication. Usually asymptomatic, but may require surgical division later.

External surgical ligation of AEAs

- Unsightly scar
- Although rare, superior oblique muscle palsy has been reported.

Angiographic embolization

- *Minor complications*: Reported rates vary significantly (2–45%) and include facial pain, jaw pain, headache, paraesthesia/anesthesia, trismus, inguinal pain, and inguinal hematoma.
- *Major complications*: Cerebrovascular accidents, blindness, ophthalmoplegia, soft tissue necrosis, facial palsy, seizures, and anaphylaxis (to the intravenous contrast) have been reported in up to 6% of patients (Vokes, et al., 2004).

Complications of Disease

Epistaxis in the setting of head injury, whether severe or mild and repetitive, should alert to the possibility of other complications.

Cerebrospinal fluid leak: Suspect in case of *skull base fractures* (Fig. 9.4).

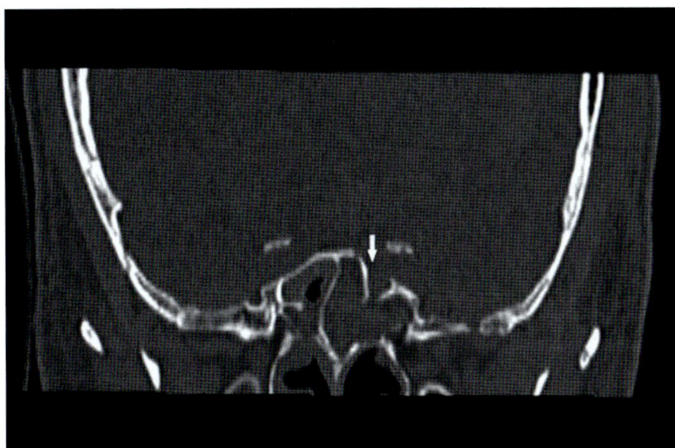

Fig. 9.4: Traumatic sphenoid fracture associated to CSF leak, caused by an altitude fall. White arrow shows the fracture in the left sphenoid roof.

Post-traumatic pseudoaneurysm: Pseudoaneurysms that present with epistaxis usually arise from the cavernous segment of the internal carotid artery or from the maxillary artery or its branches (e.g. SPA).

Epistaxis due to pseudoaneurysm rupture usually present as delayed post-traumatic bleeding. Most episodes occur within days to few weeks after the trauma, but hemorrhage can be delayed by months or years. Initial episodes of epistaxis may not be particularly impressive, but recur with increasing severity that can lead to rapid exsanguination.

Depending on their location, bony fractures on CT may increase suspicion of pseudoaneurysm formation after trauma (sphenoid sinus, sella turcica, and orbital apex). However, pseudoaneurysms may form in the absence of bony defects.

Angiography is the gold standard assessment and allows endovascular treatment. Initial angiograms may have a normal appearance and should thus be repeated within 6–8 weeks.

Hemostasis Alterations

Diagnostic Summary

Drugs
- Antiaggregants (e.g. aspirin, *clopidogrel*)
- Anticoagulants (e.g. warfarin, heparin)
- Complementary and alternative medicine (e.g. garlic, ginkgo biloba, ginseng)

Hematologic diseases
- Platelet disorders
  - Decreased production (e.g. leukemia, myelodysplastic syndrome)
  - Increased destruction (e.g. chemotherapy, immune thrombocytopenic purpura)
  - Abnormal function (e.g. Von Willebrand disease)
- Coagulation disorders
  - Hemophilias

Other diseases
- Chronic liver disease
- Chronic kidney disease

Clinical Features

Troublesome bleeding which is difficult to control despite adequate tamponade measures.

History, Examination, and Investigations

Ask family history of any bleeding disorder. Most patients taking *complementary and alternative medicine* (CAM) do not volunteer this information unless specifically asked.

Clotting screen and a full blood count (hemoglobin, platelet count, international normalized ratio, and activated partial thromboplastin time): Routine screening tests are not required for patients with minor bleeding, or those without a relevant history (e.g. those taking anticoagulants). Even when testing is performed selectively, the results are frequently normal (Awan, Iqbal and Imam, 2008). If an hematologic disease is suspected on the grounds of history and/or laboratory screening, involvement of the hematology team is helpful.

Patients with *chronic liver* disease (CLD) or *chronic renal failure* who present in the emergency room with epistaxis require routine screening tests, and liver or renal functional tests, respectively. Interestingly, these patients may experience both bleeding diathesis and thrombotic tendencies (Dasher and Trotter, 2012; Capodanno and Angiolillo, 2012).

Preferred Treatment

The current opinion is that *antiaggregant* medications prescribed for secondary prevention of cardiovascular disease or *anticoagulant* medications (within normal therapeutic levels) should not be suspended in case of mild bleeding that has been controlled. The decision to suspend medication or reverse their effect in cases of severe life-threatening epistaxis should be made in consultation with the cardiologist or hemotologist. Options include *platelet transfusion* to revert antiaggregant medications, and *fresh frozen plasma* and *vitamin K* to revert anticoagulation.

In over-anticoagulated patients, anticoagulants can be withheld until levels fall within the therapeutic range.

A wide variety of CAMs can affect coagulation or interact with conventional medications (Shakeel, et al., 2010). Thus, it is advisable to stop all CAMs until the bleeding problem has been resolved.

Treatment Outcomes

In patients with hemostasis disorders, epistaxis tends to be a recurrent problem rather than an isolated episode.

Complications of Treatment

Suspension and reversion of antiaggregant medications or anticoagulation in patients with pre-existing cardiovascular disease because of life-threatening epistaxis may lead to severe cardiovascular complications.

Complications of Disease

Hypovolemia and hypertension associated with severe bleeding may cause cardiovascular complications in patients with pre-existing disease. Hypovolemia can also cause acute decompensation of CLD or chronic kidney disease.

Sinonasal Tumors

Epidemiology and Pathogenesis

- Tumors of the sinonasal tract, nasopharynx, and adjacent skull base are a histologically diverse group of benign and malignant neoplasms that can present with different degrees of epistaxis.
- *Juvenile nasopharyngeal angiofibroma*: It is a rare benign vascular tumor that only affects males in their adolescence (an androgen related pathophysiological process is postulated) and is characterized by severe epistaxis. It accounts for 0.5% of all head and neck tumors and diagnosis is usually made during the second and third decades of life.
- Sinonasal malignant tumors account for 1% of all malignancies and 3–5% of all head and neck malignancies. Overall 75% of them occur in persons older than 50 years.

Clinical Features

Patients with sinonasal neoplasms usually present with unilateral (or at least asymmetric) symptoms. Most common symptoms are a combination of nasal obstruction, rhinorrhea, and recurrent unilateral epistaxis. Other symptoms include postnasal drip, facial pressure, headaches, and hyposmia.

Anterior rhinoscopy may reveal a mass, but nasal endoscopy is essential to view the middle meatus and postnasal space.

Advanced lesions may produce proptosis, ophthalmoplegia, facial paresthesia, and facial swelling.

Investigations

All recurrent unilateral epistaxes warrant an endoscopic evaluation of the nasal cavity and if necessary relevant imaging.

Endoscopic evaluation should be considered in patients with epistaxis who do not have an obvious site for bleeding on anterior rhinoscopy. Low threshold to decide performing it in male adolescents is recommended to rule out juvenile nasopharyngeal angiofibroma.

Computed tomography: Is often the initial imaging study performed to try and exclude the diagnosis of a tumor. It useful to determine bone erosion and is helpful in planning surgical treatment.

Magnetic resonance imaging: Is the radiological modality of choice to evaluate orbital and intracranial ivolvement. It is useful in differentiating secretions from tumor.

Biopsy of the will allow histopathologic diagnosis necessary to plan definitive reatment.

Juvenile nasopharyngeal angiofibroma are an exception as biopsy of the tumor tumor can lead to significant bleeding and is not generally necessary initially as the history and imaging should suggest the diagnosis.

Vascular Malformations

Hereditary Hemorrhagic Telangiectasia

Epidemiology and Pathogenesis

- Hereditary hemorrhagic telangiectasia (HHT), also called *Rendu-Osler-Weber syndrome*, is an autosomal dominant disorder of the development of the vasculature, characterized by the presence of multiple *arteriovenous malformations* (AVMs). Small AVMs are called telangiectases.
- It affects approximately 1 in 5,000 people, although regional variations exist.
- Affected individuals are frequently not diagnosed.
- Mutations in at least five genes are thought to result in HHT, although two frequently affected genes (ENG and ACVRL1/ALK1) are responsible for approximately 85% of cases.
- It has an age-related penetrance with increased manifestations usually developing over a lifetime. Observable manifestations can be subtle even well into adulthood.
- Arteriovenous malformations are located in characteristic sites:
  - Mucocutaneous: lips, tongue, nasal mucosa, and fingers.
  - Visceral: pulmonary, cerebral, hepatic, gastrointestinal, and spinal.

Clinical Features

Nearly all patients with hereditary hemorrhagic telangiectasia (HHT) eventually develop recurrent epistaxis. Bleeding episodes usually begin during adolescence, although the age of onset ranges from infancy to adulthood.

Nosebleeds can vary greatly in frequency and magnitude, from a couple of drops that collect within the nasal cavity to gushing, and from infrequent episodes to several per day.

As the *arteriovenous malformations* (AVMs) have thin walls and are close to the mucosal surface, bleeding episodes are often spontaneous or secondary to minimal trauma. As the vessel walls lack contractile elements, bleeding from them can be brisk and difficult to control.

Nearly all patients with HHT eventually develop telangiectases. Characteristically they are punctuate, pink to red in color, pinpoint to pinhead in size, and blanchable with pressure (Fig. 9.5). Often they are only few and quite subtle. Differential diagnosis of telangiectases includes those of CLD (spider naevi) and of elderly in sun-exposed areas.

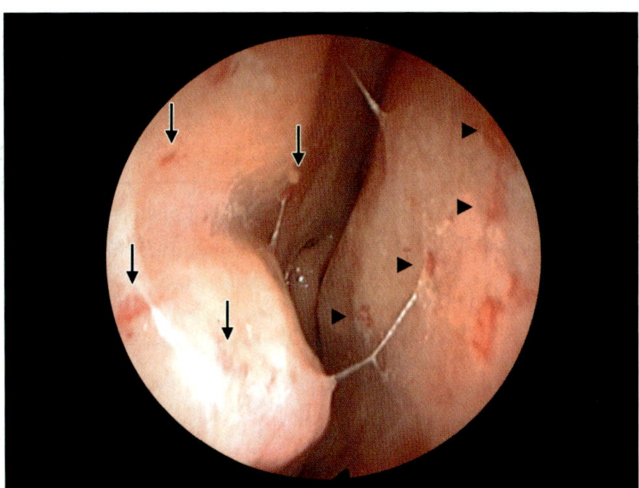

Fig. 9.5: Characteristic nasal mucosa telangiectases located in the lateral nasal wall (arrows) and septum (arrowheads) in a patient with HHT (right nasal cavity).

Investigations

The diagnosis of HHT is clinical and consensus diagnostic criteria (*Curaçao criteria*) have been described (Shovlin, et al., 2000). These include epistaxis (spontaneous and recurrent), telangiectasia (lips, oral cavity, nose, and fingers), visceral lesions, and family history (first-degree relative). The HHT diagnosis is definite if three criteria are present. With only two criteria, the diagnosis should be recorded as possible or suspected. In children, as the signs and symptoms are usually discrete or absent, the diagnosis is made by genetic testing when suspected (e.g. child of a HHT patient).

Endoscopy (upper/lower) is used to detect gastrointestinal telangiectases.

Imaging studies are used to screen for visceral AVMs.

Preferred Treatment

A graduated treatment plan is recommended (Faughnan, et al., 2011).

1. Humidification and lubrication
2. Endonasal laser therapy
3. Surgical options include *septal dermoplasty* or closure of the nasal cavity (*Young's procedure*).

Acute episodes of epistaxis in patients with HHT often require packing. Using products that are dissolvable or have a low likelihood of causing trauma on removal (e.g. lubricated low-pressure pneumatic packing) is preferred. Estrogen creams have been used with variable results.

Treatment Outcomes

Invariably, bleeding episodes recur at some point following treatment due to reformation of telangiectases (Sautter and Smith, 2012).

Nasal closure results appear to offer the best long-term control.

Complications of Treatment

- Septal perforation
- Chronic crusting from septal dermoplasty
- Complete nasal obstruction requiring obligatory mouth breathing, and loss of olfaction (Young's procedure).

Complications of Disease

- Iron deficiency anemia, sometimes requiring blood transfusion
- Gastrointestinal bleeding
- Cerebrovascular accidents: due to bleeding from cerebral AVMs or venous emboli through right to left shunting from pulmonary AVMs (more frequent)
- Increased cardiac output from hepatic and pulmonary AVMs

- Desaturation of arterial blood (right to left shunting from pulmonary AVMs)
- Pulmonary hypertension.

REFERENCES

Awan, M.S., Iqbal, M. and Imam, S.Z., 2008. Epistaxis: when are coagulation studies justified? *Emergency Medicine Journal*, 25, pp. 156-7.

Barnes, M.L., Spielmann, P.M. and White, P.S., 2012. Epistaxis: a contemporary evidence based approach. *Otolaryngologic Clinics of North America*, 45, pp. 1005-17.

Capodanno, D. and Angiolillo, D.J., 2012. Antithrombotic therapy in patients with chronic kidney disease. *Circulation*, 125, pp. 2649-61.

Dasher, K. and Trotter, J.F., 2012. Intensive care unit management of liver-related coagulation disorders. *Critical Care Clinics*, 28, pp. 389-98.

Diamantopoulos, I.I. and Jones, N.S., 2001. The investigation of nasal septal perforations and ulcers. *The Journal of Laryngology and Otology*, 115, pp. 541-4.

Elden, L., Reinders, M. and Witmer, C., 2012. Predictors of bleeding disorders in children with epistaxis: value of preoperative tests and clinical screening. *International Journal of Pediatric Otorhinolaryngology*, 76, pp. 767-71.

Faughnan, M.E., Palda, V.A., Garcia-Tsao, G., Geisthoff, U.W., McDonald, J., Proctor, D.D., Spears, J., Brown, D.H., Buscarini, E., Chesnutt, M.S., Cottin, V., Ganguly, A., Gossage, J.R., Guttmacher, A.E., Hyland, R.H., Kennedy, S.J., Korzenik, J., Mager, J.J., Ozanne, A.P., Piccirillo, J.F., Picus, D., Plauchu, H., Porteous, M.E., Pyeritz, R.E., Ross, D.A., Sabba, C., Swanson, K., Terry, P., Wallace, M.C., Westermann, C.J., White, R.I., Young, L.H. and Zarrabeitia, R.; HHT Foundation International--Guidelines Working Group., 2011. International guidelines for the diagnosis and management of hereditary haemorrhagic telangiectasia. *Journal of Medical Genetics*, 48, pp. 73-87.

Kim, S.W. and Rhee, C.S., 2012. Nasal septal perforation repair: predictive factors and systematic review of the literature. *Current Opinion in Otolaryngology and Head and Neck Surgery*, 20, pp. 58-65.

Lanier, B., Kai, G., Marple, B. and Wall, G.M., 2007. Pathophysiology and progression of nasal septal perforation. *Annals of Allergy, Asthma and Immunology*, 99, pp. 473-9.

McIntosh, N., Mok, J.Y. and Margerison, A., 2007. Epidemiology of oronasal hemorrhage in the first 2 years of life: implications for child protection. *Pediatrics*, 120, pp. 1074-8.

Murray, A. and McGarry, G.W., 2000. The clinical value of septal perforation biopsy. *Clinical Otolaryngology and Allied Sciences*, 25, pp. 107-9.

Pallin, D.J., Chng, Y.M., McKay, M.P., Emond, J.A., Pelletier, A.J. and Camargo, C.A., Jr., 2005. Epidemiology of epistaxis in US emergency departments, 1992 to 2001. *Annals of Emergency Medicine*, 46, pp. 77-81.

Qureishi, A. and Burton, M.J., 2012. Interventions for recurrent idiopathic epistaxis (nosebleeds) in children. *Cochrane Database of Systematic Reviews*, 9. p. CD004461.

Sautter, N.B. and Smith, T.L., 2012. Hereditary hemorrhagic telangiectasia-related epistaxis: innovations in understanding and management. *International Forum of Allergy and Rhinology*, 2, pp. 422-31.

Shakeel, M., Trinidade, A., McCluney, N. and Clive, B., 2010. Complementary and alternative medicine in epistaxis: a point worth considering during the patient's history. *European Journal of Emergency Medicine*, 17, pp. 17-9.

Shovlin, C.L., Guttmacher, A.E., Buscarini, E., Faughnan, M.E., Hyland, R.H., Westermann, C.J., Kjeldsen, A.D. and Plauchu, H., 2000. Diagnostic criteria for hereditary hemorrhagic telangiectasia (Rendu-Osler-Weber syndrome). *American Journal of Medical Genetics*, 91, pp. 66-7.

Vokes, D.E., McIvor, N.P., Wattie, W.J., Chaplin, J.M. and Morton, R.P., 2004. Endovascular treatment of epistaxis. *ANZ Journal of Surgery*, 74, pp. 751-3.

Walker, T.W., Macfarlane, T.V. and McGarry, G.W., 2007. The epidemiology and chronobiology of epistaxis: an investigation of Scottish hospital admissions 1995-2004. *Clinical Otolaryngology*, 32(5), pp. 361-5.

Woo, H.J., Bai, C.H., Song, S.Y. and Kim, Y.D., 2008. Intracranial placement of a Foley catheter: a rare complication. *Otolaryngology—Head and Neck Surgery*, 138, pp. 115-6.

10 Sleep-Disordered Breathing

Simon Carney, Stuart MacKay

Chapter Overview

Pearls and Pitfalls

Pearls

- The commonest cause of sleep-disordered breathing in children is adenotonsillar hypertrophy, but while examining one should always keep in mind congenital abnormalities causing sleep-disordered breathing (SDB).
- Parental history to suspect obstructive sleep apnea (OSA) in children is very important.
- Sleep study is important in diagnosis, especially when congenital abnormalities are suspected to be the cause of the obstruction.
- Obstructive sleep apnea in adults is often multifactorial and multilevel.
- Obesity is a significant cause of SDB/OSA and would need to be addressed to achieve good results in management of these cases.
- Epworth Sleepiness Score (≥10 is abnormal).
- Polysomnography is the investigation of choice for adult OSA.
- Continuous positive airway pressure remains the treatment of choice for adult sleep apnea.

Pitfalls

- Although easy to perform, overnight oximetry has a very high false negative rate.
- Addressing only one problem in adults to treat OSA often does not yield good outcome.

10.1 PEDIATRIC SNORING AND SLEEP-DISORDERED BREATHING

Epidemiology and Pathogenesis

Adenotonsillar hypertrophy: Up to 11% of all children will have some form of snoring or sleep-disordered breathing as a result of adenotonsillar hypertrophy. This may be mild or may progress toward severe obstructive sleep apnea (OSA) with failure to thrive, behavioral problems, or neurocognitive defects.

Congenital obstruction: This is common in patients with Down syndrome and other congenital forms of craniofacial abnormalities (e.g. Pierre-Robin syndrome).

Clinical Features

Features in clinical history:

- Snoring, with or without sleep apnea (maternal concern "may be obstructing at night")
- Snoring and/or obstruction may be positional or worse with upper respiratory tract infections (URTIs)

- Child may wake frequently during the night
- Restless, sweaty sleep
- Nocturnal enuresis
- Unrefreshed awakening
- Poor concentration and behavior
- Hyperactivity
- Choking on food in some cases

Typical findings on examination:

- Inspect the oropharynx paying particular attention to the size of the tonsils and position of the palate.
- If possible, examine the adenoidal pad (consider a transoral 70° endoscope or pediatric transnasal 0° or flexible endoscope). On occasion, an adenoid X-ray may be appropriate, although this will rarely change management decisions.
- Assess any tongue abnormalities such as macroglossia or lymphangioma.
- Examine the general facies for signs of fatigue (brown rings around the eyes, or general adenoidal facies).
- Examine the craniofacial pyramid for signs of mandibular and/or maxillary hypoplasia.
- High, narrow arch palate
- Malocclusion overbite
- Allergic nose/nasal features including obstructing inferior turbinates.

Investigations

Pediatric polysomnography (PSG): Sleep studies are often limited in availability due to long waiting lists, but can be important in diagnosis, especially when congenital abnormalities are suspected to be the cause of the obstruction. They are particularly useful in children less than 2 years old, cases of parental uncertainty, and for children with syndromes, neurologic conditions, or in residual symptoms after surgery.

Overnight oximetry: Although easy to perform, this investigation has a very high false negative rate. Significant desaturation is uncommon until severe obstructive symptoms develop in children. Most cases of sleep-disordered breathing or mild OSA will be missed with overnight oximetry due to its high specificity and low sensitivity.

Adenoidal X-ray: If the tonsils are small and there is doubt about the size of the adenoids, this may help in management in selected cases. If the tonsils are large and surgery is proposed, then an adenoidal X-ray probably has limited, if any, clinical value (Flowchart 10.1).

Preferred Treatment

- Total adenotonsillectomy
- Subtotal tonsillar reduction with adenoidectomy. This is frequently performed in Scandinavia and North America for children with little or no tonsillitis. There is emerging evidence that children undergoing subtotal tonsil surgery have less postoperative pain with a reduced secondary hemorrhage risk. Quality-of-life studies in Australia have shown equal benefit to full adenotonsillectomy, although a prospective randomized control trial has yet to be performed.
- Tongue reduction in selected cases of macroglossia
- Craniofacial surgery
- Tracheostomy in exceptional cases
- Continuous positive airway pressure (CPAP) in some cases with residual symptoms after adenotonsillectomy or severe disease.
- Rapid maxillary expansion or orthognathic treatment in some cases of high, narrow arch palate.

Treatment Outcomes

The vast majority of children will achieve significant improvement with adenotonsillar surgery. For patients with a congenital cause for their obstruction, outcomes from craniofacial surgery are less effective, but can make a significant difference in selected cases. For severe cases of pediatric sleep apnea, a tracheostomy may be life saving.

10.2 ADULT SLEEP-DISORDERED BREATHING

Epidemiology and Pathogenesis

With the global epidemic of obesity, OSA now affects significantly more adults than in previous decades. There is an increased prevalence in westernized countries such as the United States, Northern Europe, and Australia/New Zealand. It is estimated that 4–24% of men and 2–9% of women have OSA. It typically presents between the ages of 40 and 60 and increases with age. However, not all obese people have OSA and in adults etiology is often multifactorial and multilevel, in what is considered a heterogeneous disorder.

Clinical Features

Features in clinical history:

- Snoring that may be positional and made worse after alcohol or fatigue.

Flowchart 10.1: Pediatric sleep-disordered breathing.

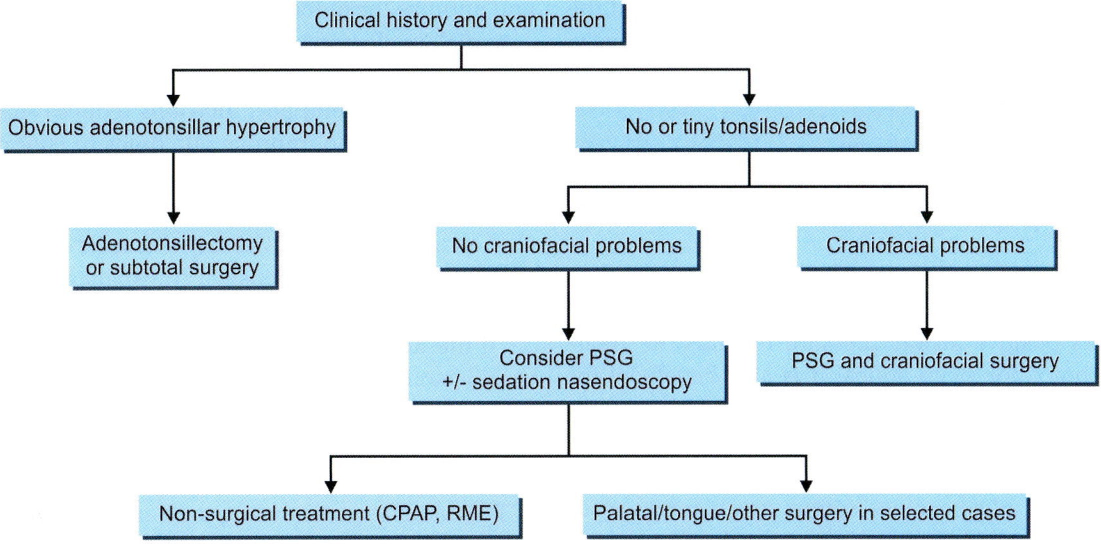

- Obstruction may be witnessed by a partner or spouse, but is not always noticed.
- Daytime fatigue/tiredness.
- Daytime sleepiness with an increase in Epworth Sleepiness Score (≥10 is abnormal).
- Low libido, impotence, and poor daytime performance/concentration.

Typical findings on examination:

- Examine the nasal cavity for signs of nasal valve collapse, septal deviation, turbinate hypertrophy, or nasal polyps. In adults, adenoidal hypertrophy can still occur.
- Examination of the palate and tonsils using the Friedman's Grading System:

  Examine the tongue
    Grade I: tonsil pillars and entire uvula visible
    Grade IIa: uvula visible
    Grade IIb: most of the soft palate and base of the uvula visible
    Grade III: some of the soft palate visible
    Grade IV: only the hard palate visible
- Flexible nasendoscopy in the erect and supine position should be performed. This can be combined with Muller's maneuver (simulated snoring on inspiration) and Woodson's hypotonic method (gentle inspiration then forced expiration once lung volume has been depleted); this will assess the degree of collapse of the retropalatal and retrolingual segments. The lingual tonsil should be assessed and structural airway abnormalities excluded.
- A jaw thrust (modified Esmarch) maneuver may be performed during the above to assess the reversibility of any retrolingual collapse and may predict response to mandibular advancement splints (MAS).
- Sleep Nasendoscopy, as circumstances warrant.

Investigations

Polysomnography is the investigation of choice: This is an overnight investigation, optimally performed in a dedicated Sleep Lab with video recording of sleep and a technician present. Airflow, electrocardiography, electroencephalography, electromyography, and electro-occulography are all measured. Chest wall movements by thermistor or transducer, capnometer CO_2, SpO_2, body position, and heart rate are all measured (oral thermistor and nasal pressure transducers are preferred). Apnea is defined as the total cessation of airflow for 10 seconds or more. The definition of a hypopnea is variable, dependent upon the type of criteria used for scoring the sleep study.

The respiratory disturbance index is defined as the number of apneas/hypopneas per hour of sleep and can also be referred to as the apnea–hypopnea index (AHI) OR may be AHI + respiratory effort-related arousals. Different staging systems are used to grade the AHI. Traditionally, AHI (Chicago) criteria were used and these were changed to the AHI (recommended) criteria in 2004. The AHI (alternate) criteria are also considered to be appropriate and it is these criteria that have been recommended by the Australian and New Zealand Sleep Association. With the increased use of thermistors, hypopneas are perhaps now documented at a greater rate than previous and the cut-off for diagnosing OSA has been adjusted accordingly.

Current interpretation of AHI (alternate) grading is generally regarded as follows:

- Mild sleep apnea: AHI 15–30
- Moderate sleep apnea: 30–45
- Severe sleep apnea: AHI 45+

Preferred Treatment

Continuous positive airway pressure remains the treatment of choice for sleep apnea. It is also beneficial for patients who snore, but may be perhaps less tolerated in patients who are not sleepy and do not have other physical symptoms and signs of OSA (Flowchart 10.2).

Mandibular advancement splints are helpful, especially in patients with isolated retrolingual collapse and normal dentition or when "coupling" advances both the retrolingual and retropalatal airway. If these are well tolerated, then they can be a simple and cost-effective way of managing simple snoring or sleep apnea. Patients need formal fitting and follow-up by expert dentist. Temporomandibular joint problems are common with prolonged use of MAS.

Lifestyle management: Weight loss, avoidance of the supine position through devices such as pillows, pillow positioning in the bed, tennis ball in a pyjama jacket, or buzz-pod vibration device may be effective in discouraging supine sleep. Avoidance of alcohol late at night and good sleep hygiene may also be beneficial.

Surgical treatment: Surgical treatment should only be considered once CPAP +/- MAS, and lifestyle measures have all been addressed, have failed, or been poorly tolerated by the patient.

For both simple snoring and OSA, it is important that comprehensive assessment of the airway for potential multilevel collapse has been performed. This can be via the airway maneuvers described above or sedation nasendoscopy (if there is any doubt as to the site of obstruction).

If the nose is blocked, nasal treatment (in the form of nasal steroids, antihistamines or "pre-phase" nasal surgery) should be performed so that the patient has a clear nasal airway. Devices and lifestyle modifications can then be tried a second time. In adults, tonsillectomy should be performed wherever tonsils remain. In patients with grade 3 or 4 tonsils, this may be all that is required to improve retropalatal obstruction. In most patients with smaller tonsils, a modified uvulopalatopharyngoplasty (mod-UPPP) should be performed. Modern modifications of UPPP address the lateral velopharyngeal ports and have been shown to reduce postoperative side effects and improve the outcomes of sleep surgery. In mod-UPPP, a partial uvulectomy or uvulopalatal flap may be performed at the same time. Mucosal preservation between the uvula and lateral port incisions reduces scarring and has been shown to improve outcomes in cohort studies.

In selected patients with a significantly posterior palate, particularly with a reduced anteroposterior dimension on assessment, or who fail after mod-UPPP with persistent retropalatal collapse, a transpalatal advancement procedure can be considered.

If the lingual tonsils are hypertrophic, then a lingual tonsillectomy can be performed using suction diathermy, argon, radiofrequency, or coblation devices. For patients with significant retrolingual collapse, reduction of the tongue bulk using either coblation tongue channeling (CTC), radiofrequency using the Somnus system, or other devices may be effective. The evidence currently favors coblation as the treatment of choice for tongue channeling. For patients with extremely large tongues or who have failed more conservative treatments, some form of midline glossectomy or submucosal lingualplasty may then be required.

Geniotubercle advancement, hyoid suspension, and hyoid advancement have largely fallen out of favor, but still remain options in selected cases. These procedures are usually reserved for patients who have failed both conservative and aggressive soft-tissue surgery (with or without palatal advancement).

For patients with marked syndromic or cephalometric abnormalities, maxillofacial surgery can provide superior outcomes in selected cases and soft tissue surgery should be regarded as having an adjunct or salvage role for most of these complex cases.

Complications of the Disease

Moderate to severe OSA is associated with significant cardiovascular morbidity and mortality when untreated. In well-designed cohort studies, patients undergoing sleep surgery demonstrated significant reduction in both morbidity and mortality—in addition to a reduction in motor vehicle accident risk and improvement in their quality of life.

Complications of Surgery

Upper airway surgery is painful and carries risk. Hemorrhage, globus pharyngeus, dysarthria, dysphagia, and dysgeusia are all symptoms experienced by a small proportion of patients. Hypernasal speech may be a complication if palatal surgery is too aggressive and nasopharyngeal

Flowchart 10.2: Adult sleep disorders.

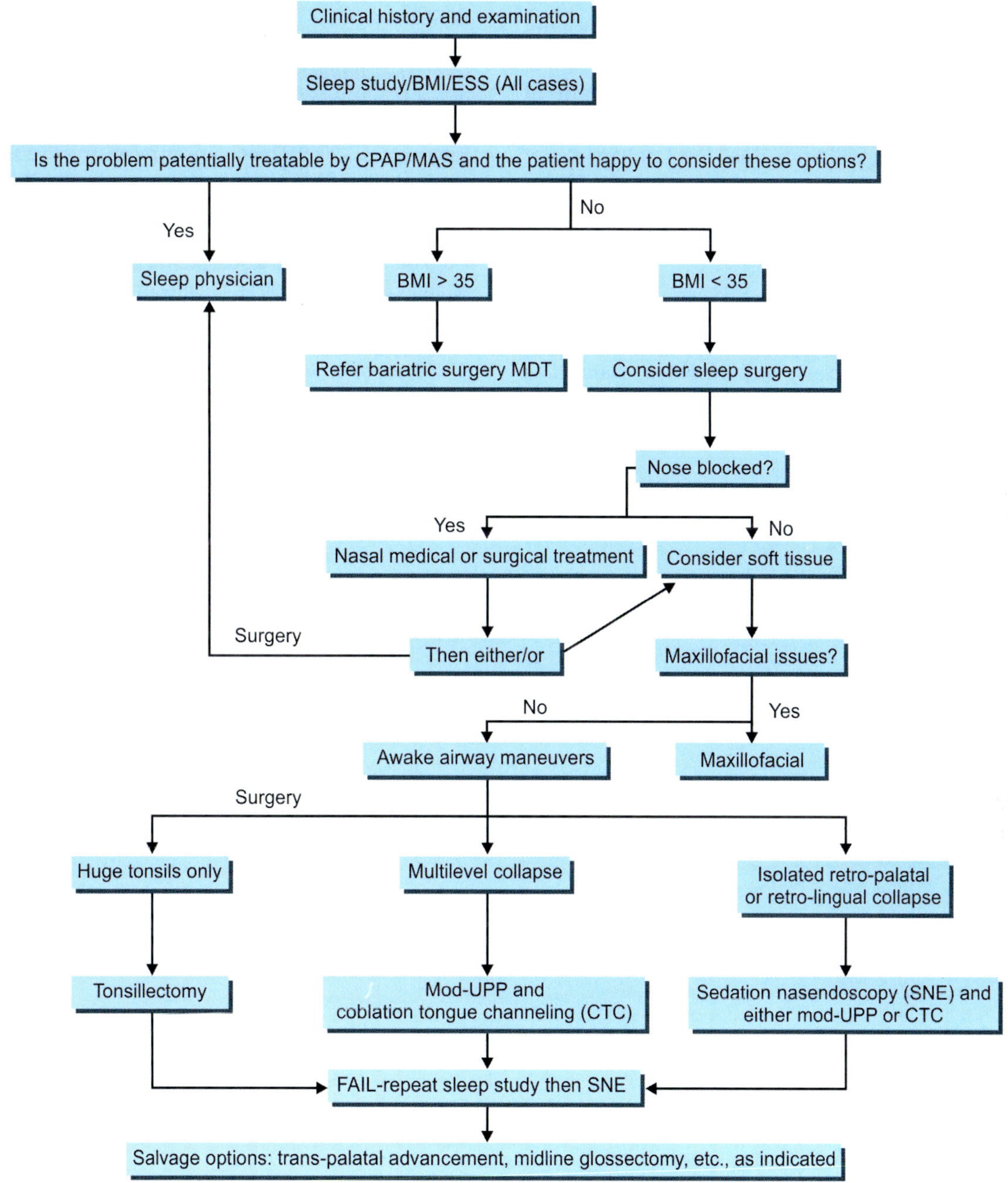

regurgitation can occur during swallowing. Severe and life-threatening hemorrhage from the lingual arteries or the palate is rare, but can occur. Airway obstruction immediately following surgery is a risk and intravenous steroid should always be given at the time of sleep surgery. Patients should be monitored in a high dependency unit or intensive care unit setting the night following surgery and airway support given where necessary. Rarely, tracheostomy can be considered to ensure safe upper airway surgery. Patients should be advised to stay close to an ENT emergency center for a minimum of 10 days following surgery.

10.3 TIPS AND PEARLS

- Surgery to the adenoids and tonsils will resolve most cases of pediatric SDB.
- Reserve pediatric PSG for complex cases or children who fail after Ts/Adenotonsillectomy.

- Always perform a sleep study on adult snorers/sleep apneic patients.
- If the nose is blocked, clear the nose and reassess the patient/retry CPAP.
- Awake airway maneuvers will allow assessment of retropalatal and retrolingual collapse.
- Most adult patients will have dual-level collapse.
- Mod UPPP and CTC now have level 2 evidence as a treatment for adult SDB.

REFERENCES

Mackay, S.G., Carney, A.S., Woods, C., Antic, N., McEvoy, R.D., Chia, M., Sands, T., Jones, A., Hobson, J. and Robinson, S., 2013. Modified uvulopalatopharyngoplasty and coblation channelling of the tongue for obstructive sleep apnoea: a multi-centre Australian trial. *Journal of Clinical Sleep Medicine*, 9(2), pp. 117-21.

Pang, K.P., Rotenberg, B.W. and Woodson, B.T., 2013. *Advanced surgical techniques in snoring and obstructive sleep apnoea.* Plural Publishing. San Diego, California.

Robinson, S., Chia, M., Carney, A.S., Chawla, S., Harris, P. and Esterman, A., 2009. Upper airway reconstructive surgery long term quality-of-life outcomes compared with CPAP for adult obstructive sleep apnoea. *Otolaryngology—Head and Neck Surgery*, 141, pp. 257-63.

Wood, J.M., Harris, P.K., Woods, C.M., McLean, S.C., Easterman, A. and Carney, A.S., 2011. Quality of life following surgery for sleep disordered breathing: subtotal reduction adenotonsillectomy vs total adenotonsillectomy in Australian children. *ANZ Journal of Surgery*, 81, pp. 340-4.

Functional and Aesthetic Analysis of the Nose

11

Pietro Palma, Iman Khodaei, Irina Vasilenko

Chapter Overview

Pearls and Pitfalls

Pearls

- Analysis comes before surgery.
- Taking standard, high-quality photographs is a sine-qua-non.
- Palpation is paramount as rhinoplasty is a tactile surgical procedure.
- Create a tailor-made operative game plan for each patient.
- Think nasal function. Operate with end aesthetic results in mind.

Pitfalls

- Not every patient asking for rhinoplasty is a good candidate for rhinoplasty.
- Overlooking nasal function.
- Not incorporating morphing into the preoperative workup.
- Telling patients that his/her surgery will be simple and 100% successful.
- "Selling" the operation.

11.1 NOSE—A COMPLEX ORGAN

The human nose performs a central role in the processing and evaluation of inspired air. It provides a first line of defense against air-borne infections, creates a database of endless number of odors, and serves as a key element in facial beauty, racial characteristics, social status, and fashion.

Surgical intervention in such a complex organ requires an in-depth knowledge of physiology, pathology, functional assessment, facial analysis, aesthetics, patient psychology, and surgical techniques. Faced with this difficult task and given the restraints placed on our clinical time and availability, the astute surgeon needs to adopt a systematic approach to evaluate the patient.

11.2 FIVE BUILDING BLOCKS OF PREOPERATIVE WORKUP

To avoid the highly undesirable outcome of an unsatisfied patient and surgeon, pay particular attention to the five building blocks of preoperative rhinoplasty planning: the medical aspects of rhinological disease, patient's psychological state, clinical assessment, functional evaluation, and aesthetic facial analysis.

The proper understanding of these highly relevant aspects will allow the surgeon to create a tailor-made, unique surgical game plan for each patient.

Medical Rhinology

A full description of the medical treatment of rhinological disease is beyond the scope of this chapter. However, the surgeon should correctly diagnose and optimize the treatment of nasal pathology before any cosmetic surgery is considered. There are two good reasons for this approach: first, medical treatment is often a long-term process, which may have to be temporarily interrupted for surgery. This can result in exacerbation of symptoms just when the patient is trying to recover from rhinoplasty. Second, an untreated nose may experience an acute exacerbation, such as seasonal allergic rhinitis in the postoperative period. The patient may then attribute these symptoms to surgery, rather than the natural cycle of rhinitis. Combining endoscopic sinus surgery with cosmetic surgery is now practiced safely in many centers and can alleviate the patient's symptoms in one sitting (Palma and Castelnuovo, 2010). Timing cosmetic procedures with medical treatment is the essence of success for these patients.

Psychological Assessment of a Patient

Surgeons receive very little education in the intricacies of managing psychological disorders. This fact is reflected in the relative paucity of articles on this subject.

Despite the cost of rhinoplasty and the current economic conditions, patients still seek to change their noses, sometimes by a matter of millimeters, for a variety of reasons (Rankin, et al., 1998; Sarwer, et al., 1998; Haraldsson, 1999; Sperry, et al., 2009). Many patients are lumbered with negative comments from their teenage years, and others are driven by dissatisfaction of their physical appearance. Although many people have cosmetic deformities, only a minority seek surgery. Although the exact motivation for undergoing surgery may not always be clear, the increasing acceptability of cosmetic procedures and the role of the media in promoting beauty through the "celebrity" culture cannot be ignored.

The patient and the surgeon both expect that an improvement in the physical appearance of the nose will help boost the patient's self-confidence and reduce social anxiety. In effect, the surgeon performs surgery to improve the patient's psyche (Hay, 1970; Robin, et al., 1988; Pruzinski and Edgerton, 1990; Cole, et al., 1994; Klassen, et al., 1996; Sheard et al., 1996; Rankin, et al., 1998; Ercolani, et al., 1999). Interestingly, when a patient desires to improve both the function and the shape of the nose, it is the latter element that leads to greater satisfaction. This happens regardless of the severity of deformity. In most patients, the desire for change, or the positive effect of rhinoplasty on others, acts as a main psychological spur. The difference between what is deemed acceptable in a particular culture or society and the patient's own unique physical features is of great importance and may explain the growth in rhinoplasty in many countries.

The timing for choosing cosmetic rhinoplasty is a little more difficult to ascertain but may be related to "doers" who seek to improve many aspects of their lives, including their appearance at a particular point in time or a general decrease in self-esteem with age (Hay and Heather, 1973; Edgerton and Langman, 1982; Shulman and Westreich, 1983; Goin and Goin, 1987; Napoleon and Lewis, 1989; Dinis, Dinis and Gomes, 1998; McKiernan, et al., 2001).

Previously, many surgeons believed that patients who seek cosmetic surgery were somehow destined for psychological disease or were already at this destination. This viewpoint has been proved to be invalid (Linn and Goldman, 1949; Hill and Silver, 1950; Hay, 1970; Wright and Wright, 1975; Marcus, 1984; Robin, et al., 1988; Goin and Rees, 1991; Sarwer, et al., 1998). Contrary to the older viewpoint, the majority of cosmetic rhinoplasty patients do not suffer from psychological disease, and the benefits gained from surgery are not fleeting. However, a minority of patients suffers from serious psychological diseases, and must be identified preoperatively before a disastrous result ruins the doctor–patient relationship, and even endangers the well-being of both parties (Zahiroddin, Shafiee-kandjani and Khalighi-sigaroodi, 2008). Referring a patient to a psychiatric specialist is not common in authors' practice, but it is highly advisable in the obvious presence of warning signs.

Body Dysmorphic Disorder (BDD)

This term strikes terror into the heart of rhinoplasty surgeons, and for very good reasons. Typically, the patient is a younger adult who experiences great distress due to an altered perception of his/her self-image. In extreme cases, this can lead to dysmorphophobia (Crerand, et al., 2005). If all three answers to the following questions are positive, then BDD can be said to exist. The Diagnostic and Statistical Manual of Mental Disorders-IV criteria that aid in the screening for BDD include (Philips, 1996; 2004):

- Are you very worried about your appearance in any way?
- Does this concern preoccupy you? That is, do you think about it a lot and wish you could worry about it less? How much time do you spend thinking about it? *(Fill in body areas of concern)*.
- What effect has this preoccupation with your appearance had on your life? Has it:
    - Significantly interfered with your social life, schoolwork, job, other activities, or other aspects of your life?
    - Caused you a lot of distress?
    - Affected your family or friends?

As up to 20% of rhinoplasty patients answer "yes" to one of these questions, referral to a psychiatrist experienced in the treatment of this condition may save the patient and the doctor unnecessary suffering in the future. While patients with milder forms of BDD may be satisfied with the surgical outcome, those suffering from severe forms should be treated under psychiatric care, before any consideration of surgery is even contemplated (Phillips, 2004).

One excellent reason for deferring any decision for surgery to a second meeting is the surgeon's own emotional response to the patient. A psychiatrist (Rohrich, 1999) summarized the role of instinct into the phrase "if you cannot elicit a smile from your patient, don't operate". The acronyms of MOSES (male, over-expectant, single, eccentric, self-lover) and SYLVANA (sensible, young, listener, verbal, attractive, nose-troubles, adult) are not helpful in the first or even second clinical encounter, as these attributes may only become apparent with time. In short, if the surgeons gut feeling is that of discomfort with the patient, it is better to defer or avoid surgery. Specialist psychiatric assistance should be sought for problematic cases.

Clinical Assessment

The process of assessment starts the moment a patient walks into the office. Their general demeanor, eye contact, greeting, and conversational skills all point toward the patient's state of mind, level of medical knowledge, and possible psychopathological state.

A detailed general ENT and rhinology history is mandatory as the first step. Ideally, a validated questionnaire such as the Sinonasal Outcome Test-22 may be employed; however, most clinicians do not have the time for this process (Abdalla, Alreefy and Hopkins, 2012). Key rhinology questions for the cosmetic patient should elucidate the presence of important symptoms, such as the pattern and duration of nasal obstruction, rhinorrhea, postnasal drip, hyposmia, facial pressure or pain, and previous sinus surgery or rhinoplasty. The clinical history must be detailed enough to distinguish between the various types of facial pain and chronic rhinosinusitis, medically amendable rhinological diseases and surgically treatable conditions such as valvular insufficiency. The surgeon should recognize psychological disturbances such as anxiety, depression, and the dreaded BDD.

Nasendoscopy is a standard practice for all patients undergoing rhinoplasty as it provides excellent information on endonasal anatomy and pathology and surgically correctable diseases. Photodocumentation of these features is very helpful for long-term follow-up. In revision cases, the effect of previous surgery on reducing the cross-sectional area of the internal valve can provide a clue regarding the sensation of a blocked nose despite an otherwise normal examination.

Palpation of the nose also provides a wealth of information about the quality and thickness of the skin and soft-tissue envelope (S-STE). Very thick skin will make even the slightest error in the technical execution of rhinoplasty a visible problem. Conversely, if the S-STE is very thick, altering the bony-cartilaginous framework may not create the desired effect. Ideally, this layer should be of intermediate thickness. Simply elevating the tip of the nose can reveal caudal subluxation of the septum. The membranous septum and the lateral crura of the lower lateral cartilages (LLCs) must also be palpated for their size, shape, and resilience to pressure. The "Tip Recoil" test will show the amount of resistance offered by the tip to digital pressure. The first author (PP) utilizes an ad hoc worksheet (Fig. 11.1) to collect relevant clinical data.

Functional Evaluation

Assessment of nasal function can also be incorporated in the first consultation. Collapse of the external valve, both static and dynamic, can be demonstrated clinically and treated surgically alongside the cosmetic procedure.

Functional studies like rhinomanometry, acoustic rhinometry, and peak nasal inspiratory flow measurements may be used to objectively measure and quantify functional impairments. In some countries, these studies are more commonly performed. This is partly due to their

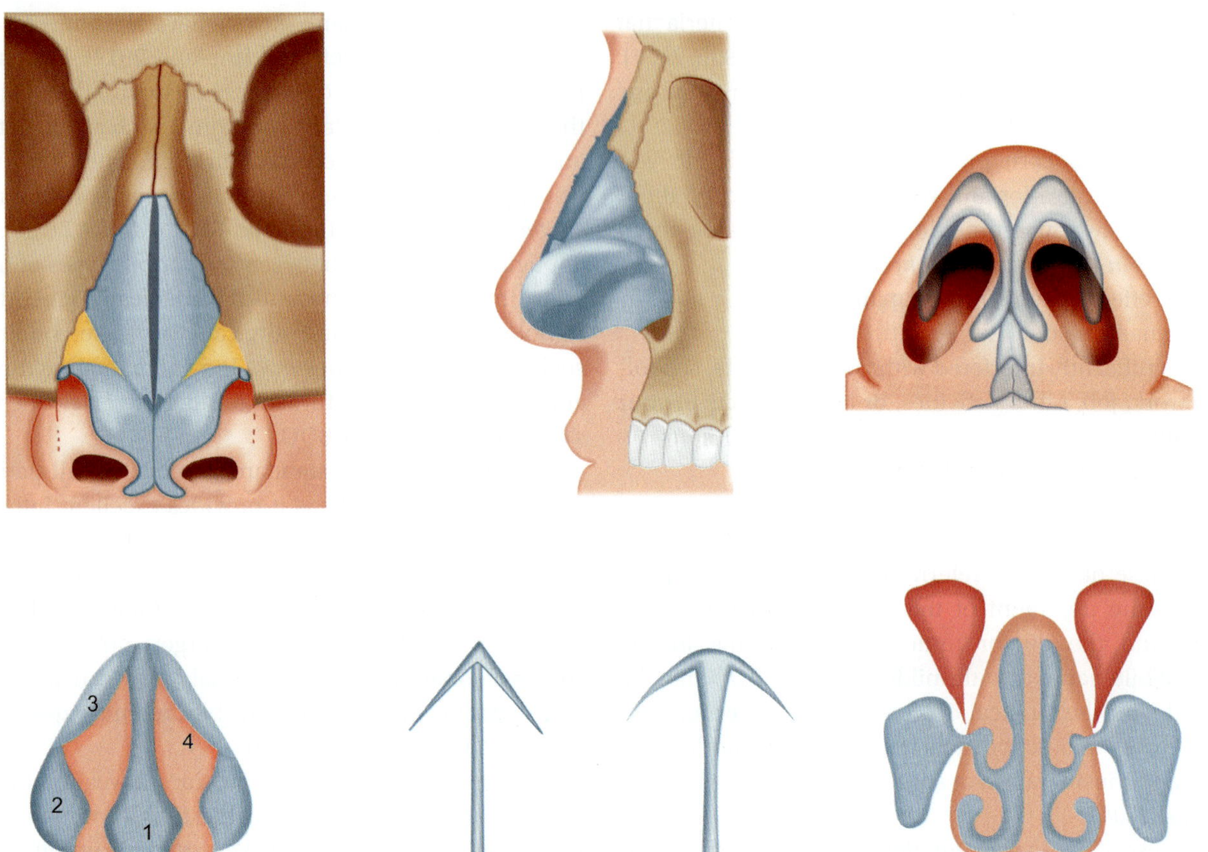

Fig. 11.1: Preoperative worksheet. (1) Nasal septum, (2) Inferior turbinate, (3) Upper lateral cartilage, (4) Internal nasal valve area.

relevance for the reimbursement of costs for the functional aspect of surgery. However, the correlation between rhinomanometric and acoustic rhinometric data and individual subjective sensation of nasal patency remains uncertain, and at present there seems to be only a limited argument for the use of rhinomanometry or acoustic rhinometry in routine rhinology practice or for quantifying surgical results. In author's practice, rhinomanometry (Fig. 11.2) is performed only in selected cases.

Furthermore, standardized tests of smell, such as the University of Pennsylvania Smell Identification Test, are now widely available and provide objective data on this increasingly important source of litigation. This test can be administered by supporting staff, and it only adds a few minutes to the overall assessment (Kimmelman, 1994).

Aesthetic Analysis

Facial analysis begins at the first encounter. The surgeon should observe the patient's face for general proportion and symmetry (Powel and Humphreys, 1984). The surgeon sits in front of the patient and shines a light directly at the midline of the nose. In a perfectly symmetrical nose, light reflects back from the center of the nose and has two areas of shadow on either side (Fig. 11.3A). The border of light and shadow demarcates two highly valuable landmarks: the brow dome line (BDL) (Palma, Khodaei and Tasman, 2011) and the nose-cheek line (NCL), both demarcating the transition between horizontal and vertical planes (Fig. 11.3B). The BDL commences at the medial head of the eyebrow, turns inferiorly and medially, and descends in parallel with its partner on the other side and ends at the dome. Superficial landmarks such as the BDLs constitute a revelation of deeper structures. A disturbance in the BDL is often associated with deviation of the septum but may also be affected by morphology of nasal bones, upper and lower cartilages, scrolls, and even the S-STE. From the frontal view, the surgeon can also appreciate the alar-columellar relationship, often described as a "gull in flight" (Fig. 11.3C). This feature depends on the orientation and the reciprocal relationships of several structures including the septum, LLCs, columella, S-STE, and previous surgery.

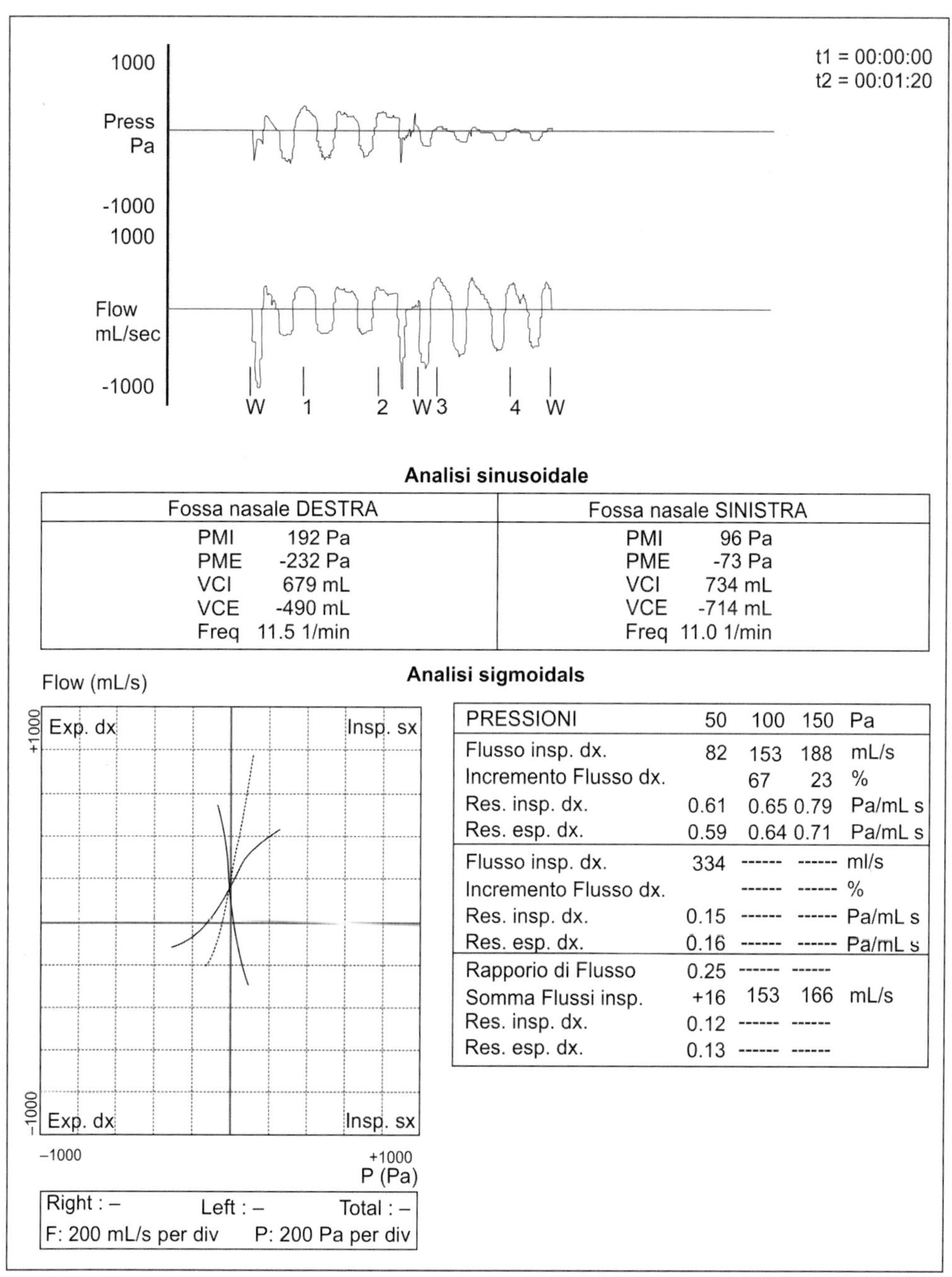

Fig. 11.2: Rhinomanometry tracing.

A simple extension of the neck will reveal shape and contour of the nasal base (Figs. 11.4A and B). Signs of previous external approach rhinoplasty such as a mid-columellar scar or sequelae of alar base surgery can be identified. *External valve collapse* may be evident when the lateral crura are cephalically malpositioned or have been excessively reduced. From the lateral view, many important landmarks such as the nasion, rhinion, point of maximal dorsal projection, anterior septal angle, rotation, projection, columellar show, nostrils axis, infratip break-point, and nasolabial junction can also be appreciated (Figs. 11.5A and B). The dorsal skin has to be thoroughly palpated to evaluate thickness and mobility of S-STE, as well as nasal framework. The surgeon should also feel for bony and cartilaginous irregularities. In revision cases, tiny spicules of bone may be palpable and represent a source of consternation for the patient, although they are not visible. The roof should be examined carefully: has

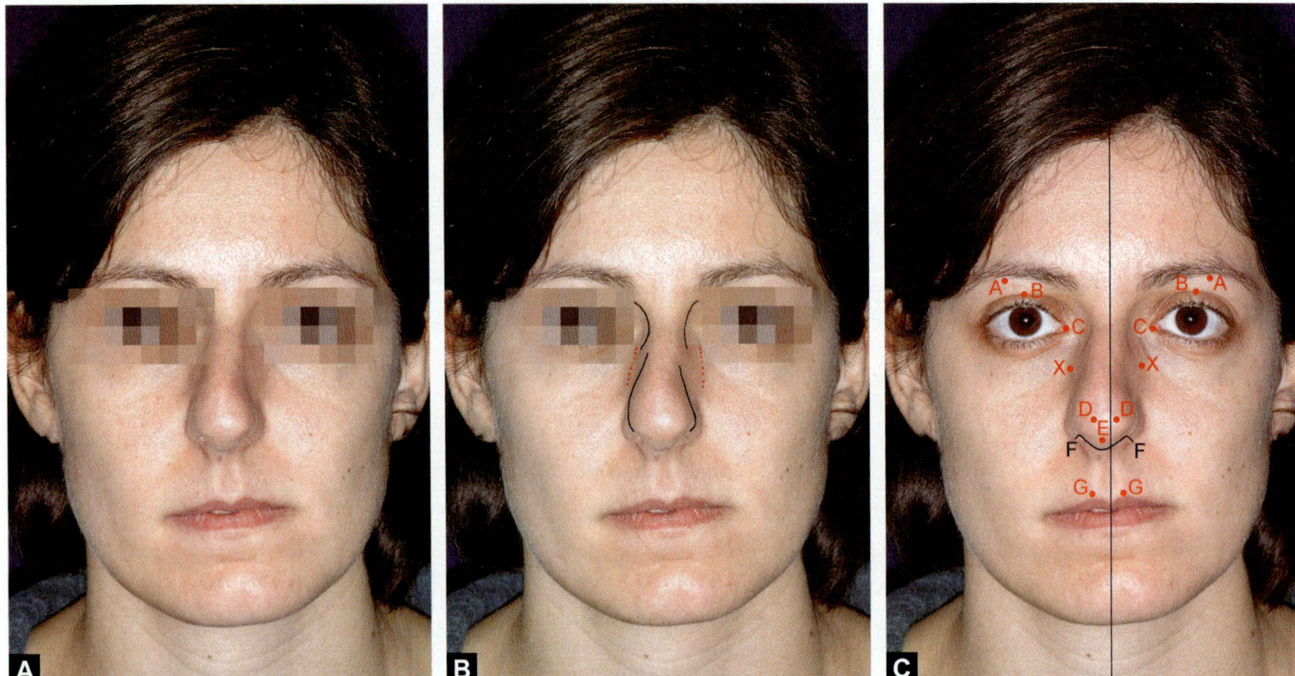

Figs. 11.3A to C: Frontal view (A) and frontal view with brow dome lines (BDLs) and nose-cheek lines (NCLs) (B). Key aesthetic landmarks on frontal view (C). Gentle downward divergence and symmetry of BDLs (black continuous lines) constitute a key feature of nasal aesthetics assessment. The NCLs (red dotted lines) provide useful information about symmetry of bony sidewalls and width of the bony base. In this actual patient, BDLs look broken, asymmetrical and excessively wide caudally. The NCLs are asymmetrical. Key landmarks on frontal view are indicated in (C): A: supraorbital notch, B: supratarsal crease, C: medial canthal point, D: tip-defining point, E: columellar break point, F: columellar–alar relationship, G: Cupid's bow (lateral borders), X-X line: width of bony base.

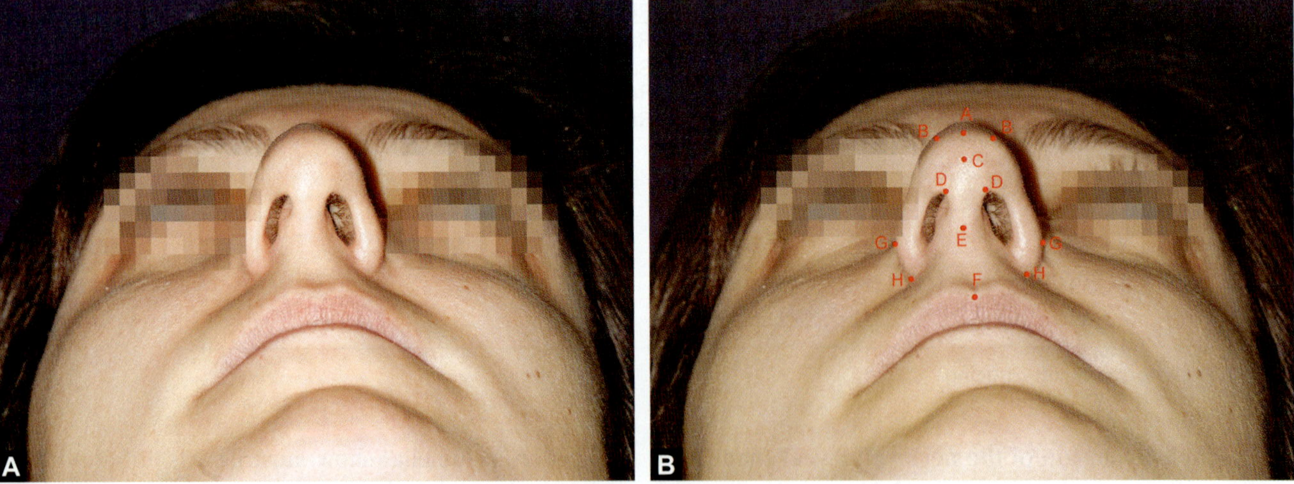

Figs. 11.4A and B: Base view (A) and key landmarks of the base view (B). A: pronasale, B: tip-defining point (right and left), C: columellar break point, D: nostril apex, E: subnasale, F: midpoint of Cupid's bow, G: maximal alar flare, H: alar crease.

it remained open after previous rhinoplasty? What is the thickness of the superficial musculoaponeurotic system over the tip? Gentle palpation of the LLCs between index finger and thumb will provide vital information on their size, resilience, and shape. The caudal and membranous septum is also palpated for orientation and relationship to the spine. In an overprojected nose, the spine can extend anteriorly into the columella.

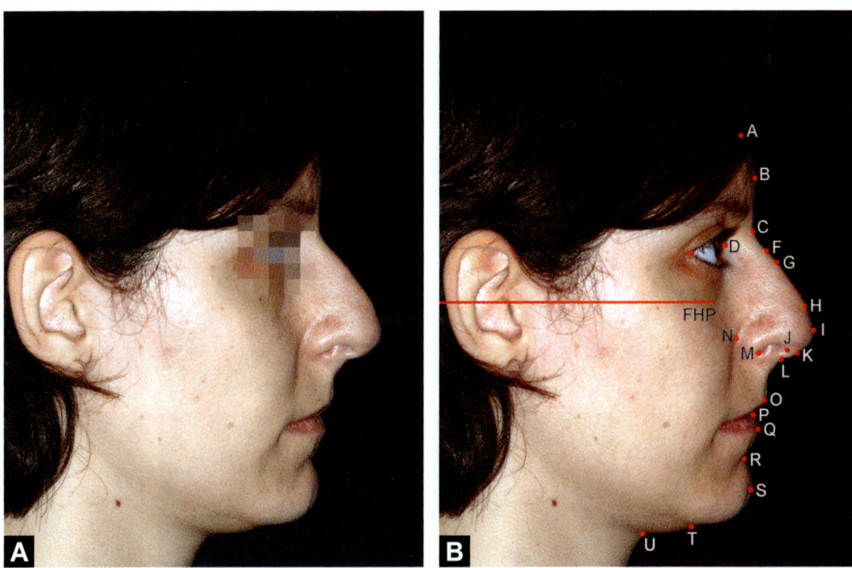

Figs. 11.5A and B: Lateral view (A) and key landmarks of the lateral view (B). A: trichion, B: glabella, C: nasion, D: corneal plane, E: lateral canthus, F: rhinion, G: point of maximal dorsal projection, H: supratip break point, I: pronasale, J: ventral nostril pole, K: columellar break point, L: subnasale, M: dorsal nasal pole, N: nasolabial fold, O: labrale superius, P: stomion, Q: labrale inferius, R: mentolabial sulcus, S: pogonion, T: menton, U: cervical point. (FHP: Frankfurt horizontal plane).

Once the clinical and functional examinations are over, standard photographs of the patient are taken with particular attention to current guidelines of facial photography. The photographic sequence and lighting should be as close as possible to these standards for good reasons: better quality films allow for more detailed analysis, and also provide the surgeon with an excellent defensive platform, should the patient forget their preoperative appearance. First author's photographic sequence includes 14 shots: frontal static and dynamic, two base-radix views, two lateral views (left and right), two dynamic lateral views (smiling and with upper lip tucked into the lower lip), two three-fourths views from each side, and one helicopter view (Figs. 11.6A to N).

It is of utmost importance to provide some breathing space for the patient and the surgeon after the initial consultation and photography. This time should be used for facial analysis and reflection on the patient's request and surgeon's emotional reactions to the encounter. Similarly, the patient is given time to consider his or her options and read material provided as literature, and possibly, the surgeon's website.

Computer-assisted facial analysis does not require the measurement of every conceivable angle, line, and asymmetry. However, there are key elements in facial analysis that are of practical importance. Basic measurements such as "the rule of fifths" or "the rule of thirds" are now considered to be not as relevant as the overall harmony and proportion of features. The surgeon must pay particular attention to the patient's ethnicity and country of residence as these parameters have an important bearing on the final decision-making process.

Measurements that provide useful practical points for analysis and surgical planning include the following. In the frontal view, a basic assessment of proportion and symmetry, with due attention to the patient's ethnicity, is an important starting point. Next, concentrate on the BDLs, the alar-columellar relationship, the width of the bony/cartilaginous dorsum (both in absolute and relative terms), the NCLs providing useful clues about symmetry and width of the bony base and the alar-cheek junction. During the frontal dynamic phase, asymmetries often become accentuated.

Base and base-radix views (Figs. 11.7A to C) provide a full view of medial (columellar) and lateral (alar) compartments of the skeleton of the nasal lower third, as well as of the various aesthetic subunits of the nasal base. The astute observer will be able to scrutinize surgically modifiable elements like caudal septum malposition, alar flare and alar width, resilience of the nostril walls, alar rim contour, flaring of the feet of the middle crura, nostrils orientation and size, reciprocal relationship between nostril height and infratip lobule, configuration and size of the soft triangles, and domal shape. Asymmetries among individual components are to be precisely identified and reported to the patient.

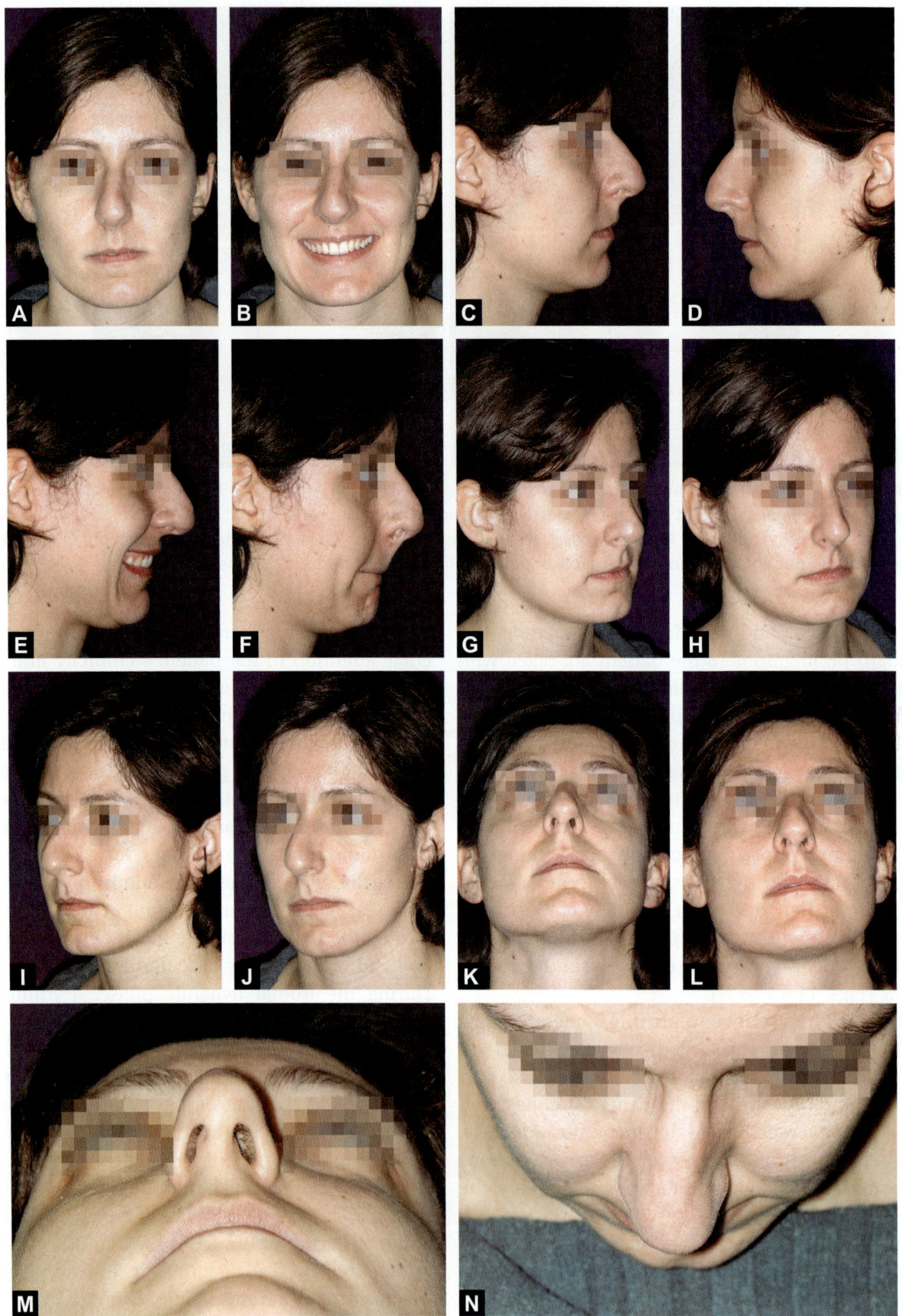

Figs. 11.6A to N: Series of 14 photographs demonstrating typical preoperative views: frontal static (A) and dynamic (B); two lateral views, right (C) and left (D); two dynamic lateral views, smiling (E) and with upper lip tucked into the lower lip (F); two three-fourths views from each side (G to J); two base-radix views (K and L); base view (M); and one helicopter view (N).

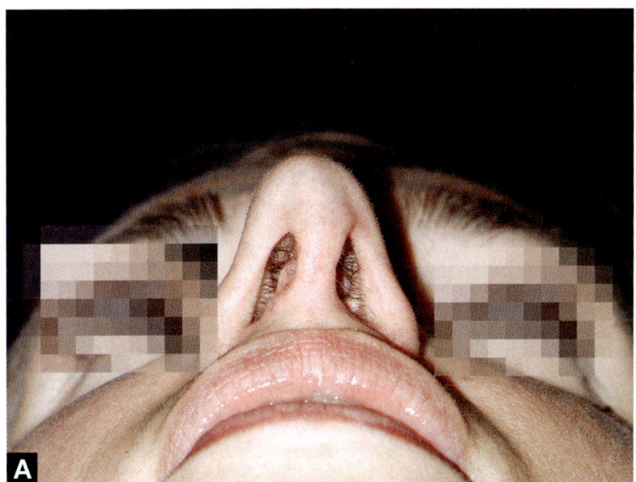

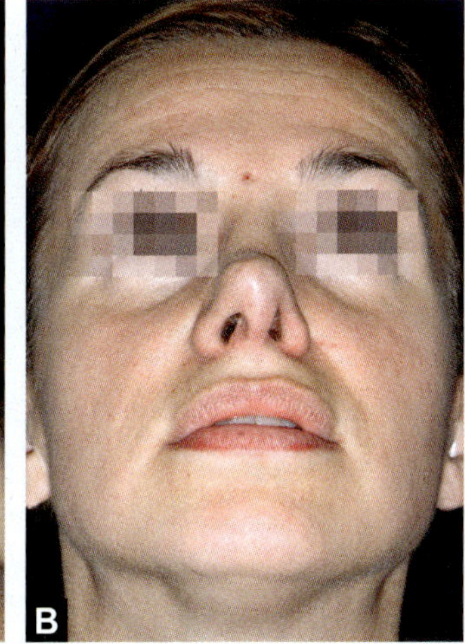

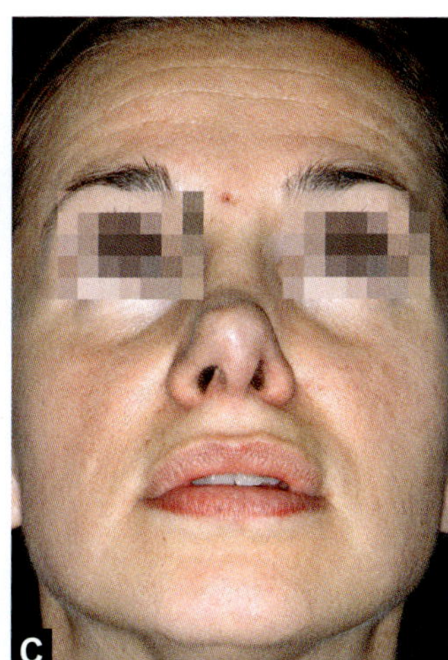

Figs. 11.7A to C: Base (A) view and base-radix views (B and C). These views provide a thorough evaluation of medial (columellar) and lateral (alar) compartments of the skeleton of the nasal lower third, as well as of the various aesthetic subunits of the nasal base.

Base-radix views are especially useful as they allow a complete view of reciprocal relationships among the three arches of the nasal pyramid as well as an unparalleled observation of the junction between tip and cartilaginous vault.

On the lateral view, in the static phase, a specific note of the nasion, rhinion, maximal dorsal height, supratip, dome, columella, columellar show, nostril poles axis, and length of the upper lip should be made. In patients with a very strong depressor nasi septi muscle, the nose derotates and the length of the upper lip reduces on smiling (Fig. 11.6E). The second dynamic view may demonstrate a prominent anterior septal angle (Fig. 11.6F). The helicopter views (Figs. 11.8A to C) are particularly useful in assessing midline position of the three arches of the nasal pyramid, showing details about the route of BDLs and the NCLs, the width of the radix area, the shape and symmetry of scroll areas, domes, peridomal areas, alar flaring, and alar base width.

The study of symmetry is also performed in every single case. Each half of the face is turned into its own mirror image and edited back onto its original half. In this way, a new face made entirely of the right half of the face and one made of the left are created (Figs. 11.9A to D). If there is a particularly attractive feature on the right half of the nose, this will be doubled on the right reconstructed view. Conversely, undesirable features are made doubly worse. This not only helps the patient to understand the principle asymmetries of the face but also allows the surgeon to plan for asymmetric surgery (Palma, Khodaei and Tasman, 2011).

Computer-assisted simulations have become increasingly popular over the past few years, as patients feel that they may predict the final outcome (Fig. 11.10A to E). Unfortunately, no software can accurately predict the final outcome, as patient's tissues do not heal in the same manner as projected on simulation surgery. Therefore, over-reliance on this technique should not be encouraged. Instead, the simulations can be used for educating patients regarding the planned surgical procedure and used as a forum for discussion.

11.3 TECHNICAL CHALLENGE

Having passed the hurdles of medical rhinology, clinical evaluation, functional testing, psychological assessment, and facial analysis, the surgeon's next task is to create a tailor-made operative game plan for each patient. This is a time-consuming and arduous task that starts and ends in a clinical setting, but it has profound, long-term repercussions. Initially, the surgeon establishes the answers to the "Four 'Ws':"

1. **W**hat specifically would the patient like the doctor to do for him or her?
2. **W**hy does the patient want this particular change?
3. **W**hy does the patient want the operation at this particular time?
4. **W**hy has the patient chosen this particular surgeon?

The result of the whole preoperative workup creates a list of surgically modifiable landmarks designed to alter the nose toward the patient's wish list for change. This unique game plan should not be repeated for another

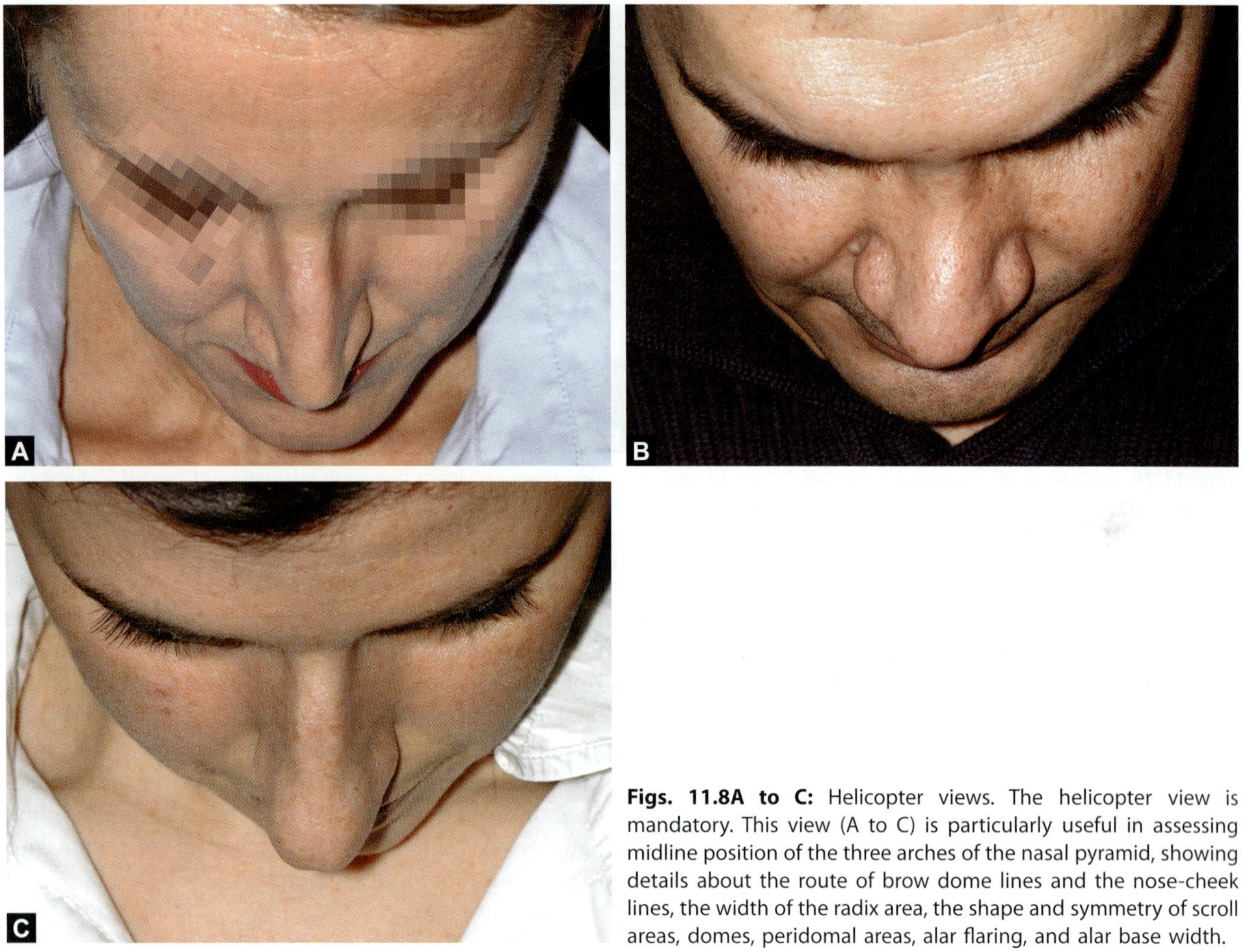

Figs. 11.8A to C: Helicopter views. The helicopter view is mandatory. This view (A to C) is particularly useful in assessing midline position of the three arches of the nasal pyramid, showing details about the route of brow dome lines and the nose-cheek lines, the width of the radix area, the shape and symmetry of scroll areas, domes, peridomal areas, alar flaring, and alar base width.

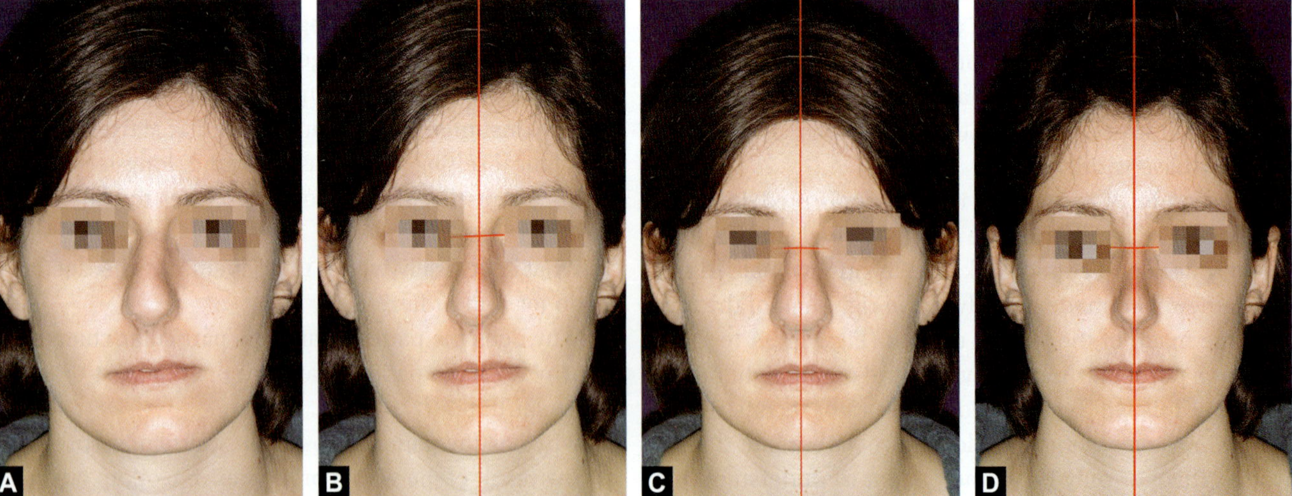

Figs. 11.9A to D: Study of symmetry. Frontal view of the actual face of the subject (A). Each half of the face (B) is turned into its own mirror image and edited back onto its original half. In this way, a new face made entirely of the right half of the face (C) and one made of the left (D) is created.

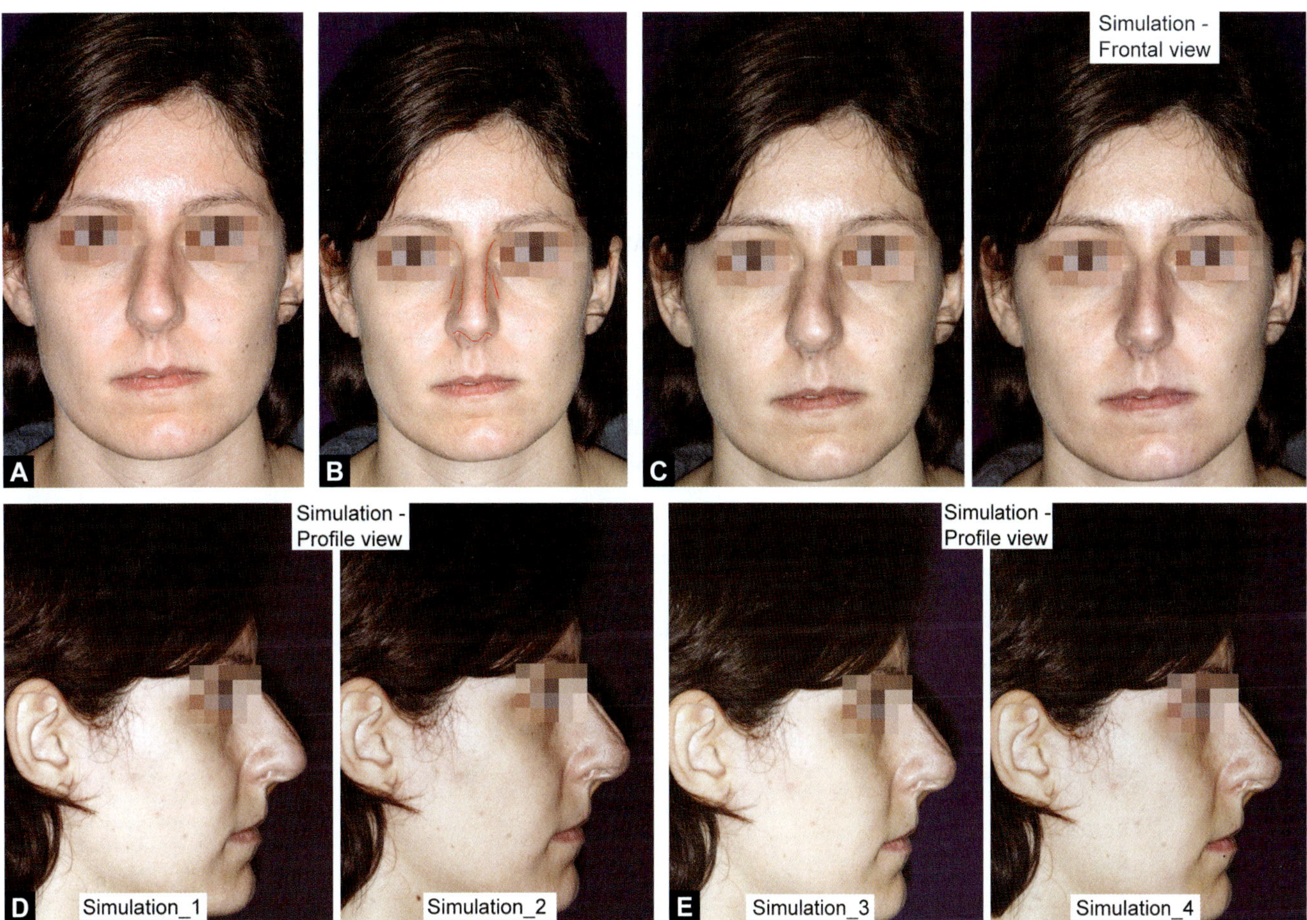

Figs. 11.10A to E: "Morphing" the preoperative photographs. On the frontal view, the actual face of the subject (A) has been manipulated to recreate a more aesthetically pleasing path of brow dome lines, nose-cheek lines, and alar–columellar relationship (B). Actual pictures and manipulated images (C to E) are used to give the patient an estimation of the finished result rather than a guarantee of the outcome.

patient. In addition to providing a series of surgical steps, facial analysis can at times also suggest auxiliary measures, such as a chin implant, botulinum toxin, and hyaluronic acid injections to improve the overall appearance of the nose. These findings are presented to the patient during a second meeting, where the patient is given ample opportunity to review the results of the facial analysis and compare them to his/her own desires. If the patient has had multiple rhinoplasty operations and still seeks further surgery, it may be wise for the less experienced surgeon to seek the opinion of a peer or a more experienced colleague.

SUMMARY

The astute surgeon starts the assessment of the nose the moment the patient walks into the office. This is a gradual, systematic, and evolutionary process that requires an in-depth knowledge of aesthetic principals, psychology, and rhinology. The first consultation establishes the patient's wish list and gleans important information from clinical examination, nasendoscopy, and functional evaluation. Clinical photography followed by facial analysis creates the solid platform for a unique, tailor-made operating plan for each patient. The second meeting allows the patient to clarify their concerns and listen to the results of the facial analysis. Photosimulations are becoming more sophisticated with time, but as they cannot predict the final outcome with absolute certainty, the patient is encouraged to think of these simulations as "a tool to understand patient's wishes and to set a tailor-made surgical plan". The game plan based on the two consultations and photographic analysis is taken into the operating room and used as a blueprint for surgery (Fig. 11.11). This game plan is never copied for another patient, as each functional and aesthetic analysis is absolutely unique.

Prof. Pietro Palma **RHINOPLASTY GAME PLAN**

Patient: .... **Date of surgery:** ....

Notes: ....

....

NASAL CAVITIES

☐ Septum

☐ Lateral wall

☐ Other

PYRAMID

APPROACH ☐ Endonasal ☐ Open

TIP

Incision Approach

Lateral Crura

☐ right ☐ left

☐ sutures

☐ grafts

☐ other

Projection = ↑ ↓ Rotation = ↑ ↓

SCROLLS

Right Left

DORSUM

Bony Dorsum

Cartilaginous Dorsum

OSTEOTOMIES

☐ No ☐ Yes

Tipology ☐ right ☐ ☐

☐ left ☐ ☐

NASO-LABIAL JUNCTION

Septum

Nasal Spine

Graft

RADIX

☐ Muscle removal ☐ Bony Remodelling

☐ Graft ☐ Type of graft

ALAR BASE ☐ No ☐ Yes ☐ Interalar Suture ☐ Weir ☐ Vestibular crescent

SUTURES ☐ ☐ ☐

NOTES

....

....

....

Fig. 11.11: The rhinoplasty game plan. This proforma based on the two consultations and the photographic analysis is taken into the operating room and used as a blueprint for actual surgery.

REFERENCES

Abdalla, S., Alreefy, H. and Hopkins, C., 2012. Prevalence of sinonasal outcome test (SNOT-22) symptoms in patients undergoing surgery for chronic rhinosinusitis in the England and Wales national prospective audit. *Clinical Otolaryngology*, 37, pp. 276-82.

Cole, R.P., Shakespeare, V., Shakespeare, P. and Hobby, J.A., 1994. Measuring outcome in low-priority plastic surgery patients using Quality of Life indices. *British Journal of Plastic Surgery*, 47, pp. 117-21.

Crerand, C.E., Phillips, K.A., Menard, W. and Fay, C., 2005. Nonpsychiatric medical treatment of body dysmorphic disorder. *Psychosomatics*, 46, pp. 549-55.

Dinis, P.B., Dinis, M. and Gomes, A., 1998. Psychosocial consequences of nasal aesthetic and functional surgery: a controlled prospective study in an ENT setting. *Rhinology*, 36, pp. 32-6.

Edgerton, M. and Langman, M., 1982. *Psychiatric considerations.* St. Louis, MO: Mosby.

Ercolani, M., Baldaro, B., Rossi, N. and Trombini, G., 1999. Five-year follow-up of cosmetic rhinoplasty. *Journal of Psychosomatic Research*, 47, pp. 283-6.

Goin, J. and Goin, M., 1987. *Psychological understanding and management of the plastic surgery patient.* Baltimore, MD: Williams & Wilkins.

Goin, M.K. and Rees, T.D., 1991. A prospective study of patients' psychological reactions to rhinoplasty. *Annals of Plastic Surgery*, 27, pp. 210-5.

Haraldsson, P., 1999. Psychosocial impact of cosmetic rhinoplasty. *Aesthetic Plastic Surgery*, 23, pp. 170-4.

Hay, G.G. 1970. Psychiatric aspects of cosmetic nasal operations. *The British Journal of Psychiatry*, 116, pp. 85-97.

Hay, G.G. and Heather, B.B., 1973. Changes in psychometric test results following cosmetic nasal operations. *The British Journal of Psychiatry*, 122, pp. 89-90.

Hill, G. and Silver, A.G., 1950. Psychodynamic and esthetic motivations for plastic surgery. *Psychosomatic Medicine*, 12, pp. 345-55.

Kimmelman, C.P., 1994. The risk to olfaction from nasal surgery. *Laryngoscope*, 104, pp. 981-8.

Klassen, A., Jenkinson, C., Fitzpatrick, R. and Goodacre, T., 1996. Patients' health related quality of life before and after aesthetic surgery. *The British Journal of Plastic Surgery*, 49, pp. 433-8.

Linn, L. and Goldman, I.B., 1949. Psychiatric observations concerning rhinoplasty. *Psychosomatic Medicine,* 11, pp. 307-14.

Marcus, P., 1984. Psychological aspects of cosmetic rhinoplasty. *The British Journal of Plastic Surgery*, 37, pp. 313-8.

McKiernan, D.C., Banfield, G., Kumar, R. and Hinton, A.E., 2001. Patient benefit from functional and cosmetic rhinoplasty. *Clinical Otolaryngology and Allied Sciences*, 26, pp. 50-2.

Napoleon, A. and Lewis, C.M., 1989. Psychological considerations in lipoplasty: the problematic or "special care" patient. *Annals of Plastic Surgery*, 23, pp. 430-2.

Palma, P. and Castelnuovo, P., 2010. *Correcting the crooked nose,* Hamilton, ON, Canada: BC Decker Inc.

Palma, P., Khodaei, I. and Tasman, A.J., 2011. A guide to the assessment and analysis of the rhinoplasty patient. *Facial Plastic Surgery*, 27, pp. 146-59.

Philips, K., 1996. *The broken mirror: understanding and treating body dysmorphic disorder.* New York, Oxford University Press.

Phillips, K.A., 2004. Body dysmorphic disorder: recognizing and treating imagined ugliness. *World Psychiatry*, 3, pp. 12-7.

Powel, N. and Humphreys, B., 1984. *Proportions of the aesthetic face.* New York, NY: Thieme Stratton Inc.

Pruzinski, T. and Edgerton, M., 1990. *Body image change in cosmetic plastic surgery.* New York: Guilford.

Rankin, M., Borah, G.L., Perry, A.W. and Wey, P.D., 1998. Quality-of-life outcomes after cosmetic surgery. *Plastic and Reconstructive Surgery*, 102, pp. 2139-45; discussion 2146-7.

Robin, A.A., Copas, J.B., Jack, A.B., Kaeser, A.C. and Thomas, P.J., 1988. Reshaping the psyche. The concurrent improvement in appearance and mental state after rhinoplasty. *The British Journal of Psychiatry*, 152, pp. 539-43.

Rohrich, R.J., 1999. Streamlining cosmetic surgery patient selection—just say no! *Plastic and Reconstructive Surgery*, 104, pp. 220-1.

Sarwer, D.B., Pertschuk, M.J., Wadden, T.A. and Whitaker, L.A., 1998. Psychological investigations in cosmetic surgery: a look back and a look ahead. *Plastic and Reconstructive Surgery*, 101, pp. 1136-42.

Sheard, C., Jones, N.S., Quraishi, M.S. and Herbert, M., 1996. A prospective study of the psychological effects of rhinoplasty. *Clinical Otolaryngology and Allied Sciences*, 21, pp. 232-6.

Shulman, J. and Westreich, M., 1983. Rhinoplasty update: preoperative evaluation of 4,040 cases. *Aesthetic Plastic Surgery*, 7, pp. 227-32.

Sperry, S., Thompson, J.K., Sarwer, D.B. and Cash, T.F., 2009. Cosmetic surgery reality TV viewership: relations with cosmetic surgery attitudes, body image, and disordered eating. *Annals of Plastic Surgery*, 62, pp. 7-11.

Wright, M.R. and Wright, W.K., 1975. A psychological study of patients undergoing cosmetic surgery. *Archives of Otolaryngology*, 101, pp. 145-51.

Zahiroddin, A.R., Shafiee-Kandjani, A.R. and Khalighi-Sigaroodi, E., 2008. Do mental health and self-concept associate with rhinoplasty requests? *Journal of Plastic, Reconstructive & Aesthetic Surgery*, 61, pp. 1100-3.

Trauma to Nose 12

Stephen Lo

Chapter Overview

Pearls and Pitfalls

Pearls

- Thorough clinical examination and nasal endoscopy are essential to diagnose the extent of nasal injury, its associated complications, and the persistent functional and cosmetic deformity.
- The surgical approach should be determined by the severity of the nasal bone fracture, involvement of other major components of the nose, presence of other facial fractures, and patient compliance.
- Obtain informed consent and be prepared to proceed to septorhinoplasty in patients with severe external nasal or septal deviation, caudal or dorsal septal deviation, or narrowing of the internal nasal valve angle.

Pitfalls

- Failure to address nasal septal deviation at the time of manipulating the nasal bones may result in persistent external nasal deformity.

12.1 NASAL ANATOMY

The external nose consists of the following structures from superficial to deep:

1. Skin and subcutaneous fat
2. Nasal muscles (four groups)

- These are located deep to the skin and interconnected to each other by the nasal superficial musculoaponeurotic system, a continuous fibrous sheet from the frontal area to the alar margin (Saban, et al., 2008)
  - Elevators—procerus and levator labii superioris alaeque nasi
  - Depressors—alar nasalis and depressor septi nasi
  - Compressor—transverse nasalis
  - Dilators—dilator naris anterior and posterior

3. Bones (three pairs, two midline):

- Nasal bones, syndesmose to four other bones:
  - Nasal process of frontal bone superiorly
  - Frontal process of the maxilla laterally
  - Perpendicular plate of the ethmoid and vomer posteriorly (nasal septum)

4. Cartilages (three pairs, one midline):

- Quadrangular cartilage
  - Quadrangular-shaped midline-supporting structure of cartilaginous portion of nasal septum is attached to the confluence of the nasal bones (rhinion)

superiorly and perpendicular plate of ethmoid posteriorly. The quadrangular cartilage then sits via fibrous connections into a bony groove in the vomer and premaxilla inferiorly, and is attached to the anterior nasal spine via fibrous connections anteroinferiorly. It is separated from the medial crura of the lower lateral cartilages by the membranous septum caudally. It is thickest where it is attached to the nasal bones.

- Upper lateral cartilages
  - Paired
  - Fused to the dorsum of the septal cartilage in the midline
  - Attached to the bony margin of the pyriform aperture laterally by loose ligaments and areolar tissue
  - Cephalic margin is attached to the undersurface of the nasal bones through tough fibrous connections. The caudal margin is attached to the lateral crus of the lower lateral cartilage in the scroll area through varied configurations
- Accessory (sesamoid) cartilages
  - Found variably
  - Located lateral to the upper lateral cartilages in fibroareolar connective tissue
- Lower lateral cartilages (alar cartilages)
  - Paired
  - Support the nasal tip
  - Consist of three parts: medial crura (caudal to septum), middle crura (dome of nasal tip), and lateral crura (caudal to the upper lateral cartilages).

Nerve Supply

Trigeminal Nerve

- V1
  - Infratrochlear nerve provides sensation to the upper part of nasal dorsum.
  - Anterior ethmoidal nerve supplies the lower dorsum and nasal tip through its external nasal branch.
- V2
  - Infraorbital nerve supplies the lower part of lateral nose (nasal side wall and ala).
  - Nasopalatine nerve carries sensation from nasal septum and anterior hard palate.

Arterial Supply

The superficial arterial supply of the nose is contributed by branches from both the internal and the external carotid arteries (Flowchart 12.1 and Figs. 12.1 to 12.3).

12.2 APPLIED ANATOMY

Skin and Soft Tissues

The thickness of the skin/soft tissue envelope of the nose differs in the upper, middle, and lower third. This must be appreciated when dealing with traumatic nasal injuries that alter the lateral profile of the nose.

The skin is thick and mobile over the underlying structures in the upper third of the nose. It then becomes thin but remains mobile in the middle third and finally transitions to become thick, sebaceous, and adherent to the underlying nasal tip structures in the lower third. The skin becomes very thin over the margin of the nares and columella.

Where reconstruction of nasal skin is anticipated, the external soft tissue can be divided into subunits. For best cosmetic outcome, reconstruction should occur within the subunit involved if <50% of the subunit is affected. Replacement of the whole subunit gives better cosmetic results if >50% of the subunit is lost.

Internal Nasal Valve Area

- Internal nasal valve area is the narrowest part of the nasal airway.
- It is bounded anteriorly by the caudal part of upper lateral cartilage, septum medially, nasal floor posteriorly, and head of the inferior turbinate laterally.
- The septum and upper lateral cartilage form an internal angle of 15° in Caucasians and 20° in Asians.
- Narrowing of the nasal valve area or angle leads to a sensation of nasal obstruction.

Keystone Area (Rhinion)

- Keystone area is formed at the junction of the bony (nasal bones, bony septum) and cartilaginous (septal cartilage, upper lateral cartilages) framework of the nose.
- Fracture dislocation of this junction leads to loss of dorsal height, saddle deformity, and nasal tip numbness as the external branch of the anterior ethmoidal nerves can be damaged when they emerge between the nasal bones and upper lateral cartilages.

Tip Support Mechanism

The structural support mechanisms and dynamics of the nasal tip are based on Anderson's tripod theory (Anderson, 1970). Subsequently, this has been refined

Flowchart 12.1: Diagrams showing the blood supply of the external nose.

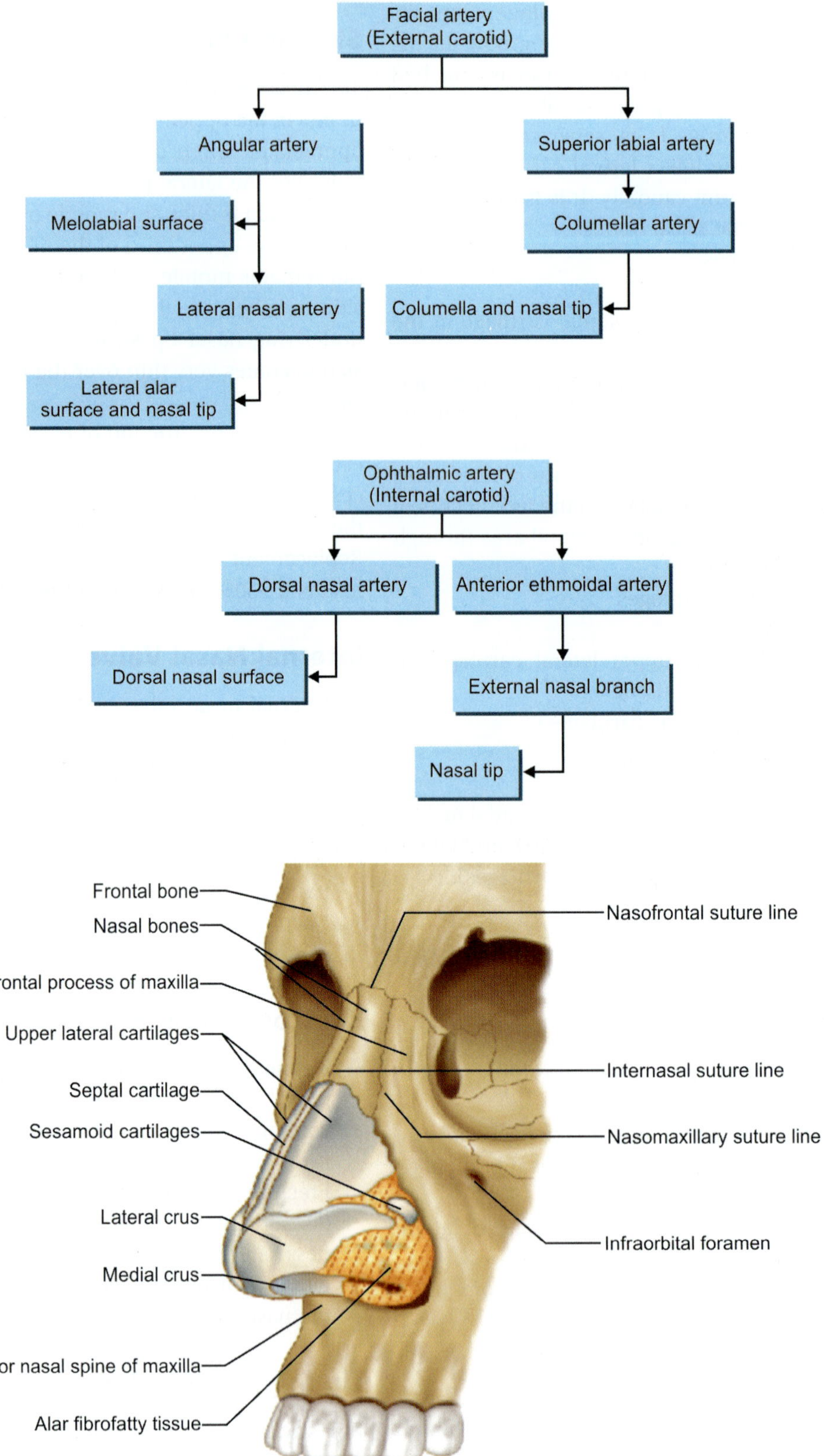

Fig. 12.1: External anatomy of the nose.

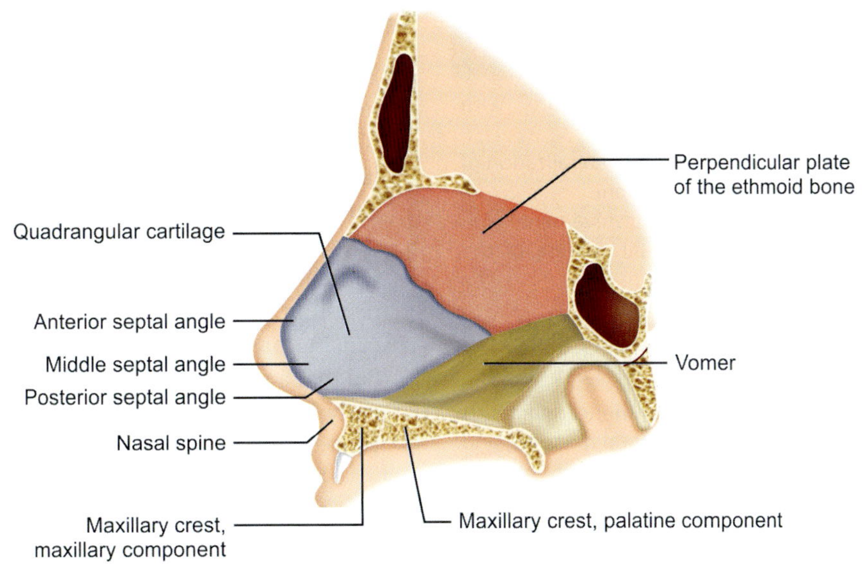

Fig. 12.2: Anatomy of the nasal septum.

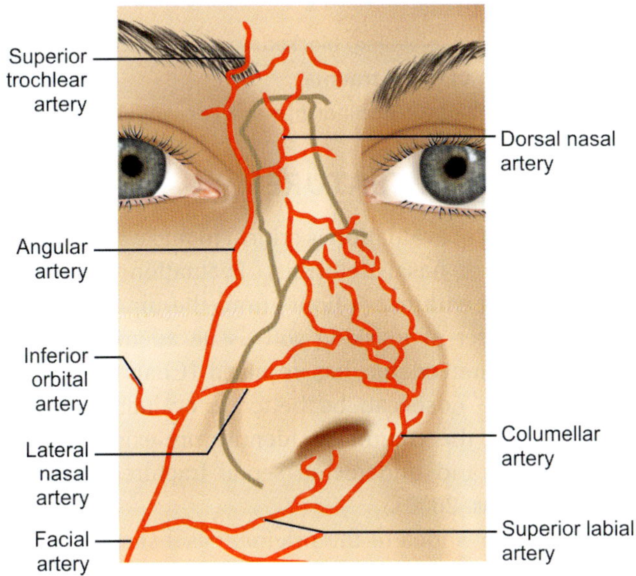

Fig. 12.3: Blood supply of external nose.

into three major and three minor tip support mechanisms (Tardy and Brown, 1990). Nasal trauma affecting these components will cause deformity of the nasal tip.

Major Tip Support Mechanisms

- Inherent strength and integrity of lower lateral cartilages
- Attachment of the upper lateral cartilages to the lower lateral cartilages (scroll region)
- Fibrous attachment between feet of medial crura and caudal septum.

Minor Tip Support Mechanisms

- Interdomal ligament
- Anterior nasal spine
- Attachments of the lower lateral cartilages to overlying skin.

12.3 EPIDEMIOLOGY

Nasal fractures are the most common fractures of the face (Rhee, et al., 2004), occurring in almost four out of 10 patients with maxillofacial fractures (Haug and Prather, 1991). The peak incidence occurs from adolescence to middle age, with males being affected more often than females. Motor vehicle accidents, sport injuries, assaults, and personal accidents are the most common causes of nasal fractures (Rubinstein and Strong, 2000). Among children and elderly however, most nasal fractures are related to falls and accidents (Karagama, et al., 2004).

12.4 PATHOPHYSIOLOGY OF NASAL TRAUMA

Many classification systems exist to describe nasal fractures; Stranc's classification has been described in Table 12.1.

- The lower part of the nasal bone is thin and broad and more susceptible to fracture (Mondin, et al., 2005).
- Fracture of the thicker bone at the nasal root is usually associated with fractures of the other facial bones. Sutures between bones are usually not involved.

Table 12.1: Stranc's classification of nasal fractures (Stranc and Robertson, 1979).

Lateral oblique	• Unilateral nasal bone fracture with depression of bone • Unilateral depression and lateralization of the contralateral nasal bone • Bilateral nasal bone involvement with fracturing of the frontal process of the maxilla
Frontal	• *Type 1*: Does not extend posterior to a line drawn from the lower nasal bones to the maxillary spine • *Type 2*: Flattening of the cartilaginous and bony structures, septal fractures, and intranasal mucosal injuries • *Type 3*: Severe collapse of the nasal bones and upper lateral cartilages with telescoping of the septum. Associated intracranial and orbital injuries may occur

- Up to 80% of nasal fractures occur at the junction of the nasal bones and upper lateral cartilages. Freeing of the upper lateral cartilages from the septum may be necessary to fully mobilize both cartilages during surgical correction (Converse, 1974; Fernandes, 2004).
- Caudal septum deviation may affect the positioning of the lower lateral cartilages leading to nasal tip deformity, if not properly addressed (Natvig, et al., 1971; Rohrich and Adams, 2000). Similarly, dorsal septal deviation secondary to fracture of quadrangular cartilage needs to be addressed to achieve a straight midline nasal dorsum. High dorsal deviation in the area of the anterior septal angle will lead to the lower third being deviated to one side.
- Over 90% of simple nasal bone fractures are associated with septal fractures (Rhee, et al., 2003). Low-velocity injuries usually lead to septal fractures or dislocations along the vomer bony groove. High-velocity or frontal impacts result in more extensive septal fractures through the thin central region of the quadrangular cartilage (Rohrich and Adams, 2000). Elasticity of the septal cartilage results in C-shaped fracture of the quadrangular cartilage, with overlapping fracture edges (Murray, et al., 1984).
- A fractured septum affects the alignment of the nasal bones during healing and should be addressed during the management of nasal fractures to minimize the potential for secondary deformity (Gunter and Rohrich, 1988; Mondin, et al., 2005).

Septal Hematoma

- Nasal injuries are associated with formation of septal hematoma, which may develop into a septal abscess. If left untreated, avascular necrosis of the septal cartilage may follow, leading to perforation of the septal cartilage, retracted columella, or a saddle nose deformity.
- Untreated septal hematoma may become organized, resulting in subperichondrial fibrosis and thickening causing nasal airway obstruction. Hence, it is essential that a septal hematoma be recognized and treated early by immediate evacuation and drainage to prevent complications from developing.

12.5 SYMPTOMS

Bone and/or cartilage
Pain, blocked nose, and external nasal deformity
Skin and soft tissue
Swelling, bruising, bleeding, blocked nose, and numbness
Complications of nasal trauma
Cerebrospinal fluid (CSF) rhinorrhea and telecanthus

12.6 CLINICAL FEATURES

- The timing of evaluation is critical to make an accurate diagnosis of nasal deformity. Evaluation should be performed within 2–3 hours from the time of injury, before onset of masking soft tissue edema, or after 5 days when edema has resolved (Chan and Most, 2008). The nose can be better re-evaluated several days after the trauma to identify pre-existing nasal deformity and undetected septal fractures (Rohrich and Adams, 2000).
- The patient's idea of the original nasal shape is often inaccurate in determining recent deviation (Murray, et al., 1984). Hence, the surgeon should instruct the patient, whenever possible, to bring photographs taken prior to injury showing the frontal, oblique, and profile views.

Typical Findings on Examination

- Soft tissue
  - *External*: Edema, ecchymosis, subcutaneous emphysema, skin laceration
  - *Internal*: Epistaxis, septal hematoma, mucosal tear
- Bone deformity
  - Upper third deviation, depression, protuberance

- Cartilaginous deformity
  - *External*: Middle third deviation, depression, tip deviation, tip asymmetry
  - *Internal*: Septal deviation, nasal valve collapse.

12.7 INVESTIGATIONS

Conventional Radiography

Water and lateral views have low sensitivity and accuracy in diagnosing isolated nasal bone fractures, cartilaginous fractures, and other facial bone abnormalities. It is the author's view that conventional facial radiographs have limited clinical value (Sharp and Denholm, 1994) and have no place in the decision-making process in the management of nasal trauma (Logan, et al., 1994).

Computed Tomography

Computed tomography (CT) scan is the gold standard investigation for detecting facial bone fractures. It may however be unable to detect fine nasal bone fracture lines (Hong, et al., 2007). It is also unable to predict the severity of septal fractures and cannot be relied upon to determine whether septal surgery is required (Rhee, et al., 2004). The decision to perform septal surgery is therefore based on the patient's complaint of nasal obstruction, which is then corroborated with finding of a deviated septum.

High-Resolution Ultrasound

High-resolution ultrasound has been reported to have a 100% sensitivity and accuracy in detecting nasal bone fractures (Lee, et al., 2009), and is able to show a nasal fracture of 0.1 mm width (Hirai, et al., 1996). It can identify subperiosteal hematomas (Mohammadi, et al., 2009), but is unable to identify septal and other facial bone fractures. It is able to show septal deformity, but its role in making management decisions is unproven. Hence, the author does not recommend its routine use for patients with nasal bone fracture (Hong, et al., 2007).

Nasal Endoscopy

Nasal endoscopy is mandatory for internal anatomical and functional assessments of the nose. The site and severity of nasal septal deviation and its impact on the nasal airway should be documented. Particular attention should be paid to the presence of caudal and dorsal septal deviation and the resulting narrowing of the external nasal valve, internal nasal valve angle, and nasal valve area (Fernandes, 2004; Rohrich and Adams, 2000).

12.8 TREATMENT

Timing of Treatment

- Immediate treatment is performed under the following circumstances:
  - A patient is seen shortly (within 2–3 hours) after trauma, before significant edema develops
  - There is presence of skin and soft tissue lacerations with exposure of the underlying skeletal or cartilaginous structures
  - There is presence of a septal hematoma that requires immediate drainage
- Generally treatment within 3 weeks is considered acceptable, beyond 3 weeks the nasal bones may heal in an abnormal position, which requires a septorhinoplasty for correction. Surgical management of nasal fractures within 10 days of injury is less likely to require revision septorhinoplasty since significant scarring is less likely to have occurred (Fernandes, 2004). However, in a proportion of patients with severe external nasal deviation and fracture of nasal septum, a septoplasty may need to be performed at the time of manipulation and reduction in nasal bones to help in their midline alignment.

Closed Reduction

Under Local Anesthesia

- Manipulation and reduction in nasal bones can be performed under local anesthesia as an office procedure. It is indicated in the presence of nasal bony deviation with no or minimal septal or nasal tip displacement. Compared to general anesthesia, manipulation under local anesthesia is more convenient, less time-consuming, and cost-effective (Chegar and Tatum, 2005; Murray and Maran, 1980; Rajapakse, et al., 2003). There is no evidence suggesting that it results in inferior cosmetic outcome or nasal airway patency (Cook, et al., 1990; Cook, et al., 1992; Jones and Nandapalan, 1999; Khwaja, et al., 2007). Subsequent septorhinoplasty rates are also similar to manipulation and reduction under general anesthesia (Khwaja, et al., 2007). However, patients with post-traumatic septal deformity and nasal tip deviation are more likely to have persistent postoperative nasal deformity when manipulation of nasal bones is done under local anesthesia (Khwaja, et al., 2007). This is probably because most surgeons do not address the nasal septal deviation at the same time as nasal bone manipulation and reduction under local anesthesia. Persistent septal deviation in these cases then leads to external nasal deviation of the middle and lower third of the nose.

- No major adverse effects from using local anesthesia for nasal manipulation have been reported. Minor complaints include vasovagal episodes, and rarely, epistaxis (Cook, et al., 1992; Green, 2001; Jones and Nandapalan, 1999).
- Postoperative pain is similar to general anesthesia (Khwaja, et al., 2007; Rajapakse, et al., 1980).

Under General Anesthesia

- Closed reduction under general anesthesia is preferred in patients with deviation of nasal septum and gross external nasal deformity.
- Nasal septal fracture and dislocation commonly accompany nasal bone fractures. An untreated septal fracture unfavorably affects the alignment of the nasal bone during the healing process (Mondin, et al., 2005; Rhee, et al., 2004), and the persistent septal deviation is an important cause of secondary nasal deformity and obstruction (Rhee, et al., 2004). Concurrent septoplasty should be performed if the fractured cartilaginous septum cannot be reduced or a dislocation cannot be replaced back onto the nasal crest of the maxilla.
- If the deviated septum interferes with repositioning of nasal bones back to their native position, the surgeon may need to carry out a septorhinoplasty (Fattahi, et al., 2006). If there is suspicion of disruption of the tip support mechanisms (e.g. nasal tip cartilage fracture), septorhinoplasty should be considered.

Septorhinoplasty

- The main advantage of septorhinoplasty is that it can address deformities of both the bony and cartilaginous components, thus avoiding the need for future secondary procedures (Huizing and De Groot, 2003; Konstantinidis, et al., 2011; Mondin, et al., 2005; Reilly and Davison, 2007; Stucker, et al., 2009)
- Indications for primary septorhinoplasty include:
  - Nasal pyramid deviation exceeding one half of the width of the nasal bridge
  - Extensive fracture-dislocation of the nasal bones and septum
  - Fracture and dislocation of the caudal or dorsal septum
  - Closed septal fracture in the presence of nasal pyramid deformity
  - Open trauma at the columella and the quadrangular cartilage
  - Separation of cartilaginous vault from the bony pyramid
  - Significant internal valve collapse
  - Nasal tip deformity.

Open- versus Closed-Approach Septorhinoplasty

Compared to closed approach, open approach has the following features:

- Superior access to middle vault and nasal tip
- Lower rate of postoperative septal deviation and lower rate of revision surgery (Reilly and Davison, 2007).

12.9 HOW I DO IT?

- In the author's practice, imaging is not routinely requested for patients with only suspected nasal bone fractures. The author requests a CT scan in patients with a CSF leak and a CT with three-dimensional reconstruction in patients with facial bone fractures.
- A nasal bone radiograph is undertaken in the presence of medical legal reasons (e.g. assault, workplace related injury, road traffic accident).
- General anesthesia is always offered as first line regardless of mode of treatment. Closed reduction is indicated in the presence of nasal bone deviation with minimal/or no associated septal or nasal tip displacement. All other remaining cases of nasal bone fracture with additional involvement of one or more of other parts of the nose (e.g. internal valve, septum, nasal tip) are offered open approach septorhinoplasty. Closed reduction is attempted for dubious cases, but in patients where a satisfactory functional or aesthetic result is not achieved the author has a low threshold for immediately proceeding to open septorhinoplasty during the same anesthetic setting.

REFERENCES

Anderson, J.R., 1970. The dynamics of rhinoplasty. Presented at: Proceedings of the Ninth International Congress in Otorhinolaryngology; August 10–14, 1969; Mexico City,

Mexico. Amsterdam, the Netherlands: Excerpta Medica, *International Congress Series*, p. 206.

Chan, J. and Most, A.P., 2008. Diagnosis and management of nasal fractures. *Operative Techniques in Otolaryngology*, pp. 263-66.

Chegar, B.E. and Tatum. S.A., 2005. Nasal fractures. In: Cummings, C.W., Gaughey, B.H., Thomas, J.R., et al., eds. *Otolaryngology head and neck surgery*. 4th ed. St Louis, MO: Mosby-Yearbook Inc. pp. 963-80.

Converse, J.M., 1974. *Surgical treatment of facial injuries*. 3rd ed. Baltimore: Williams & Wilkins.

Cook, J.A., McRae, R.D., Irving, R.M. and Dowie, L.N., 1990. A randomized comparison of manipulation of the fractured nose under local and general anaesthesia. *Clinical Otolaryngology and Allied Sciences*, pp. 343-6.

Cook, J.A., Murrant, N.J., Evans, K. and Lavelle, R.J., 1992. Manipulation of the fractured nose under local anaesthesia. *Clinical Otolaryngology and Allied Sciences*, pp. 337-40

Fattahi, T., Steinberg, B., Fernandes, R., et al., 2006. Repair of nasal complex fractures and the need for secondary septorhinoplasty. *Journal of Oral and Maxillofacial Surgery*, pp. 1785-9.

Fernandes, S.V., 2004. Nasal fractures: the taming of the shrewd. *Laryngoscope*, pp. 1587-92.

Green, K.M., 2001. Reduction of nasal fractures under local anaesthetic. *Rhinology*, pp. 43-6.

Gunter, J.P. and Rohrich, R.J., 1988. Management of the deviated nose: the importance of septal reconstruction. *Clinical Plastic Surgery*, pp. 43-55.

Haug, R.H. and Prather, J.L., 1991. The closed reduction of nasal fractures: an evaluation of two techniques. *Journal of Oral and Maxillofacial Surgery*, pp. 1288-92.

Hirai, T., Manders, E.K., Nagamoto, K. and Saggers, G.C., 1996. Ultrasonic observation of facial bone fractures. *Journal of Oromaxillofacial Surgery*, pp. 776-9.

Hong, H.S., Cha, J.G., Paik, S.H., et al., 2007. High-resolution sonography for nasal fracture in children. *American Journal of Roentgenology*, 188, pp. W86-W92.

Huizing, E. and De Groot, J., eds, 2003. *Acute nasal trauma in functional reconstructive nasal surgery*. New York: Thieme Publishers.

Jones, T.M. and Nandapalan, V., 1999. Manipulation of the fractured nose: a comparison of local infiltration anaesthesia and topical local anaesthesia. *Clinical Otolaryngology and Allied Sciences*, pp. 443-6.

Karagama, Y.G., Newton, J.R. and Clayton, M.G.G., 2004. Are nasal fractures being referred appropriately from the accident and emergency department to ENT? *Injury*, pp. 968-71.

Khwaja, S., Pahade, A.V., Luff, D., Green, M.W. and Green, K.M., 2007. Nasal fracture reduction: local versus general anaesthesia. *Rhinology*, pp. 83-8

Konstantinidis, I., Malliari, H. and Metaxas, S, 2011. Nasal trauma: primary reconstruction with open rhinoplasty. *Canadian Journal of Plastic Surgery*, pp. 108-10.

Lee, M.H., Cha, J.G., Hong, H.S., Lee, J.S., Park, S.J., Paik, S.H. and Lee, H.K., 2009. Comparison of high-resolution ultrasonography and computed tomography in the diagnosis of nasal fractures. *Journal of Ultrasound in Medicine*, pp. 717-23.

Logan, M., O'Driscoll, K. and Masterson, J., 1994. The utility of nasal bone radiographs in nasal trauma. *Clinical Radiology*, pp. 192-4.

Mohammadi, A., Javadrashid, R., Pedram, A. and Masudi, S., 2009. Comparison of ultrasonography and conventional radiography in the diagnosis of nasal bone fractures. *Iranian Journal of Radiology*, pp. 7-11.

Mondin, V., Rinaldo, A. and Ferlita, A., 2005. Management of nasal bone fractures. *American Journal of Otolaryngology*, pp. 181-5.

Murray, J.A. and Maran, A.G., 1980. The treatment of nasal injuries by manipulation. *Journal of Laryngology and Otology*, pp. 1405-10.

Murray, J.A.M., Maran, A.G.D., Mackenzie, I.J., et al., 1984. Open vs. closed reduction of the fractured nose. *Archives of Otolaryngology*, pp. 797-802.

Natvig, P., Sether, L.A., Gingrass, R.P., et al., 1971. Anatomical details of the osseous-cartilaginous framework of the nose. *Plastic and Reconstructive Surgery*, pp. 528-32.

Rajapakse, Y., Courtney, M., Bialostocki, A., et al., 2003. Nasal fractures: a study comparing local and general anaesthesia techniques. *ANZ Journal of Surgery*, pp. 396-9.

Reilly, M.J., Davison, S.P., 2007. Open vs closed approach to the nasal pyramid for fracture reduction. *Archives of Facial Plastic Surgery*, pp. 82-6.

Rhee, S.C., Kim, Y.K., Cha, J.H., et al., 2004. Septal fracture in simple nasal bone fracture. *Plastic and Reconstructive Surgery*, pp. 45-52.

Reilly, M.J. and Davison, S.P., 2007. Open vs closed approach to the nasal pyramid for fracture reduction. *Archives of Facial Plastic Surgery*, pp. 82-6.

Rohrich, R.J. and Adams, W.P., 2000. Nasal fracture management: minimizing secondary nasal deformities. *Plastic and Reconstructive Surgery*, pp. 266-73.

Rubinstein, B. and Strong, E.B., 2000. Management of nasal fractures. *Archives of Family Medicine*, pp. 738-42.

Saban, Y., Andretto Amodeo, C., Hammou, J.C., Polselli, R., 2008. An anatomical study of the nasal superficial musculoaponeurotic system: surgical applications in rhinoplasty. *Archives of Facial Plastic Surgery*, pp. 109-15.

Sharp, J.F. and Denholm, S., 1994. Routine X-rays in nasal trauma: the influence of audit on clinical practice. *Journal of the Royal Society of Medicine*, pp. 153-4.

Stranc, M.F. and Robertson, G.A., 1979. A classification of injuries of the nasal skeleton. *Annals of Plastic Surgery*, pp. 468-74.

Stucker, F., de Souza, C., Kenyon, G., Lian, T., Draf, W. and Schick, B., eds. 2009. *Rhinology and facial plastic surgery*. New York: Springer.

Tardy, M.E. and Brown, R., 1990. *Surgical anatomy of the nose*. New York, NY: Raven Press.

13 Crooked Nose

Hemal Raja, Julian M Rowe-Jones

Chapter Overview

Pearls and Pitfalls

Pearls

- Ensure you understand your patient's hopes and concerns and that you can meet their expectations.
- It is important to recognize intrinsic curvature in the cartilaginous septum, as this will not be corrected by releasing the quadrilateral cartilage inferiorly and posteriorly with a swing door technique. If this intrinsic curvature affects the caudal and dorsal edges, it will have esthetic as well as functional consequences.
- When performing incisions for septal curvature release that are full thickness through the cartilaginous septum and extend to either the caudal or dorsal free margin, fix the bracing baton graft to the septum, across the incision at one end of the graft first, prior to completing the incision. When the incision has been completed, the septum strut either side of the incision is very mobile and it is technically demanding to align and suture the graft accurately if one end has not been fixed.
- In cases of facial asymmetry aim to align the nose in the frontal view with the nasion, as it is a fixed point and cannot be moved, rather than with the position of the columella.
- Intraoperatively pause to reassess the anatomy with the better exposure afforded, and in the light of the findings reassess your primary operative plan.
- Recognize lateral wall asymmetries and concavities and disguise with onlay grafts if necessary. Out fracture of the medialized lateral nasal wall may not maintain a lateralized position for the bone.

Pitfalls

- Recognize facial asymmetry preoperatively and bringing it to patient's attention as a limiting factor in achieving a straight nose after surgery. Patients will accept less than perfect result if asymmetry is pointed out preoperatively. Otherwise the patient will consider the modest result as surgical failure.
- Recognize the crooked nose associated with tension nose deformity. These cases have short nasal bones, thin mid thirds and are over projected with excess development of the quadrilateral cartilage. Dorsal reduction to correct the lateral profile and to allow tip retroprojection, when performed with osteotomies to straighten the nose, and septal incisions to correct the quadrilateral cartilage carry a high risk of septal disarticulation.

13.1 INTRODUCTION

The *crooked nose* is not one deformity and therefore it must not be assumed that there is one surgical technique or set of surgical steps that can be universally applied. Analysis is therefore of fundamental importance with regard to understanding the patients anatomy. It is important to recognize that the crooked nose can often be associated with complex deformity involving multiple components of the:

- Nasal skeleton
- Skin soft tissue envelope
- Mucosal lining

These anatomical elements may not just be *displaced* but also *remodeled* if there is a history of trauma. Furthermore, patient's expectations can also not be assumed in advance. Functional as well as aesthetic improvement may need to be addressed. Motivation for surgery in the patient may also be complex. Special attention should be given to psychological issues not only in the patient requesting cosmetic change for congenital nasal deformity but also in those who've had nasal trauma, perhaps due to assault, and hope for return of their pretraumatic nasal appearance. The surgeon therefore must be sensitive to patients psychological concerns, must be capable of recognizing and understanding a wide range of anatomical deformities, and must be competent with a wide range of surgical techniques for all elements of the nasal skeleton and soft tissues.

13.2 HISTORY

The history should start with an open question asking the patient what they expect to achieve from the consultation and from any future surgery. It is important to establish what the patients' main hopes are. Subsequently, the patient can be guided with questions specifically addressing their aspirations and expectations with regard to both nasal function and appearance and their expectations as to how surgery will help them make progress generally. It is also important to ask the patients about their concerns and worries. Whether previous nasal trauma (including iatrogenic) has occurred should be investigated as this may warn the surgeon of increased unpredictability during any subsequent rhinoplasty. It should, however, be remembered that trauma could have occurred in childhood and the patient may have no recollection of this event. If the patient presents after trauma, it is important to ascertain whether the patient is hoping for their preinjury nasal shape and function to be restored or whether they're looking for additional improvement (Roofe and Murakami, 2006). Preinjury photographs can be helpful in understanding what the patient wants. If the patients' nasal deformity was acquired through trauma, it is important to determine whether there is any continuing litigation, frustration, or anger present in the patient, as this could adversely affect the current doctor patient relationship and potentially even lead to transference of anger and disenchantment. As with any surgery that plans to change the shape of the nose, it is important to be sure there is no significant psychological morbidity or personality disorder. Even though at this stage, the patient may not know what is possible from surgery; it is important to reflect on whether the patients expectations are generally reasonable and whether they are embracing surgery as a positive step or not.

13.3 PHYSICAL EXAMINATION AND ANALYSIS

The purpose of examination and analysis is to recognize, understand, describe, and record:

- The shape and position of each external and intranasal anatomical component
- A comparison of the symmetry of paired right and left anatomical components
- Potential anatomical pitfalls related to surgery
- Abnormal nasal function
- Pathology of the nasal mucosa
- Facial asymmetry
- Other associated deformities such as a saddle nose or dorsal hump.

The authors like to assess the nose externally as upper, middle, and lower thirds and in the following views:

- Frontal
- Half basal and full basal
- Head down
- Right and left oblique
- Right and left lateral

Endoscopy can aid intranasal examination particularly when functional symptoms are present. Computed tomography can help determine the nature of any bony deformity. The authors find good photography with appropriate lighting and background essential for analysis. Careful study of the photographs reinforces the initial understanding of the nose gained from examination. The author finds it helpful in assessing nasal asymmetry and deviation to use computerized photographic tools that can split the frontal view and recompose the face using two right half images and two left half images.

13.4 PREOPERATIVE PLANNING

The operation plan should take into account foremost the patient's aims. These must be considered alongside the surgical options and possibilities with their risks

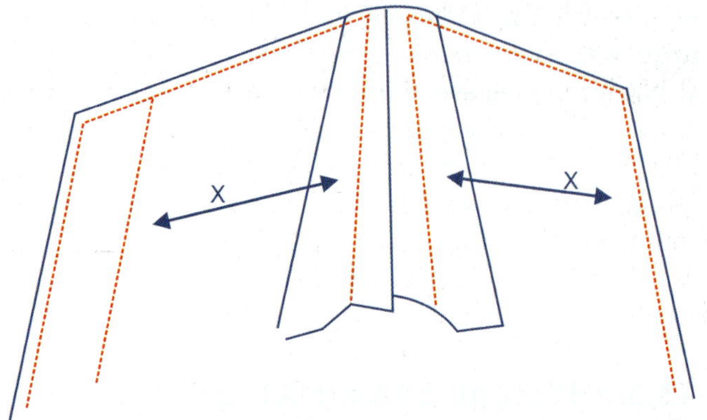

Fig. 13.1: The right lateral nasal wall is longer from the dorsum to the face. Bilateral medial osteotomies, low-to-low lateral osteotomies flush with the face, superior transverse osteotomies and an additional right intermediate osteotomy are shown. The right intermediate osteotomy is shown measured equidistant from the midline as the left lateral osteotomy.

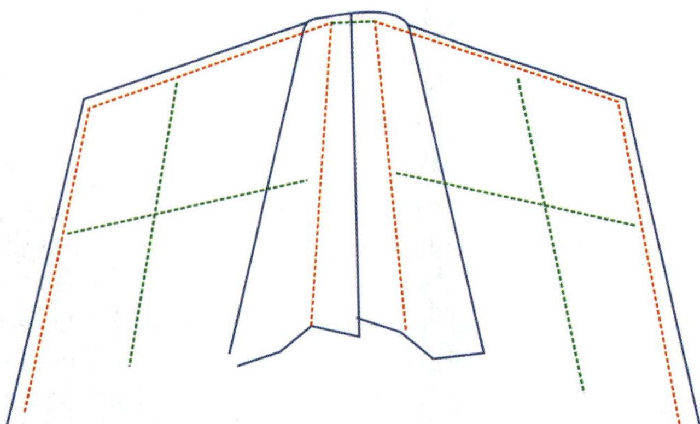

Fig. 13.2: Bilateral lateral, superior transverse and medial osteotomies are shown in red. A single midline cephalic root osteotomy and bilateral dorsal to ventral and caudal to cephalic intermediate osteotomies are shown in green.

and limitations and the surgeon's level of experience. Aesthetically special attention is given individually to the

- Dorsum
- Lateral nasal walls.

The authors aim to correct the position of the dorsum with regard to the midline and the shape of the dorsum if curved. Symmetry of the dorsum is also carefully assessed, with consideration given to correction of bony and cartilaginous humps and irregularities. The length of the nasal bones is assessed. Short nasal bones increase the risk of septal disarticulation with osteotomies. The relationship of the dorsum to the lateral wall, both bony and cartilaginous, is determined. The contour of the lateral walls is determined, as is their width from the dorsum to the junction with the face. The wider lateral wall from dorsum to face wall in a deviated nose may need an additional, intermediate osteotomy for correction. A convex lateral wall may also need an intermediate osteotomy to break the curvature. The position of the lateral walls in relation to the midline is assessed when deciding on lateral, superior transverse, and medial osteotomies (Figs. 13.1 to 13.3). The half basal view is helpful in analyzing the contour and position of the lateral nasal walls and the head down view is very helpful for assessing the position and shape of the dorsum.

13.5 SEPTUM

Septal surgery is invariably necessary in the treatment of the crooked nose for functional and aesthetic reasons. When planning septal correction, particular attention is given to the position and shape of the caudal and dorsal edges of the quadrilateral cartilage. These edges with their contiguous 10–12 mm of cartilage should not be resected, if straight. They may need repositioning and reshaping, if deviated. In cases of severe deviation of the caudal and dorsal edges, these may need to be excised and reconstructed. In cases of nasal blockage, particular attention must be given to the internal nasal valves (Daniel, 2010). Narrowing at this site will require high dorsal septal and upper lateral cartilage reconstruction. The position of the bony septum must be noted during planning, as deviation here will influence the position of the quadrilateral cartilage. Care must be taken in planning for bony septum resection especially if bony hump reduction and osteotomies are required as the risk of septal disarticulation is higher. As mentioned above, this risk is greater in the presence of short nasal bones.

13.6 NASAL TIP

The position and symmetry of the tip cartilages are also noted. Deviation of the tip may be intrinsic requiring surgery to the lower lateral cartilages or it may be extrinsic due to displacement secondary to septal deviation. Planning for correction of tip cartilage asymmetries must consider resection of segments of excessively long crura or grafting of short crura. Repositioning sutures may be required, as may onlay grafts inserted into pockets to camouflage depressions.

In most cases, the authors use an open approach as it is felt that this is the best way to diagnose accurately

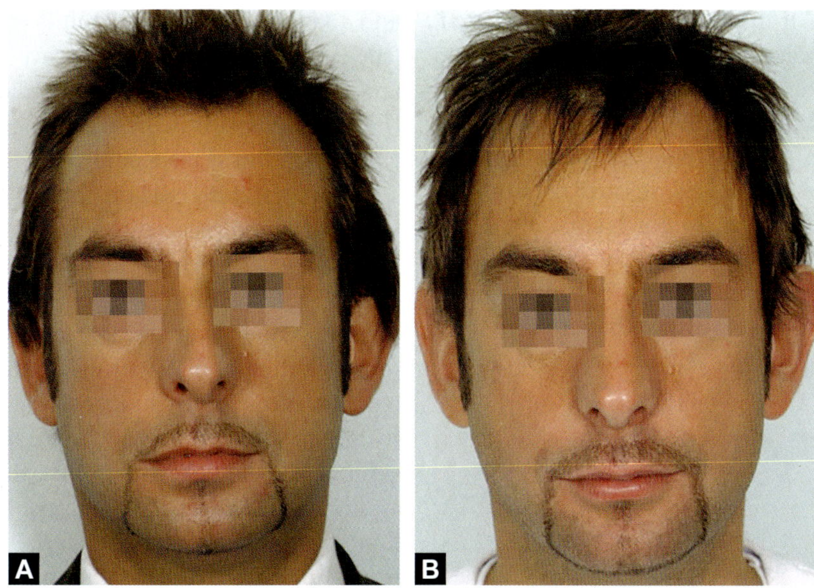

Figs. 13.3A and B: (A) Preoperative frontal view. (B) Postoperative frontal view. A swing-door septoplasty and bilateral medial, superior transverse, low-to-low lateral, and a right intermediate osteotomies were performed.

the anatomical deformities particularly those of the septum. The authors always write each anticipated step of the surgical procedure in the notes, after consultation and when photographic analysis is complete. This plan is reviewed with the patient when informed consent for surgery is taken, and in the operating theater with photograph review prior to the commencement of surgery.

The surgical plan may be modified during surgery and it is important to understand that planning is a dynamic process and continues during surgery when it is possible to understand nasal anatomy better. The authors find taking intraoperative photographs from several positions and viewing them on the camera's liquid crystal display during surgery very helpful in increasing their appreciation of the patient's anatomy.

13.7 CONTRAINDICATIONS

The main contraindications to surgery are psychological. If the patient's expectations cannot be met or the patient cannot accept the risks of surgery, then these must be considered absolute contraindications. If the patient has a sense of bitterness or unfairness about considering surgery or has an excessive sense of importance and entitlement, then these may be relative contraindications to surgery. The entitled patient may feel even more embittered if they have any amount of adverse outcome. The crooked nose is often associated with complex nasal and septal deformity and surgical inexperience is therefore also a relative contraindication to surgery. As with any elective operation, the patient's general health must also be considered.

13.8 SURGICAL TECHNIQUES

Surgery is performed under general anesthesia with a laryngeal mask in the author's practice. A hypotensive technique is used complemented by a reverse Trendelenberg patient position. The nasal and facial skin and nasal lining are prepared with aqueous chlorhexidine and the patient is draped. The nose is marked as necessary to aid incisions and recognition of anatomical features and infiltrated with 2–4 mL of 1:80,000 adrenaline with 2% xylocaine. In most cases, an open approach is used and the tip cartilages are separated to allow bilateral septal flap elevation and a full view of the entire quadrilateral cartilage. This is further enabled by release of the upper lateral cartilages flush with the quadrilateral cartilage (Fig. 13.4).

A step-wise approach is taken to septal correction. Initially, the ventral edge of the quadrilateral cartilage is released from the maxillary crest and vomer while preserving the attachment of the posterior septal angle to the anterior nasal spine if both are in the midline. This and release of the soft tissues may allow the cartilage to sit straight and in the midline with no tension. It is important to maintain at least a 1 cm connection between the ethmoid plate and the posterior edge of the quadrilateral cartilage at the K area. If the ethmoid plate is deviated, the author prefers to release the bony septum with an osteotome or the Becker-Caplan scissors from the floor of the nose and to fracture it to the midline, rather than resecting bone. If the quadrilateral cartilage remains intrinsically curved, the authors excise cartilage from the body of septum but ensure at least a 1 cm caudal and dorsal strut remains. Curves in these struts are corrected by incision through the maximum points of curvature and splinting of the cartilage pieces with a batten of excised cartilage (Figs. 13.5 and 13.6) or ethmoid plate (Figs. 13.7 and 13.8). If the cartilage graft is curved, its concave surface is placed against the concave surface of the septum and sutured with 4/0 or 5/0 polydioxanone (PDS) suture (Figs. 13.9A to F). If these cartilage batten grafts, which when paradorsal in position may also be considered as spreader grafts, do not straighten a deformity, then it may be necessary to excise the deformed piece of cartilage and replace it with harvested straight cartilage or bony septum grafts (Figs. 13.10A and B). In severe cases of deformity, the entire quadrilateral cartilage may need to be excised, remodeled, and reconstructed on the back table and replaced. This is the extracorporeal septoplasty technique (Gugisch, Constantinescu, 1999). It is important that the septum is fixed well at 2 points, these being at least the anterior nasal spine and the upper lateral cartilages at the K area. If insufficient graft material is available for harvest from the septum, then additional cartilage can be taken from the ear or rib or the reconstructed pieces of septum can be stabilized on polydioxanone foil (Tweedie, Lo and Rowe-Jones, 2010). More recently the authors have found some anecdotal evidence of increased infection rates in cases where PDS foil has been used and at this stage caution has been advised.

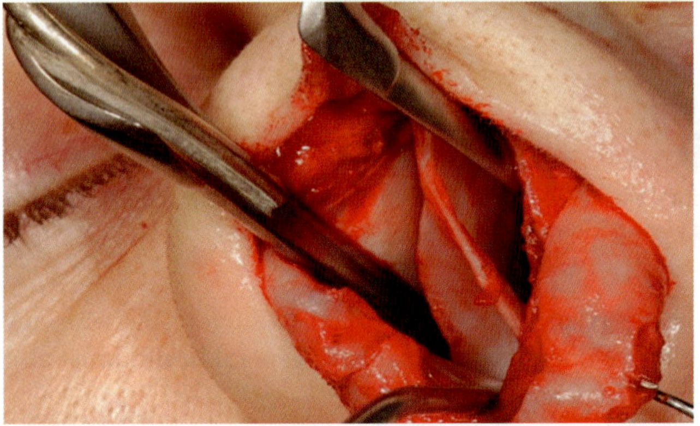

Fig. 13.4: An open approach with separation of the lower lateral cartilages, elevation of bilateral septal mucoperichondrial flaps and release of the upper laterals from the quadrilateral cartilage gives an excellent view of multiple curvatures in the quadrilateral cartilage.

Osteotomies are required to reposition and improve symmetry in the external bony nose. If the entire bony vault is deviated but the slope of each lateral wall is symmetrical in its relationship with the dorsum, then low to low lateral and superior transverse osteotomies may be

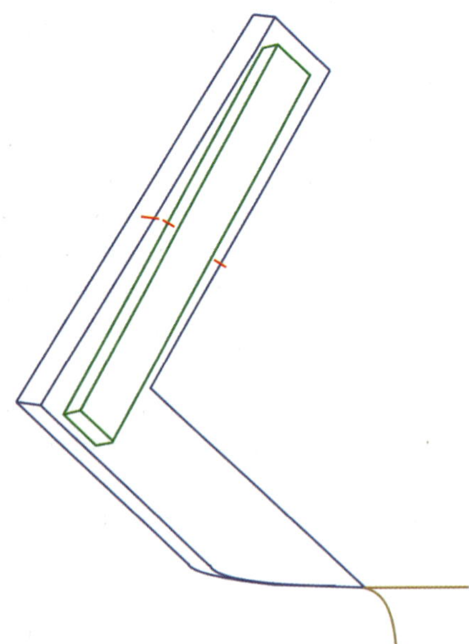

Fig. 13.5: Incision through the dorsal strut stabilized on a left spreader graft.

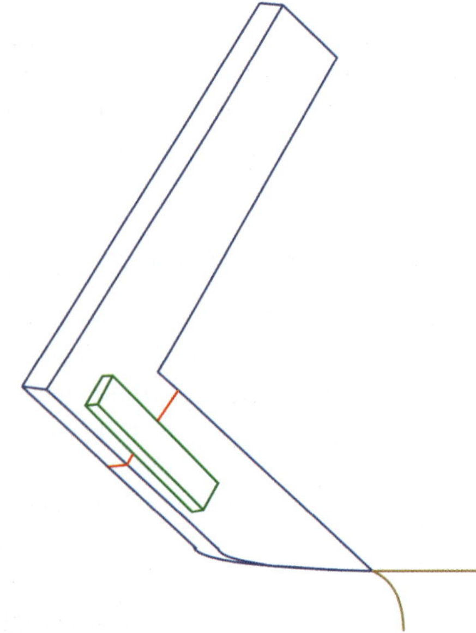

Fig. 13.6: Incision through the caudal strut stabilized on a linear batten graft.

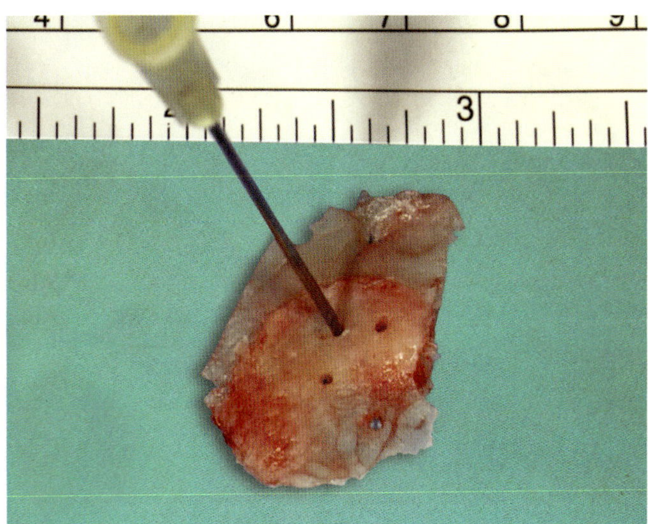

Fig. 13.7: Holes made in ethmoid plate with a 19 gauge needle to enable suturing of this graft across curved septal cartilage. The graft stabilizes and straightens incised septum.

all that is necessary without necessitating medial osteotomies. The entire vault is then repositioned en bloc. If there is reluctance of the bony vault to move, then it may be necessary to use an additional midline nasal root osteotomy at the nasion.

However, if one lateral wall is excessively medialized, it may be necessary to perform a medial osteotomy to enable out fracture of this bone. If one bony lateral wall is wider than the other side (measured from the dorsum to the face), or is excessively convex, an intermediate osteotomy may also be necessary (Figs. 13.1 and 13.3). If an excess of length is present with a dorsal hump, asymmetric hump reduction with more hump removed from the longer side may be considered.

Bony asymmetries due to callous formation may need to be rasped and cartilage irregularities shaved. Asymmetries due to depressions may be disguised with onlay grafts inserted into precise pockets. These grafts can be of shaved, softened, crushed, or diced cartilage.

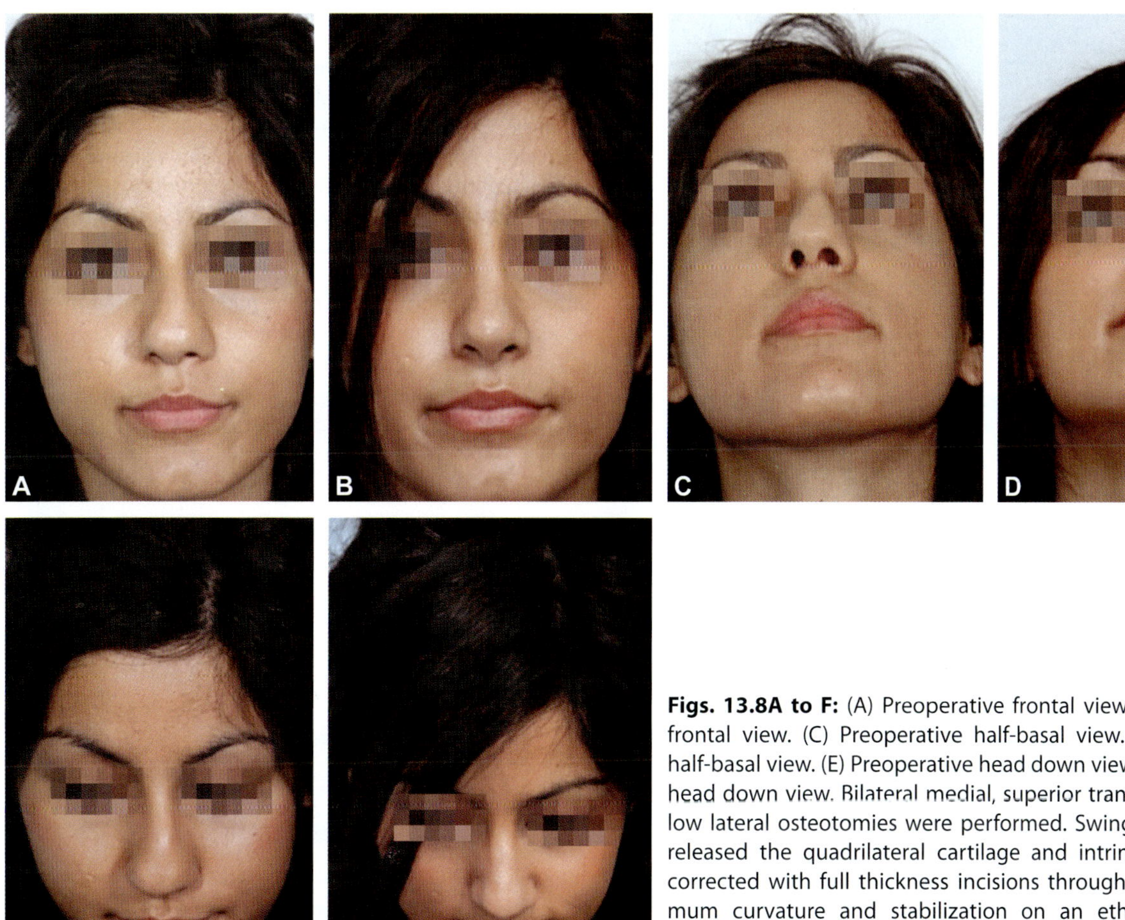

Figs. 13.8A to F: (A) Preoperative frontal view. (B) Postoperative frontal view. (C) Preoperative half-basal view. (D) Postoperative half-basal view. (E) Preoperative head down view. (F) Postoperative head down view. Bilateral medial, superior transverse and low to low lateral osteotomies were performed. Swing door septoplasty released the quadrilateral cartilage and intrinsic curvature was corrected with full thickness incisions through the axes of maximum curvature and stabilization on an ethmoid plate graft. Bilateral dome creation and a dome equalization sutures were used to correct tip asymmetry and improve definition. A right alar rim support graft was also used.

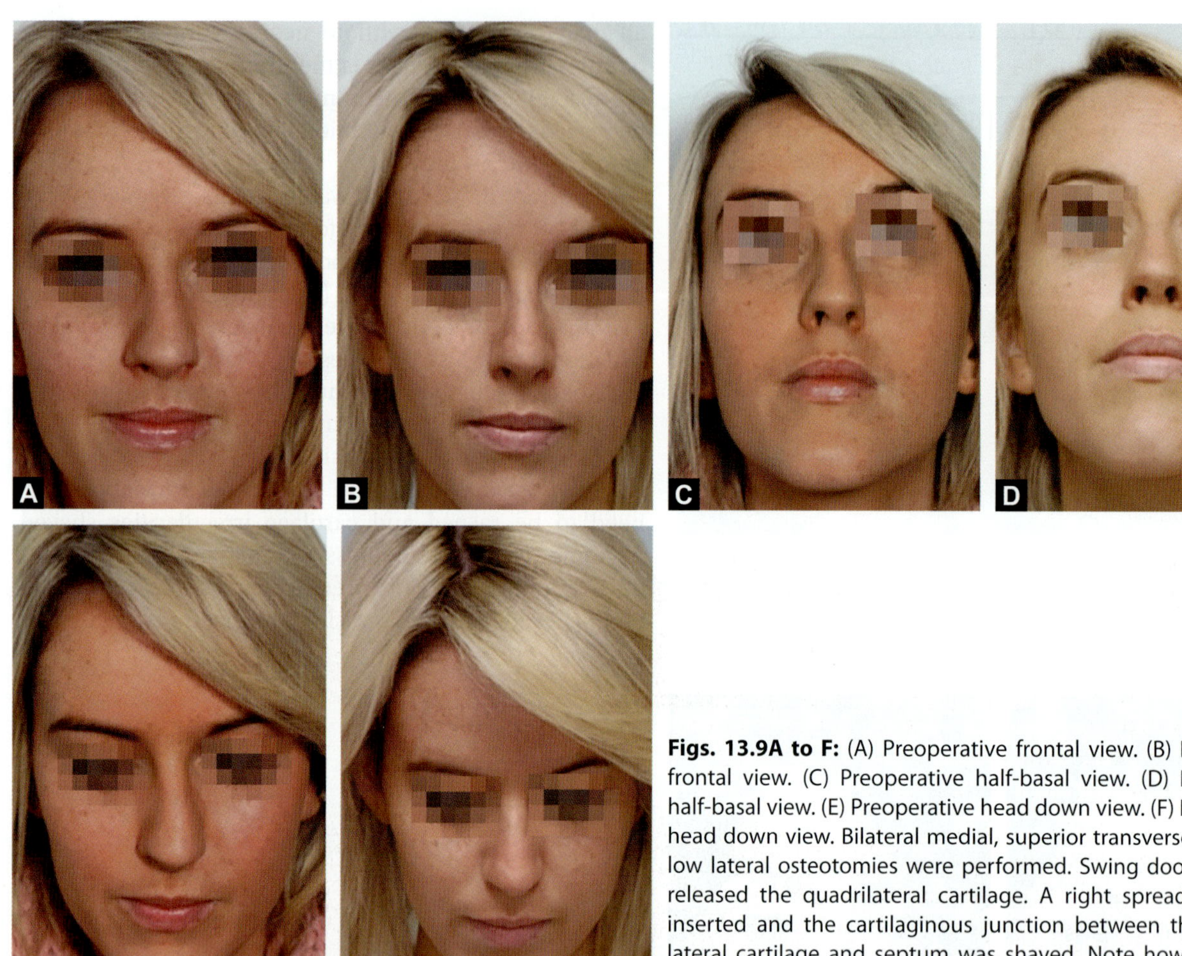

Figs. 13.9A to F: (A) Preoperative frontal view. (B) Postoperative frontal view. (C) Preoperative half-basal view. (D) Postoperative half-basal view. (E) Preoperative head down view. (F) Postoperative head down view. Bilateral medial, superior transverse and low-to-low lateral osteotomies were performed. Swing door septoplasty released the quadrilateral cartilage. A right spreader graft was inserted and the cartilaginous junction between the left upper lateral cartilage and septum was shaved. Note how the menton and philtrum are still to the right of the midline but straightening the nose leads to an improved appearance.

Figs. 13.10A and B: (A) 1 = new caudal septal strut, 2 = right spreader graft. Extracorporeal construction of a new caudal septal strut with incorporated right spreader graft. (B) 1 = new caudal septal strut; 2 = right spreader graft; 3 = remaining dorsal septal strut after caudal resection; 4 = upper lateral cartilages. The construction in situ. The new caudal strut is positioned to overlap the remaining dorsal strut on its right side. This dorsal strut was curved to the right prior to insertion of the grafts.

Table 13.1: Complications associated with septorhinoplasty for the crooked nose.

Primary reactionary hemorrhage
Secondary hemorrhage which may occur up to 2 weeks after surgery
Infection
New or residual aesthetic deformity
New or residual functional disorder
Visible scars
Persistent skin-soft tissue swelling
Skin changes
Septal perforation
Psychological morbidity

The authors close columella incisions with 6/0 Vicryl rapide and marginal incisions with 5/0 monocryl. The septum is quilted with 4/0 Vicryl rapide. Intranasal packs are not routinely used. The nose is dressed with an external splint of melolin, Steri-Strips, plaster of Paris, and micropore. The patient is recovered sitting-up initially with the laryngeal mask still in place until fully conscious.

13.9 POSTOPERATIVE MANAGEMENT

The patient remains in hospital for 6 hours postoperatively, as this is the period during which reactionary hemorrhage is most likely. The patient is discharged with an oral broad-spectrum antibiotic such as co-amoxiclav 625 mg 8 hourly for a week and instructed to perform careful toilet of the nares and columella, nasal vestibules, and any external incisions. This is performed with 3% hydrogen peroxide solution and topical antibiotics including mupirocin ointment and ciprofloxacin two to three times daily for a week. The patient is reviewed 1-week postoperatively for the removal of external nasal dressings and nasal sutures. The patient is advised to avoid vigorous exercise for the first 2 weeks postoperatively and contact sports for 6 weeks at least. Strong sunlight on the nose should be avoided for 3 months and the use of sun block on any scars is recommended.

13.10 COMPLICATIONS

The complications are listed in Table 13.1. Complications are minimized by exacting and careful analysis and operative planning, careful patient selection, and comprehensive preoperative discussion explaining the risks limitations and unpredictability of surgery. Careful tissue handling, meticulous dissection, and good exposure aided by hypotensive anesthesia are essential. Exacting intraoperative anatomical assessment and surgical techniques that embrace reconstruction rather than resection with the maintenance of good caudal and dorsal septal struts and augmentation of tip support mechanisms with sutures and grafts are vital. Rarely does the patient with a crooked nose need any net loss of nasal skeleton tissue. Any cartilage removed that is not used for grafting and strengthening should be shaved and divided if necessary to straighten and replaced between the septal mucosal flaps. In our last rhinoplasty series, our postoperative hemorrhage rate was 1.4% and our infection rate was 0.7%.

REFERENCES

Daniel, R.K., 2010. Functional factors. In: R.K. Daniel, ed. *Mastering rhinoplasty*. 2nd ed. Berlin: Springer-Verlag. pp. 183-224.

Gubisch, W. and Constantinescu, M.A., 1999. Refinements in extracorporeal septoplasty. *Plastic Reconstruction Surgery*, 104(4), pp. 1131-40.

Roofe, S.B. and Murakami, C.S., 2006. Treatment of the post-traumatic and postrhinoplasty crooked nose. *Facial Plastic Surgery Clinics of North America*, 14(4), pp. 279-90.

Tweedie, D., Lo, S. and Rowe-Jones, J., 2010. Reconstruction of the septum using perforated and non-perforated polydioxanone foil. *Archives of Facial Plastic Surgery*, 12(2), pp. 106-13.

Saddle Nose 14

Amit D Bhrany, Craig S Murakami

Chapter Overview

Pearls and Pitfalls

Pearls

- The saddle nose deformity represents a spectrum of dorsal nasal depression with varying degrees of structural loss and functional compromise. A thorough preoperative evaluation to determine the extent of deficit is required for optimal reconstruction.
- Saddle nose deformity may be secondary to systemic diseases like Wegener's granulomatosis, sarcoidosis, and malignancy. It is important to treat these underlying conditions before initiating treatment for saddling.
- Saddle nose deformity may be associated with severe collapse/contracture of the internal and/or external nasal valve. In such patients nasal framework reconstruction with replacement of all three nasal layers is the appropriate treatment to correct the form and function of the nose.

Pitfalls

- Failure to recognize the functional impact of saddle nose deformity and treating it solely as an aesthetic deformity will lead to suboptimal nasal function and an unhappy patient.

14.1 INTRODUCTION

The saddle nose deformity refers to the collapse and depression of the nasal dorsum when viewed in profile, resembling the depression in a horse's saddle. It develops from a loss of dorsal and septal structural support beneath the nasal soft-tissue envelope. The deformity may vary from a slight supratip depression to loss of projection along the entire nasal dorsum depending on the extent of nasal skeletal deficiency. As the severity of framework weakness progresses, collapse and widening of the middle vault concavity are hallmarks followed by columellar retraction, tip rotation, deprojection, widening of the alar base, and the appearance of a short nose. Functionally, nasal valve compromise of the internal and external nasal valves leads to nasal obstruction.

14.2 ETIOLOGY AND PREOPERATIVE EVALUATION

Although congenital causes of saddle deformity exist, iatrogenic and incidental trauma are the most common etiologies. Excessive resections of the dorsum and/or septum are common reasons for saddle deformity in postsurgical patients. For patients who have not sustained any trauma or previous nasal surgery, septal destruction from chronic vasoconstrictor use (oxymetazoline, cocaine), long-term topical steroid use or systemic disease (Wegener's granulomatosis, sarcoidosis, infection, malignancy) should be considered.

As with most rhinoplasty patients, a complete history and physical examination are critical for successful evaluation and treatment of the patients with a saddle nose

Table 14.1: Classification of saddle nose deformities (Alsarraf and Murakami, 1999).

	External deformity	*Nasal airway*
Type 1	Mild supratip saddle	Normal
Type 2	Moderate depression of dorsal septum and upper lateral cartilages	Mild nasal valve collapse
Type 3	Moderate depression of dorsal septum and upper lateral cartilages	Nasal stenosis with mucosal contracture
Type 4	Depression of the bony and cartilaginous nose	Severe nasal stenosis
Type 5	Massive depression of the bony and cartilaginous nose	Minimal or no septum and severe nasal stenosis

deformity. Specific attention should be paid to elucidating the timing and onset of presentation, rate of progression, presence of any associated epistaxis, crusting, nasal obstruction, and history of any previous nasal surgery or trauma. Physical examination initiates with inspection of the external nose at rest and upon inspiration to evaluate for dynamic collapse of the nasal valves. Palpation assesses the status of the septum, bony pyramid, upper and lower lateral cartilages, and tip. Particular attention should be paid to thoroughly palpate the dorsal and caudal septal struts. The relative profile of the bony and cartilaginous dorsum must be determined as it is possible that a small saddle deformity confined to only the cartilaginous portion of the nose is accentuated by an adjacent bony hump deformity. The converse is also common where a small traumatic dorsal hump is in reality a subtle saddling of the cartilaginous dorsum. The Cottle maneuver using lateral cheek retraction can help identify nasal valve compromise. Providing support intranasally with a cotton swab or ear curette can help specify internal versus external nasal valve collapse. Intranasal examination provides information on the presence of septal perforation, mucosal crusting or ulceration, and degree of valve compromise. In addition to loss of cartilage support, there may be additional airway compromise caused by internal nasal lining stenosis (contracture). When a septal perforation is present, a low threshold for biopsy should be present to rule out an inflammatory or neoplastic process causing the saddle deformity.

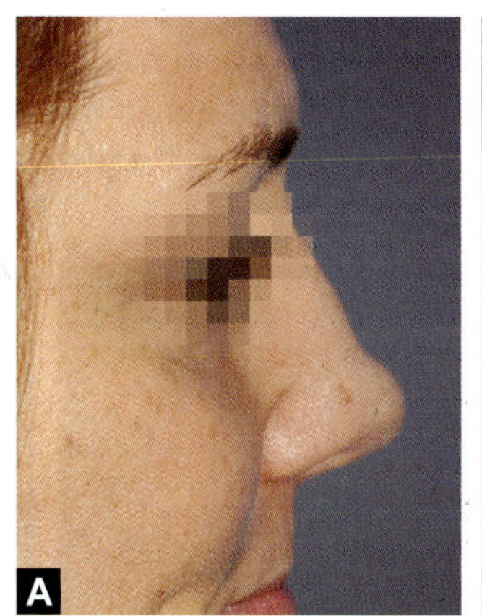

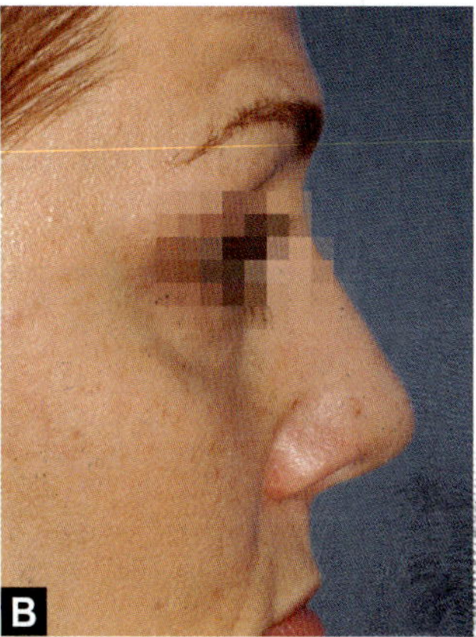

Figs. 14.1A and B: (A) Preoperative view of patient with supratip type 1 saddle depression. (B) Four months postoperative after correction with onlay conchal cartilage graft.

14.3 CLASSIFICATION AND TREATMENT

Once the assessment is complete, the severity of the saddle deformity should be classified because the approach for correction differs based on the degree of deformity. Numerous classification schemes of saddle deformity have been described and are useful in surgical planning (Sessions and Stallings, 1972; Tardy, Schwartz and Parras, 1989; Alsarraf and Murakami, 1999; Daniel and Brenner, 2006). Alsarraf and Murakami describe the external and nasal airway impact of the deformity (Table 14.1).

Type 1

Type 1 saddle deformities are the least severe, with only a mild supratip saddle and a normal nasal airway. Dorsal and caudal septal support is intact with a normal or near-normal tip position. Nasal length to the subnasale is normal. Generally, there is no columellar retraction and loss of tip projection. A simple onlay camouflage graft of autogenous cartilage or temporalis fascia is typically adequate for reconstruction (Figs. 14.1A and B). A columellar strut is useful in the rare occasion when patients also have decreased tip projection and columellar retraction. Graft placement is often achievable into precise pockets through intranasal incisions. Occasionally, a coexisting bony hump deformity accentuates as small supratip saddle. An acceptable profile may be achieved with bony dorsal hump correction alone as opposed to camouflage or augmentation of the saddle deformity itself.

Type 2

Type 2 deformities have moderate depression of the dorsal septum and upper lateral cartilages with mild nasal valve collapse. There is loss of nasal length, decreased middle third and tip projection, and some degree of columellar retraction. A more extensive reconstruction is required with an external approach. The upper lateral cartilages are separated from the dorsal septum leaving the septal mucosa intact. Once the upper lateral cartilages have been mobilized and elevated back into normal position, an onlay spreader graft is placed straddling the depressed dorsal septum and sutured between the upper lateral cartilages. The graft is approximately 4 mm in width at its cephalic end widened to 6 mm at its caudal end and approximately 2 cm in length. Such a graft simultaneously elevates the dorsum and opens the nasal valves bilaterally (Figs. 14.2A to E). Septal cartilage is preferred, but if deficient, either autologous rib or conchal cartilage is used. Fixation of the conchal cartilage graft to a polydioxanone plate can strengthen grafts giving them rigidity similar to septal cartilage. Another technique is to use bilateral spreader grafts as opposed to the onlay spreader graft. An additional onlay graft is required for correction of the dorsal depression. This decision is based on the degree of airway compromise in the area of the internal valve.

Type 3

Type 3 saddle deformities have severe depression of the dorsal septum and upper lateral cartilages with significant

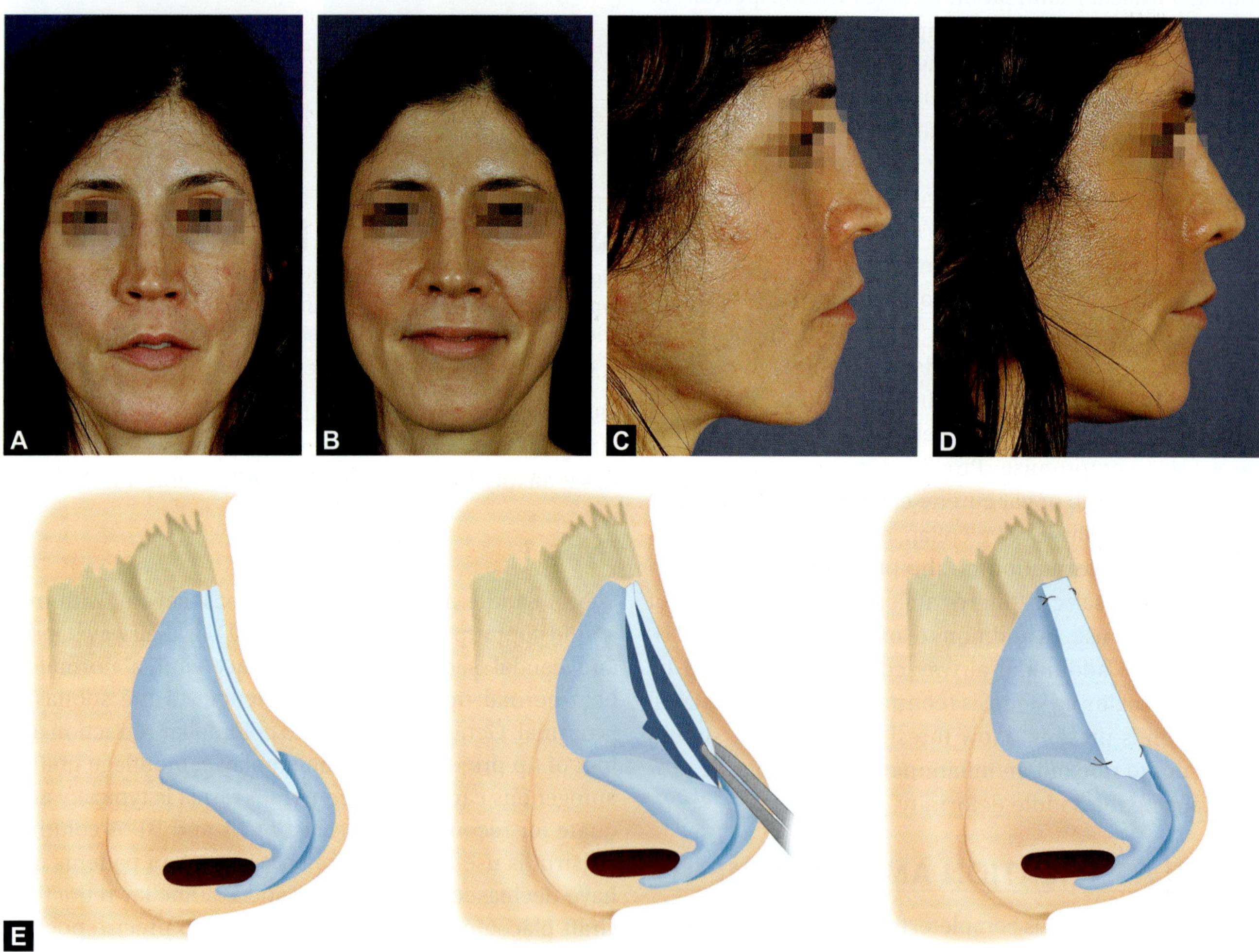

Figs. 14.2A to E: (A and C) Preoperative views of patient with type 2 saddle deformity. The patient underwent repair with a dorsal onlay spreader graft and a columellar strut to improve mild columellar retraction and tip support. (B and D) Fifteen-month postoperative views. (E) Schematic of saddle deformity correction with dorsal onlay spreader graft.

Source: With permission from Murakami, C.S. and Guida. R., 1998. Saddle deformity. In: R. Gates, ed. *Current therapy in Oto/HNS*. St. Louis: Mosby. p. 170.

nasal valve stenosis. There is total loss of septal support for the middle third, tip, and nasal valves. The vestibular mucosa may also be contracted, further worsening nasal valve compromise. Repair is taken through an approach similar to repair for type 2 deformities. The extent of the defect typically requires autologous rib cartilage for placement of onlay spreader graft or extended bilateral spreader grafts. A strong columellar strut fixed to the anterior nasal spine and spreader grafts augments tip support and helps in repair of nasal valves. If the contracted internal nasal lining is contributing to nasal valve compromise, the nasal mucosa can be elevated medially along the septum and laterally beneath the upper lateral cartilages. If the mucosa is immobile, it can be incised to open nasal valve stenosis. An elliptical composite graft (conchal cartilage and skin) can be placed, straddling the dorsal septum similar to the butterfly graft described by Clark (Alsarraf and Murakami, 1999; Clark, 2002). The skin on the graft is incised vertically to create two separate islands that line each nasal valve region. Additional onlay or tip grafts may be needed for further projection (Figs. 14.3A to F).

Type 4

Type 4 deformities have progressed to the end stage of septal collapse with depression of both the bony and cartilaginous dorsum (Fig. 14.4A). Severe contraction of the internal nasal lining with an associated septal perforation is often present. There is columellar shortening, loss of tip projection, increased tip rotation, with a widened alar base, and broad nostrils. The nose is shortened with an acute nasolabial angle. There is significant nasal valve compromise and nasal obstruction. A dorsal graft of autologous rib or split calvarium is required for structural

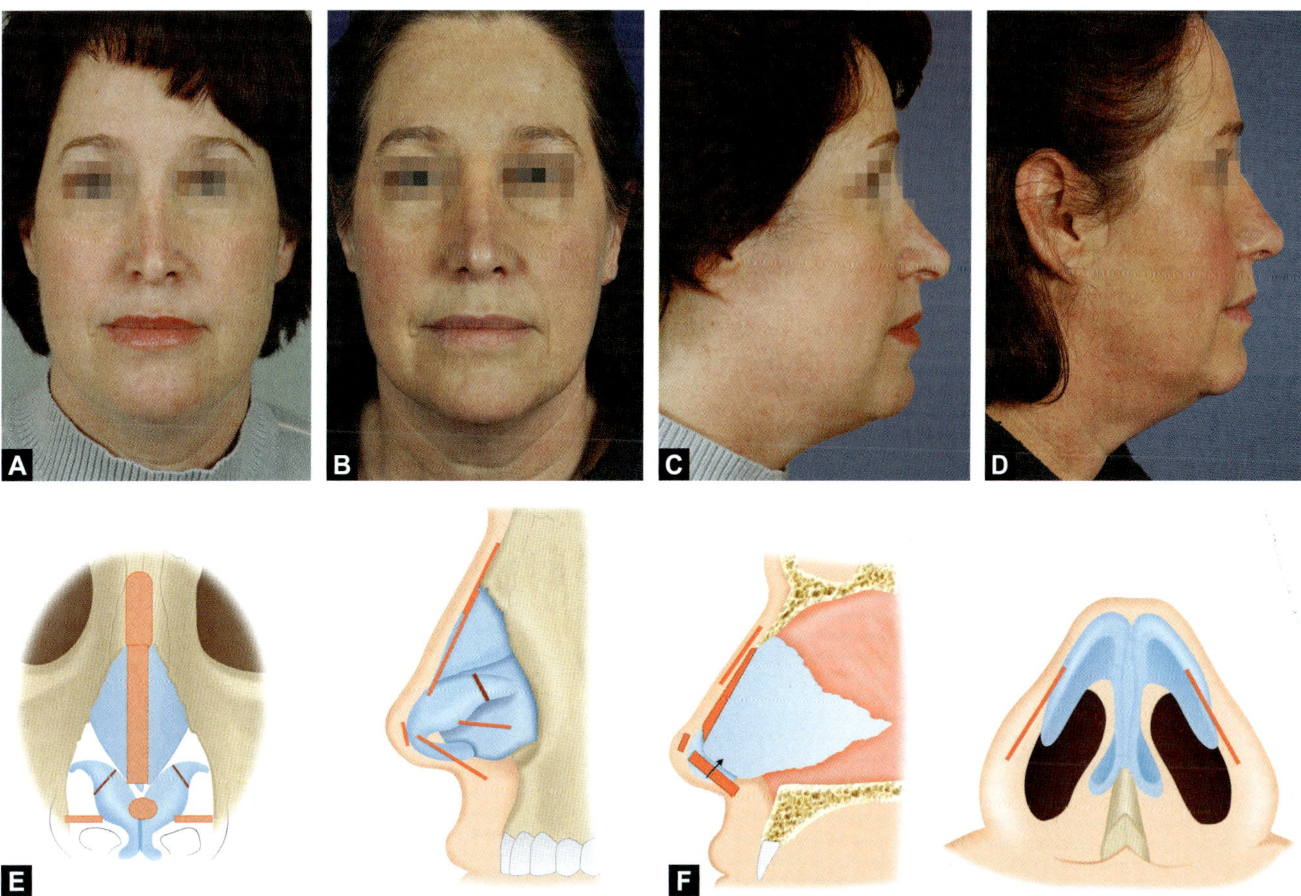

Figs. 14.3A to F: (A and C) Preoperative views of patient with type 3 saddle deformity. (B and D) Eight-year postoperative views. (E and F) Schematic diagrams demonstrating dorsal onlay spreader graft with additional cartilage augmentation of the dorsum for saddle deformity. Lateral crural overlay, a columellar strut, and a tip cap graft provided additional tip rotation, projection, and definition. Bilateral alar rim grafts were placed to correct the alar–columella disproportion.

support (Figs. 14.4A and B). The graft is placed in a precise subperiosteal pocket and cantilevered from the remaining bony nasal dorsum, often secured with a single fixation screw. If an osseocartilaginous rib graft is being used, the bony portion of the graft is placed cephalically at the nasal bones to facilitate integration. The caudal end of the dorsal graft is secured to a columellar strut that is fixed to the anterior nasal spine. If minimal periosteal tissue is present along the nasal spine, a hole can be drilled in the spine to permit fixation. The upper lateral cartilages can be elevated to the dorsal graft to improve nasal valve compromise. Attempts are made to elevate the domes of the lower lateral cartilages over the caudal end of the dorsal graft and columellar strut to improve the external valves. Alar batten and possibly rim grafts are placed for further support of the external nasal valves.

Figs. 14.4A and B: (A) Preoperative views of patient with type 4 saddle deformity associated with septal perforation from Wegener's granulomatosis. Patient underwent dorsal cantilevered calvarial bone graft and extended columellar strut fixed to anterior nasal spine. (B) Three-month postoperative views.

Type 5

Type 5 deformities are catastrophic and represent massive dorsal depression with a complete loss of nasal support and lack of a nasal septum. The overlying soft tissue and internal nasal lining are often scarred and contracted due to major resections and postoperative radiation therapy for sinonasal malignancies. Composite grafts, inferior turbinate mucosal flaps, melolabial flaps, or a forehead flap may be necessary for internal coverage of multiple grafts required for total nasal reconstruction (Murakami, Kriet and Ierokomos, 1999; Parikh, Futran and Most, 2010) (Figs. 14.5A to D). Free tissue transfer reconstruction such as with a radial forearm flap can be used for extremely large defects and when no local options exist (Antunes and Chalian, 2011).

SUMMARY

The saddle nose deformity represents a spectrum of dorsal nasal depression with varying degrees of structural loss and functional compromise. A thorough preoperative evaluation to determine the extent of deficit is required for optimal reconstruction. Repair necessitates placement of a number of grafts that not only augment the dorsum but also open the nasal airway.

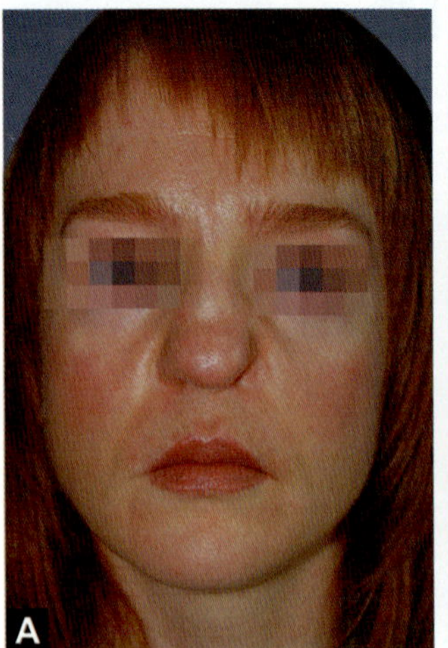

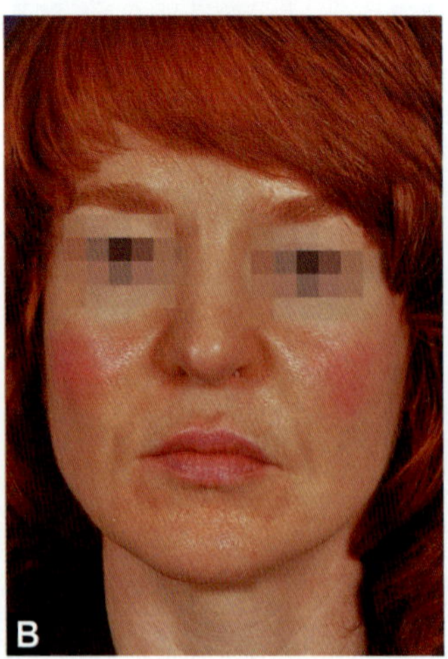

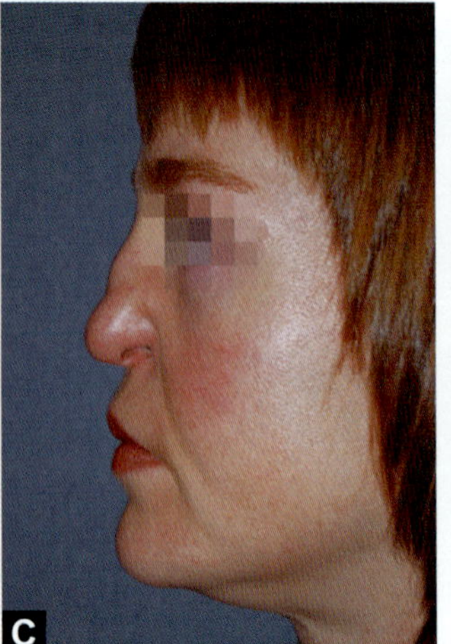

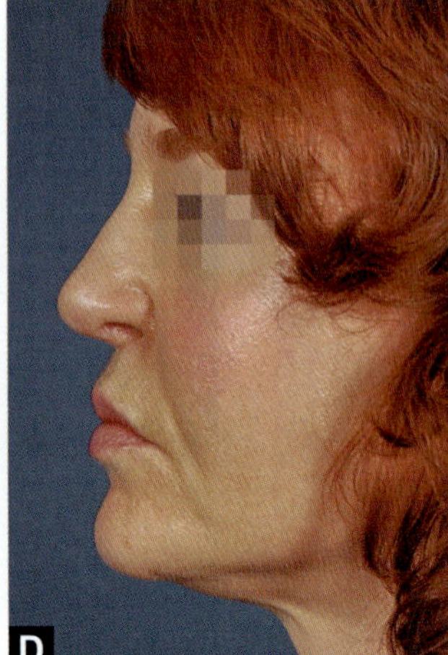

Figs. 14.5A to D: (A and C) Preoperative views of patient with type 5 saddle deformity associated with total septal perforation. Patient underwent dorsal cantilevered rib graft with extended columellar strut. Severe left alar retraction reconstructed at second stage with a composite conchal cartilage graft. (B and D) Eight-month postoperative views.

REFERENCES

Alsarraf, P. and Murakami, C.S., 1999. The saddle nose deformity. *Facial Plastic Surgery Clinics of North America*, 7, p. 303.

Antunes, M.B. and Chalian, A.A., 2011. Microvascular reconstruction of nasal defects. *Facial Plastic Surgery Clinics of North America*, 19, pp. 157-62.

Daniel, R.K. and Brenner, K.A., 2006. Saddle nose deformity: a new classification and treatment. *Facial Plastic Surgery Clinics of North America*, 14, pp. 301-12, vi.

Murakami, C.S., Kriet, J.D. and Ierokomos, A.P., 1999. Nasal reconstruction using the inferior turbinate mucosal flap. *Archives of Facial Plastic Surgery*, 1, pp. 97-100.

Parikh, S., Futran, N.D. and Most, S.P., 2010. An alternative method for reconstruction of large intranasal lining defects: the Farina method revisited. *Archives of Facial Plastic Surgery*, 12, pp. 311-4.

Sessions, D.G. and Stallings, J.O., 1972. Correction of saddle nose deformity. *Laryngoscope*, 82, pp. 2000-7.

Tardy, M.E., Jr., Schwartz, M. and Parras, G. 1989. Saddle nose deformity: autogenous graft repair. *Facial Plastic Surgery*, 6, pp. 121-34.

The Patient Wanting to Alter Asian Nose

15

Ian Loh, Jung Dong Hak

Chapter Overview

Pearls and Pitfalls

Pearls

- Oriental ideals for the nose differ significantly from Caucasian populations. An appreciation of these norms is necessary for a good outcome when performing rhinoplasty for the Oriental patient.
- The radix is significantly lower with a more obtuse nasofrontal angle, whereas the nasolabial angle is also more acute.
- The nasal tip is less projected and bulbous, whereas the alar base is wider.
- Most Oriental patients will require augmentation rhinoplasty: with dorsal augmentation, increased tip projection with control of tip rotation, reduction in tip bulbosity, and alar base surgery to reduce alar base width.
- The need for significant augmentation material in the Oriental patient, combined with smaller septal cartilages available for autologous harvest, often results in the need for alloplastic material to be used for dorsal augmentation.

Pitfalls

- Control of tip rotation with structural tip grafting is important while projecting the Oriental nasal tip to prevent creation of a "short nose".
- Scarring and soft-tissue complications are more common in the thicker and more sebaceous Oriental skin.
- Suture techniques, which may work well for the Caucasian nose, have limited effect on the Oriental nasal tip. Tip projection and definition are best achieved with structural tip grafting coupled with onlay tip grafting.

15.1 INTRODUCTION

Asia is region of great ethnic diversity. Although it is impossible to speak of a standard ideal for the nose across all racial groups that exist in Asia, the following chapter will focus chiefly on the *Oriental nose* and *Oriental rhinoplasty*. The term "Asian" has thus been used interchangeably with "Oriental" in this chapter.

15.2 ANATOMY

The Asian nose varies greatly from its Caucasian counterpart. Appreciation of these differences helps the rhinoplasty surgeon to refine the nose while retaining its ethnicity. These differences will be highlighted using Caucasian norms for comparison (Sim, Smith and Chan, 2000).

Frontal View

The bridge of the nose and nasal base is wider in the Asian patients. Vertical lines drawn tangential to the Asian alar facial groove are often lateral to the medial canthus. Tip bulbosity is more pronounced and is due to a combination of weaker, more flared lower lateral cartilages (LLCs) and thicker, more sebaceous nasal tip skin. Asian nasal

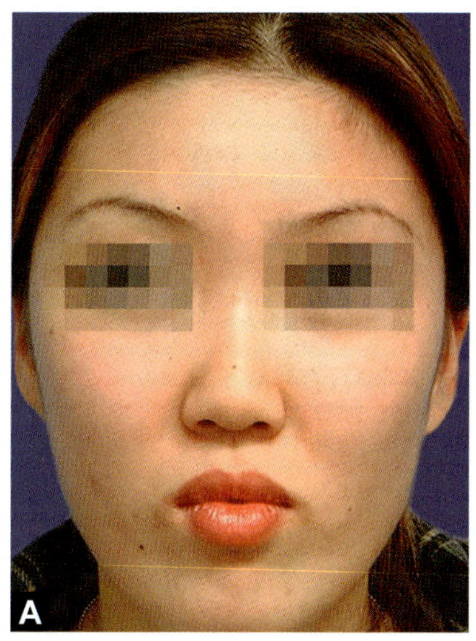

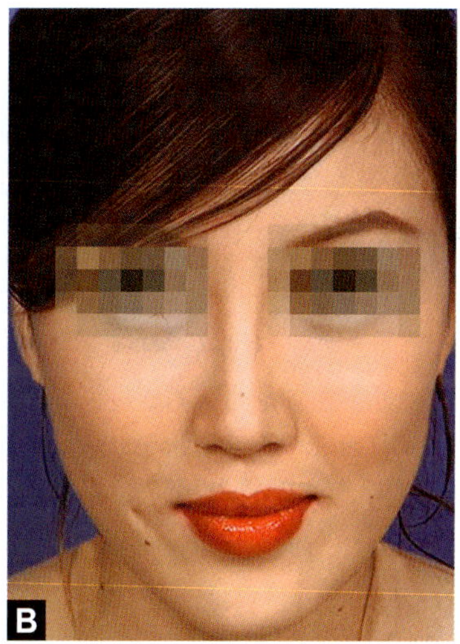

Figs. 15.1A and B: (A) Typical Asian nose demonstrating low-lying radix and dorsum. The tip is underprojected, excessively rotated, and bulbous. The columella is retracted. The prominent nasolabial folds, concavity of the paranasal region, and appearance of a protruding mouth reflect a bony deficiency in the paranasal area. This patient also had significant hypertelorism. (B) Same patient after augmentation rhinoplasty and *paranasal augmentation* resulting in improved facial aesthetic. Augmentation and accentuation of the radix have also resulted in an apparent reduction in hypertelorism and narrowing of the nasal dorsum.

tips also have a rounder less defined configuration when compare with Caucasian nasal tips (Figs. 15.1A and B).

Profile View

The Asian radix, dorsum, and nasal tip tend to be underprojected. In Caucasians, the nasion lies between the superior eyelash and supratarsal crease, whereas the vertical level of the nasion is often lower in Orientals. This should lie between the interpupillary line and upper eyelid crease in Orientals (the upper eyelid crease is also lower in the Asian eyelid).

The Asian nasal tip is underprojected and often overrotated. The combination of a low radix and over-rotated tip results in a "short nose" where the overall dorsal nasal length is reduced.

The ideal nasofrontal angle for Asians is between 135° and 140°, whereas the ideal nasolabial angle is between 90° and 95°. This differs significantly from Caucasian norms, where the ideal nasofrontal angle is more acute at 115°–130°, and the nasolabial angle is greater at 90°–105°.

The supratip break is also less obvious in Orientals; this is often small or absent and very often less than the 1–2 mm quoted for Caucasian norms.

Alar-Columella Relation

The Asian columella tends to be retracted. Certain ethnic groups, such as Southern Chinese and people of South East Asian descent, exhibit the hanging columella deformity.

Basal View

The Asian alar base is wider, and the alar sidewalls are thicker and more flared than the Caucasian noses (Figs. 15.2A and B). This results in larger appearing nostrils. The nostril axis is more horizontally oriented and the tip lobule tends to be smaller as compared to alar lobule. The tip tends to be more bulbous and less well defined.

Asian Skin

Oriental skin is darker, thicker, and more sebaceous than Caucasians and hence more prone to poorer scars and hyperpigmentation after surgery.

Thick nasal skin reduces the effectiveness of onlay tip grafts and makes it more challenging to increase nasal tip projection. Thicker tip skin also tends to camouflage attempts to define the tip using suture techniques and onlay tip grafts. The surgeon often needs to use multiple tip grafts stacked on top of each other to improve tip projection and definition.

Septal Cartilage

Asian septal cartilage is markedly smaller, weaker, and thinner than Caucasian septal cartilage (Fig. 15.3). Due to the inherent weakness of the cartilage, at least 1.5 cm caudal and dorsal struts should be left in situ when harvesting septal cartilage in Asian patients (in comparison

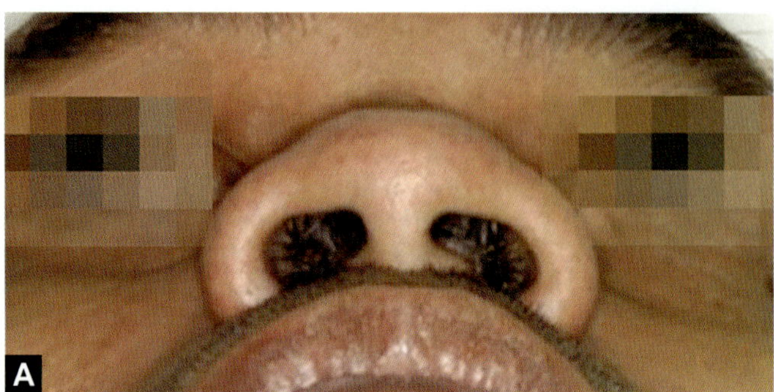

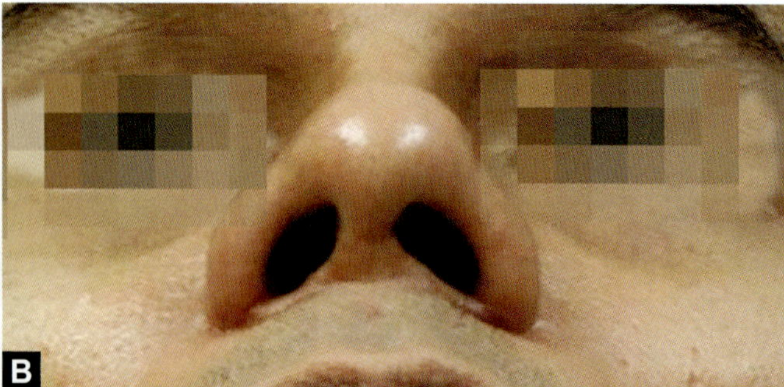

Figs. 15.2A and B: (A) Basal view of an oriental male patient with an extremely bulbous tip, flared alar sidewalls, and wide alar base. (B) Same patient after tip-plasty and alar base surgery.

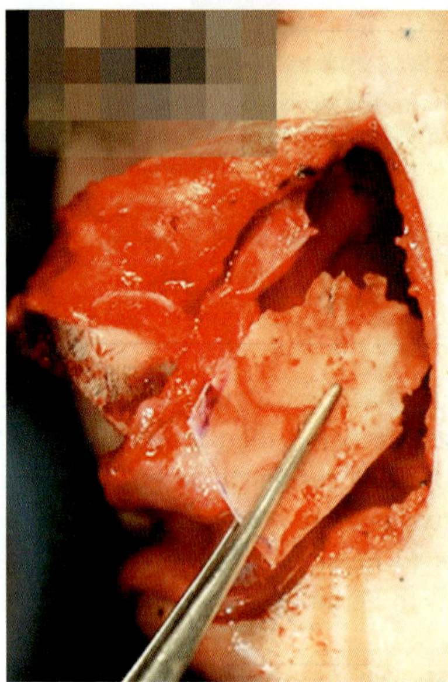

Fig. 15.3: Maximal septal cartilage harvest in preparation for nasal reconstruction in an oriental female patient after partial rhinectomy. At least 1.5-cm-caudal and dorsal septal struts have been left in situ. The bony septum has been left attached to the septal cartilage rostrally. The size of the septal cartilage and thickness of the cartilage is less as compared to Caucasian norms.

to 1 cm struts in Caucasian patients) to prevent postoperative saddle nose deformity, columellar retraction, and reduced tip projection. However, this reduces the amount of cartilage available for harvesting and makes obtaining adequate material for structural grafting and augmentation a challenge in Asian rhinoplasty (Kim, et al., 2010).

Internal Nasal Valve (INV)

The Asian INV angle is often wider (20°) as compared to Caucasian noses (15°) and results in a more flared and obtuse nasal dorsum (Suh, Jin and Kim, 2008). This widened INV, and the tendency toward smaller dorsal humps in Asians (*see* Section Humpectomy), often eliminates the need for spreader graft placement to maintain nasal patency following surgery to the nasal dorsum.

Associated Structures

The Asian patient also has a relative *midface deficiency*, most pronounced in the premaxillary and paranasal areas. This is sometimes in combination with a *bimaxillary protuberance*, which gives the appearance of a protruding mouth and facial concavity in the lateral view.

Deficiency of the mentum (chin) is a common Asian problem and should always be addressed along with any augmentation rhinoplasty; otherwise, augmentation rhinoplasty will accentuate any underlying deficiency of the chin.

The ideal Caucasian chin should touch a vertical line dropped from the lower vermillion border with the face in the Frankfort plane in males, or be just behind this in females. The ideal Asian chin is significantly less projected than this and should lie behind this line in both genders. Asian females consider a less projected chin to be aesthetically more pleasing and desirable.

An *epicanthal fold* is a feature of the Asian eyelid. *Medial epicanthoplasty* (effacement of the medial epicanthal fold) in conjunction with augmentation of the radix can be considered to improve the appearance of hypertelorism in Oriental patients.

15.3 PRINCIPLES IN ASIAN RHINOPLASTY

The typical Asian nose requires augmentation rhinoplasty. The radix, dorsum, and tip require increased projection. In general, autologous cartilage is used for structural grafting and tip surgery while alloplastic materials can be considered for augmenting the dorsum and radix.

The nasal tip often needs reduction in bulbosity, increased projection, and derotation. The need for a combination of increased tip projection and derotation requires the use of structural tip grafts (Toriumi and Pero, 2010).

Alar base surgery is used to reduce alar flaring and nasal base width; this should be carefully planned and resection minimized in the Asian patient. Scar-related complications could give poor results in Asian patients. Hence, radical alar base resections carried high into the alar groove are best avoided in the Asian patient.

Columella lengthening and reduction in the hanging ala are occasionally required in appropriate patients.

Chin and paranasal augmentation along with blepharoplasty with medial epicanthoplasty are important adjunct procedures to be considered in Asian patients.

Increased tip projection will accentuate a pre-existing hypoplastic mentum. Paranasal augmentation should be considered for patients with a deficiency in this area. This manifests as a depression in the area of the alar facial groove. Augmentation will greatly improve the result of the rhinoplasty in appropriate patients, especially improving the profile view.

Blepharoplasty and medial epicanthoplasty, together with radix augmentation, will result in an apparent narrowing of the intercanthal distance, which is useful in a patient with far spaced eyes.

15.4 SPECIFIC SURGICAL TECHNIQUES

Radix and Dorsal Augmentation

Alloplastic, autologous, and homologous material can all be considered for augmentation. Silicone in particular has a long history of use in the Asian patient. With a thicker soft-tissue envelope, the incidence of extrusion and obvious implant show may occur less often than in the Caucasian patient with much thinner skin. However, problems with soft-tissue contracture and shortening of the nose remain a long-term concern (Jung, et al., 2004b). The author's choice of material for dorsal augmentation in Asian patients is autologous graft (cartilage or fascia lata/temporalis fascia) (Jung, et al., 2012; Tay, Tan and Loh, 2013), donor-irradiated fascia lata (Tutoplast processed fascia lata), or expanded polytetrafluoroethylene (Jang, et al., 2009).

Unless the patient is willing to accept rib cartilage harvesting or cadaveric donor grafting, alloplastic material is often needed for dorsal augmentation; this is due to the scarcity of septal cartilage in the Asian rhinoplasty patient, coupled with the need for significant full length dorsal augmentation in most Asian patients (Jung, et al., 2004a).

Regardless of choice of material, dorsal implants should maintain the same configuration as those in Caucasian patients. However, the width of the "rhinion" portion of the implant should be made less prominent in Asian patients, and the nasion vertical level should be placed slightly lower than in Caucasian patients. When the implant's cross section is examined, the dorsum of the implant should also be made more obtuse, reflecting the natural appearance of the Asian dorsum.

Humpectomy

Dorsal humps in Asian patients are smaller and require less resection of bone and cartilage. Very often, after humpectomy, there is preservation of the mucosa and a minimal or no open roof deformity. This is especially possible if the bony portion of the hump has been removed in a gradual manner using a rasp. In these instances, there will be no necessity to perform osteotomies to medialize the nasal bones.

Intermediate Osteotomies in Asians

Nasal bones are intrinsically smaller and thinner in the Asian patient. Consequently, contour deformities of the nasal bones are also less obvious, and the indications for intermediate osteotomy are less frequent in the Asian patient. If intermediate osteotomies are used to correct these contouring deformities, uncontrolled fracturing and shattering of the nasal bones can occur. The smaller nasal bones also result in less soft-tissue contact with the overlying skin, and consequently a higher risk of bony pyramid collapse into the nasal cavity following osteotomies.

Because of the above-mentioned reasons, the authors prefer the use of onlay camouflage grafts to correct any concave contouring deformities of the nasal bones. With intermediate osteotomies reserved for patients with severe contour defects, the intermediate osteotomy is performed percutaneously to avoid injury to the keystone area and collapse of the bony pyramid. When possible, the intermediate osteotomy is performed unilaterally on the convex side, as convex deformities are more amenable to correction with intermediate osteotomies.

Spreader Grafts

The Asian INV is wider in comparison to the Caucasian INV (15° vs 21°) (Suh, et al., 2008). Consequently, INV obstruction occurs less frequently in the Asian patient. This is important to consider when determining the cause of nasal obstruction in patients undergoing *functional septorhinoplasty*.

The combination of smaller humpectomies and intrinsically wider INVs in Asians also reduces the need for routine bilateral spreader graft placement after humpectomy or dorsal resection of the LLCs.

Tip Surgery and Structural Grafting

Anderson's tripod theory states that any increase in tip projection will secondarily result in increased tip rotation. This presents a challenge for the Asian nasal tip. The need for increased tip projection with derotation in Asian nasal tips requires structural tip grafting to control the secondary tip rotation that occurs naturally with increasing tip projection.

Ideal structural tip grafts include extended spreader grafts or *caudal septal extension grafts*. An *extended spreader graft* is often coupled with a modified or floating *columella strut* in the author's practice (Jung and Loh, 2011). A structural graft serves as an extension of the cartilaginous septum. The LLCs are sutured to this fixed structure to affect changes in the tip.

Full mobilization of the LLCs from the overlying skin, septum, and upper lateral cartilages is a prerequisite prior to mounting the LLCs to the structural graft. This may involve a conservative cephalic trim and dissection of the scroll area to mobilize the scroll area completely, allowing the LLCs to be transposed caudally and dorsally to achieve tip projection and derotation. Once mobilization is complete, the LLCs are then mounted onto the structural tip graft using polydioxanone sutures (PDS).

Additional tip projection and derotation are achieved through placing shield and cap grafts after this step. Cap grafts often need to be stacked in the Asian patient as the thick-soft-tissue covering decreases graft show significantly. Cap grafts for the Asian tip are routinely made rounder and broader than those used in Caucasian patients to give a more natural, roundish nasal tip in the author's practice.

Reducing the Bulbous Asian Tip

The combination of flared and weak LLCs and a thick-soft-tissue envelope makes the correction of tip bulbosity a challenge in the Asian rhinoplasty patient.

Because of the thick Asian skin and soft-tissue envelope, domal sutures, when used in isolation, only have a modest effect on changing the Asian tip. Often, a combination of methods must be used to improve tip bulbosity including domal sutures (transdomal, interdomal and lateral crural spanning sutures), cephalic trim of the LLC, thinning of the overlying skin and soft-tissue envelope, and multiple stacked cap and shield grafts (Fig. 15.4).

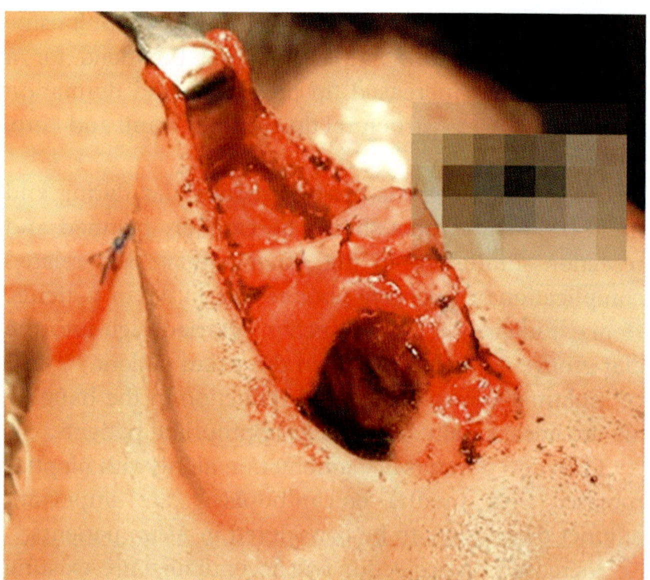

Fig. 15.4: Structural tip grafting through use of an extended spreader graft coupled with a columella strut has been used in this case to achieve projection and derotation of the nasal tip. The lower lateral cartilages have been mounted on this graft after determining the ideal tip projection and rotation. Multiple stacked cap grafts have also been used.

Projecting the tip through structural tip grafting also produces an apparent narrowing of the tip. Structural tip grafting should also be performed to prevent subsequent tip drooping and splaying of the medial crural footplates; this occurs principally with the placement of multiple stacked onlay tip grafts, resulting in gradual tip ptosis after surgery.

Alar Base Surgery

A modified Weir excision, excising a portion of the sill and alar sidewall while preserving the curved portion of the lateral nostril is most commonly used in the Asian patient. This reduces both the alar flaring and the width of the nasal base. A figure of 8 PDS suture is placed through the premaxillary soft tissue as a tension suture to reduce tension on the skin closure (Fig. 15.5).

Retracted Columella

A columella strut displaces the medial crura caudally and increases columella show in patients with a retracted

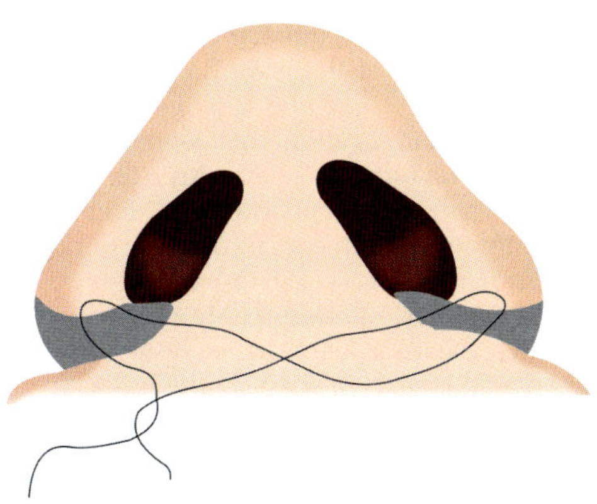
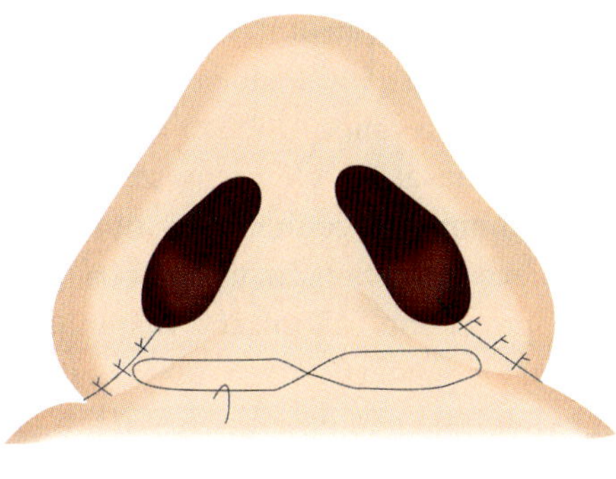

Fig. 15.5: A modified Weir excision technique is used to reduce alar flaring and nasal width. A figure of 8 polydioxanone suture is then passed through the alar base soft tissue to maintain a tension free closure while the excision site heals.

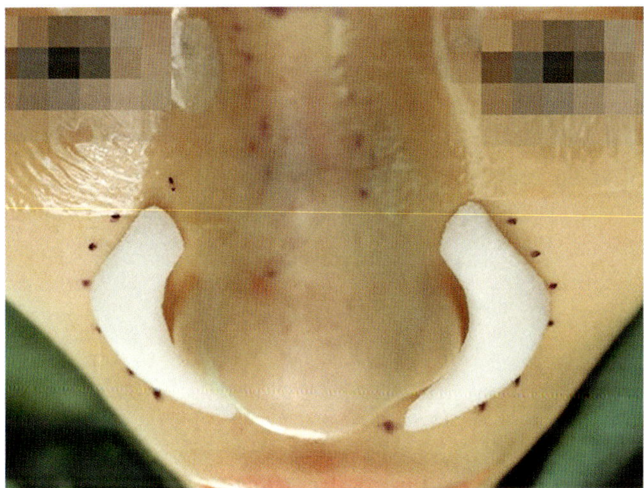

Fig. 15.6: Intraoperative photographs demonstrating the correct placement of bilateral Medpor paranasal implants. These are inserted transorally through small sublabial incisions.

columella. In severe cases, an extended caudal septal extension graft can be used to project the medial crura of the LLCs further caudally to increase columella show.

Hanging Ala

A "sail incision" within the vestibular skin can be used to elevate the alar sidewall to improve a hanging ala deformity. The incision is closed within the vestibule to hide any scarring (Yap, 2012).

Paranasal Augmentation

The concavity caused by paranasal hypoplasia can be addressed through facial skeletal surgery or augmentation using autologous bone, cartilage, or alloplastic material. The authors routinely use silicone or Medpor implants (Fig. 15.6) for this purpose and have achieved good results with a very low complication rate.

The implants are inserted through a 1.5 cm vestibular incision placed on either side of the frenulum. Subperiosteal pockets are created lateral to the pyriform aperture, and the implants are inserted under direct vision. The dissection pockets are kept small to prevent implant migration. Fixation is not necessary.

Skin Thickness

Reducing the soft-tissue thickness of the Asian nasal tip skin is sometimes required to decrease tip bulbosity and to increase definition. This is performed by the authors only after all onlay grafts have been placed on the tip, and additional tip definition is still required. Thinning of the nasal tip skin carries potential complications of skin necrosis, dermal injury, and skin discoloration, which are difficult to remedy, and should only be performed when necessary.

A pair of blunt-tipped scissors is used to make shallow perpendicular cuts on the undersurface of the skin flap, and the direction of the scissors is then changed to a plane parallel to the skin flap and used to trim the undersurface of the soft-tissue flap under tension. The process is performed under tactile feedback from the surgeon's nonoperating hand, and the skin thickness is checked intermittently to avoid injury to the dermis. This process is repeated carefully until adequate definition is attained, taking care not to over-thin the skin.

CONCLUSION

Asian rhinoplasty has different objectives from the typical Caucasian rhinoplasty. A clear understanding of the differences between Caucasian and Asian aesthetic norms is important in obtaining good results.

Augmentation is a key aim of Asian rhinoplasty, and surgery of the Asian nasal tip often requires strong structural grafting, combined together with multiple other methods to achieve reduction in tip bulbosity and tip derotation with projection. Alloplastic material is often required for dorsal augmentation.

Paranasal hypoplasia and deficiencies of the mentum are common and should be addressed at the same time to achieve ideal results.

REFERENCES

Jang, T.Y., Choi, J.Y., Jung, D.H., Park, H.J. and Lim, S.C., 2009. Histologic study of Gore-Tex removed after rhinoplasty. *Laryngoscope*, 119, pp. 620-7.

Jung, D.H., Choi, S.H., Moon, H.J., Chung, I.H., Im, J.H. and Lam, S.M., 2004a. A cadaveric analysis of the ideal costal cartilage graft for Asian rhinoplasty. *Plastic and Reconstructive Surgery*, 114, pp. 545-50.

Jung, D.H., Moon, H.J., Choi, S.H. and Lam, S.M., 2004b. Secondary rhinoplasty of the Asian nose: correction of the contracted nose. *Aesthetic Plastic Surgery*, 28, pp. 1-7.

Jung, D.H. and Loh, I., 2011. The "X-graft" for nasal tip surgery. *Plastic and Reconstructive Surgery*, 128, pp. 79e-80e.

Jung, D.H., Valse, D., Chang, G.U., Loh, I. and Park, K.M., 2012. New grafting technique to correct alar retraction. *Plastic and Reconstructive Surgery*, 130, pp. 221e-3e.

Kim, J.S., Khan, N.A., Song, H.M. and Jang, Y.J., 2010. Intraoperative measurements of harvestable septal cartilage in rhinoplasty. *Annals of Plastic Surgery*, 65, pp. 519-23.

Sim, R.S., Smith, J.D. and Chan, A.S., 2000. Comparison of the aesthetic facial proportions of southern Chinese and white women. *Archives of Facial Plastic Surgery*, 2, pp. 113-20.

Suh, M.W., Jin, H.R. and Kim, J.H., 2008. Computed tomography versus nasal endoscopy for the measurement of the internal nasal valve angle in Asians. *Acta Otolaryngologica*, 128, pp. 675-9.

Tay, V.S., Tan, K.S. and Loh, I.C., 2013. Minimally invasive fascia lata harvest: a new method. *Plastic and Reconstructive Surgery Global Open*, 1(1), pp. e7-e8.

Toriumi, D.M. and Pero, C.D., 2010. Asian rhinoplasty. *Clinics in Plastic Surgery*, 37, pp. 335-52.

Yap, E., 2012. Improving the hanging ala. *Facial Plastic Surgery*, 28, pp. 213-7.

Prominent Nose 16

Pietro Palma, Iman Khodaei, Irina Vasilenko

Chapter Overview

Pearls and Pitfalls

Pearls

- Sharpen your analytical skills.
- Treat septum first, then re-evaluate the lateral profile.
- Do not forget depressor septi nasi and nasal spine.
- Do not think in terms of humpectomy. Manage the whole profile!
- Final refinements do matter.

Pitfalls

- Not every tension nose is a true tension nose.
- Failing to see relevant anatomy.
- Overlooking stable repositioning of the tip.
- Being surgically aggressive when it is not necessary.
- Repeating the same haggard technique for every patient.

16.1 INTRODUCTION

The term *tension nose* conveys the image of a very prominent narrow nose. In essence, a tension nose is the result of an overprojection of the middle third of the nose that looks too massive for that particular individual's nasal and facial proportions. While this is somewhat true, as surgeons we need to define the clinical presentations, the specific anatomical factors that contribute to the nasal size and shape, and specific surgical options.

16.2 DEFINITION AND CLINICAL PRESENTATIONS

The common denominator in prominent or the tension nose deformity is an overprojection of the cartilaginous pyramid from the anterior septal angle to the point of maximal dorsal projection. This cartilaginous prominence leads to some secondary changes that have different expression in different patients, such as stretching of the soft-tissue envelope, narrowing of the *internal nasal valve*, apparently malpositioned lower lateral cartilages (LLCs), thin and weak alar walls, and slit-like opening of the external nostrils. These findings are often accompanied by an overprojection of the inferior–anterior nasal spine and hyperactivity of the depressor septi nasi muscle. Nasal valvular dysfunction often results due to narrowing of the internal valve angle and the distortion of the upper and LLCs (Barelli, 1982; Sputh, 1985).

The term "tension nose" is inappropriate to describe a nose where the LLCs are disproportionately large and/or malpositioned, but the septum is moderately sized. The authors classify tension nose in three basic variations, depending on the following surface landmarks: nasion, anterior septal angle, pronasale in static and dynamic state, alar rim configuration, and subnasale. However, it is important to realize that any of these three categories may be found in various combinations with each other. The surgeon must take into account the patients unique features both in formulating the game plan and executing surgery. Tension nose may be classified into three groups:

1. *Type A*: This type of tension nose is characterized by prominent, often cephalically positioned nasion, overprojection of the three arches of the nasal pyramid (bony vault, cartilaginous vault, tip), prominent nasal spine, crowded columella–lip junction, short upper lip, and tip animation.
2. *Type B*: The relevant anomalies are represented by overprojection of the cartilaginous framework that may or may not be associated with overprojection of the bony vault, relative/absolute underprojection and/or under-rotation of the nasal tip, and acute columellar–labial angle.
3. *Type C*: This third clinical situation presents deep and caudal nasion causing a low radix appearance, underprojection of the upper part of the bony vault, overprojection of the cartilaginous vault, underprojection and/or under-rotation of the nasal tip, acute columellar–labial angle. It is the paradigmatic "pseudohump" trap.

These three types of tension nose deformities need distinct surgical techniques for correction of form and function.

16.3 CLINICAL ASSESSMENT

A nose that is too large for the patient's face represents the most obvious and characteristic feature in tension nose patients. This fact is immediately obvious as soon as the patient walks into the consultation room.

Patients with this condition often reveal a state of profound psychological distress, as they have been the objects of negative remarks from their peers. This acts as a strong motivating factor to ask for rhinoplasty. Obtaining an improvement in the physical appearance of the nose is more important to these patients than the functional aspect when these two factors coexist in the same individual (Hay and Heather, 1973; Dinis, Dinis and Gomes, 1998; McKiernan, et al., 2001). It is of paramount importance to exactly establish what the patient wants in terms of cosmetic and functional change. It is important that the surgeon discusses the issue of the balance between functional improvement and aesthetic appearance with the patient and formulates the surgical plan accordingly. In authors' experience, this discussion should be with the patient at the earliest possible opportunity during the initial consultation. In a significant number of cases, grafting procedures are indicated for functional purposes that may ultimately result in widening of the midnose and/or alar sidewalls. In authors' patient population, a significant proportion of individuals, especially women, dislike this "swollen" appearance of the inferior nasal two thirds and often discard the option of structural, supporting grafts in these critical areas despite the beneficial functional impact that might result. These aspects are to be clearly reviewed during the second meeting and reported in detail on the consent form.

Inspection

The following systematic examination of the nose is designed to glean as much information as possible in a relatively short period. Begin by assessing the brow dome lines (BDLs) (Palma and Khodaei, 2010; Palma, Khodaei and Tasman, 2011). Sit in front of the patient and analyze the light/shade interplay on both the midline of the patient's nose and at the nose–cheek junction. Ideally, you will notice a central area of light reflection, with a light-shadow border on each side. These two borders are the actual BDLs. Lateral to each BDL, there will be an area of shadow on the nasal sidewalls up to the transition with the periorbital/cheek area.

The alar–columellar relationship should lead to a "gull in flight" appearance in an aesthetically pleasing nose. This orientation depends on the size and orientation of the LLCs, caudal septum position and length, position and orientation of the middle crura, and position/size of the nasal spine. In a tension nose, the LLCs are often distorted due to the large septum pushing them from a posterolateral position. This may create the illusion that the altered LLCs configuration represents a major deformity of the tip, rather than a consequence of the protruding septum. It is the authors' policy to primarily execute a significant septoplasty that will alleviate LLCs distortion and then plan specific surgery on the tip cartilages. From the lateral viewpoint, the overprojection of the nose is immediately obvious. Often, the lateral view of the face reveals the effects of an over-active depressor nasi septi muscle when the patient smiles: the upper lip shortens and the tip de-rotates. The nose should always be carefully inspected for signs of previous surgery, such as a columellar or alar scar as some tension nose patients have had previous surgery but are not fully satisfied with the results.

Observe the patients in quiet respiration with their mouth closed and watch for evidence of collapse of the lateral walls of the cartilaginous pyramid. Then perform the forced inspiration test by asking the patient to obstruct each nostril gently and only breathe through the not-obstructed side. This forces a larger amount of air to traverse the external valve and makes its dysfunction more pronounced. Lifting the cheek laterally can improve the airflow and is known as a positive Cottle's sign. The surgical implication of a positivity of the *Cottle's sign* is generally overestimated as it does not provide a clear indication about the anatomical site of dynamic obstruction. On the contrary, the "wax curette test" is much more specific in defining the location of collapsible areas: a wax curette is introduced inside the mid-lower nose and gently pushed outward when the patient inspires. The patient is asked to precisely indicate the location(s) where outward pull significantly ameliorates inspiratory breathing difficulty. This test is routinely repeated immediately before surgery, and the areas of major collapsibility are carefully outlined over the external skin with a marking pen. These areas will need structural support.

Palpation

Palpation of the nose is extremely important, as rhinoplasty is mainly a "tactile" surgery. The surgeon must manually assess quality and thickness of the soft-tissue envelope; size, firmness, and orientation of both upper lateral cartilages (ULCs) and LLCs; position, shape, and thickness of the caudal septum as well as its relation with membranous septum and nasal spine. Patients with a tension nose often do not suffer from a thick soft-tissue envelope. On the contrary, the excessively large septum is said to contribute to a thinning of the skin, and even the mucosa. Gently press on the nasal tip and release the pressure while looking and feeling for the response of the tissues under your finger. This "tip recoil" test differs greatly depending on the type of tension nose: type A will not show a weakness or delay in response, whereas it will reveal a weak and delayed reaction in type C. In these patients, the nasal spine has to be systematically evaluated. Usually, the spine can be palpated with the ventral aspect of the examiner's thumb as it makes its way into the base of the columella. When the spine is large, it may even reach half way up the columella. This fact needs to be noted for the surgical game plan.

Nasal Endoscopy

All rhinoplasty patients need to be examined with a nasal endoscope prior to surgery. There are several good reasons for this policy: rhinosinusitis is a prevalent disease that regularly occurs in ENT clinics. Signs of coincidental disease, such as early nasal polyposis or past surgery, should not be missed; the angle of the internal valve may have already been altered by trauma or distorted by an overly large septum. Pay specific attention to the cicatricial sequelae of past surgery: webbing, circumferential stenosis along the contour of the internal nasal valve. Scarring at the level of previous infracartilaginous incisions must be systematically searched for and reported on the preoperative worksheet. Finally, endoscopy provides the surgeon with vital photodocumentation to investigate the effects of surgery postoperatively. Photodocumentation of these findings is now readily available through adaptors for smart phones and should be made part of the patient's notes.

16.4 FACIAL PHOTOGRAPHY

There are many fine texts on the subject of taking photographs; however, obtaining consistently excellent photographs requires skill, patient, practice, and a systematic approach. The authors take photographs in the following sequence as their analysis leads to surgically relevant conclusions: frontal static, frontal dynamic (patient smiles), base/radix, base, lateral static, lateral dynamic (patient smiles), second lateral dynamic to show the prominence of the anterior nasal spine (patient pulls the upper lip downward), 2 three-quarter views from each side, and two helicopter views.

16.5 SURGICAL PLANNING

The wealth of information obtained during the first consultation, examination, and photography is analyzed to create a unique game plan for surgery. Photographic analysis concentrates on surgically relevant and useful landmarks as measuring every single possible angle and line is neither productive nor helpful. The findings of the photoanalysis and first meeting are described to the patient in a compulsory second consultation. Performing rhinoplasty based on a single meeting is a recipe for disaster. Once the surgical goals have been agreed upon, the operation can go ahead.

16.6 SURGICAL SOLUTIONS

The patient's photographs, facial analysis results, and game plan are taken into the operating room. While the main aims of surgery (deprojection, re-establishing surface aesthetics, and possible increased tip rotation) may also be achieved by an external approach (Johnson and Godin, 1995), authors manage tension nose patient's endonasally (Tasman and Palma, 2008), without outside incisions, thus avoiding the remote chance of an unsightly scar (Figs. 16.1 to 16.3).

After administration of general anesthesia, the patient is draped, and the head of the bed is elevated by 30° to decrease venous pressure in the face. Use of local anesthesia with adrenaline is limited to the infraorbital nerve, osteotomy lines, caudal septum, and premaxillary region. Distortion of the tip and dorsum by injecting are undesirable. Use of bipolar diathermy is limited to the depressor septi nasi muscle as this minimizes postoperative upper lip contusion and hematoma.

Septum surgery forms the most important part of the rhinoplasty in these patients and needs detailed attention. First, expose the caudal septum and raise submucoperichondrial flaps to expose the bony-cartilaginous

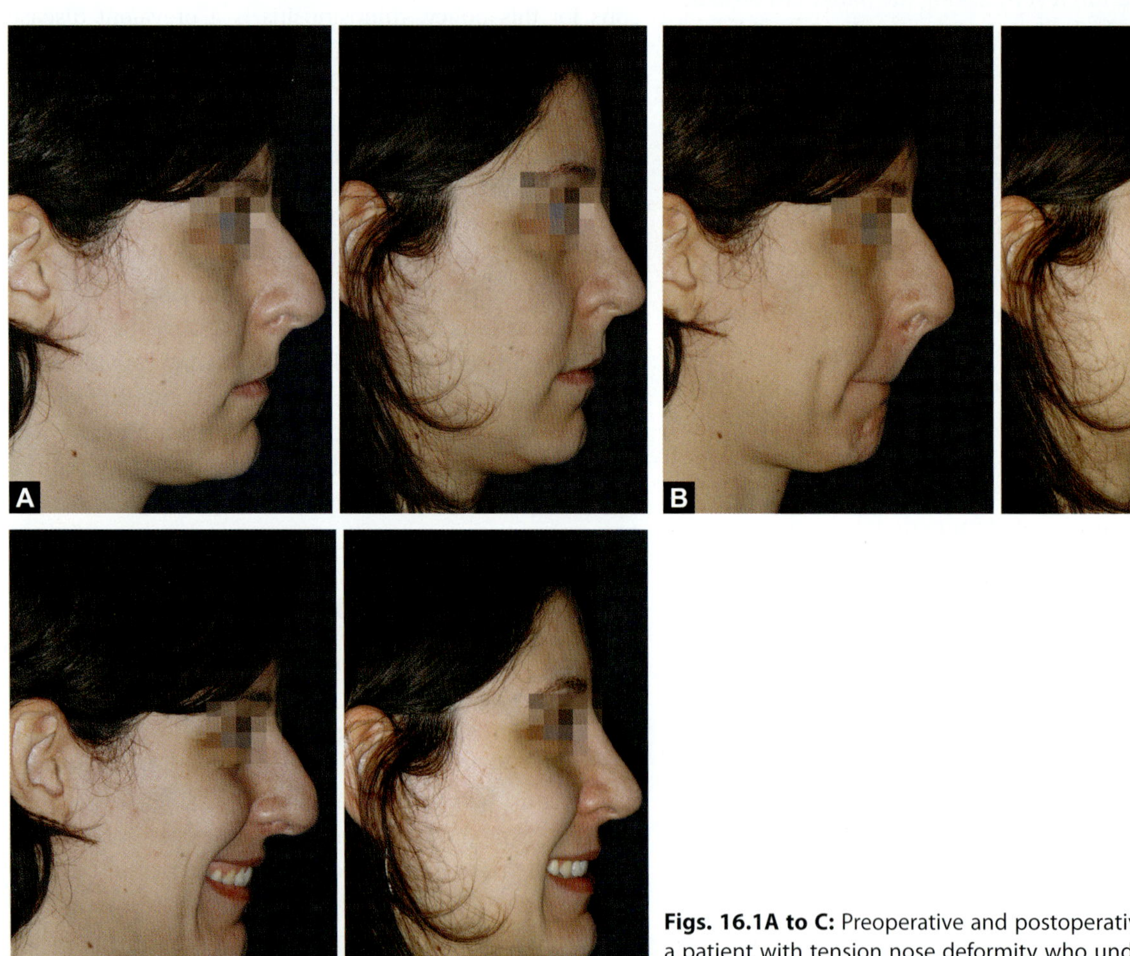

Figs. 16.1A to C: Preoperative and postoperative photographs of a patient with tension nose deformity who underwent endonasal septorhinoplasty. Note the improvement in dorsal profile and, nasolabial angle.

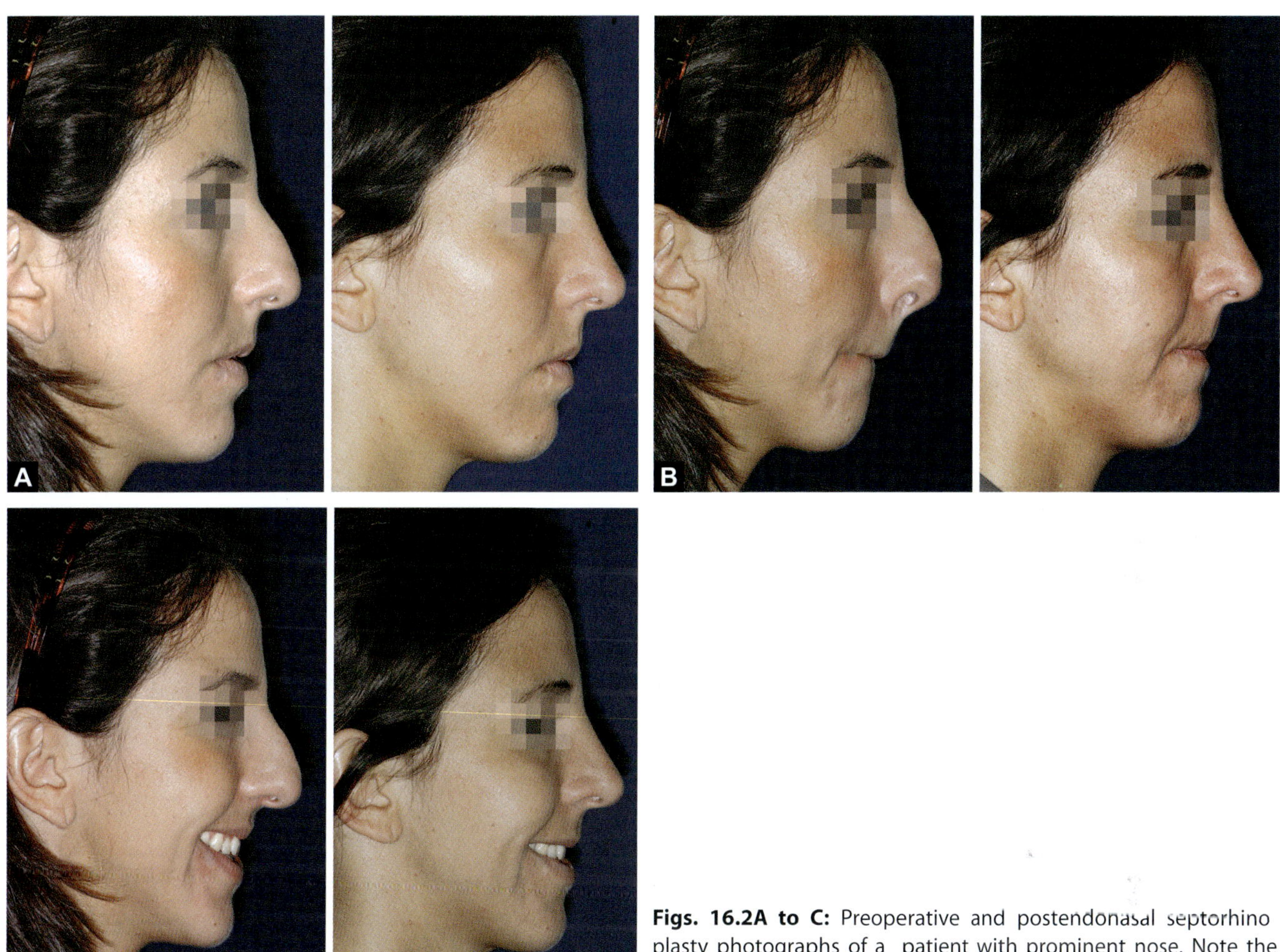

Figs. 16.2A to C: Preoperative and postendonasal septorhino plasty photographs of a patient with prominent nose. Note the correction of static and dynamic dorsum and tip deformities.

junction between the septum and adjacent bony structures. In revision cases when finding the correct plane may be difficult, use magnification with loops and approach the septum inferocaudally (Fig. 16.4) realizing a pocket in front of the nasal spine, severing scar tissue and exposing the most constant structures- nasal spine and medial aspect of pyriform aperture (Figs. 16.5 and 16.6). The size of the spine should already be known from the clinical examination of the patient. A spine and its wings need to have appropriate size and orientation. Both of these factors can be corrected surgically by gently rasping when appropriate, or at times by more rigorous excision if necessary. In authors' experience, reduction in the spine is an important first step in deprojecting a tension nose, together with well-planned and precisely executed inferior and posterior chondrotomies (Fig. 16.7) of the quadrangular cartilage. The combination of these maneuvers will allow the posterior septal angle to be repositioned onto the nasal spine so that the septum may be returned to its new, more anatomically appropriate position. Re-evaluate the lateral profile at this point: the reduction in projection will be immediately apparent. Also the frontal view should be re-evaluated at this point: most of the times, the resizing of the quadrangular cartilage (through ad hoc horizontal and longitudinal wedge resections) will correct the malposition of the cartilaginous pyramid. The explanation for such a dramatic change lies in the native imbalance between the oversized cartilaginous septum and its mucoperichondrial envelope. The septal cartilage is stretched inside a relatively small envelope, which produces a distortion of the quadrangular cartilage resulting in a C-shaped or inverted C-shaped configuration. This may have the secondary effect of causing deviation of the cartilaginous dorsum.

The next task is reconstruction of the intermediate and anterior septal angles. This can be achieved by excising a

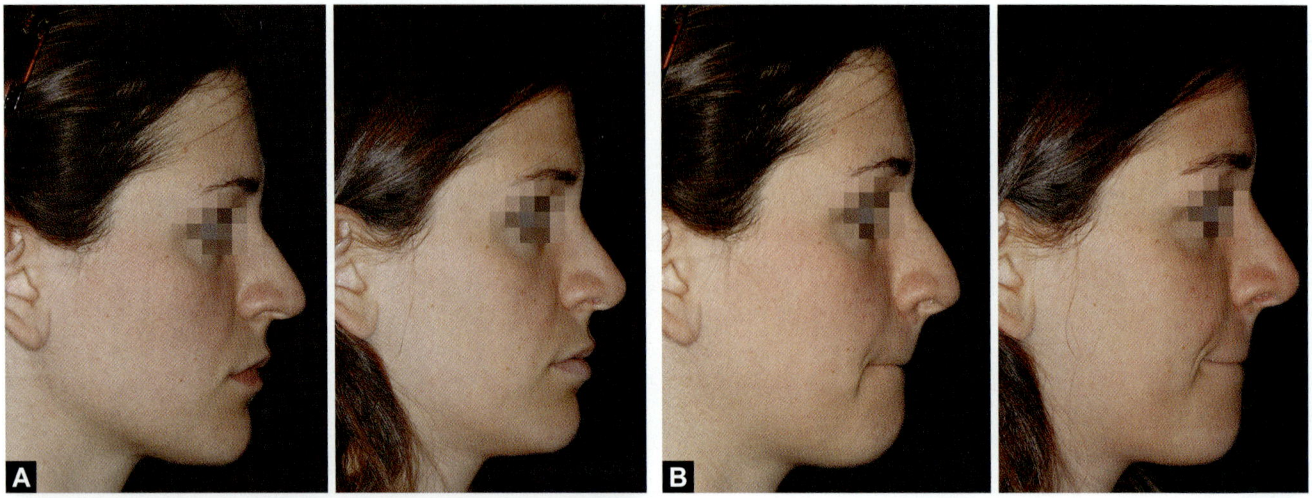

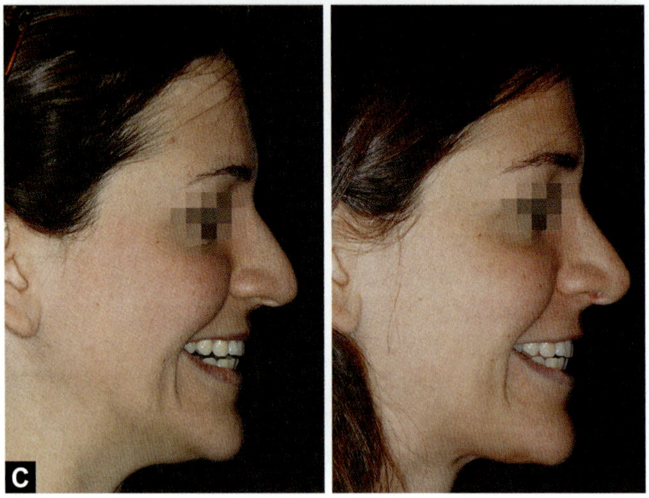

Figs. 16.3A to C: Preoperative and postendonasal septorhinoplasty photographs of a patient showing correction of dynamic tip ptosis and dorsal hump.

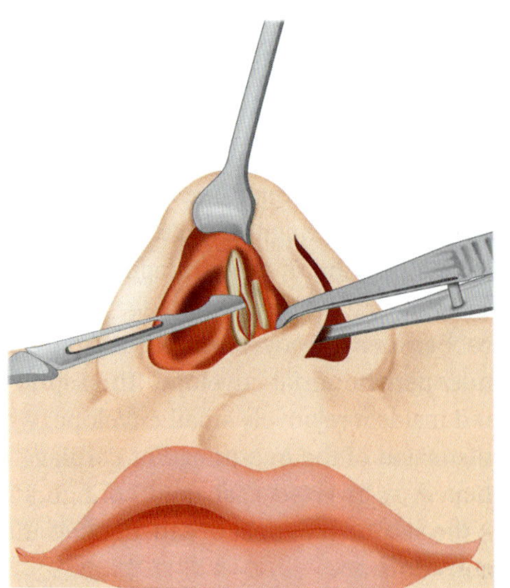

Fig. 16.4: Inferocaudal approach to the septum through hemitransfixion incision.

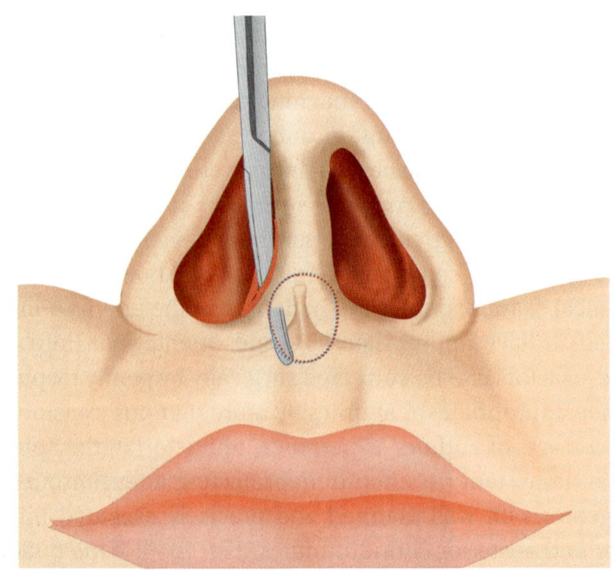

Fig. 16.5: Exposure of the spine and premaxilla via hemitransfixion incision.

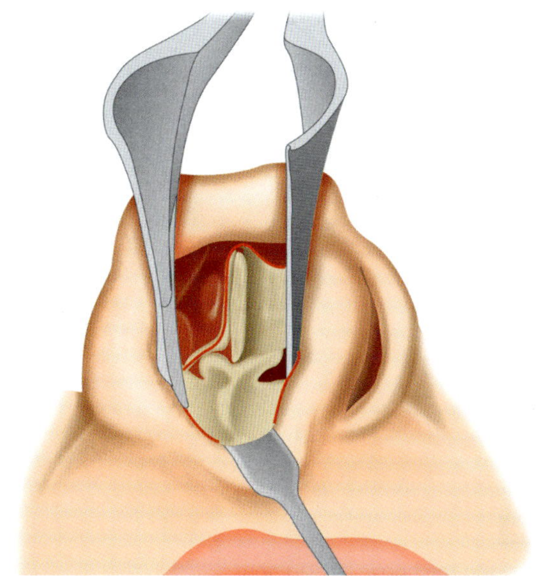

Fig. 16.6: Endonasal access to the septum-spine area.

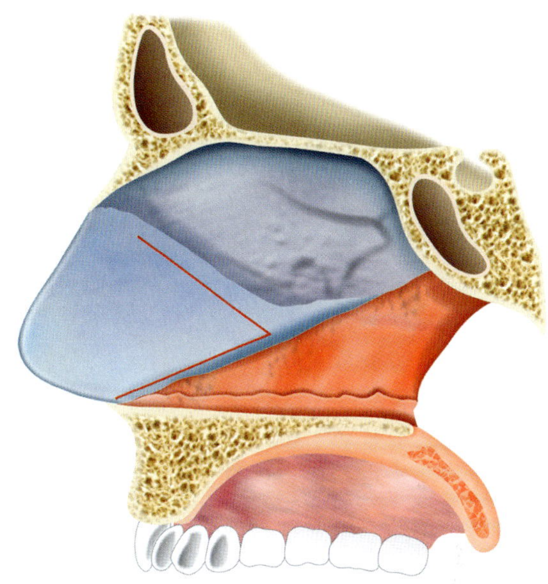

Fig. 16.7: Posterior and inferior chondrotomies.

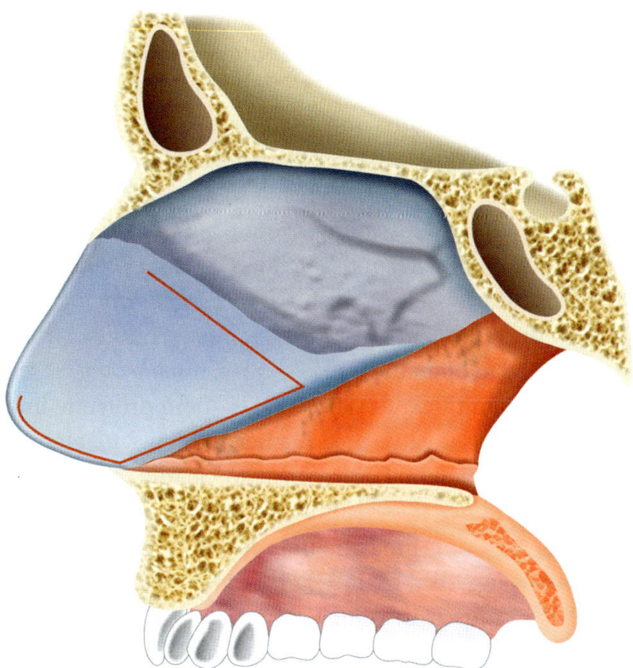

Fig. 16.8: "U-shaped" modeling of the caudal septum aimed to recontour the three septal angles.

"U"-shaped piece of caudal septum (Fig. 16.8) that starts at the newly created posterior septal angle, and continues anteriorly to include the intermediate septal angle, and then climbs superiorly to reduce the height of the anterior septal angle. The level of the newly created anterior septal angle shows significant gender differences: a light supratip dip is specially desired by most of the authors' female patients.

The intermediate septal angle is often overlooked, although it plays a significant role in the aesthetic contour of the columella-upper lip junction. Standard use of columellar strut tends to flatten and straighten the contour of the caudal septum. Endonasal surgery provides a more flexible way to deal with such a relevant aesthetic landmark. Lost intermediate angle must be recreated in both male and female patients with gently crushed cartilage at the end of surgery; otherwise, the columella will look unnaturally straight.

Reassess the size and projection of the nose again. This second step will reduce the undesirable parameters even more. Finally, if the above two steps have not been enough, a posterior chondrotomy can radically deproject the nose and should be used with great care. The junction of the cartilaginous and bony septum is confirmed by sight and palpation. Using a Freer's elevator, start the separation of cartilage from bone inferiorly and ascend toward the junction of the ULC with the nasal bones without ever reaching it. The amount of deprojection gained is proportional to the amount of vertical ascent along the bony-cartilaginous junction: the greater the dissociation, the larger the amount of deprojection gained in the long term. The endonasal aspect of the keystone area must never be violated so posterior chondrotomy should

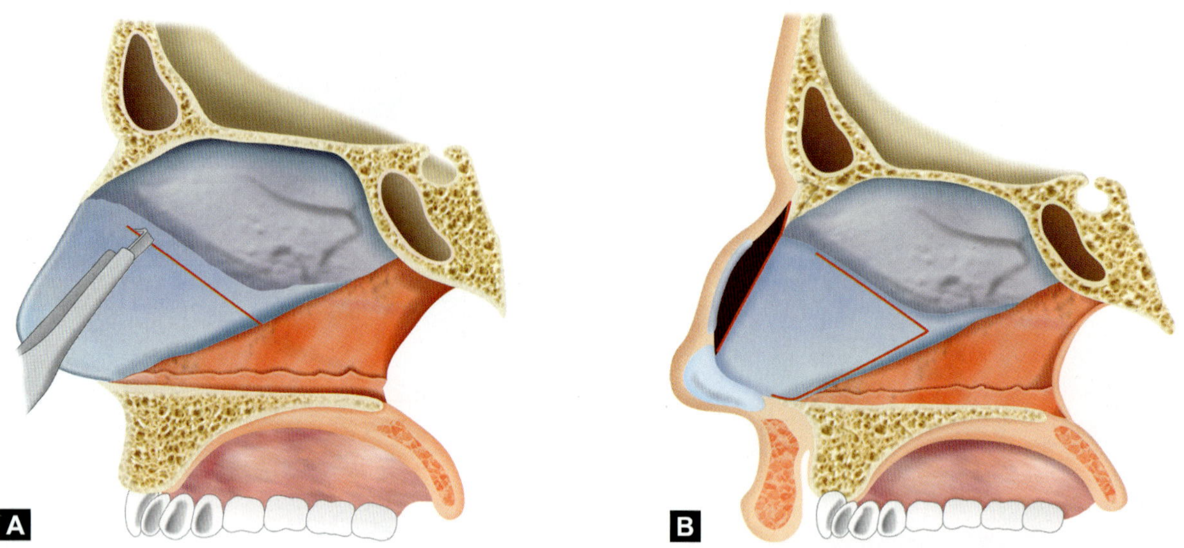

Figs. 16.9A and B: Posterior chondrotomy. (A) The amount of vertical ascent along the bony–cartilaginous junction should be carefully planned and executed. (B) The 1 cm of untouched bony–cartilage connection of the septum is to be considered also in relation to the amount of hump to be removed.

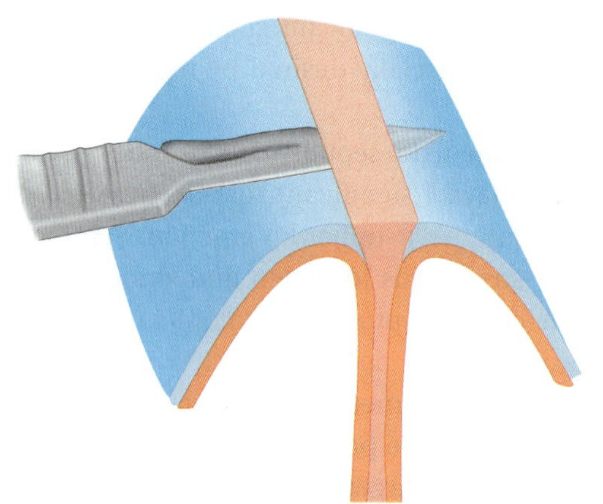

Fig. 16.10: Longitudinal splitting of the upper lateral cartilages–septum junction.

always keep 1 cm of untouched assembly between quadrangular cartilage and perpendicular plate (Figs. 16.9A and B).

From the previous discussion, it becomes apparent that there are two pivot points that are vital for septal stability: the spine and the keystone area. The spine may be carefully altered while maintaining a close relation with the posterior septal angle that should ideally rest on the nasal spine without surpassing it. The keystone area is definitely the core problem in the management of the tension nose.

Many tension nose patients require dorsal humpectomy, which can result in dissociation of the ULCs from the septum and the central portion of the overlying nasal bones (Fig. 16.10). Before routinely splitting the full thickness of the septum-ULC junction and placing a spreader graft, consider the implications of these steps. In many cases, the amount of cartilaginous hump to be removed is not so massive to result in a complete separation of the natural "spreading relation" of the septolateral cartilaginous unit. Second, spreader grafts broaden the dorsum of the nose and distort the BDLs, which many patients do not desire. Moreover, spreader grafts, which are intended to open the internal valve, must be harvested with significant thickness. This makes them protrude into the internal nasal valve area further reducing its already narrow cross-sectional area. Instead, a fold of mucosa released from the ULC-septum junction ("extramucosal" technique by Robin) may be interposed between the two structures (Figs. 16.11A to C). This latter technique will produce a softer spreading effect helping to prevent a decrease in the vital angle of the internal valve, without causing the potential problems due to spreader graft positioning.

In an attempt to prevent inverted V deformity, the authors prefer to minimize the dissection over the bony-cartilaginous vault junction and bony vault (Fig. 16.12). In these cases, the dissection is just above the periosteum and is strictly limited to the area of the hump to be removed. Preservation of the junction between ULCs and nasal bones lateral to be hump is critical. For the same

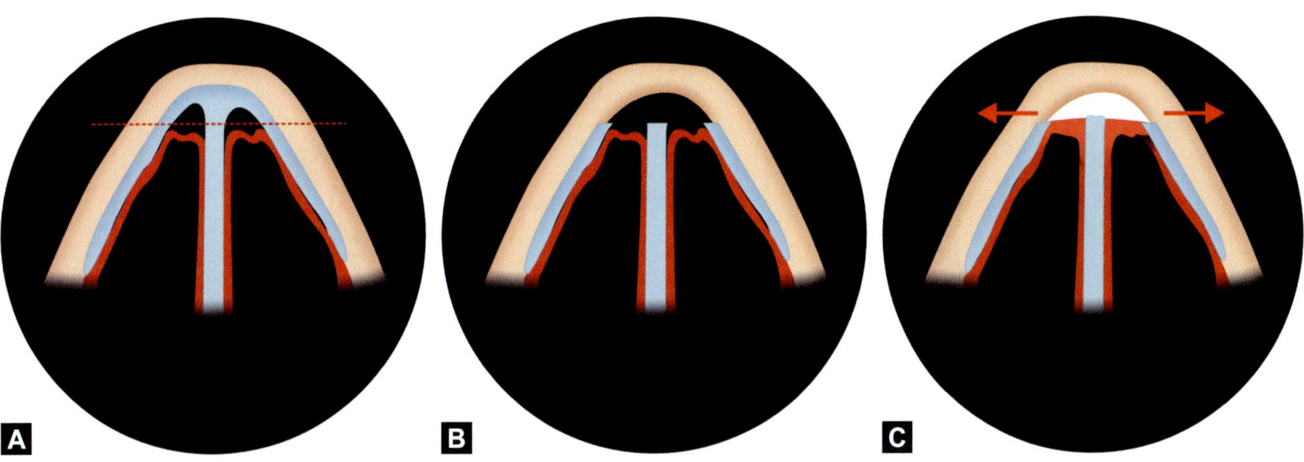

Figs. 16.11A to C: Middle vault protection.

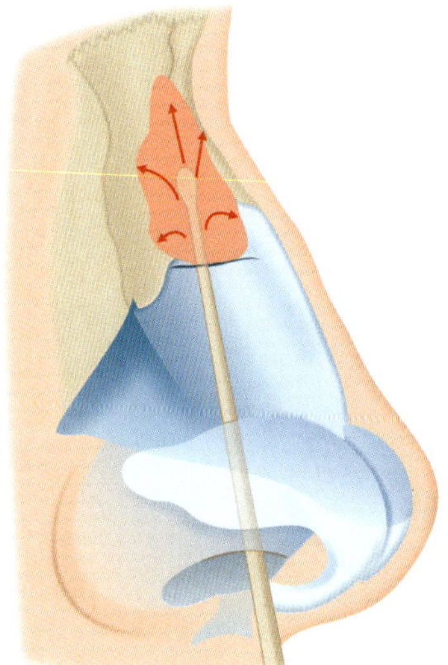
Fig. 16.12: Limited supraperiosteal elevation.

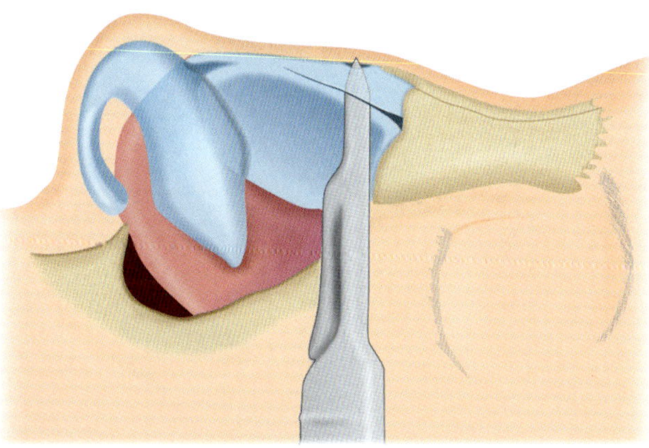
Fig. 16.13: Dorsal resection. First step: cartilaginous humpectomy.

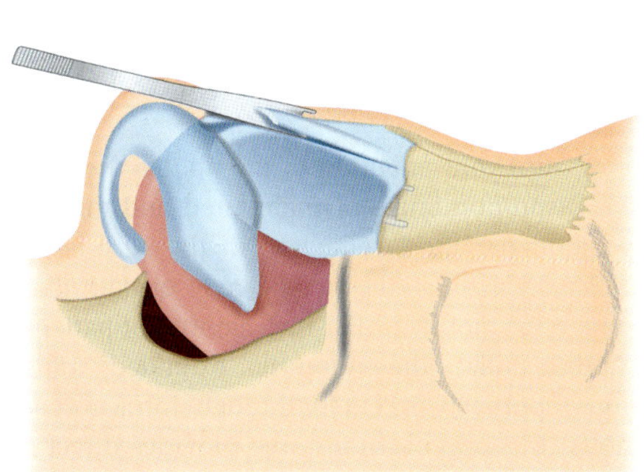
Fig. 16.14: Dorsal resection. Second step: bony humpectomy.

reason, the use of a perfectly sharpened osteotome for removing the bone is by far preferable to rasps whose up-and-down movements can easily jeopardize the integrity of the bony-cartilaginous vault junction. Hump removal is executed sequentially, first cartilage (Fig. 16.13) and then bone (Fig. 16.14), but in one piece as it guarantees a smooth transition at the rhinion area.

The pattern of osteotomies is dictated by the facial photographic analysis. As the vast majority of noses are asymmetrical, osteotomies should reflect this point. Internal basal osteotomies start just above the head of the inferior turbinate and follow a high-low-high pattern up to the junction with the frontal bone. The thick, solid

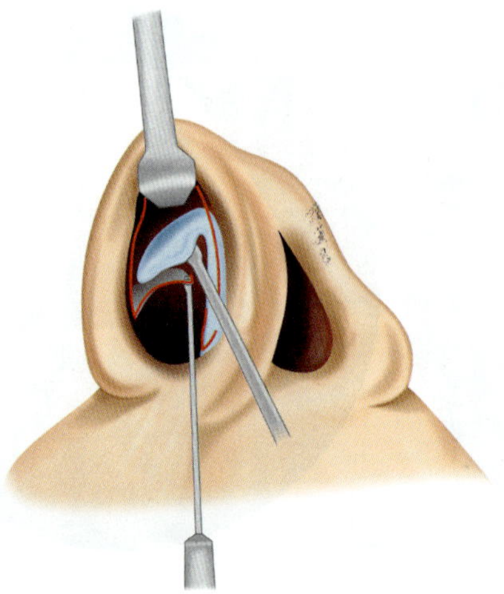

Fig. 16.15: Extramucosal tunneling through intercartilaginous incision.

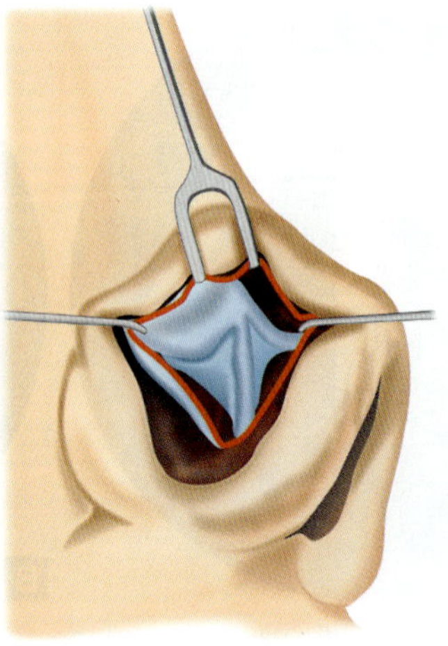

Fig. 16.16: Endonasal extramucosal approach to the vault through the hemitransfixion incision.

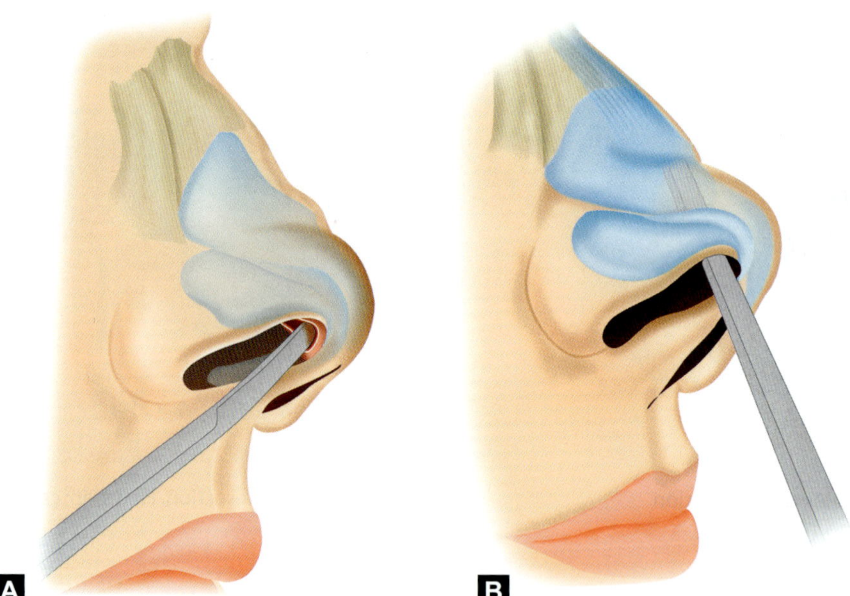

Figs. 16.17A and B: Access to the dorsum through the hemitransfixion incision.

frontal bone represents the pivot point where a medial-downward rotation of the hand creates a back fracture and mobilizes the bony wall so to close the open roof. This osteotomy sequence makes paramedian osteotomies unnecessary in most of the cases. Should an osteotomy result in inadequate infrastructure, a superiorly placed transverse osteotomy may also be required. Gentle use of fingers in performing in-fracture maneuvers is important in order not to detach the ULCs from the overlying bones lateral to the area of hump removal.

Now, turn your attention to the tip. Do the LLCs still appear disproportionate or malrotated and the alar rim malpositioned? Often, reduction in the very large septum gets rid of this illusion and may obviate the need for surgery or modify it. For the majority of patients, the first author utilizes the endonasal "extended" transcartilaginous approach executed through intracartilaginous incisions. This approach not only provides direct access to the areas of the lateral crura that need resculpting but also for refining the scrolls as required. Endonasal

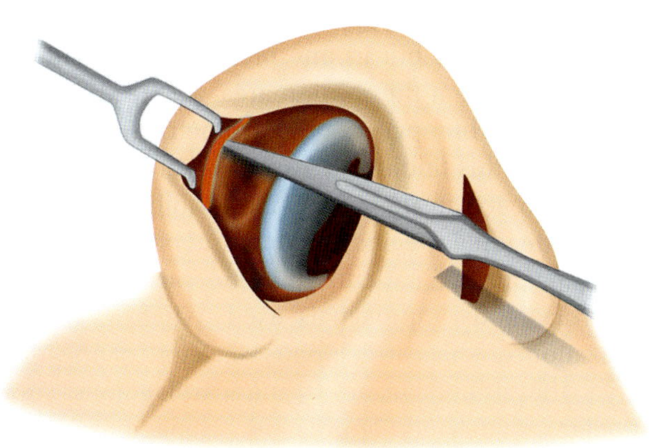
Fig. 16.18: Access to the lateral aspect of the ala through lateral "slot" marginal incision.

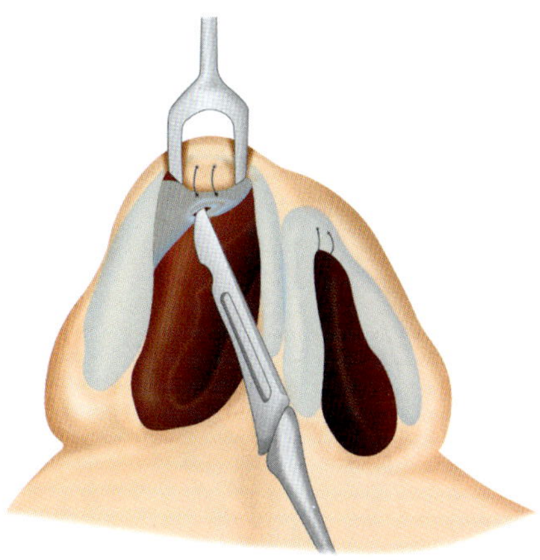
Fig. 16.19: Access to the domes area through medial "slot" marginal incision.

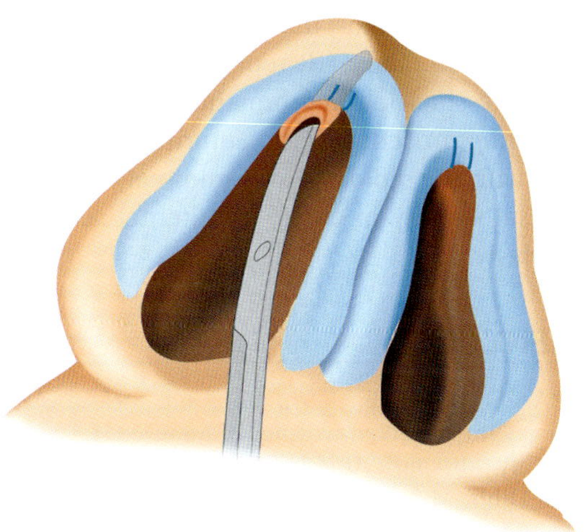
Fig. 16.20: Access to the domes area through medial "slot" marginal incision. The plane of dissection is shown here.

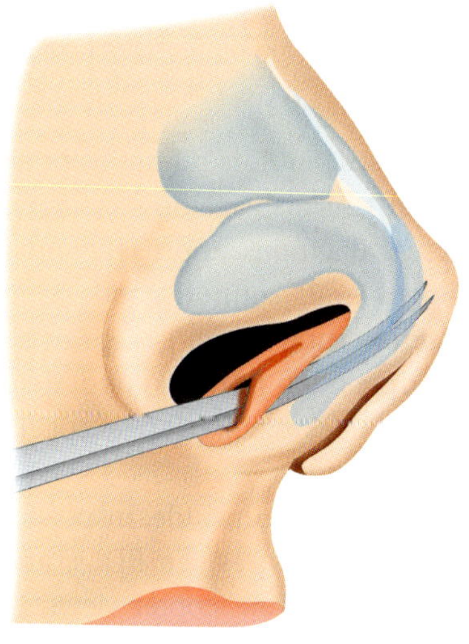
Fig. 16.21: Dissection plane between the medial crura is utilized for placement of columellar strut.

intercartilagenous extramucosal approach (Fig. 16.15) and hemitransfixation incisions (Figs. 16.16 and 16.17) may also be used to expose the nasal dorsum. Many sutures and grafts can be used through the transcartilaginous approach and concurrent endonasal incisions (hemitransfixion, partial infracartilaginous, or slot (Figs. 16.18 to 16.20) "custom-made" incisions). Such an "extended" transcartilaginous approach allows for greater flexibility in dealing with complex tip problems and the recreation of surface aesthetics. When a complete visualization of the cartilaginous skeleton of the tip is needed, the authors resort to infracartilaginous, transvestibular, or delivery approaches.

The "type C" tension nose poses special problems that require a change in strategy. After the septum has been addressed, the tip is approached before dealing with the dorsum. This is done because repositioning and stabilization of the pronasale will dictate the degree of dorsal reduction. The main tool used to stabilize the tip position is the intracolumellar strut (Figs. 16.21 and 16.22) that is positioned through the hemitransfixion incision. At the end of the operation, the tongue-in-groove suture helps achieve further stabilization. Special attention needs to be paid to the alar rim that may present an unsightly "Chinese hat" configuration. This can be part of the picture of the so-called cephalic malposition of the lateral

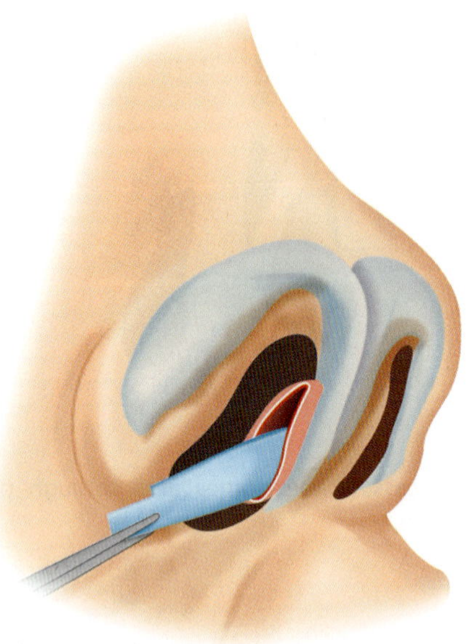

Fig. 16.22: Endonasal placing of intercrural columellar strut.

crura. In these cases, authors refrain from aggressive surgery. The caudal rim displacement is managed through a partial infracartilaginous approach and utilization of a custom-shaped graft sutured caudally to the arched part of the lateral crura, which is kept in a more caudal position, after dissection from the underlying superficial musculoaponeurotic system, with a specially designed infracartilaginous suture.

A final check of the nose includes inspection of the major lines of importance, such as the BDLs, and symmetries from frontal, lateral, and helicopter views. Using crushed cartilage in precise slots restores surface aesthetics.

SUMMARY

Treatment of a tension nose depends on adequate preoperative diagnosis of features that create the impression of a "large nose". Clinical and photographic assessment will clearly show the guilty culprit and direct the specific surgical game plan toward the septum as the main cause of the problem. Septoplasty is the key to a successful outcome, but it needs to be done in a stepwise manner. The refashioned septum needs to support the tip and projects itself onto the midline of the two parallel BDLs and recreates a proportionate alar–columellar relationship.

Whenever possible, the unity of the septolateral cartilage is maintained, and extramucosal approach represents the workhorse for managing the cartilaginous vault. Hump removal is executed sequentially, first cartilage and then bone but in one piece as it guarantees a smooth transition at the rhinion area. As the vast majority of noses in rhinoplasty are asymmetric, osteotomies should reflect this finding.

The approach to the tip needs flexibility taking into account individual specific anatomy and patient's desires. For the majority of patients, the endonasal "extended" transcartilaginous approach is used. When a complete visualization of the cartilaginous skeleton of the tip is needed, the authors resort to infracartilaginous, transvestibular, or delivery approaches, depending on the techniques to be used. A variety of sutures can be used through these different approaches.

Grafts are utilized judiciously. In most of the cases, their use is aimed to recreate surface aesthetic lines and soften contours. Sometimes they are to be employed to regain structural firmness. The tension nose represents the typical paradigm for the use of endonasal hybrid rhinoplasty (EHR). The EHR represents the best of both worlds: the lessons learnt from the external approach, mainly grafting procedures and suturing techniques, are combined with the philosophy of minimal tissue damage of endonasal surgery to create an alternative third path for rhinoplasty.

REFERENCES

Barelli, P.A., Loch, W.E.E., Kern, E.R., and Steiner, A. (Eds.), Rhinology. The collected writings of Maurice H. Cottle, M.D. Kansas City, Missouri: American Rhinologic Society, 1987.

Dinis, P.B., Dinis, M. and Gomes, A. 1998. Psychosocial consequences of nasal aesthetic and functional surgery: a controlled prospective study in an ENT setting. *Rhinology*, 36, pp. 32-6.

Hay, G.G. and Heather, B.B. 1973. Changes in psychometric test results following cosmetic nasal operations. *British Journal of Psychiatry*, 122, pp. 89-90.

Johnson, C.M., Jr. and Godin, M.S. 1995. The tension nose: open structure rhinoplasty approach. *Plastic and Reconstructive Surgery*, 95, pp. 43-51.

Mckiernan, D.C., Banfield, G., Kumar, R. and Hinton, A.E. 2001. Patient benefit from functional and cosmetic rhinoplasty. *Clinical Otolaryngology and Allied Sciences*, 26, pp. 50-2.

Palma, P. and Khodaei, I. 2010. Hybrid rhinoplasty: the 21st century approach to remodeling the nose. *Archives of Facial Plastic Surgery*, 12, pp. 412-4.

Palma, P., Khodaei, I. and Tasman, A.J. 2011. A guide to the assessment and analysis of the rhinoplasty patient. *Facial Plastic Surgery*, 27, pp. 146-59.

Sputh, C.B. 1985. The tension nose. *Rhinology*, 23, pp. 79-80.

Tasman, A.J. and Palma, P. 2008. The infracartilaginous approach revisited. *Archives of Facial Plastic Surgery*, 10, pp. 370-5.

Nasal Valve Collapse

17

W Heppt, T Hildebrandt, Julia Vent

Chapter Overview

Pearls and Pitfalls

Pearls

- The nasal valve is the key zone of airstream regulation, acting as an accelerator and diffuser of air. Despite its importance in physiology and pathology of nasal airflow, it is one of the least understood fields in rhinology.
- The assessment of nasal valve dysfunction/compromise (NVC) causing breathing and ventilation problems is limited to patients' symptoms, external inspection with and without forced inspiration, palpation and nasal endoscopy.
- Nasal valve surgery is only indicated when all conservative means have failed.
- Nasal valve dysfunctions are the main cause for breathing problems after previous functional and esthetic surgery of nose.
- The main sites for surgical correction are the nasal septum, turbinates, nasal isthmus, lateral and medial crura of the lower lateral cartilages (LLCs), and the nasal tip.

Pitfalls

- The indication for surgery should not be based on rhinomanometric or acoustic rhinometric measurements, but on clinical symptoms alone.
- There is no standard technique for nasal valve surgery, but rather a myriad of single procedures designed for the correction of different anatomical deformities. The selection of suitable surgical techniques is unique to an individual patient and dictated by the anatomical variations and pathology encountered.
- Every aspect of nasal valve surgery from diagnosis to surgical planning and execution is challenging and should only be embarked upon by experienced surgeons.

17.1 INTRODUCTION

Despite its clinical importance, the *nasal valve* is one of the least understood fields in rhinology. Lacking evidence-based investigations, even today the nasal valve resembles a "black box" full of hidden secrets. The nasal valve is a "playground" reserved for the most creative surgeons and scientifically interested clinical researchers.

First described by Mink in 1903 (Mink, 1903), the *nasal valve area* represents the caudal part of the nose beginning from the nostrils up to the isthmus nasi, which is composed of the caudal border of the upper lateral cartilage and the septum (Figs. 17.1A and B). This area is called the internal nasal valve, whereas the *external nasal valve* accounts for the alar region. The teardrop-shaped isthmus nasi is the narrowest part of the nasal valve.

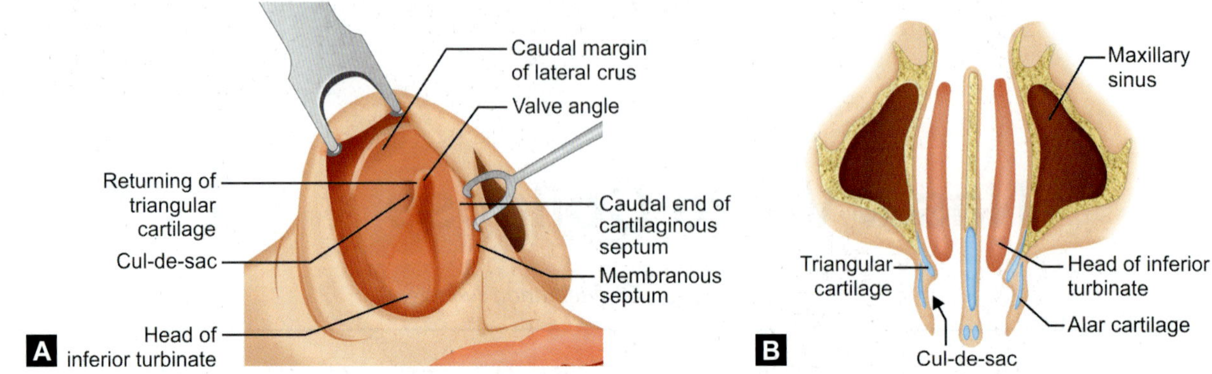

Figs. 17.1A and B: The nasal valve area. Illustrations demonstrate (A) endoscopic view and (B) axial cross section.

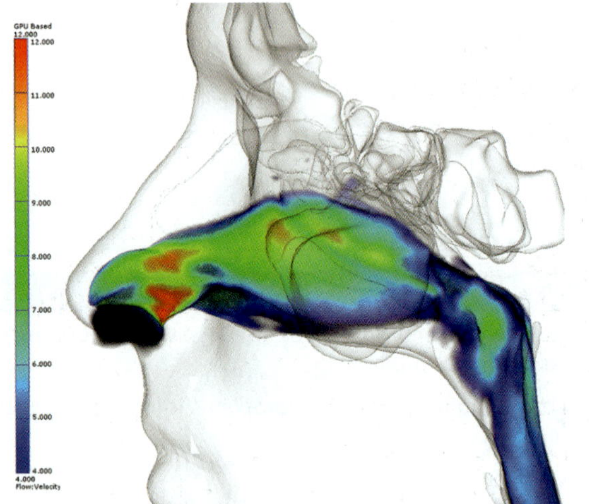

Fig. 17.2: Intranasal inspiratory flow evaluated through computational fluid dynamics program (CFD) (Hildebrandt, et al., 2013).

It has an average size of 50–70 mm^2 and an angle of 10–15° opening at its apex (*internal nasal valve angle*) (Huizing and de Groot, 2002).

According to Wexler (2004), the nasal valve accounts for up to 80% of the nasal resistance (Wexler and Davidson, 2004). Considering its characteristic features, the nasal valve is supposed to be the key area in understanding and treating nasal breathing impairment.

17.2 PHYSIOLOGY

The nasal valve is the key zone of airstream regulation, acting as an accelerator and diffusor, concentrating the inspired air into the middle meatus. Due to the Bernoulli effect, air velocity may reach up to 12–18 m/s in the isthmus area (Fig. 17.2) (Huizing and de Groot, 2002). This acceleration is associated with a concomitant reduction of static pressure, leading to an inward directed negative pressure on the ala during inspiration (Venturi effect, which means reduction in flow pressure resulting from a flow through a constricted section). The situation is different during expiration, when air is also distributed to the upper and lower nasal meati and the nasal valve is stented by the positive static pressure transmitted from the lungs. The whole process is determined by resilience and shape of the lateral nasal wall, the geometry of nasal isthmus and downstream nasal cavity, nasal resistance factors such as septal deviations, hyperplastic turbinates, activity of nasal muscles, and the force of respiration. Asymmetry of both nasal cavities may interfere with different flow characteristics and reflex mechanisms such as the nasal cycle.

The isthmus is the narrowest part of the nasal valve and of major importance when one is trying to identify the cause of NVC. According to Hagen–Poiseuille's law (volume of a homogeneous fluid passing per unit time through a capillary tube is directly proportional to the pressure difference between its ends and to the fourth power of its internal radius, and inversely proportional to its length and viscosity of the fluid, $V = \mathrm{d}V/\mathrm{d}t = \left(\frac{\pi . r^4}{8 . \eta} \frac{\Delta p}{l}\right)$, even minor constrictions of the airflow may result in a disproportionately high increase in resistance. The complexity of all valve-determining factors clearly reveals the difficulty in assessment of the individual etiology of NVC.

17.3 ETIOLOGY

Nasal valve compromise can have many etiologies, congenital, traumatic, or iatrogenic (Table 17.1), and may be differentiated into mucosal, skeletal, or cartilaginous according to the offending tissue. If nasal airstream is changed by obstruction from laminar to turbulent flow,

Table 17.1: Common etiologies of nasal valve compromise.

Caudal septal deflection
Hypertrophy of the inferior turbinates
Weakness, malformation, and malposition of lower lateral cartilages
Weakness, excessive elongation, and upward rotation of upper lateral cartilages
Pyriform aperture narrowing
Ptotic nasal tip

the sensation of nasal blockage occurs as a chief complaint (Hornung, et al., 1987). However, patients can also suffer from the sensation of nasal blockage if the trigeminal receptors of intranasal mucosa are decreased, as is the case in empty nose syndrome or in patients with chronic rhinosinusitis (Wrobel and Leopold, 2005).

Among all anatomic pathologies, caudal septal deflections, hypertrophy of the inferior turbinates, weakness, malformation, and malposition of the LLCs, as well as weakness, excessive elongation and upward rotation of upper lateral cartilages, pyriform aperture narrowing, and the ptotic nasal tip are most frequently observed. However, even rare causes such as facial nerve palsy, leading to loss of function of nasal dilator muscles, should be considered. Each of these components plays a different role in nasal deformity and consequently has to be addressed individually.

17.4 DIAGNOSIS

Despite its pivotal importance in the regulation of airstream, there is no generally accepted method to meaningfully measure the impact of functional and morphologic nasal valve disorders on nasal airflow to date. Neither *Cottle's test* (pulling the skin of the cheek laterally to open the valve), nor opening the valve by placement of a small cotton tip at the internal nasal valve's apex, or raising the ala using a curette from the nasal vestibule have been found to be reliable means to distinguish normal from pathologic nasal valve function. This is also true for the columella narrowing test (where the base of the columella is approximated by the gentle use of a forceps), active anterior rhinoresistomanometry (Siegert and Balczun, 2010), 4-phase rhinomanometry (Vogt, et al., 2010), acoustic rhinometry (Vidyasagar, et al., 2005), and computed tomography (CT) and magnetic resonance imaging (MRI) scan (Rhee, et al., 2010). However, in the last decade, computational fluid dynamic (CFD) programs have become a promising tool to calculate nasal airflow. Based on CT-originated three-dimensional geometric models and calculation of various flow parameters by CFD programs, this technique allows for analysis of isthmus deformities and alignment of anatomical structures with the functional isthmus of the nasal cavity (Hildebrandt, et al., 2013). Nevertheless, until the validation of reliable clinical applications of CFD methods, nasal valve pathology assessment is limited to taking a thorough history, external inspection with and without forced inspiration, palpation of the cartilaginous framework, nasal endoscopy, and photographic documentation (Table 17.2).

Table 17.2: Value of different parameters in diagnosing nasal valve problems (++ high value, + moderate value, -/+ questionable value).

Method	*Diagnostic value*
Patient's history	++
Palpation of cartilaginous framework	+
External inspection with and without forced inspiration	++
Nasal endoscopy	++
Cottle's maneuver	+
Cotton ball test, Curette test	+
Columella narrowing test	-/+
Active anterior rhinoresistomanometry	-/+
Four-phase rhinomanometry	-/+
Acoustic rhinometry	-/+
Computed tomography, magnetic resonance imaging	-/+
Computational fluid dynamic programs	-/+

17.5 TREATMENT

Conservative

The possibilities of nonsurgical treatment of nasal valve stenosis are limited. There are intranasal stents such as Nasanita (Fig. 17.3A) (Zumegen, Schneider and Michel, 2001; Riechelmann, et al., 2010), Nozovent, and AlaxoLito Nasal Stent (Fig. 17.3B), devices which splint the anterior nasal vestibule, or externally applied tape-strips such as Breathe-right (Peltonen, et al., 2004; Latte and Taverner, 2005; Raudenbush, 2011), which enlarge the diameter of the nasal valve region by lateralizing and stabilizing the nasal alae. However, these devices do not cure the underlying problem, and might cause mucosal or cutaneous irritation with long-term use.

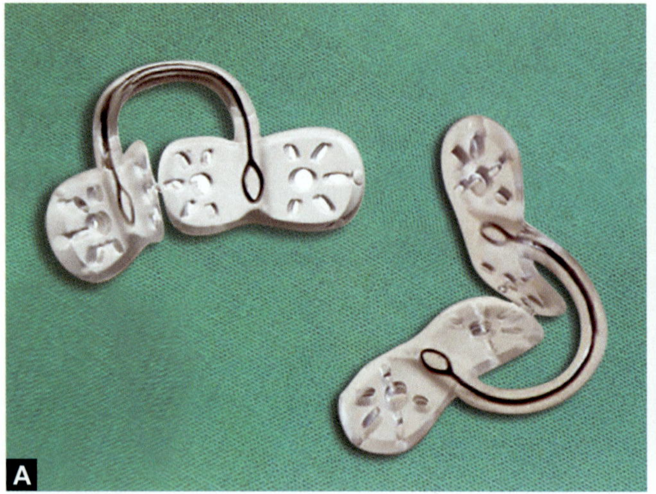
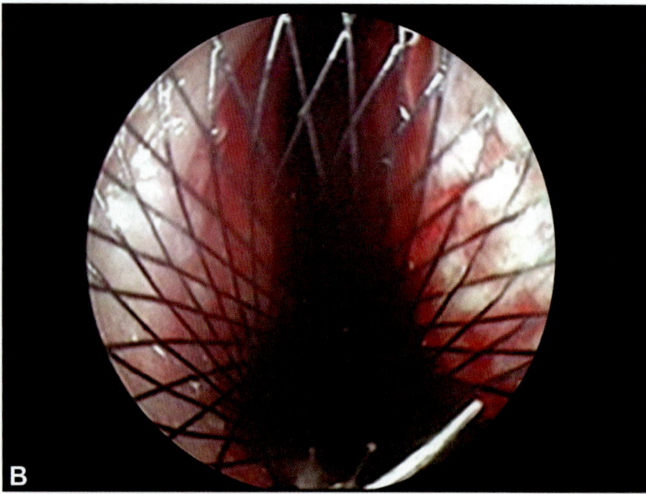

Figs. 17.3A and B: Intranasal stents for nasal valve stenosis. Nasanita (A) and AlaxoLito Nasal Stent (B).

If hyperplastic inferior turbinates are the major cause for nasal valve collapse, nasal decongestants followed by topical steroids may be helpful.

Surgical Principles

If allergic and nonallergic inflammatory processes are ruled out as underlying causes of nasal obstruction, and all conservative means have failed to improve breathing, surgical options for symptomatic NVC should be considered (Table 17.3).

This requires a thorough evaluation based on history, inspection, palpation, and endoscopic findings. Surgical correction of nasal valve dysfunction is based on determining the principal dysfunctional spot, be it a *static obstruction* of the nasal valve, e.g. due to a septal deviation or a crooked nose or a *dynamic collapse* of the flexible cartilaginous framework during respiration (Ballert and Park, 2006).

In general, surgery aims to widen the nasal base and pyriform aperture, straighten the septum, and reduce the bulk of the turbinates to improve nasal air pressure characteristics and thus the airflow. Reinforcement and reconstruction of the nasal alae helps to support them during inspiration and prevents collapse in the area that spans the isthmus.

Spreader grafts, flaring sutures, butterfly grafts, and intranasal flaps or skin-cartilage composite grafts are used to widen and support the narrow isthmus area. Alar batten grafts, lateral crural underlay (Timmer, et al., 2013), or strut grafts (Gunter and Friedman, 1997), and lateral crural turn-in flaps (Apaydin, 2012) are appropriate to correct dynamic obstruction caused by a malformed or easily collapsing lateral crura thus supporting the nasal sidewall (Ballert and Park, 2006). Correction of dynamic collapse from paradoxical concavity of the lateral crura may be obtained from the lateral crural flip-flop graft or by reconstructing the lateral crura using cartilage grafts.

The general principles for rotating the nasal tip upward include removing the factors that resist the rotation of the LLCs, creating space to accommodate them, rotating the LLCs into the desired position, and stabilizing the cartilages in the desired position (Bohluli, et al., 2013).

The following paragraphs provide an overview of the various techniques in detail.

First-Line Treatment of NVC

Septoplasty and *turbinoplasty* are the most frequently performed first line treatments of NVC in order to compensate for isthmus stenosis and nasal valve collapse. Straightening of caudal septal deflections using stabilizing batten grafts (Figs. 17.4A to D) and extracorporeal reconstruction procedures have been found to be most effective (Heppt and Gubisch, 2011). Alignment of the septum in the valve area results in a reduction of undesirable, asymmetrical flow characteristics, subsequently leading to a reduced tendency for collapse of the lateral nasal wall. Similarly, reduction in inspiratory transmural pressure is achieved by a reduction in the bulk of hyperplastic turbinates causing nasal obstruction. Preservation of mucosal physiology is best achieved when turbinoplasty is carried out using mucosa-sparing techniques like submucous reduction, high frequency, or shaver technology (Figs. 17.5A to D).

Table 17.3: Nasal valve surgery at a glance. Location and origin of nasal valve stenosis and the appropriate techniques to correct them.

Main dysfunctional spot	*Surgical technique*
Septum, turbinates	Septal correction, reduction of the turbinates
Isthmus nasi	Spreader technique
	Spreader graft, spreader flap
	Upper lateral splay grafts
	Butterfly grafts
	Silicon and titanium implants
	Flaring sutures
	Suspension sutures
	Intranasal flaps
	M plasty
	Z plasty
	Osteotomy of pyriform aperture stenosis
Nasal ala	Lateral crura of lower lateral cartilage (LLC)
	Grafts
	Alar batten grafts
	Alar rim grafts
	Lateral crural strut grafts
	Lateral crural spanning grafts
	Lateral crural underlay spring grafts
	Flipping over technique
	Correction of malposition
	Lateral crural turn-in flap
	Spanning and suspension sutures
Medial crura of LLC	Footplate resection
	Approximation of both footplates
	Intercrural soft tissue excision
	Repositioning of the footplates
	Caudal septoplasty.
Nasal tip	Septal reconstruction
	Columella strut
	Cephalic trimming
	Suspension sutures
	Lateral crural overlay technique
	External rhinolift

Isthmus Nasi Corrections

The nasal isthmus presents the main airstream regulator of the upper respiratory tract. The isthmus functions as a Starling resistor, which is able to control the flow relatively independent of the downstream pressure.

Spreader Techniques

The use of *spreader grafts* (Sheen, 1984) or *spreader flaps* have proved to be an effective method for reconstructing the roof of the middle nasal vault (Figs. 17.6A to D). These techniques are widely accepted as part of the component dorsal hump resection for correction of tension nose deformities. Using these techniques, the cross-sectional area of the nasal isthmus is increased by lateralizing the insertion of the upper lateral cartilages. Out of the two techniques, spreader flaps seem to be more appropriate because of their lower tendency to create a constriction in the valve area. By bending, inward rotation and refixation of the mobilized upper lateral cartilages to the septum, a more physiological stabilization and widening of the isthmus is achieved.

Upper Lateral Splay Grafts

Islam (Islam, et al., 2008) and Guyuron (Guyuron, Michelow and Englebardt, 1998) described the technique of upper lateral splay grafting. In this technique, conchal cartilage is placed underneath the caudal portion of the upper lateral cartilage as a splay graft. In the butterfly graft technique (Figs. 17.7A to C), described by Clark and Cook (Clark and Cook, 2002), conchal cartilage is sutured to the outer surface of the upper lateral cartilages and underneath the cephalic portion of LLCs to widen the isthmus and the adjacent middle vault. Both techniques deliver more reliable results than the spreader graft procedures. Although there is a slight increase in the width of the middle third of the nasal dorsum with these techniques, many patients are satisfied with the appearance of the nose after surgery (Friedman and Cook, 2009).

In the event of failure, alloplastic implants made of reinforced silicone (Deva, Merten, Chang, 1998) or titanium (Wengen, 2012) may be used; however, this option should be used as a last resource since these implants have a higher rate of extrusion and infection compared to autologous grafts.

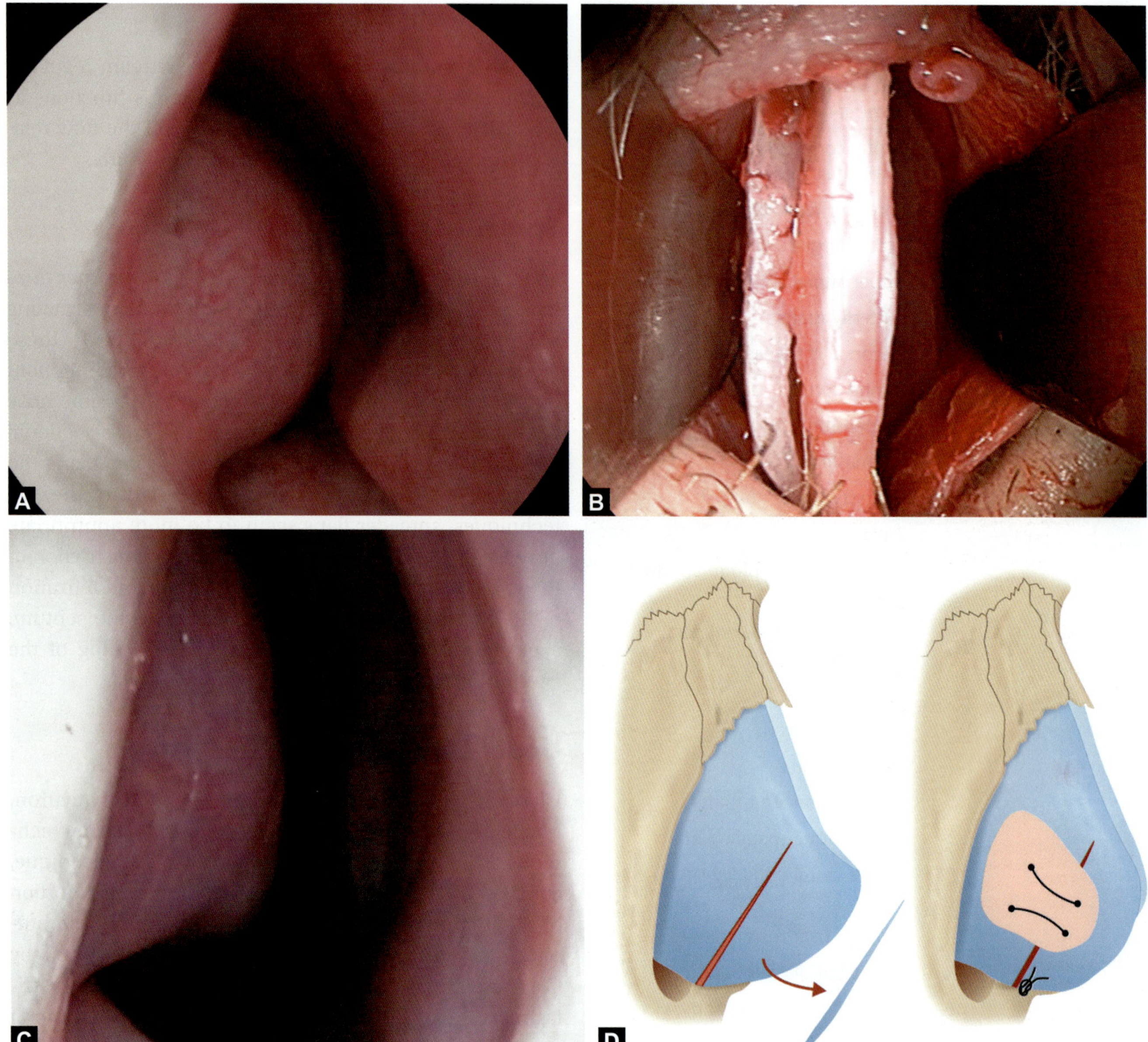

Figs. 17.4A to D: Correction of caudal septal deflection using a batten graft. (A) Preoperative endoscopy showing caudal septal deviation causing narrowing in the isthmus area. (B) Alignment of the caudal septum in the midline using a septal batten graft. (C) Postoperative endoscopy showing improvement of nasal airway in the internal nasal valve area. (D) Illustration demonstrating the surgical principle.

Flaring and Suspension Sutures

The splaying effect of inserted conchal cartilages may be increased by placement of *flaring sutures* (Fig. 17.8A) in a mattress fashion, running between both upper lateral cartilages over the nasal dorsum (Park 1998). Tightening the suture pulls the upper lateral cartilages laterally, resulting in widening of the nasal valve angle. Another option for widening of the isthmus angle is *suspension sutures* placed from the caudolateral border of the upper lateral crus (ULC) to the periosteum or the bone of the infraorbital rim (Paniello, 1996). These sutures are powerful not only in correcting stenosis of the isthmus but also for correcting alar collapse. However, the indication should be critically evaluated because of the potential for discomfort and fullness of the nasofacial groove by these permanent stitches. A less invasive method of opening the isthmus is

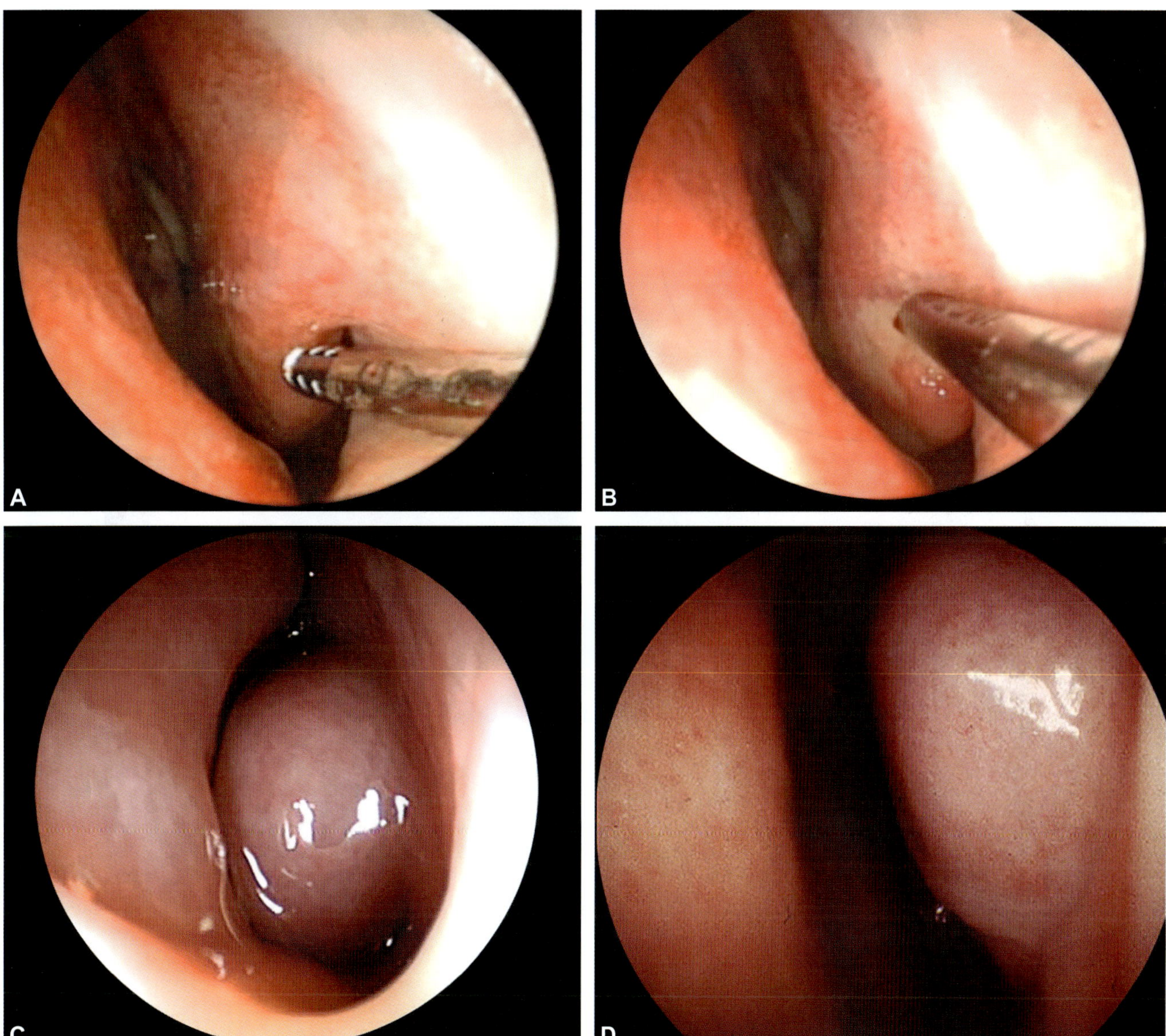

Figs. 17.5A to D: Shaver-technique for reduction of hypertrophic inferior turbinates (A and B). (C) Endoscopy of a patient with hypertrophy of the inferior turbinate before surgery. (D) The same patient after Shaver-turbinoplasty.

subcutaneous placement of Polydioxanone (PDS) sutures designed with cone anchors (Fig. 17.8B) (Saban, Braccini and Polselli, 2006; Saban, di Benito and Massa, 2014).

Intranasal Flaps

Opening of the isthmus may also be achieved by shortening the caudal end of the upper lateral cartilages and trimming of excess vestibular skin (Figs. 17.9A to E). Due to the intercartilaginous incision running into the hemitransfixion on both sides, the technique was named intranasal M plasty by Lopez Infante (Kasperbauer and Kern, 1987). Alternatively, a medially based skin and cartilage containing flap of the cephalic portion of the lateral crus may be raised and swung between ULC and septum, resulting in an intranasal Z plasty (Figs. 17.10A and B) (Dutton and Neidich, 2008). Large cartilages are a prerequisite for these techniques to prevent development of unpleasant post-operative cephalic alar retractions.

Opening of Pyriform Aperture Stenosis

Pyriform aperture stenosis (PAS) may occur in childhood, causing nasal respiratory distress to varying degrees. It

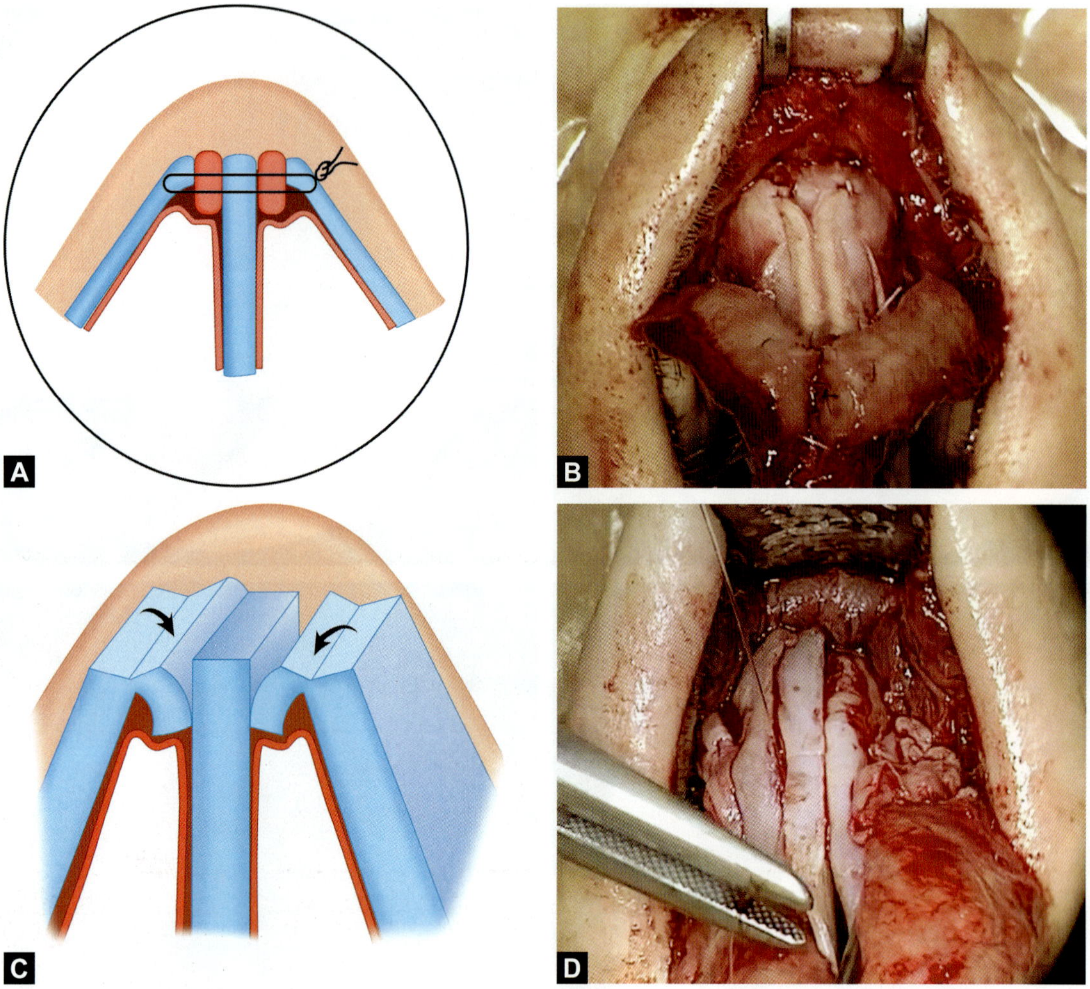

Figs. 17.6A to D: Increase in the cross-sectional area of the nasal isthmus by the use of spreader grafts (A and B) and spreader flaps (C and D).

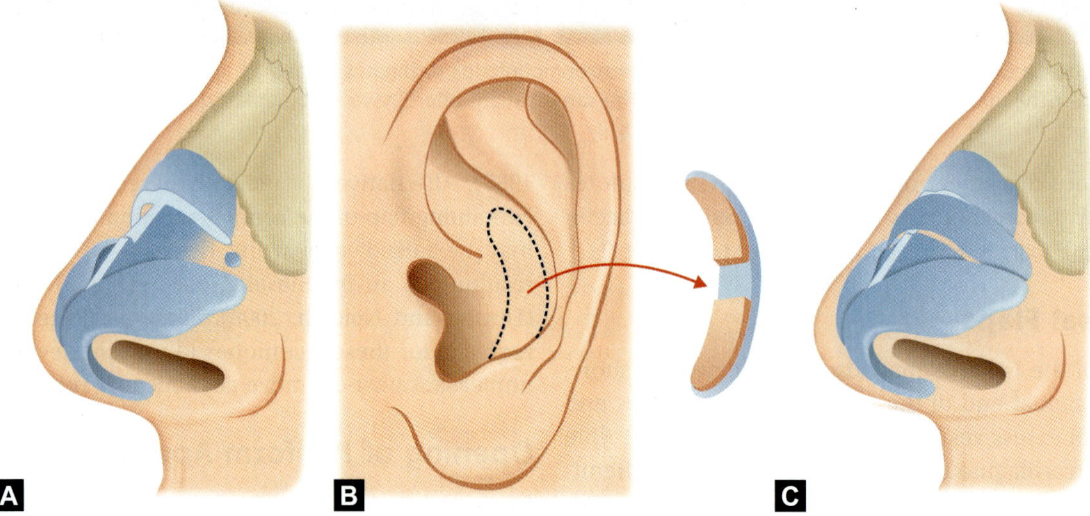

Figs. 17.7A to C: Butterfly graft fashioned from a composite skin-conchal cartilage graft used for widening the isthmus.

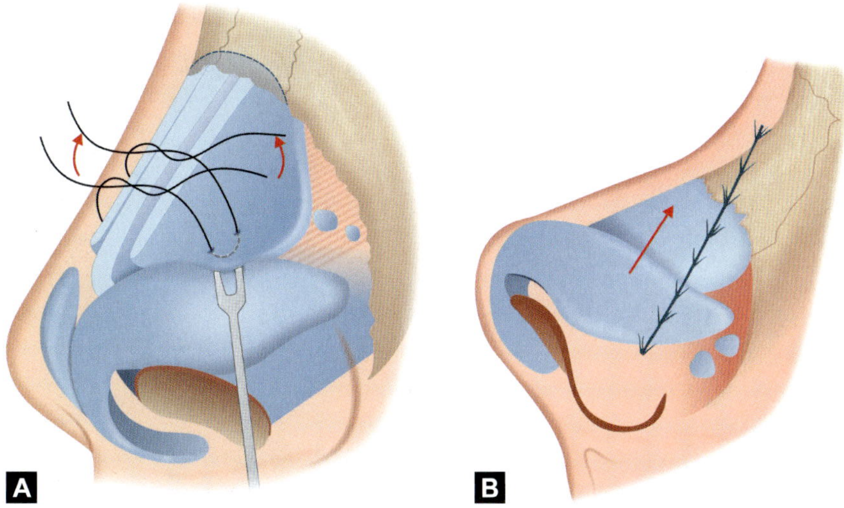

Figs. 17.8A and B: Suture techniques to open the isthmus. Flaring sutures through both upper lateral cartilages (A) and subcutaneously placed PDS suspension threads (B).

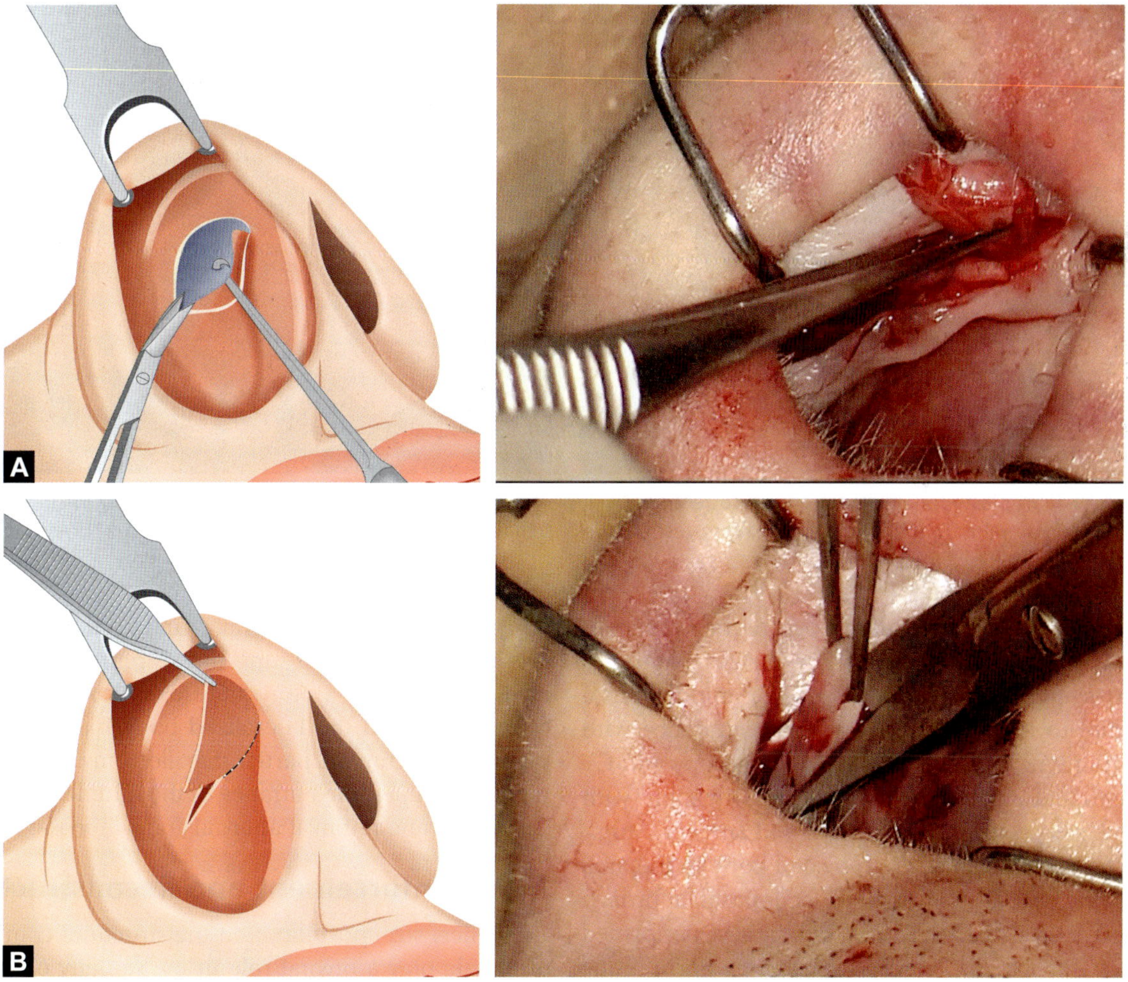

A

B

Figs. 17.9A and B

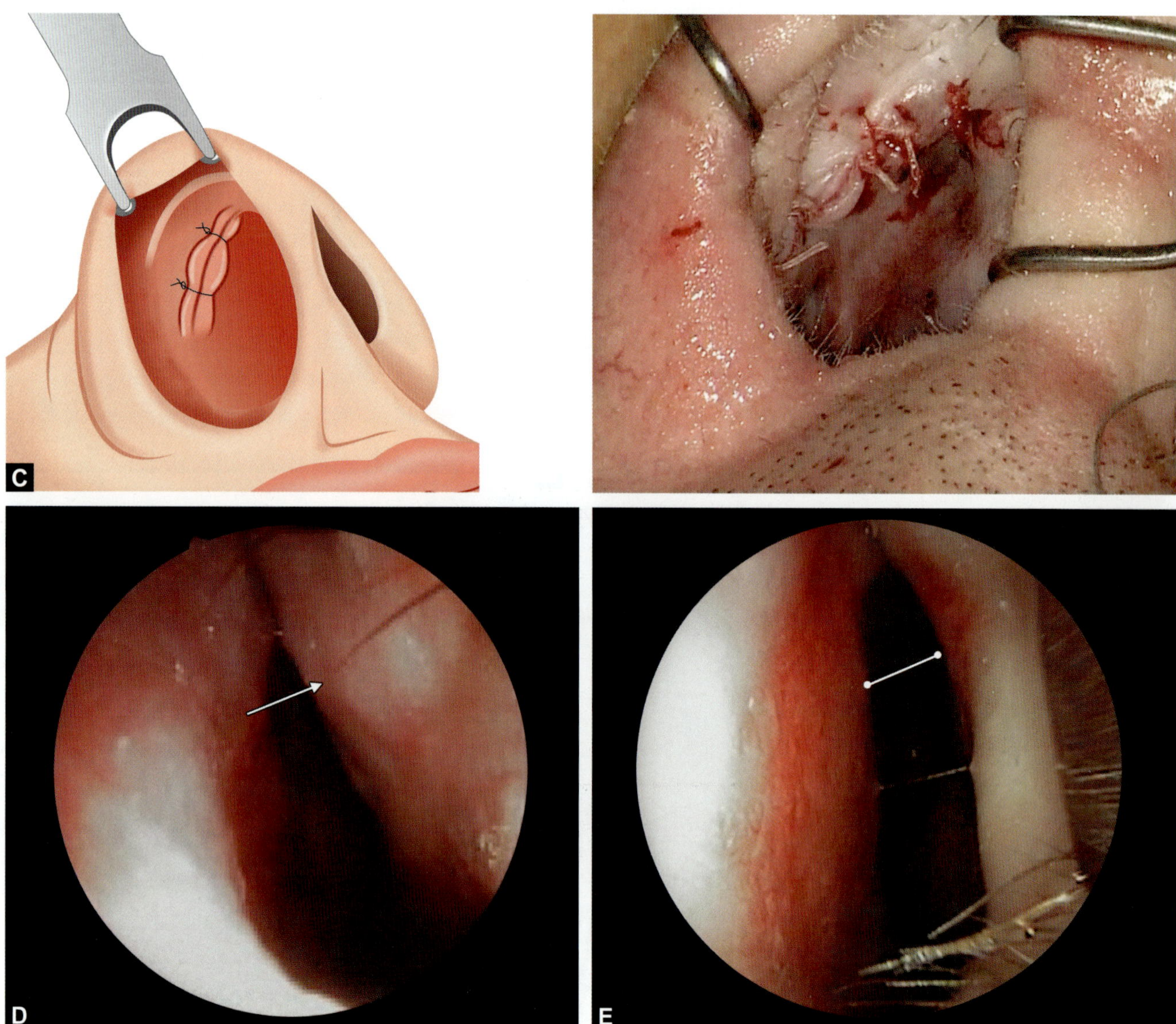

Figs. 17.9A to E: M plasty for isthmus stenosis correction. (A) Resection of a 2–3 mm triangular shaped strip of cartilage from the elongated upper lateral crus. (B) Trimming of excess vestibular skin. (C) Closure. (D) Isthmus before and (E) after correction.

may be congenital or traumatic in origin and is characterized by a narrowing of the outer pyriform aperture with narrowing of the entrance of the middle nasal meatus due to maxilla overgrowth. In accordance with the extent of PAS, diagnosed by nasal endoscopy and CT scan, treatment options include nasal irrigation with hypertonic saline, topical ointments, and surgery. Surgical management is aimed at removal of bone in the area of narrowing via a sub labial or endonasal approach with the use of a diamond drill. This is best performed by door wing like osteotomies of the pyriform bone through an endonasal approach (Figs. 17.11A to D). The bony insertion of the lateral crural complex should be preserved. To minimize the risk of remedialization, it is advisable to place a bony graft taken from the posterior septum between the lateralized bony fragment and the pyriform aperture. A partial maxillectomy is also recommended to open the entrance of the middle meatus, consisting of bone removal after raising a mucosal local flap.

Alar Reinforcement and Reconstruction

Resilience, size, position, and the structural composition of the ala play a pivotal role in the stability of the lower lateral nasal wall. Combined with the nasal isthmus, the

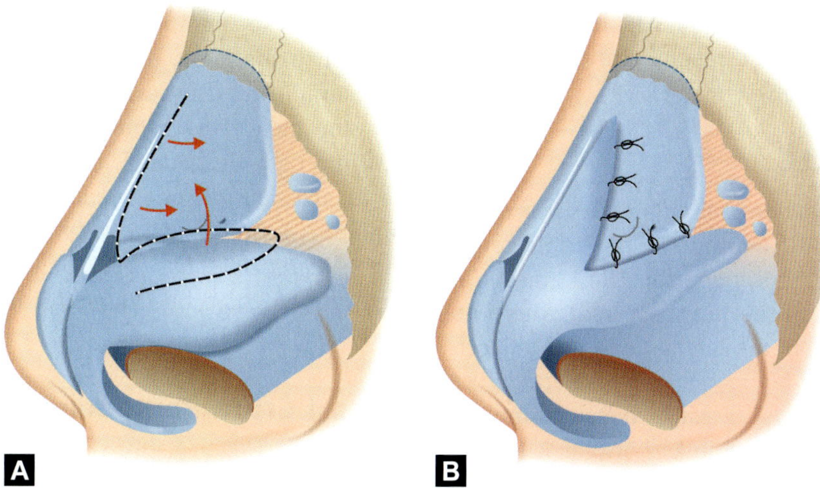

Figs. 17.10A and B: Z plasty to open a stenotic isthmus. (A) Dissection of a medially based skin and cartilage containing flap of the lower lateral cartilage and separation of upper lateral crus (ULC) from the septum. (B) Upward rotation of the flap and its placement between septum and ULC produces a splay effect to widen the isthmus.

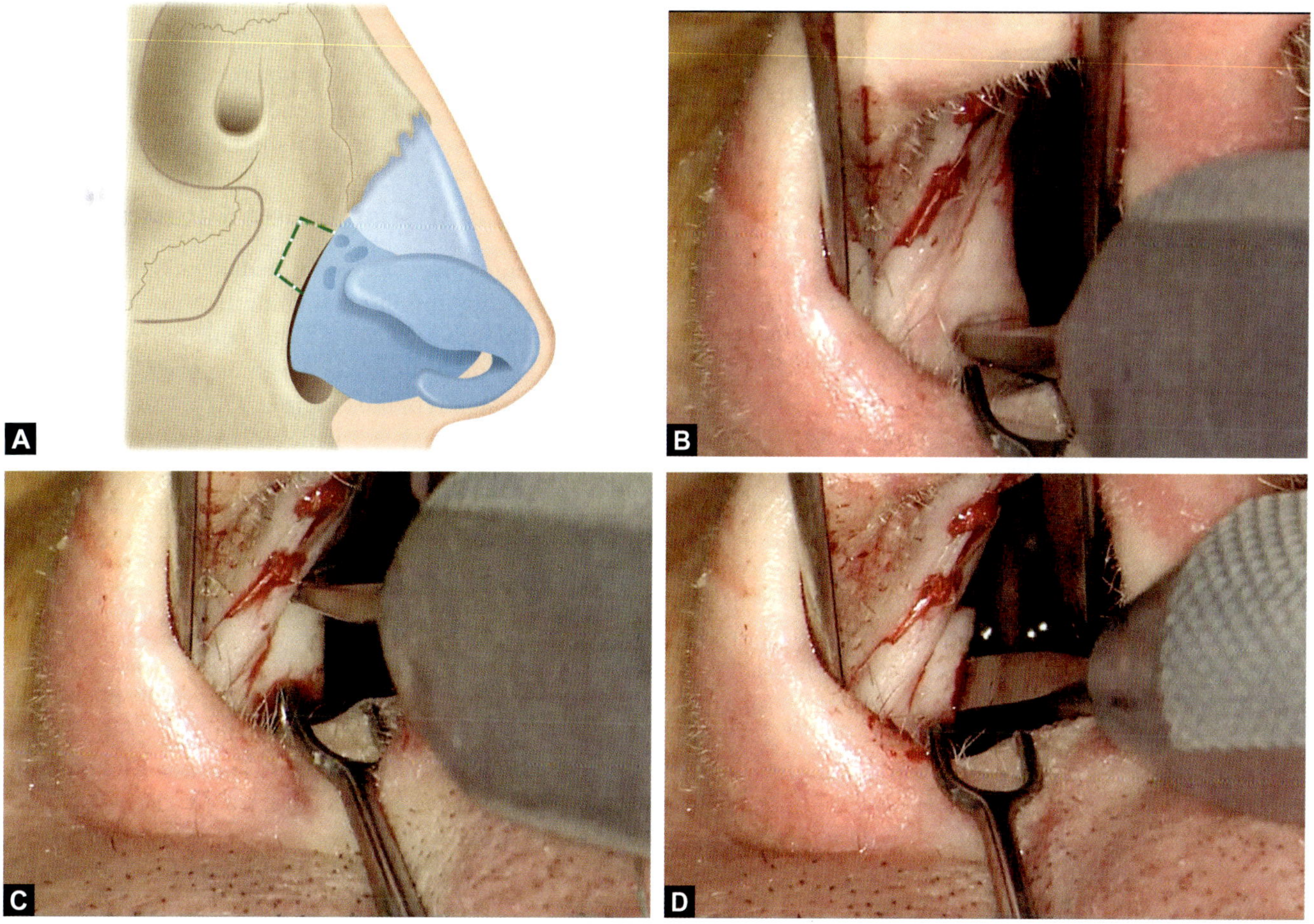

Figs. 17.11A to D: Door wing like osteotomies to address pyriform aperture stenosis (A). Caudally (B), cranially (C), and medially (D) performed miniosteotomies are used to lateralize the bone next to the isthmus.

alae determine the bias of developing an alar collapse. Out of the three segments of the LLC (defined by tip, ala, and columella), the lateral and medial crura are particularly important in nasal valve surgery.

Lateral Crura of LLC

The usually convex-shaped lateral crus varies from 16 to 30 mm in length and 6 to 16 mm in height. In its course from medial to lateral, it overlaps the ULC running in a laterosuperior vector to the bony pyramid where the pyramid ligament anchors the lateral crus and adjacent accessory cartilages to the maxilla. The lateral crural complex connects to the ULC through dense connective tissue fibers. Connective tissue links between ULC and LLC in the overlapping zone known as the scroll area are as important for stability of ala as shape, resilience, and position of the lateral crura (Koppe, Giotakis and Heppt, 2011).

Alar Grafts

Alar batten grafts (Figs. 17.12A and B) harvested from the septum, cavum conchae or rib are effective in reinforcing the lateral wall, which has a tendency to collapse (Tardy, 2004; Toriumi, et al., 1997). Most frequently placed in the supra-alar groove or caudal to the lateral crura, they increase the cartilaginous resilience of the lateral crura and counteract negative pressure forces during inspiration. The grafts usually measure 10–15 mm in length and 4–8 mm in width, and are placed into precise pockets or suture fixated on top of the relevant areas. If the surgeon seeks even greater support for the ala, grafts may be tailored in an oblong fashion in order to rest on the pyriform aperture laterally. The *lateral crural strut graft* (Figs. 17.12C and D) is positioned under the cephalic portion of the lateral crus of the LLC and fixated with mattress stitches (Gunter and Friedman, 1997). It is a powerful graft, commonly used in a variety of alar reshaping procedures, as well as in isthmus stenosis due to malformations in the scroll area or around the lateral crural complex. Supported laterally at the pyriform aperture, lateral crural strut grafts are also indicated for correction of instabilities of the lateral crural complex. On the other hand, *lateral crural spanning grafts* (Teichgraeber and Wainwright, 1994) and *lateral crural underlay spring grafts* (Figs. 17.12E to H) (Timmer, et al., 2013), increase sidewall tension and rigidity while increasing the nasal valve angle and cross-sectional area. Consistent and satisfactory results have also been obtained with *alar spreader grafts* supporting lateralized and caudally mobilized lateral crura after complete release (Kim, et al., 2012). In contrast to the latter, *alar rim grafts* are less functional than contouring. They are inserted into pockets along the alar rim, measuring about 2–3 mm in width and 10–15 mm in length. In general, the use of alloplastic materials in alar reinforcement such as porous polyethylene implants (Romo, Sclafani and Sabini, 1998; Romo, Litner and Sclafani, 2003) has been abandoned, because of their high rate of extrusion (Ramakrishnan, Danner and Yee, 2007).

Lateral Crura Remodeling

Nasal valve compromising concavities or other irregularities of the LLC may be corrected by *flipping over* the lateral crus ipsi- or contralaterally (Fig. 17.13A), fixation of a convex-shaped *onlay graft* to the lateral crus (Figs. 17.13B to D), or by *repositioning of an alar malposition* after complete dissection and reinforcement with additional use of a *lateral crural strut graft* (Figs. 17.12C and D). The *lateral crural turn-in flap* provides a gentle method to reshape and strengthen the lateral crura when the cephalic portion is large enough and cephalic trimming is carried out for tip refinement (Apaydin, 2012).

Spanning and Suspension Sutures

For the treatment of weak and medially displaced lateral crura, widening and strengthening may be achieved by a *lateral crus pull-up* carried out with permanent submucosal spanning sutures between the pyriform aperture and the lateral part of the LLC (Fig. 17.14) (Menger, 2006). The same effect may be achieved by the use of lateral expansion sutures taking both lateral crura and running over the septum (Mendelsohn and Golchin, 2006) and to a lesser extent by subcutaneous PDS suspension sutures (Fig. 17.8B) (Saban, di Benito and Massa, 2014).

Medial Crura of LLC

The medial crus of the LLC is composed of two segments, the vertically orientated columellar segment and the diverging footplate segment (Koppe, Giotakis and Heppt, 2011). Asymmetries and widely diverging footplates compromise the cross-sectional area of the nostrils, leading to an increased risk of alar collapse. The surgical options for narrowing a broad columella are effected by various parameters such as the degree of footplate divergence, the projection of the tip, shape and position of the

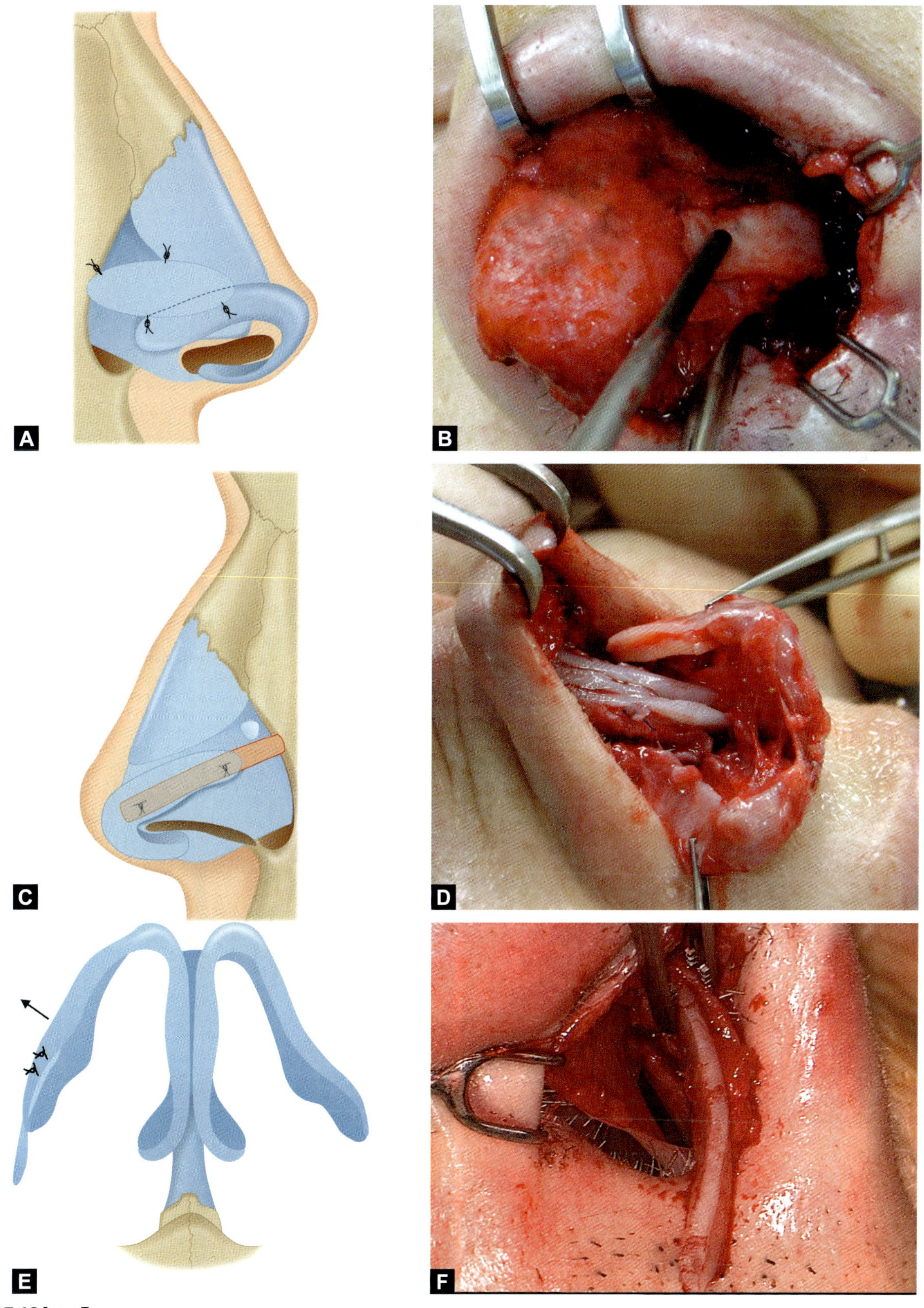

Figs. 17.12A to F

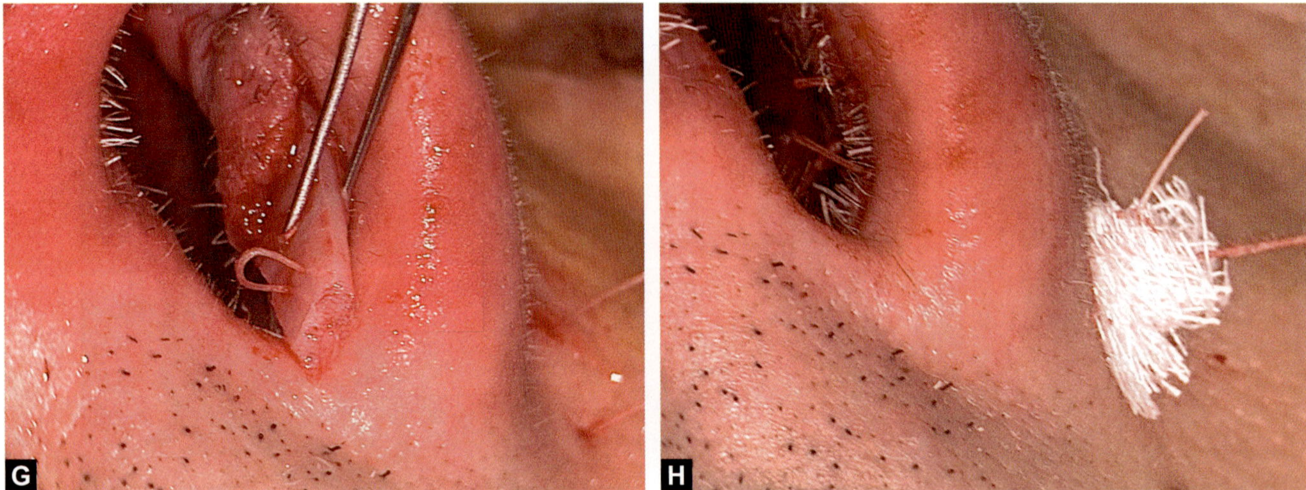

Figs. 17.12A to H: Alar grafts in nasal valve surgery. Alar batten grafts (A and B), lateral crural strut grafts (C and D), and lateral crural underlay spring grafts (E to H) are effective in reinforcing the nasal side wall that has a tendency to collapse, as well as in the correction of malpositioned lateral crura.

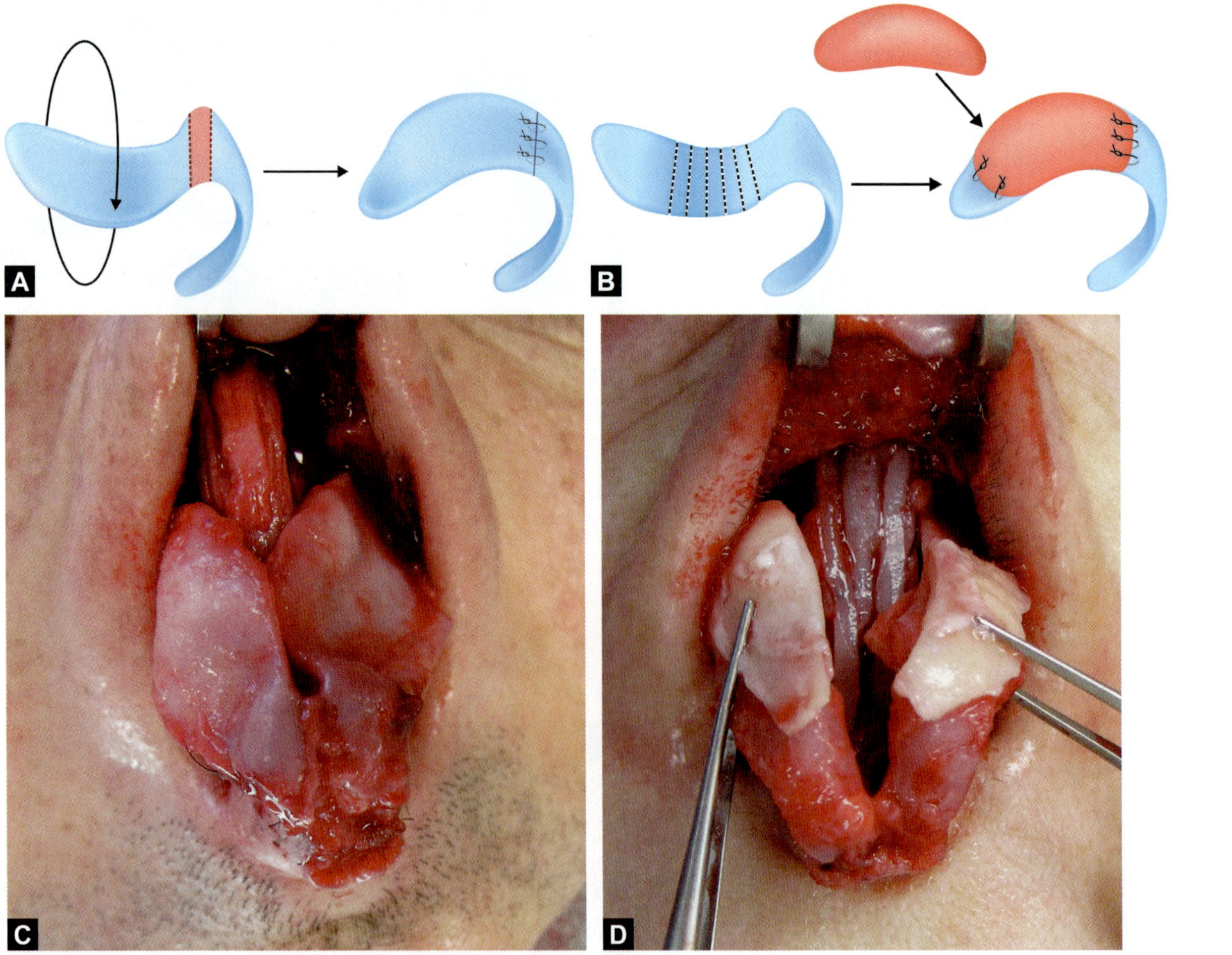

Figs. 17.13A to D: Correction of lateral crus concavity. Correction with flip-flop technique (lateral crural turnover flap) (A) and onlay graft (B to D).

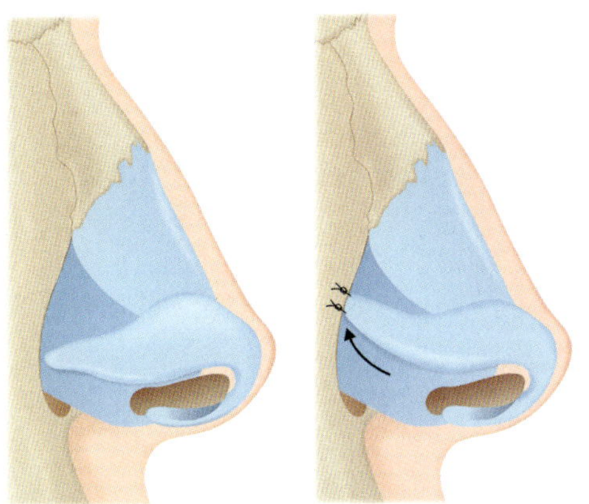

Fig. 17.14: Lateral crus pull-up technique with sutures between the pyriform aperture and the lateral part of the lower lateral cartilage.

subnasal and the columellar base, and deviation of the caudal septum. Also, reduction can improve nasal ventilation by opening the inner nasal valve angle (Tardy, Patt and Walter, 1993; Becker, et al., 1997).

Footplate Reshaping

Simple resection of the lateral part of the divergent footplates of medial crura narrows the columellar base and decreases tip projection in tension nose deformities, whereas approximation of both footplates increases tip projection and the subnasal volume (Figs. 17.15A to E). The need for intercrural soft tissue excision depends on columellar base conditions. It is indicated for columellar base protrusion but not for its retraction.

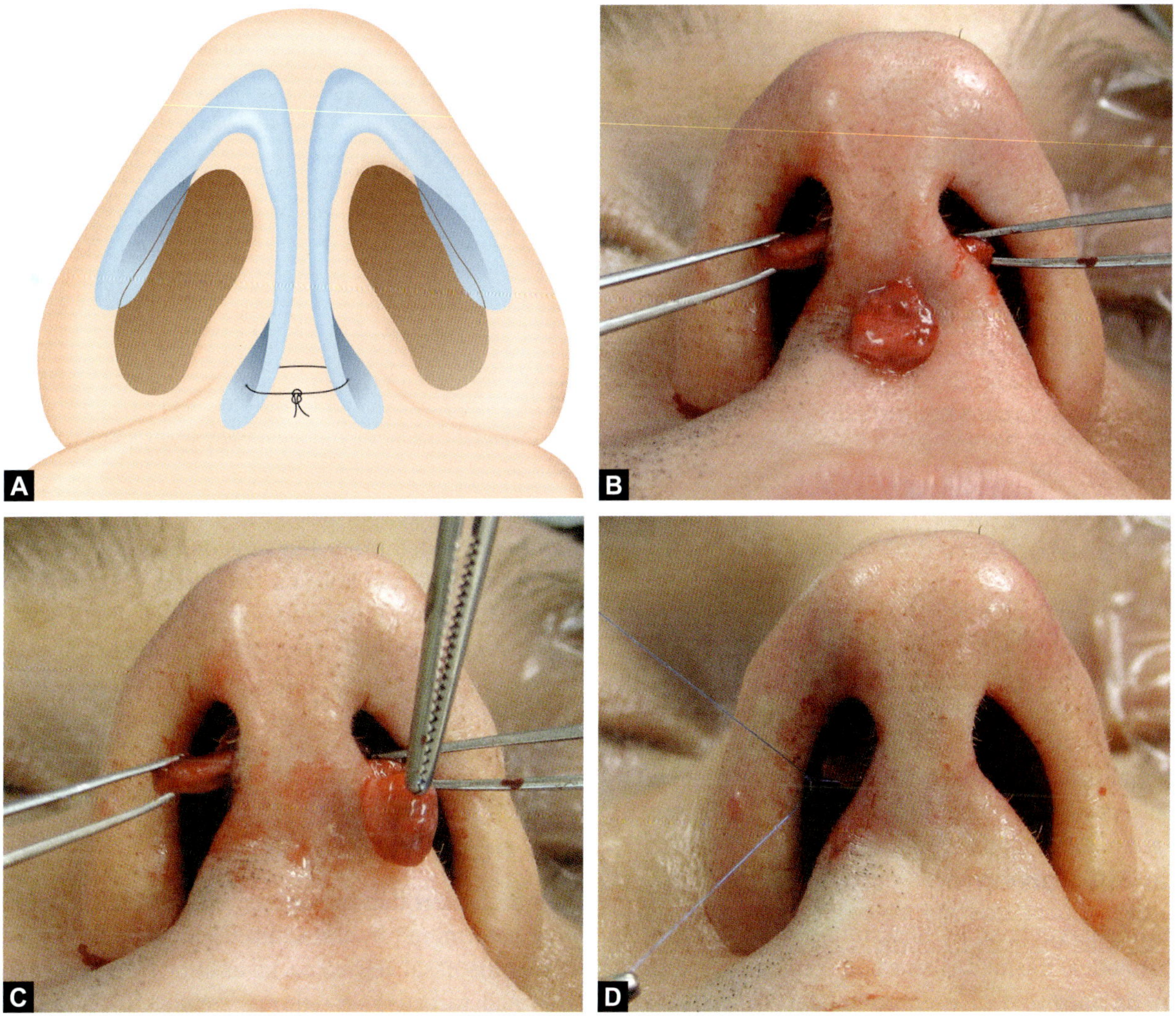

Figs. 17.15A to D:

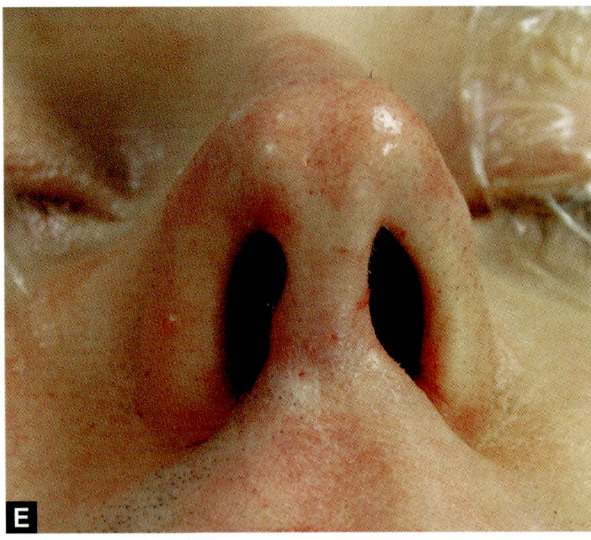

Figs. 17.15A to E: Approximation of diverging footplates using mattress sutures (A). Dissection of the medial crura and excision of intercrural soft tissue (B), narrowing of the columellar base by a mattress suture placed under the mucosa (C to E).

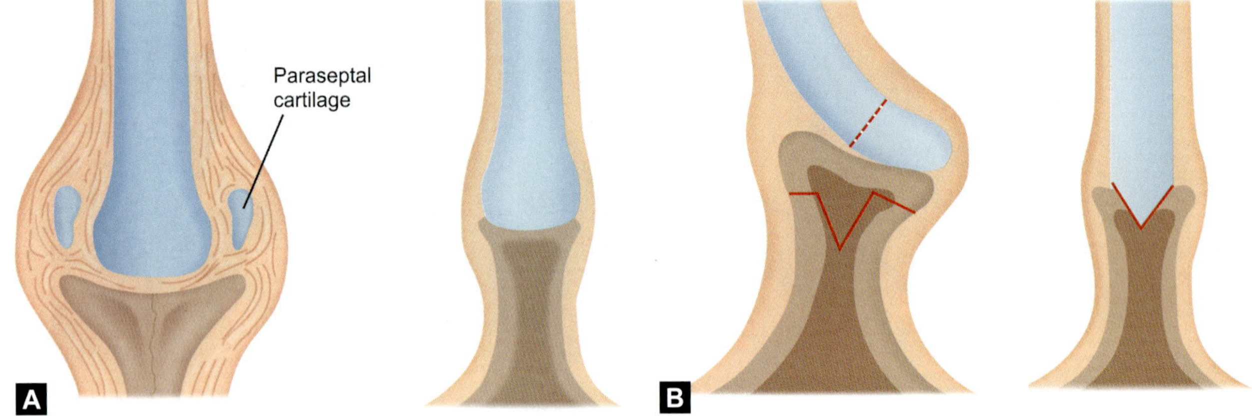

Figs. 17.16A and B: Narrowing of the caudal septum by removal of paraseptal cartilages and alignment of the premaxilla (A) and by placement of the shortened inferior septum into a premaxilla groove (B).

Caudal Septoplasty

Septal deviations may also create malformations of the footplates. They might need a combined procedure of repositioning of the footplates and caudal septoplasty. This includes techniques such as straightening of the septum correcting a caudal deflection or subluxation, removal of paraseptal cartilages and premaxilla crests or the alignment of a deviated anterior nasal spine (Figs. 17.16A and B).

Nasal Sill Correction

The nasal sill is defined as the intranostril region between the footplate of the medial crus and the alar facial groove. It may be narrowed or even obliterated congenitally or after trauma or infection. Depending on the type and nature of the deformity, the surgeon may choose between a Z plasty (Day and Stucker, 1994) and a Y-to-V advancement technique (Burm and Yang, 2011). The insertion of a free composite graft of the cavum conchae (Figs. 17.17A to D) has proven useful in severe cases with recurrent scar contracture, but even this method requires the long-term use of custom made intranasal stents to prevent restenosis (Daya, 2009).

The Ptotic Tip

Due to the fact that impairment of nasal breathing is not only determined by the width but also by the cross section of the nasal valve area, an existing tip ptosis is always assumed to cause an isthmus stenosis by lowering the dorsal indentation of the airflow space. The influence of

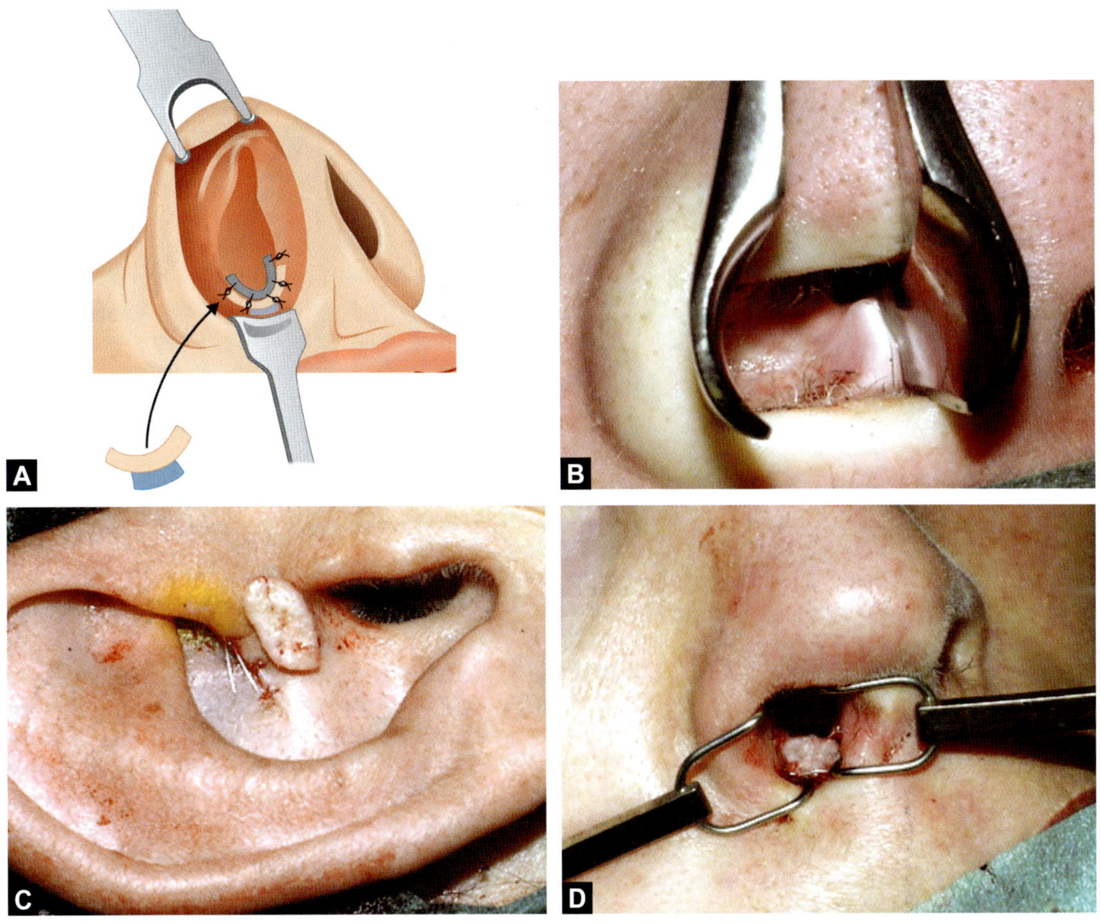

Figs. 17.17A to D: Free composite graft of the concha is being used for correction of nasal sill stenosis (A). Traumatic sill stenosis (B), harvesting of an auricular composite graft (C), graft sutured in place (D).

a ptotic tip on the direction of inspired air and the consequent compromise in nasal breathing is likely to be a rather minor effect according to the authors. Even so, elevation of the tip using septal reconstruction (Heppt and Gubisch, 2011), insertion of a columella strut (Figs. 17.18A to D) (Glasgold, 1988), PDS suspension sutures (Figs. 17.19A to C) (Daniel, 2014; Saban, di Benito and Massa, 2014) or the lateral crural overlay technique (Kridel and Konior, 1991) help to improve nasal breathing and ventilation. An additional effective option for treating ptotic tips in the aging nose is the *external rhinolift* (Slavit, et al., 1990). In this technique, the tip rotation is increased by rhombic resection of excess skin at the radix. This and the other tip elevating procedures are indicated in patients with tip ptosis and concomitant alar collapse resulting from inadequate cartilaginous support. All techniques are aimed at the restoration of the "cul-de-sac" area in the nasal vestibule, which is defined by the relationship between the caudal border of the ULC and the cephalic margin of the LLC. Elevation of the cephalic margin of the LLC to a position superficial to the ULC restores the normal position of these two structures. Both cartilages then assist in stenting the nasal vestibule, and thereby improve nasal breathing.

CONCLUSION

Even though the nasal valve forms one of the most important control elements of the upper respiratory tract, major details of physiology, diagnostics, and therapy are still unsolved and undiscovered. This chapter maps out the most important developments of conservative and surgical procedures of the last decade, focusing on pragmatic possible solutions for differentiated nasal valve pathologies. A concise workup of all techniques is given in Table 17.3.

In the end, the experienced surgeon will have to determine which method or combination of methods is most

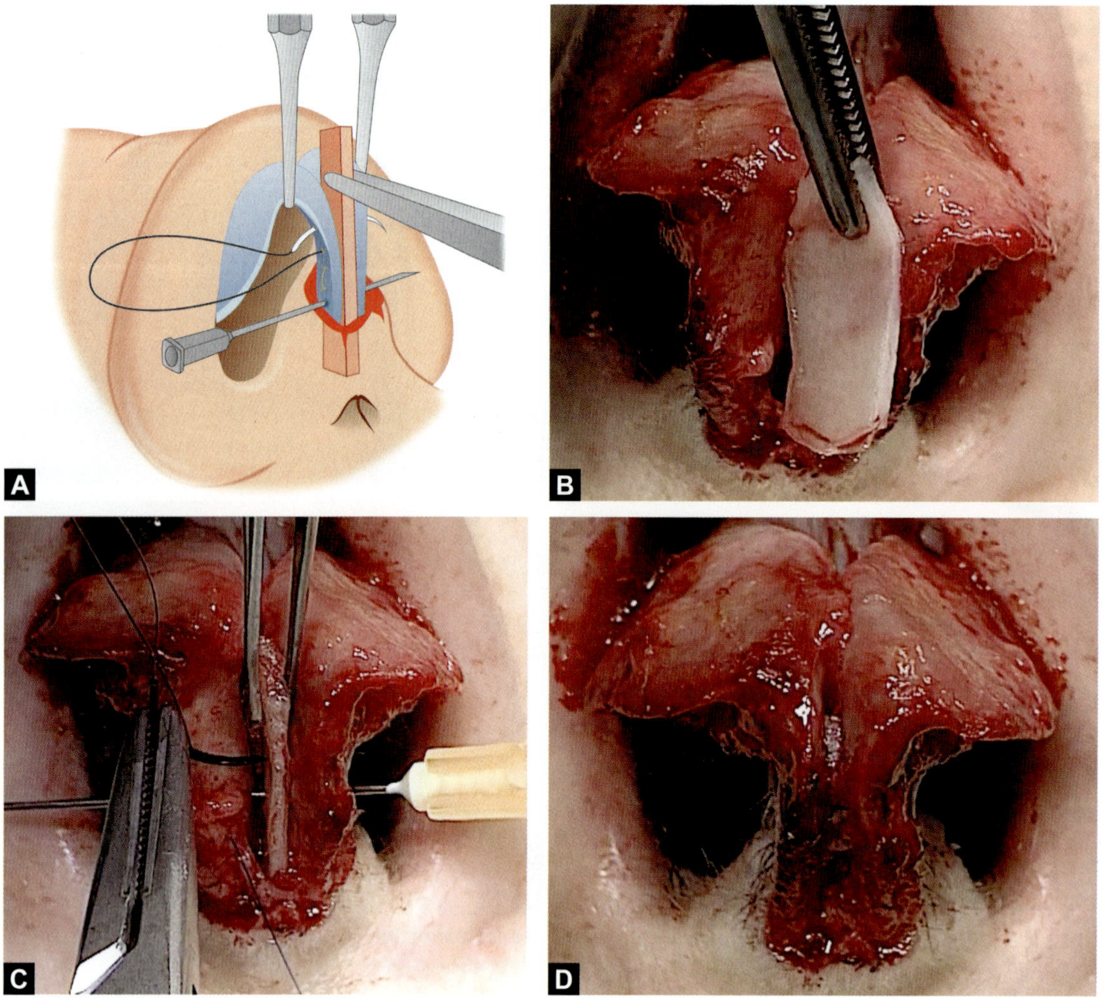

Figs. 17.18A to D: Support and elevation of the nasal tip by insertion of a columella strut.

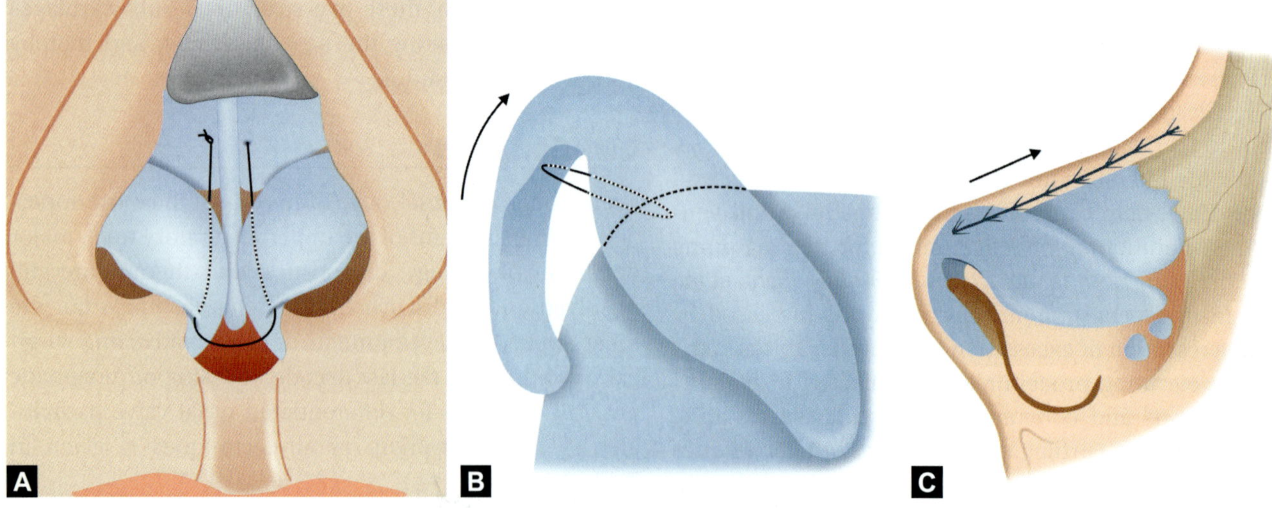

Figs. 17.19A to C: Elevation of the nasal tip by application of a suspension suture, taking both medial (A) or intermedial crura (B) or by the use of subcutaneously placed PDS threads (C).

suitable for the individual patient in order to achieve the most satisfactory functional and esthetic result.

ACKNOWLEDGMENT

Illustrations in Figures 17.1A and B, 17.16A and B, and 17.17A have been modified after Huizing E and de Groot J, *Functional Reconstructive Nasal Surgery*, New York, Thieme, 2003.

All illustrations were sponsored by Karl Storz (Tuttlingen, Germany).

REFERENCES

Apaydin, F., 2012. Lateral crural turn-in flap in functional rhinoplasty. *Archives of Facial Plastic Surgery*, 14(2), pp. 93-6. Available from: PM:22006234.

Ballert, J.A. and Park, S.S., 2006. Functional rhinoplasty: treatment of the dysfunctional nasal sidewall. *Facial Plastic Surgery*, 22(1), pp. 49-54. Available from: PM:16732504.

Becker, D.G., Weinberger, M.S., Greene, B.A. and Tardy, M.E., Jr., 1997. Clinical study of alar anatomy and surgery of the alar base. *Archives of Otolaryngology—Head and Neck Surgery*, 123(8), pp. 789-95. Available from: PM:9260542.

Bohluli, B., Varedi, P., Nazari, S. and Bagheri, S.C., 2013. Lateral crural suspension flap: a novel technique to modify and stabilize the nasolabial angle. *Journal of Oral and Maxillofacial Surgery*. Available from: PM:23769462.

Burm, J.S. and Yang, W.Y., 2011. Modification of running Y-V plasty to correct bilateral nostril stenosis with a circular, linear contracture. *Journal of Plastic, Reconstructive and Aesthetic Surgery*, 64(12), pp. 1665-8. Available from: PM:21628106.

Clark, J.M. and Cook, T.A., 2002. The "butterfly" graft in functional secondary rhinoplasty. *Laryngoscope*, 112(11), pp. 1917-25. Available from: PM:12439155.

Daniel, R.K., 2014. *Mastering rhinoplasty: a comprehensive atlas of surgical techniques with integrated video clips*. 2nd ed. Springer: Berlin.

Day, T.A. and Stucker, F.J., 1994. Regional and distant flaps in nasal reconstruction. *Facial Plastic Surgery*, 10(4), pp. 349-57. Available from: PM:7713452.

Daya, M., 2009. Nostril stenosis corrected by release and serial stenting. *Journal of Plastic, Reconstructive and Aesthetic Surgery*, 62(8), pp. 1012-9. Available from: PM:18515201.

Deva, A.K., Merten, S. and Chang, L., 1998. Silicone in nasal augmentation rhinoplasty: a decade of clinical experience. *Plastic and Reconstructive Surgery*, 102(4), pp. 1230-37. Available from: PM:9734450.

Dutton, J.M. and Neidich, M.J., 2008. Intranasal Z-plasty for internal nasal valve collapse. *Archives of Facial Plastic Surgery*, 10(3), pp. 164-8. Available from: PM:18490542.

Friedman, O. and Cook, T.A., 2009. Conchal cartilage butterfly graft in primary functional rhinoplasty. *Laryngoscope*, 119(2), pp. 255-62. Available from: PM:19160388.

Glasgold, A.I., 1988. The technique and clinical application of the columella strut. *Laryngoscope*, 98(7), pp. 789-90. Available from: PM:3386388.

Gunter, J.P. and Friedman, R.M., 1997. Lateral crural strut graft: technique and clinical applications in rhinoplasty. *Plastic and Reconstructive Surgery*, 99(4), pp. 943-52. Available from: PM:9091939.

Guyuron, B., Michelow, B.J. and Englebardt, C., 1998. Upper lateral splay graft. *Plastic and Reconstructive Surgery*, 102(6), pp. 2169-77. Available from: PM:9811019.

Heppt, W. and Gubisch, W., 2011. Septal surgery in rhinoplasty. *Facial Plastic Surgery*, 27(2), pp. 167-78. Available from: PM: 21404159.

Hildebrandt, T., Goubergrits, L., Heppt, W.J., Bessler, S. and Zachow, S., 2013. Evaluation of the intranasal flow field through computational fluid dynamics.*Facial Plastic Surgery*, 29(2), pp. 93-8. Available from: PM:23564240.

Hornung, D.E., Leopold, D.A., Youngentob, S.L., Sheehe, P.R., Gagne, G.M., Thomas, F.D. and Mozell, M.M., 1987. Airflow patterns in a human nasal model. *Archives of Otolaryngology—Head and Neck Surgery*, 113(2), pp. 169-72. Available from: PM:3801173.

Huizing, B.H. and de Groot, J.A.M., 2002. *Functional reconstructive nasal surgery*, 1st ed. New York, Stuttgart: Thieme.

Islam, A., Arslan, N., Felek, S.A., Celik, H., Demirci, M. and Oguz, H., 2008. Reconstruction of the internal nasal valve: modified splay graft technique with endonasal approach. *Laryngoscope*, 118(10), pp. 1739-43. Available from: PM:18622313.

Kasperbauer, J.L., and Kern, E.B., 1987. Nasal valve physiology. Implications in nasal surgery. *Otolaryngologic Clinics of North America*, 20(4), pp. 699-719. Available from: PM:3320865.

Kim, J.H., Park, S.W., Oh, W.S., and Lee, J.H., 2012. New classification for correction of alar retraction using the alar spreader graft. *Aesthetic Plastic Surgery*, 36(4), 832-41. Available from: PM:22538276.

Koppe, T., Giotakis, E.I. and Heppt, W., 2011. Functional anatomy of the nose. *Facial Plastic Surgery*, 27(2), pp. 135-45. Available from: PM:21404156.

Kridel, R.W. and Konior, R.J., 1991. Controlled nasal tip rotation via the lateral crural overlay technique. *Archives of Otolaryngology—Head and Neck Surgery*, 117(4), pp. 411-15. Available from: PM:2007012.

Latte, J. and Taverner, D., 2005. Opening the nasal valve with external dilators reduces congestive symptoms in normal subjects. *The American Journal of Rhinology*, 19(2), pp. 215-19. Available from: PM:15921224.

Mendelsohn, M.S. and Golchin, K., 2006. Alar expansion and reinforcement: a new technique to manage nasal valve collapse. *Archives of Facial Plastic Surgery*, 8(5), pp. 293-9. Available from: PM:16982983.

Menger, D.J., 2006. Lateral crus pull-up: a method for collapse of the external nasal valve. *Archives of Facial Plastic Surgery*, 8(5), pp. 333-7. Available from: PM:16982991.

Mink, J., 1903. Le nez comme voie respiratoire. Brussels, Belgium, *Presse Otolaryngol.*

Paniello, R.C., 1996. Nasal valve suspension. An effective treatment for nasal valve collapse. *Archives of Otolaryngology—Head and Neck Surgery*, 122(12), pp. 1342-6. Available from: PM:8956747.

Park, S.S., 1998. The flaring suture to augment the repair of the dysfunctional nasal valve. *Plastic and Reconstructive Surgery*, 101(4), pp. 1120-22. Available from: PM:9514349.

Peltonen, L.I., Vento, S.I., Simola, M. and Malmberg, H., 2004. Effects of the nasal strip and dilator on nasal breathing—a study with healthy subjects. *Rhinology*, 42(3), pp. 122-5. Available from: PM:15521663.

Ramakrishnan, J.B., Danner, C.J. and Yee, S.W., 2007. The use of porous polyethylene implants to correct nasal valve collapse. *Otolaryngology—Head and Neck Surgery*, 136(3), pp. 357-61. Available from: PM:17321859.

Raudenbush, B., 2011. Stenting the nasal airway for maximizing inspiratory airflow: internal Max-Air Nose Cones versus external Breathe Right strip. *The American Journal of Rhinology and Allergy*, 25(4), pp. 249-51. Available from: PM: 21819762.

Rhee, J.S., Weaver, E.M., Park, S.S., Baker, S.R., Hilger, P.A., Kriet, J.D., Murakami, C., Senior, B.A., Rosenfeld, R.M. and DiVittorio, D., 2010. Clinical consensus statement: Diagnosis and management of nasal valve compromise. *Otolaryngology—Head and Neck Surgery*, 143(1), pp. 48-59. Available from: PM:20620619.

Riechelmann, H., Karow, E., DiDio, D., and Kral, F., 2010. External nasal valve collapse—a case-control and interventional study employing a novel internal nasal dilator (Nasanita). *Rhinology*, 48(2), pp. 183-8. Available from: PM:20502758.

Romo, T., III, Litner, J.A., and Sclafani, A.P., 2003. Management of the severe bulbous nasal tip using porous polyethylene alloimplants. *Facial Plastic Surgery*, 19(4), pp. 341-8. Available from: PM:14737703.

Romo, T., III, Sclafani, A.P. and Sabini, P., 1998. Use of porous high-density polyethylene in revision rhinoplasty and in the platyrrhine nose. *Aesthetic Plastic Surgery*, 22(3), pp. 211-21. Available from: PM:9618188.

Saban, Y., Braccini, F. and Polselli, R., 2006. Rhinoplasty: morphodynamic anatomy of rhinoplasty. Interest of conservative rhinoplasty. *Revue De Laryngologie Otologie Rhinologie*, 127 (1-2), pp. 15-22. Available from: PM:16886524.

Saban, Y., di Benito, J. and Massa, M., 2014. Nasal lift: nasal valve lift and nasal tip lift. *Facial Plastic Surgery*.

Sheen, J.H., 1984. Spreader graft: a method of reconstructing the roof of the middle nasal vault following rhinoplasty. *Plastic and Reconstructive Surgery*, 73(2), pp. 230-39. Available from: PM:6695022.

Siegert, R. and Balczun, J., 2010. Diagnosis of nasal valve stenosis via anterior rhinomanometry using a nasal valve dilatator. *Laryngorhinootologie*, 89(6), pp. 334-37. Available from: PM:20539947.

Slavit, D.H., Lipton, R.J., Kern, E.B. and McCaffrey, T.V., 1990. Rhinolift operation in the treatment of the aging nose. *Otolaryngology—Head and Neck Surgery*, 103(3), pp. 462-7. Available from: PM:2122379.

Tardy, M.E., Jr. 2004. Graduated sculpture refinement of the nasal tip. *Facial Plastic Surgery Clinics of North America*, 12(1), pp. 51-80. Available from: PM:15062238.

Tardy, M.E., Jr., Patt, B.S. and Walter, M.A., 1993. Alar reduction and sculpture: anatomic concepts.*Facial Plastic Surgery*, 9(4), pp. 295-305. Available from: PM:8181769.

Teichgraeber, J.F. and Wainwright, D.J., 1994. The treatment of nasal valve obstruction. *Plastic and Reconstructive Surgery*, 93(6), pp. 1174-82. Available from: PM:8171137.

Timmer, F.C., Roth, J.A., Borjesson, P.K. and Lohuis, P.J., 2013. The lateral crural underlay spring graft. *Facial Plastic Surgery*, 29(2), pp. 140-45. Available from: PM:23564247.

Toriumi, D.M., Josen, J., Weinberger, M. and Tardy, M.E., Jr., 1997. Use of alar batten grafts for correction of nasal valve collapse. *Archives of Otolaryngology—Head and Neck Surgery*, 123(8), pp. 802-8. Available from: PM:9260543.

Vidyasagar, R., Friedman, M., Ibrahim, H., Bliznikas, D. and Joseph, N.J., 2005. Inspiratory and fixed nasal valve collapse: clinical and rhinometric assessment. *American Journal of Rhinology*, 19(4), pp. 370-74. Available from: PM:16171171.

Vogt, K., Jalowayski, A.A., Althaus, W., Cao, C., Han, D., Hasse, W., Hoffrichter, H., Mosges, R., Pallanch, J., Shah-Hosseini, K., Peksis, K., Wernecke, K.D., Zhang, L. and Zaporoshenko, P., 2010. 4-Phase-Rhinomanometry (4PR)—basics and practice 2010. *Rhinology: Supplement*, 21, pp. 1-50. Available from: PM:20649107.

Wengen, D.F., 2012. Alternatives to flaring spreader flaps and upper lateral advancement for the internal nasal valve. *HNO*, 60(7), pp. 595-6. Available from: PM:22763765.

Wexler, D.B. and Davidson, T.M., 2004. The nasal valve: a review of the anatomy, imaging, and physiology. *American Journal of Rhinology*, 18(3), pp. 143-150. Available from: PM:15283487.

Wrobel, B.B. and Leopold, D.A., 2005. Olfactory and sensory attributes of the nose. *Otolaryngologic Clinics of North America*, 38(6), pp. 1163-70. Available from PM:16326176.

Zumegen, C., Schneider, D. and Michel, O., 2001. Influence of an internal nasal dilator (Nasanita) on nasal flow in healthy adults. *Laryngorhinootologie*, 80(12), pp. 704-7. Available from: PM:11793265.

18 Septoplasty

Robert Almeyda, Humera Babar Craig, Huib van Waegeningh, Hade Vuyk

Chapter Overview

Pearls and Pitfalls

Pearls

- Time spent with thorough preoperative assessment will be saved at surgery through a more efficient surgical procedure.
- Be respectful of the nasal valve.
- One size does not fit all. Failure to tailor surgical techniques to the anatomical pathology will lead to a poor outcome.
- The cartilage at the posterior septal angle should be reattached to the anterior nasal spine to prevent loss of tip projection and reduction of dorsal height due to posterior rotation of septal cartilage.

Pitfalls

- Resection in the keystone area will lead to saddle nose deformity.
- Resection of caudal septal cartilage may lead to columellar retraction or loss of tip projection.

18.1 INTRODUCTION

Septoplasty is one of the most commonly performed surgical procedures in otolaryngology and its evolution has led from a technique of cartilage excision, as seen with submucous resection, to techniques with emphasis on reshaping, repositioning, and restructuring with conservation of cartilage. This chapter discusses assessment, anatomy, and modern surgical techniques for correction of nasal septal deviation.

18.2 ETIOLOGY AND PREVALENCE OF SEPTAL DEVIATION

Nasal septal deviation is common. Pediatric and adult anatomical studies have found its prevalence to be between 30% and 40% (Gray, 1978). However, the percentage of anterior cartilaginous deformity is much lower.

Septal deviation can be acquired in the form of injury to the quadrilateral cartilage, or developmental deformity. Deformity secondary to injury can occur at any age but often leads to a more complicated deformity in the younger prepubescent age group (Gray, 1978). Developmental deformity can also result in septal deviation. Many associations have been suggested including contralateral concha bullosa and maxillary molding during parturition.

18.3 INDICATIONS

Septoplasty is indicated in following cases:

- Correction of septal deviation causing nasal obstruction

- Correction of external nasal deviation
- Improving access for endoscopic sinus surgery
- Donor tissue harvesting for nasal reconstruction, augmentation, or endoscopic skull base repair
- Repair of septal perforation.

18.4 DIAGNOSTIC ASSESSMENT

- Nasal analysis requires an assessment of both external and internal components to define areas of nasal septal deviation causing narrowing or obstruction of the nasal airway and/or external nasal deviation. Anterior rhinoscopy can visualize the anterior septum and internal nasal valve but care must be taken to avoid anatomical distortion with the nasal speculum, particularly around the internal nasal valve region.
- Nasal endoscopy is essential to assess all areas of the nasal septum and to exclude sinonasal disease as a cause of patient's symptoms. Nasal mucosal decongestion can be helpful in differentiating mucosal and structural etiologies. It can also be informative to palpate the nasal septum with a cotton-tipped applicator to assess the amount and location of residual septal cartilage, particularly if previous septal surgery has been performed.
- It is important to assess the extent of caudal and dorsal septal deviation and the narrowing of the internal nasal valve angle and area. Patients with these structural deformities may not benefit from standard septoplasty techniques and often require more advanced techniques like replacement of caudal or dorsal septal strut, extracorporeal septoplasty, or spreader grafts for correction of nasal obstruction. To evaluate the potential benefit of surgery in the nasal valve region, an instrument such as the handle of an otolaryngology mirror may be placed vertically as a wedge in between the intact septum and nasal valve, or a modified Cottle's maneuver may be performed to support the more lateral components of the nasal valve area during inspiration. This can demonstrate to the patient the expected functional improvement and the potential broadening of the middle and lower third of the nose that may result from the proposed surgery.
- Objective assessment can be achieved with acoustic rhinometry and rhinomanometry but these investigations are not widely used in clinical practice due to expense and poor correlation with subjective symptoms (Andre, et al., 2009). This absence of objective assessment has led to the evolution of various validated scoring systems to measure the severity of patient's symptoms and their effect on the quality of life. The nasal obstruction septoplasty effectiveness (NOSE) scale is one such validated example that has been shown to correlate symptoms of nasal obstruction with surgical outcome (Stewart, et al., 2004).
- It is important to recognize that nasal septal deflection can be developmental and a manifestation of nasal and facial asymmetry, or acquired following direct injury. In cases without a history of injury, assessment of facial asymmetry should be undertaken.
- Informed consent should include discussions regarding the expected outcome and the risk of potential complications like hemorrhage, infection, septal hematoma/abscess, septal perforation, nasal shape change, and numbness to palate and upper incisors. Taking all surgical techniques into account, a perceived improvement in symptoms is expected in >75% of cases. It should be emphasized to the patient that there is an unpredictable correlation between subjective and objective outcomes (Andre, et al., 2009).

18.5 SURGICAL ANATOMY

- The nasal septum is a vertical osseocartilaginous plate separating the left and right nasal cavities. Anteriorly, it is comprised of the quadrilateral cartilage caudally, which joins with the perpendicular plate of the ethmoid cephalically. The inferior portion of the septum is made up of the maxillary crest caudally, and the vomer and perpendicular plate of the palatine bone cephalically. The tough fibrous covering over this structure has important significance when it comes to performing surgery (Fig. 18.1). This structure comprises perichondrium over the cartilaginous septum and periosteum over the bony components. There is significant decussation of fibers between the perichondrial and periosteal layers over the quadrilateral cartilage and the maxillary spine, respectively. These fibers need to be dissected sharply to facilitate flap elevation. This is demonstrated in Figure 18.2. Failure to do so will often result in a tear in the elevated flap.
- The quadrilateral cartilage has important embryological development, which requires deliberation when considering pediatric septal surgery. Nasal growth continues well after puberty and in general should not be considered complete until the patient is 16-year-old (males 16–18 years, females 14–16 years)

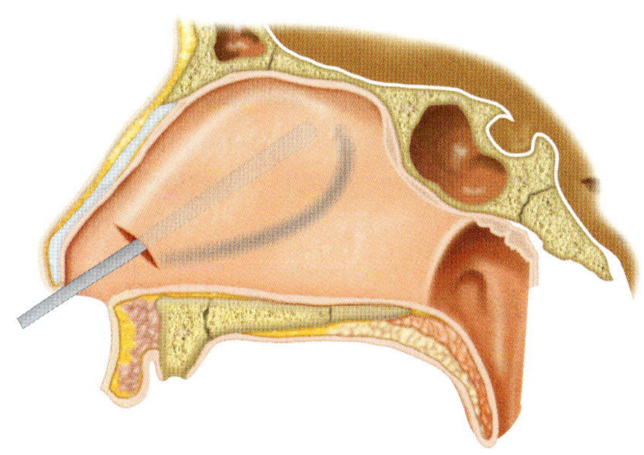

Fig. 18.1: Diagram showing the use of Freer elevator for elevating a mucoperichondrial flap through a hemitransfixion incision.

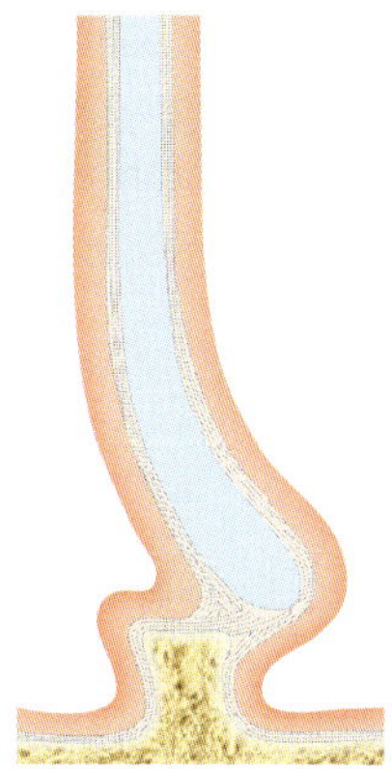

Fig. 18.2: Diagram showing the complex arrangement of decussating fibers between perichondrium above and periosteum below. Care must be taken to avoid flap tears in this region.

(Verwoerd and Verwoerd-Verhoef, 2005). There are two growth centers within the quadrilateral cartilage, sphenodorsal, and sphenospinal. The sphenodorsal extends from the sphenoid toward the nasal dorsum and the sphenospinal extends from the sphenoid toward the anterior nasal spine. Disruption to these areas during development can result in retroposition of the anterior nasal spine and maxilla, which can be extremely challenging to correct in later life (Verwoerd and Verwoerd-Verhoef, 2005).

- The anterior cartilaginous nasal septum has a structural supportive function for the lower two-thirds of the nose. This can be demarcated by drawing a vertical line from the anterior-most part of the nasal bone, so-called "keystone area", to the anterior nasal spine. Cartilage anterior to this imaginary line provides major stability to the nose and a strong L-shaped midline structure (1.5 cm dorsal and caudal strut) is essential to maintain support, function, and aesthetics (Scheithauer, et al., 2006).
- The quadrilateral cartilage is fused with the upper lateral cartilages by fibrous connective tissue to form a functional unit, the internal nasal valve. The normal internal nasal valve angle is about 15° in Caucasians and 20° in Asians and Africans. This junction of upper lateral cartilages and nasal septum provides significant nasal resistance and its assessment is important when considering septal surgery. In patients with a narrow nasal valve angle and nasal obstruction, the angle between the septum and upper lateral cartilages can be increased using spreader grafts to reduce inspiratory nasal resistance. This is demonstrated in Figure 18.3.

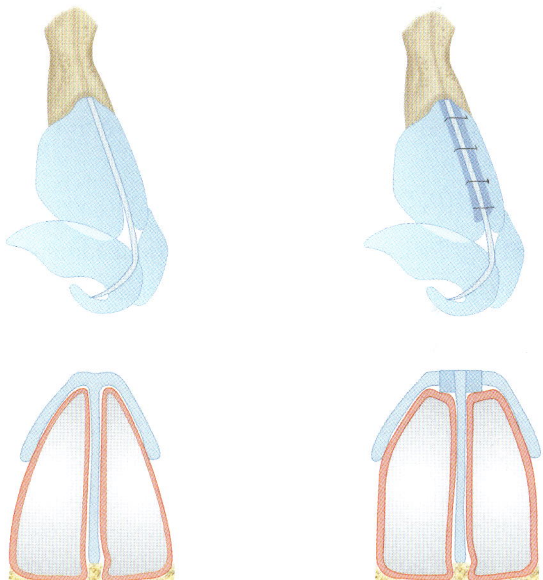

Fig. 18.3: Diagram showing the placement of spreader grafts between the upper lateral cartilages and the nasal septum. The increase in nasal valve angle can be appreciated.

18.6 SURGICAL TECHNIQUE

Preparation

Septoplasty requires appropriate nasal decongestion and vasoconstriction prior to surgery. Numerous topical solutions have been used with various means of application, ranging from atomized spray to cotton pledgets. The authors favor a combination of atomized topical Moffett's solution (2 mL 10% cocaine solution, 1 mL of 1:1,000 adrenaline, and 3 mL 8.4% bicarbonate) and local anesthetic infiltration with 2% lignocaine and adrenaline

1:80,000 into the septal mucosal flap. This, along with hypotensive anesthesia, gives an excellent surgical field. General anesthesia is preferable, but local anesthetic procedures are well described.

Surgical Approaches

Killian Incision

A vertical incision into the septal mucosa 1.5 cm from the caudal septal border allows relatively easy elevation of the mucoperichondrial flap to allow access to most areas of the septum apart from the anterior septal angle, columella, and anterior nasal spine regions. A Killian incision is generally advocated for harvesting cartilage, correcting deformities of the perpendicular plate of the ethmoid, and removing vomerine spurs. Raising only one mucosal flap has a risk of mucosal tearing and subsequent long-term perforation. Contralateral flap elevation is recommended around spurs. This approach does not yield enough surgical exposure for very anterior deflections of the septum.

Hemitransfixion Incision

This vertical incision is placed along the leading edge of the caudal septum down to the nasal spine. This is best done by stretching the skin over the caudal edge of the septum. This produces tension on the vestibular skin that allows for a clean incision. Although the incision gives excellent exposure to the whole septum, the perichondrium at this point is tightly tethered to the underlying cartilage making subperichondrial flap elevation technically difficult. Flap elevation is made easier by elevation of a mucosa only flap for 3–4 mm using sharp scissors followed by precise perichondrial incision using a number 15 blade. Making to-and-fro movements along the perichondrial incision (using the tips of a sharp curved iris scissors) can then be used to enter the correct subperichondrial plane. This helps elevate the perichondrium from the underlying cartilage.

External Approach

An external approach provides complete exposure of the nasal septum both caudally and anteriorly. It comprises a horizontal broken columella incision combined with marginal incisions to allow the dorsal skin and soft tissue envelope to be elevated. The lower and upper lateral cartilages can then be separated exposing the complete cartilaginous septum. This approach is indicated for most dorsal and caudal septal deviations specifically when the internal nasal valve apex region is involved. The external approach allows for subtotal septal reconstruction to address patient's aesthetic and functional concerns resulting from extensive septal deviation (Andre and Vuyk, 2006).

Septoplasty Techniques

The classical swing door technique can be used to mobilize the septum allowing it to be repositioned in the midline. Initial surgical steps require a nasal speculum, headlight, and Freer elevator. Once a mucosal flap has been elevated, either an endoscope or headlight can be used to continue the dissection (Fig. 18.1). The nasal speculum is positioned on either side of the caudal edge of the septum to stretch the mucosa allowing visualization of layers of soft tissue overlying the cartilage. These layers can then be dissected carefully with a scalpel down to the cartilage. The correct dissection plane can be identified by the bluish-white appearance of the cartilage. Elevation of the mucoperichondrial flap continues with an elevating instrument such as a Freer or Cottle elevator beyond the septal deviation, preferably to the perpendicular plate of the ethmoid. The contralateral side is then elevated to avoid tears in the mucosa at the stage when cartilage is resected. Failure to elevate the flap bilaterally prevents the cartilage from being repositioned in the midline. This happens because the attachment between the mucoperichondrium and cartilage on one side tends to maintain the septum in the deviated position.

A strip of cartilage is usually excised along the floor of the septum separating it from the maxillary crest and vomer. It is important to try and leave the attachment of the nasal septum to the anterior nasal spine intact. The surgeon must be aware that any resection here can lead to loss of dorsal height and columella retraction. If it is mobilized off the anterior nasal spine, it must be reattached with a polydioxanone suture (PDS) following septal work. A posterior chondrotomy is then made at the osseocartilaginous junction, maintaining the attachment at the keystone area superiorly. This then forms a "swing door", which when gently moved to one side enables visualization of any posterior bony deviation. This can then be resected with an instrument such as a Blakesley or Tilley forceps. Care must be taken when performing this maneuver as excessive twisting of the bone can cause a fracture at its attachment to the cribriform plate resulting in cerebrospinal fluid (CSF) leak. At this stage, the

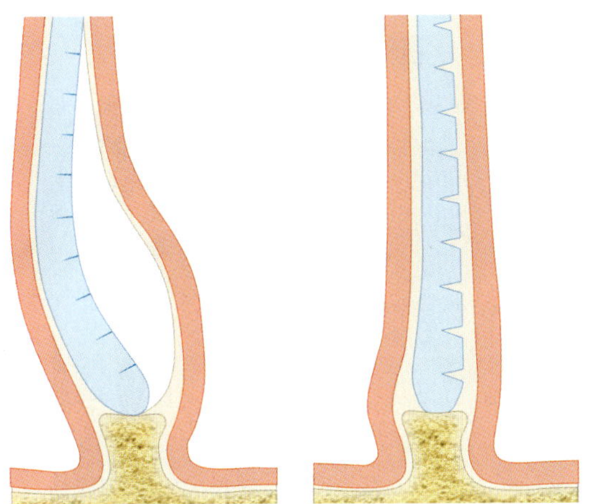

Fig. 18.4: Diagram showing the effect of scoring the concave surface of septal cartilage to reduce its memory and facilitate its straightening.

septum is free to be repositioned into the midline with only limited peripheral bony tethering in the keystone area and via its attachment to the upper lateral cartilages.

This basic technique might be appropriate when dealing with an essentially straight septal cartilage plate, which is held off the midline. However, when the septal cartilage is vertically curved, the "swing door" release and repositioning technique do not always lead to straightening of the cartilage.

The next step in the surgical ladder is to appreciate and subsequently preserve an anterior and caudal L-shaped cartilaginous structure with a width of 1.5 cm anchored at the keystone area and anterior nasal spine. Cartilaginous and bony deflections posteriorly can then be resected, straightened, and reinserted if required. The L-shaped strut can be weakened and straightened with scoring, sutures, and batten grafts (Andre and Vuyk, 2006).

Scoring vertically or horizontally with a scalpel can weaken and eliminate cartilaginous memory thus allowing repositioning with sutures to be facilitated (Fig. 18.4). Scoring should be performed on the concave surface. If unsuccessful, through and through noncommunicating incisions may be necessary to facilitate straightening. However, the surgeon should be aware that scoring and incisions into cartilage can lead to unpredictable results and should not be relied upon alone for correction of septal deformities. In all these scenarios, sutures and battens should be used to keep the cartilage in place.

Spreader grafts have dual functions. They first widen the nasal valve angle and thus the nasal valve cross-sectional area and also act as battens to straighten any septal curvature in the nasal dorsum (Weeks, Walker and Dutton, 2012). These grafts can be positioned on one or both sides of the septum. Spreader graft size is advocated to be approximately 15 × 2 × 3 mm (Fig. 18.3). Wider grafts may improve the nasal valve cross-sectional area further but the tradeoff will be to the detriment of aesthetic appearance. Although this technique can be performed by an endonasal approach (Andre, Paun and Vuyk, 2004), an external approach will allow more precise placement and fixation of the grafts. The surgeon should avoid using bulky battens to straighten the caudal septum as these can impinge on the nasal valve area.

As modern septoplasty techniques advocate repositioning and conservation of cartilage, any resected cartilage should be straightened or morcellized and reinserted into the septum between the two mucoperichondrial layers to maintain integrity and reduce the risk of septal perforation.

Specific Problems

Caudal Septal Deviation

A very anterior septal deviation can cause an external deviation of the nose by dislocating the leading edge of the septum out of the columella and into the nasal cavity. To access such a deviation, a hemitransfixion incision will be needed to expose the caudal septal leading edge and allow retrograde dissection of the columella to create a pocket into which the septum can be repositioned, once straightened. Minor septal deflections have often been dislocated alongside the premaxilla and protruded into the nasal vestibule. These can either be carefully shaved off or mobilized and repositioned onto the nasal spine. The cartilage is then secured with slow-dissolving sutures such as PDS applied between the anterior nasal spine periosteum and posterior caudal septal leading edge. Some surgeons prefer to drill a hole in the anterior nasal spine for a more secure assembly. Major deflections may require a vertical-strip incision into the fracture line to allow the cartilage to swing back into the midline. Care must be taken, however, that the septum is not transected completely at this point as this could facilitate retrograde migration or overlap of the septal fragments, leading to operative failure with external cosmetic deformity.

Deviation of the caudal septal leading edge can be further splinted straight using a "caudal batten graft". A small piece of cartilage can be harvested from the posterior septum and secured to the anterior leading edge of the septum to maintain a straightened position.

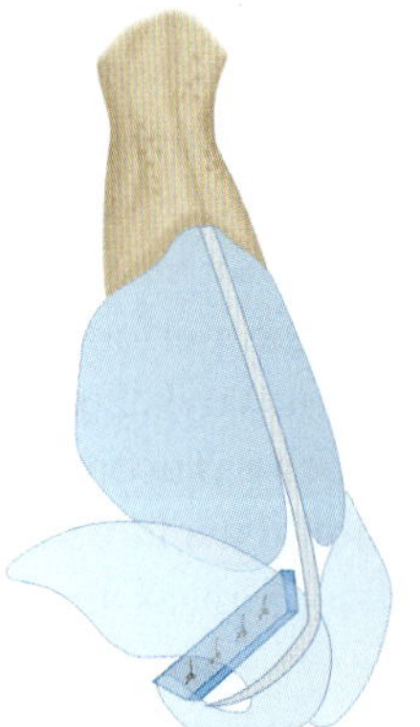

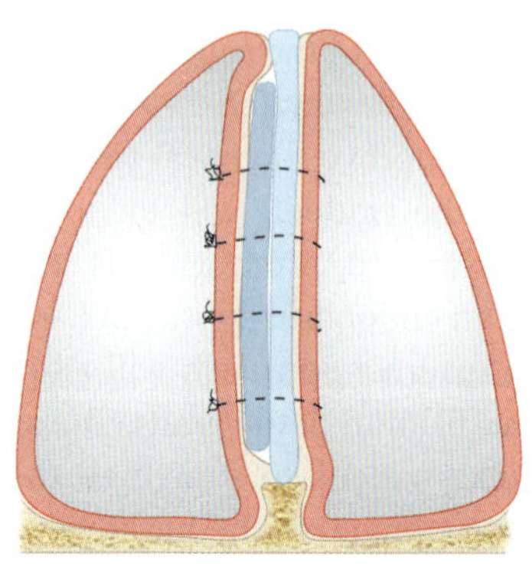

Fig. 18.5: Diagram showing the placement of a caudal septal batten. This helps to strengthen the cartilage especially following scoring and ensures a more predictable result.

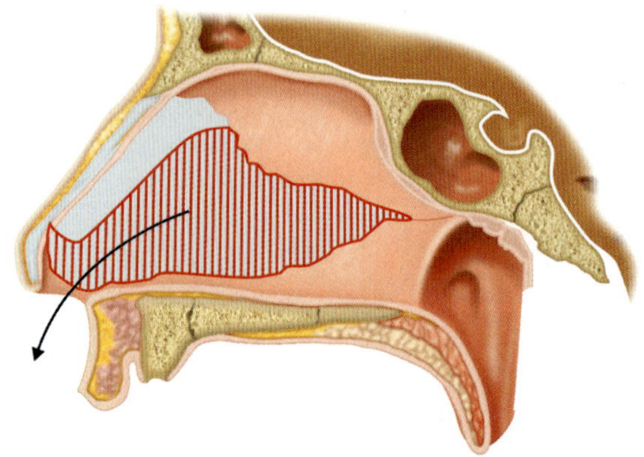

Fig. 18.6: Diagram showing the subtotal removal of the cartilaginous septum. Note the keystone area remains untouched allowing for anchoring of the neoseptum to this region.

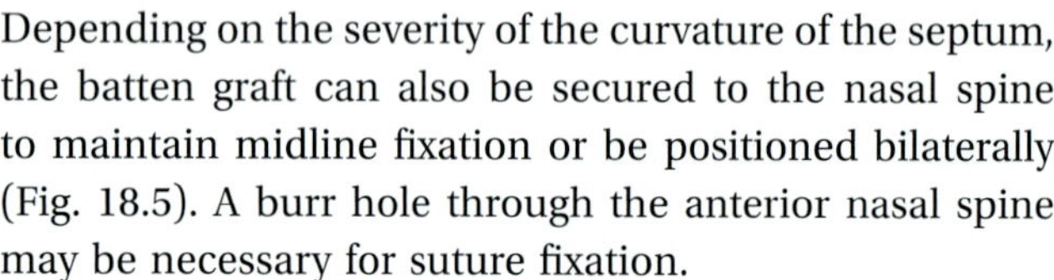

Depending on the severity of the curvature of the septum, the batten graft can also be secured to the nasal spine to maintain midline fixation or be positioned bilaterally (Fig. 18.5). A burr hole through the anterior nasal spine may be necessary for suture fixation.

Alternatively, if only the most caudal part of the septum is deviated off the midline, it is possible to judiciously resect the deviation and reproduce the support by insertion of cartilage into a columella pocket. This technique should be used with caution.

High Dorsal Deflection

High dorsal deflections are an indication for an external approach and often require subtotal septal reconstruction. Only very rarely, however, do the authors feel that it is necessary to take the whole septum out to reshape it extracorporeally prior to replacement. In cases of subtotal reconstruction, all but a 1 cm dorsal strip attached to the perpendicular plate of the ethmoid in the keystone area can be resected (Fig. 18.6). A straight part of the resected cartilage can be selected and used to reconstruct the dorsal septum. Fixation is required at the anterior nasal spine and keystone area. At the anterior nasal spine, burr holes will need to be drilled into the anterior nasal spine and premaxilla to facilitate suture fixation. The graft is then fixed with sutures to the upper lateral cartilages and dorsal cartilaginous remnant in the keystone area (Fig. 18.7). Spreader grafts should be inserted here to improve both dorsal support and nasal valve angle. Usually, this neoseptum will lie in a more caudal position than the original septum. This can be advantageous, allowing the medial crura to be fixed to the septum in a "tongue in groove" fashion. Thus nasal tip repositioning is possible. In some scenarios, it may be impossible to fashion a suitable piece of cartilage to act as an L strut. In this scenario, a 0.15 mm perforated PDS foil may be used as a splint onto which fragments of straight cartilage can be attached to facilitate reconstruction of the neoseptal plate. Alternatively, an autologous or cadaveric rib cartilage can be harvested if insufficient septal cartilage is available.

This method facilitates straightening of high dorsal deviations with reconstitution of a straight septal plate. Camouflage grafts may then be necessary to ensure that the profile and frontal view is aesthetically pleasing.

Closure

Once surgical correction of the deviated septum has been performed, it is vital to approximate the mucoperichondrial flaps to the reconstructed cartilaginous septum adequately, thus reducing any dead space. Failure to do so can lead to septal hematoma and abscess formation, which will decrease the vitality of the underlying cartilage.

Closure of the mucoperichondrial flaps can be achieved with an absorbable suture such as 4/0 Vicryl Rapide. Multiple quilting passes are required, covering all quadrants of the septum (Fig. 18.8). The caudal portion is the most important area to quilt adequately to prevent excessive thickening in this region during the healing process.

Formal nasal packing may not be required following septoplasty if adequate quilting is performed, but can be employed to prevent bleeding in the postoperative period.

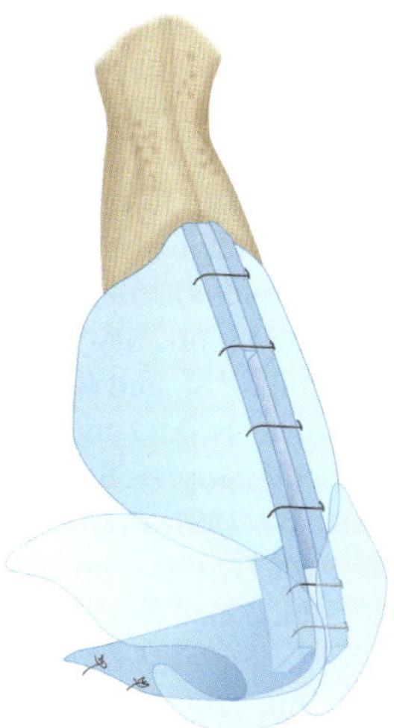

Fig. 18.7: Diagram showing L-strut being sutured to the anterior nasal spine and upper lateral cartilages during subtotal septal reconstruction.

18.7 COMPLICATIONS

Septal Hematoma/Abscess

Septal hematoma formation postoperatively is rare when adequate quilting sutures are used. Some surgeons have used silastic splints in the past to try and prevent this complication. However, splints are uncomfortable for the patient, may induce infection, and can hide a small hematoma from the clinician.

The presence of a hematoma or abscess is an emergency and should be suspected in all cases with increased pain and fever postoperatively. Early incision and drainage can prevent avascular necrosis of the septal cartilage and its subsequent long-term sequelae including saddle nose deformity and septal perforation.

Septal Perforation

With the evolution of cartilage-preserving techniques for septal deviation correction, perforation rates are <5%. In traditional submucosal resection of nasal septum, perforation rates have been reported to be as high as 25% (Schwab and Pirsig, 1997). Bilateral, adjacent mucosal tears during surgery, especially if cartilage has been resected, will usually result in a perforation. Repair at the time of surgery, with careful cartilage or temporalis fascia interposition to close defects, may prevent perforations from arising. The authors advocate "bruising" and reinsertion of spare cartilage fragments between any bare mucosa-mucosa pockets that may be evident at the end of the septal correction.

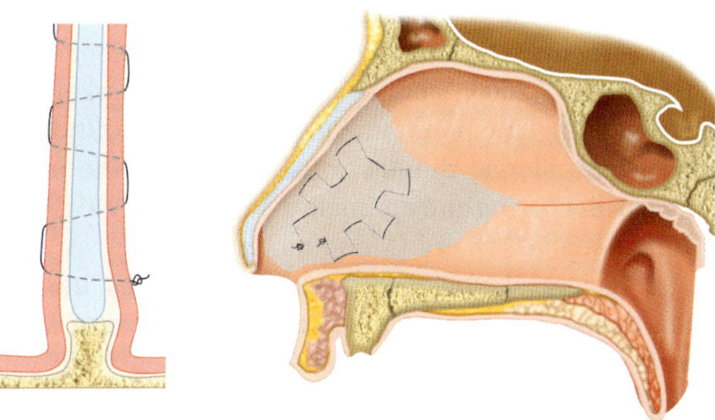

Fig. 18.8: Diagram showing the principle of multiple quilting to reduce dead space between the mucoperichondrial flaps and the septum.

Saddle Deformity

It has been estimated that approximately 20% of patients have subtle aesthetic changes to the nasal shape following septoplasty. Significant postoperative changes occur in <1% of cases (Vuyk and Langenhuijsen, 1997).

Over-resection of cartilage with disruption to either the keystone area or the caudal or dorsal 1 cm strip of cartilage may result in a saddle deformity. Similarly, failure to reattach the septal cartilage to the anterior nasal spine may cause posterior rotation of the caudal septum, leading to decrease in nasal tip projection. This will be evident at the time of surgery or may develop a few months following surgery due to destabilization of the septal support areas. Repair will require revision surgery with repositioning of the nasal septum where possible, but may require reconstruction with cartilage grafts (harvested from rib or auricular cartilage) inserted via an external approach to support and camouflage any deformity.

CSF Leak

The perpendicular plate of the ethmoid attaches to the skull base. Aggressive manipulation may result in a CSF leak. This is a very rare complication but may be more prevalent if septal deformity is associated with extensive facial trauma. Persistent CSF leaks would require a formal endoscopic skull base repair.

18.8 RESULTS

With objective clinical assessment of nasal obstruction routinely unavailable to the clinician, it can be difficult for the surgeon to identify those who would benefit most from septoplasty. Despite this, quality of life assessment tools such as the NOSE and RhinoQol consistently show improvement in symptom scores following septoplasty (Siegel, et al., 2000; Stewart, et al., 2004; Toyserkani and Frisch, 2012). One poor outcome predictor is found to be concurrent allergic rhinitis, which highlights the importance of identifying and optimally treating mucosal disease prior to septal surgery (Mondina, et al., 2012). A systematic review of objective outcome measures has also demonstrated improved nasal patency following septoplasty suggesting symptom score assessments are valid (Moore and Eccles, 2011). However, a further review has highlighted that correlation between objective and subjective outcome measures remains uncertain (Andre, et al., 2009). Failure to recognize and correct dorsal septal deviation and narrowing of the nasal valve may contribute to poorer postoperative results. Vigilance in identifying these preoperatively and addressing them concurrently with septal surgery help improve the surgical success rate.

REFERENCES

Andre, R., Paun, S. and Vuyk, H., 2004. Endonasal spreader graft placement as treatment for internal valve insufficiency. *Archives of Facial Plastic Surgery*, 6, pp. 36-40.

Andre, R. and Vuyk, H., 2006. Reconstruction of dorsal and/or caudal nasal septum deformities with septal battens or by septal replacement: an overview and comparison of techniques. *Laryngoscope*, 116(9), pp. 1668-73.

Andre, R., Vuyk, H., Ahmed, A., Graamans, K. and Nolst, T., 2009. Correlation between subjective and objective evaluation of the nasal airway. A systematic review of the highest level of evidence. *Clinical Otolaryngology*, 34, pp. 518-25.

Gray, L., 1978. Deviated nasal septum. Incidence and aetiology. *Annals of Otology, Rhinology, and Laryngology*, Suppl 50, pp. 3-20.

Mondina, M., Marro, M., Maurice, S., Stoll, D. and de Gabory, L., 2012. Assessment of nasal septoplasty using NOSE and RhinoQoL questionnaires. *European Archives of Otorhinolaryngology*, 269, pp. 2189-95.

Moore, M. and Eccles, R., 2011. Objective evidence for the efficacy of surgical management of the deviated septum as a treatment for chronic nasal obstruction: a systematic review. *Clinical Otolaryngology*, 36, pp. 106-13.

Scheithauer, M.O., Kirkland, P.M. and Rettinger, G. 2006. Septal reconstruction. In: Vuyk, H.D., Lohuis, P.J.F.M., eds. *Facial Plastic and Reconstructive Surgery*. Edward Arnold Publishers.

Schwab, J.A. and Pirsig, W., 1997. Complications of septal surgery. *Facial Plastic Surgery*, 13(1), pp. 3-14.

Siegel, N.S., Gliklich, R.E., Taghizadeh, F., Chang, Y., 2000. Outcomes after nasal septoplasty. *Otolaryngology—Head and Neck Surgery*, 122(2), pp. 228-32.

Stewart, M.G., Smith, T.L., Weaver, E.M., et al., 2004. Outcomes after septoplasty: results from the nasal obstruction septoplasty effectiveness (NOSE) study. *Otolaryngology—Head and Neck Surgery*, 130(3), pp. 217-21.

Toyserkani, N.M. and Frisch, T., 2012. Are too many septal deviations operated on? A retrospective patient's satisfaction questionnaire with 11 years follow-up. *Rhinology*, 50(2), pp. 185-90.

Verwoerd, C.D.A. and Verwoerd-Verhoef, H.L., 2005. Rhinosurgery in children. Developmental and surgical aspects. In: Nolst Trenite G.J., ed. *Rhinoplasty. A Practical Guide to Functional and Aesthetic Surgery of the Nose*, 3rd edition. Kugler Publications.

Vuyk, H. and Langenhuijsen, K., 1997. Aesthetic sequelae of septoplasty. *Clinical Otolaryngology and Allied Sciences*, 22, pp. 226-32

Weeks, D., Walker, D. and Dutton, J., 2012. Anatomical comparison of minimally invasive nasal valve procedures. *Archives of Facial Plastic Surgery*, 14, pp. 189-92.

19 Septal Perforation

Ullas Raghavan

Chapter Overview

Pearls and Pitfalls

Pearls

- Asymptomatic septal perforation does not need treatment.
- Try to find the cause for the perforation, still some will remain idiopathic.
- Tension free closure of mucosal flaps is essential.
- Vertical mattress sutures ensure close approximation of raw mucosal surfaces.
- Posterior sutures are difficult to insert, do these first.
- Interposition graft is essential, at least till the mucosal flaps heal.
- Once the flaps are sutured the nasal cavity will appear small. In four weeks the mucosa will reline the nasal floor and upper lateral cartilage and the nasal cavity will get back to its normal dimensions.

Pitfalls

- Repairing mucosal flaps only on one side will almost always fail.
- Septal perforation secondary to septal surgery during which mucoperichondium had been excised leads to excessive scarring, making it difficult to raise flaps, and compromises the repair.
- Do not use crushed cartilage as interposition graft.
- Do not use quilting sutures as they may compromise vascularity.

19.1 ANATOMY OF NASAL SEPTUM

- The nasal septum forms the partition between right and left nasal cavities.
- Anterior two-thirds is cartilaginous and posterior one-third is bony.
- Cartilage is the quadrangular-shaped piece of hyaline cartilage with a small contribution caudally by the medial crura of the lower lateral cartilages (Fig. 19.1).
- A small area of connective tissue forms the membranous septum between medial crura and caudal border of the quadrangular cartilage.
- Bony septum is formed by the perpendicular plate of ethmoid, vomer, nasal crest of maxillary bone, nasal crest of palatine bone, and the rostrum of sphenoid (Fig. 19.1).
- Either side of the cartilaginous and bony framework of the septum is covered with mucoperichondrium and mucoperiosteum, respectively.

- Facial artery, which is a branch of the external carotid artery, supplies the anterior part of the nasal septum through the septal branch of superior labial artery. The posterior part of the septum is supplied by the posterior septal branch of sphenopalatine artery and the ascending branch of the greater palatine artery, both of which are branches of the internal maxillary branch of the external carotid artery. Internal carotid artery supplies the septum through anterior and posterior ethmoidal branches of the ophthalmic artery. All the arteries anastomose in the Little's area to form Kiesselbach's plexus. The venous drainage is through facial, sphenopalatine, and ophthalmic veins.
- The ordinary sensations of touch, pressure, and temperature are carried by the anterior ethmoidal branch of the ophthalmic nerve (V1), and greater palatine and nasopalatine branches of the pterygopalatine ganglion (V2). The posterosuperior part of the nasal septum contains olfactory mucosa, with the sensation of smell being carried by the olfactory nerve. Parasympathetic preganglionic nerve fibers are carried from the brain to the nose via the facial nerve, greater petrosal nerve, nerve of the pterygoid canal, and pterygopalatine ganglion, where they synapse. Sympathetic preganglionic nerve fibers leave the upper thoracic spinal cord, traverse white rami communicans, ascend the cervical sympathetic chain, and finally synapse in the superior cervical sympathetic ganglion. The postganglionic nerve fibers follow the internal carotid artery and then the nerve of the pterygoid canal to reach the pterygopalatine fossa. These postganglionic nerve fibers pass through the ganglion without synapsing to join branches of the maxillary nerve and artery to reach the nasal mucosa.

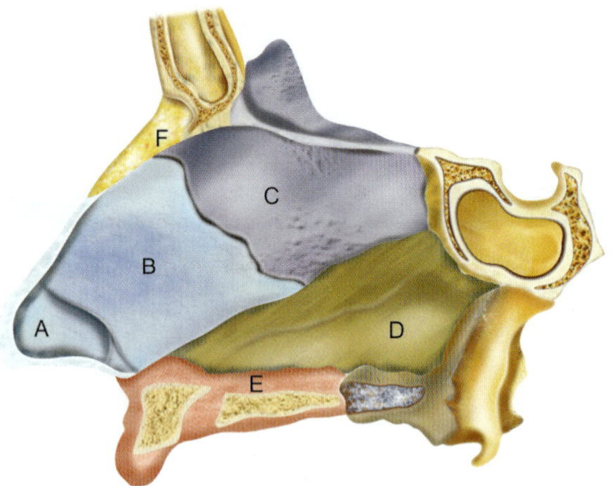

Fig. 19.1: Nasal septum. A—lower lateral cartilage, B—septal cartilage, C—perpendicular plate of ethmoid, D—vomer, E—maxillary crest, F—nasal bone.

19.2 ETIOLOGY

Various causes of septal perforation are summarized in Table 19.1.

19.3 SYMPTOMS OF NASAL SEPTAL PERFORATION

- Asymptomatic
- *Whistling*: Caused by high-velocity airflow through small anterior perforations (Grutzenmacher, et al., 2002) and possibly because of cross-flow from high-flow rate to low-flow rate nostril (Lee, et al., 2010).

Table 19.1: Causes of nasal septal perforations compiled from world literature.

Trauma	*Chemicals*	*Inflammatory*	*Neoplastic*	*Idiopathic*
Septal surgery	Cocaine	Wegener's, ulcerative colitis, Crohn's disease, rheumatoid arthritis, Takayasu's arteritis, lupus vulgaris, relapsing polychondritis, lupus erythematous, sarcoidosis, cryoglobulinemia, antiphospholipid syndrome, pyoderma gangrenosum	Squamous cell carcinoma	
Intentional piercing	Chromium	Tuberculosis, *Mycobacterium kansasii*, invasive fungal sinusitis, AIDS	Malignant melanoma	
Nose picking	Nickel	Rhinitis medicamentosa	Lymphoma	
Cautery to both sides	Methotrexate			
Long-term use of oxygen cannula	Button batteries			
	Bevacizumab			

(AIDS: Acquired immunodeficiency syndrome).

- *Crusting*: Caused by reduced humidity in the area of the perforation due to altered airflow (Lindemann, et al., 2001) and reduced air conditioning (Pless, et al., 2004). The reduction in crusting following successful surgical closure of septal perforation is related to improved humidification of the inspired air (Lindemann, et al., 2004).
- *Nasal blockage*: Because of crusting, turbulent nasal airflow, or lack of sensation of air movement in case of large perforations.
- *Epistaxis*: This may be because of the high air velocity and wall shear stress found near the downstream region of the septal perforation (Lee, et al., 2010).
- Collapse of the nose and/or nasal valve in case of large anterior and dorsal perforations.

Majority (62%) of nasal septal perforations are asymptomatic (Newton, White and Lee, 2003). All patients presenting with nasal septal perforation should be investigated to find a cause for the perforation. Whistling is almost always seen only in anterior septal perforation measuring about 0.5 × 0.5 cm, and noticed on deep inspiration (Grutzenmacher, et al., 2002). Perforation of the nasal septum interrupts the normal smooth flow of nasal mucus posteriorly. This stagnation and reduced humidity cause nasal mucus to dry along the posterior margin of the septal perforation forming crusts. Presence of crusts causes inflammation of the underlying mucosa, which may then bleed from trauma resulting from forceful dislodgement of the crust. Large crusts lead to nasal blockage and occasional complaints of foul smell from the nose. Large septal perforation can weaken the dorsal support of the nose, causing collapse and resultant supra tip depression and associated internal nasal valve collapse.

19.4 INVESTIGATIONS

- Erythrocyte sedimentation rate
- Cytoplasmic antineutrophil cytoplasmic antibody

Both tests help in diagnosing vasculitis, especially Wegener's granulomatosis.

- Biopsy (Murray and McGarry, 2000) is recommended to rule out malignancy or to diagnose vasculitis. History of septal surgery or other trauma, use of cocaine, exposure to chemicals like chromium, or presence of inflammatory diseases known to cause septal perforations is usually diagnostic. It is advisable to biopsy any nasal septal perforation with granulations along the margins to rule out the possibility of malignancy. There is no diagnostic advantage of obtaining a biopsy in every patient with nasal septal perforation. In a previously published research, all of the 88 patients who underwent a biopsy of the septal perforation were diagnosed as having chronic nonspecific inflammation (Murray and McGarry, 2000).

19.5 TREATMENT

If patients with nasal septal perforation are asymptomatic, no further treatment is required provided the investigations have ruled out any significant pathology.

Conservative Treatment

- *Alkaline nasal douching and application of topical cream*: This helps to reduce crusting that is the main cause of most of the symptoms associated with nasal septal perforation.
- *Obturators*: These are made from acrylic (Purna, et al., 2013) or silicone to close the perforation and reduce whistling. There is also a report of using acrylic intranasal stent in one nostril, which will act as an obturator for large nasal septal perforations (Goyal and Goyal, 2011). Osma, et al. (1999) have shown that obturators help to reduce the symptoms of epistaxis, whistling during inspiration, and nasal obstruction, but do not control crusting around the margins of the perforation. Sometimes, crusting can get worse because the obturator itself causes increased nasal secretions and traps the mucus causing further crusting. Only 50% of patients with an obturator derive long-term benefit (Metzinger, 2005). Al Kadah, et al. (2012) reported a statistically significant improvement in all symptoms more so for respiratory noise and nasal obstruction followed by epistaxis, pain, and crusting.

Septal buttons need to be replaced periodically for cleaning purpose and this can be painful and may cause the perforation to get bigger (Federspil and Schneider, 2006; Teschner, Willenborg and Lenarz, 2012). A study from Norway with 45 patients and a mean follow-up of 13 years reported 67% removal rate of silicone prosthesis, 11% considered obturators as optimal, and remaining preferred to have surgery if possible (Dosen and Haye, 2008). Almost similar rate of removal of obturators was reported by Blind, Hulterstorm and Breggren (2009). However, there are also reports of better tolerance and almost complete control of symptoms with obturators (Facer and Kern, 1979; Federspil and Schneider, 2006;

Mullace, et al., 2006). It is the author's practice not to use the silicone splints or any form of obturators unless the patient is unwilling or medically unfit for surgery, or is asymptomatic with the use of douching and creams.

Surgical Treatment

Surgical options for repair of septal perforations include:
- Local mucosal flaps alone
- Local mucosal flaps with interposition grafts
- Distant flaps, e.g. oral mucosal flaps
- Implants (Daneshi, et al., 2010; Deng, et al., 2006)

A wide variety of surgical procedures is described for closing nasal septal perforations (Goy and Husain, 2007; Meyer, 1994; Tardy, 1976) (Table 19.2). Surgical closure can be challenging due to limited availability of healthy local tissue to close the perforation. The presence of so many surgical techniques points to the fact that none of them have given consistently good results. A brief description of the various surgical techniques is given below with a more elaborate description of the author's favored technique, which has given consistently good results.

Islam, et al. (2009) have suggested that highest success rate in closure of perforation is achieved when local advancement and rotation flaps are used. Moon, et al. (2011) have suggested that bilateral closure of the perforation with flaps is the most important predictive factor for repair of the perforation. They also pointed out that there is a negative correlation between symptom control and size of perforation and previous trauma including surgery.

Surgical repair can be done endoscopically (Ayshford, et al., 2003; Castelnuovo, et al., 2011; Chen, et al., 2012; Giacomini, et al., 2011; Lee, et al., 2012; Ma, et al., 2011; Tastan, et al., 2012), endonasally (Chhabra and Houser, 2012; Fairbanks and Fairbanks, 1994; Neumann, Morales-Minovi and Schultz-Coulon, 2011; Rokkjær, Barrett and Petersen, 2010), or through the external approach (Foda, 1999; Romo, et al., 1999; Wong and Raghavan, 2010; Yenigun, et al., 2012). Use of pedicled oral mucosal flap through an incision in the gingivolabial sulcus was described by Tardy (1976). Meyer (1994) described a staged procedure involving pedicled buccal flap and conchal cartilage.

Newton, White and Lee (2003) achieved 90% success in closing nasal septal perforations using unilateral bipedicled flaps and temporalis fascia. Retrospective telephone questionnaires were used to assess preoperative and postoperative symptom scores using linear analogue scores. They achieved a statistically significant improvement in symptom score after closure of septal perforation.

Foda (1999) used an open rhinoplasty approach for closing nasal septal perforations in 20 patients and achieved 90% success. He used reduction rhinoplasty techniques to increase the availability of tissue for designing the flaps. Bipedicled and advancements flaps were used on both sides. Symptoms completely resolved in 80% and partially in the remaining 20%.

Kridel, Foda and Lunde (1998) described surgical septal perforation repair with bipedicle flaps and acellular human dermal allograft in 12 patients. They managed to achieve a 91% success rate in patients by placing acellular human allograft between flaps. Of the 12 patients, seven had closure of flaps on both sides and four had closure on one side.

Pedroza, Patrocinio and Arevalo (2007) used both external and endonasal approach using temporalis fascia, conchal cartilage, and mastoid cortical bone either in isolation or combination concomitantly and achieved a success rate of 97% in closing the perforation. All patients with complete closure of septal perforation had improvement in symptoms.

Woolford and Jones (2001) used local mucosal flap and composite conchal cartilage graft in 11 patients for closing septal perforation. They suggested that composite cartilage graft is preferred to fascia as it provides greater strength and support. They explain that the role of skin in the composite graft is less clear as sometimes it forms a yellow-looking covering that can take weeks to re-epithelialize, while on other occasion the graft takes immediately. All but one of their patients was asymptomatic postoperatively.

Surgical Technique

The author prefers to use bilateral advancement nasal flaps, which have consistently given 97% success in closure of septal perforation with statistically significant improvement in nasal symptoms. So far 88 patients have been operated using this technique and the result of the first 28 patients has already been published (Wong and Raghavan, 2010). The maximum size of the nasal septal perforation, the author has successfully repaired, was 3.5 cm in the vertical dimension. The vertical dimension (Fig 19.2A) of the perforation is deemed to represent a greater surgical challenge than the horizontal dimension (Fig. 19.2B). As the vertical length increases, there is less nasal mucous membrane available to mobilize for closing

Table 19.2: Surgical techniques and results.

Authors	*Technique*	*Surgery*	*Size of perforation*	*Number of patients*	*Follow-up*	*Symptom control*	*Success in closure*
Park, J.H., Kim, D.W., Jin H.R., et al. (2013)	Local mucosal flaps with or without interposition grafts	Bilateral advancement with or without rotation flaps with or without conchal, septal cartilage or bone	5–27 mm	14	36 +/- 18 months	Obstruction, crusting, epistaxis, whistling. 92.9% improvement	85.5% (12/14) Failure in two large perforations, no interposition grafts
Chen, F.H., Deng, J., Wen, Y.H., Xu, G., Shi, J.B. (2012)	Local mucosal flaps with interposition grafts	Bone, cartilage, and fascia lata as interposition with free middle turbinate mucosa	10–20 mm	13	3 months	Obstruction, epistaxis, dryness	92.3%
Raol, N., Olson, K. (2012)	Local flaps	One side superior and other side inferior advancement flaps	6–16 mm	7	3 years	Not mentioned	100%
Lee, D.H., Yoon, T.M., Joo, Y.E., et al. (2012)	Local flaps	Anterior pedicled inferior turbinate flaps	5–18 mm	6	2–6 years	Not mentioned	83.3%
Tastan, E., Aydogan, F., et al. (2012)	Inferior turbinate composite graft, local flaps	Inferior turbinate composite grafts with or without bipedicled flap	3–26 mm	27	1–3 years	6–30 months	88.8%
Chhabra, N., Houser, S.M. (2012)	Local mucosal flap and interposition	Unilateral rotational mucosal flap and acellular dermal interposition grafts	<10–>20 mm	20	Mean 5 months	19/20 complete symptom control	85%
Yenigun, A., Meric, A., Verim, A., et al., (2012)	Free graft	Conchal graft with perichondrium on both sides	1.86 +/- 0.78 cm	15	6 months	Crust, epistaxis, blockage and whistling—statistically significant improvement	93.3%
Dosen, L.K., Haye, R. (2008)	Local flaps	Bilateral posterior based mucoperichondrial flaps with or without conchal cartilage	Vertical diameter <15 mm	104	6 months–10 years	Not mentioned	82%

Contd...

Contd...

Authors	*Technique*	*Surgery*	*Size of perforation*	*Number of patients*	*Follow-up*	*Symptom control*	*Success in closure*
Ma, Y.X., Tao, A.Z., Lu, C., Tian, H., Dong, B.C. (2011)	Local flap and interposition graft	Unilateral local mucosal flap and acellular dermal matrix interposition	10–23 mm	12	3 months–4 years	Crusting and obstruction	92%
Castelnuovo, P., Ferreli, F., Khodaei, I., Palma, P. (2011)	Local flap	Unilateral anterior ethmoidal artery based mucosal flap	10–25 mm	11	12–132 months	Obstruction, crusting, epistaxis, whistling, rhinorrhea	100%
Teymoortash, A., Hosch, S., Eivazi, B., Werner, J.A. (2011)	Local mucosal flap	Unilateral local mucosal flap	11–38 mm	55	3.3–18 months	Not mentioned	94%
Taskin, U., Yigit, O., Sisman, S.A. (2011)	Local mucosal flap and interposition graft	Bilateral nasal floor flap and conchal cartilage	Anteroposterior: 20–38 mm; vertical: 20–27 mm	17	9–28 months	Obstruction, crusting, epistaxis, whistling	94%
Li, F., Liu, Q., Yu, H., Zhang, Z. (2011)	Local flaps and interposition graft	Unilateral pedicled local mucosal flap and autogenous interposition graft	10–20 mm	28	7–39 months	Not mentioned	92.9%
Giacomini, P.G., Ferraro, S., Di Girolamo, S., Ottaviani, F. (2011)	Local mucosal flaps and interposition graft	Bilateral horizontal bipedicled mucosal advancement flap and conchal interposition graft	20–40 mm	14	12–36 months	Crusting, epistaxis, whistling, headache	85.7%
Mansour, H.A. (2011)	Local mucosal flaps	Inferior turbinate-free graft	Horizontal: 10–25 mm; vertical: 5–15 mm	6	6–24 months	Crusts, obstruction, cacosmia, epistaxis	83%
Rokkjaer, M.S., Barrett, T.Q., Petersen, C.G. (2010)	Local flaps and interposition grafts	Bilateral bipedicled mucosal flap and septal/conchal cartilage graft	3–25 mm	19	6–164 weeks	Nasal obstruction, crusting, epistaxis, whistling	84%

Contd...

Contd...

Authors	*Technique*	*Surgery*	*Size of perforation*	*Number of patients*	*Follow-up*	*Symptom control*	*Success in closure*
Wong, S., Raghavan, U. (2010)	Local mucosal flap and interposition graft	Bilateral superior and inferior mucosal flap and porcine collagen interposition	Horizontal: 10–35 mm; vertical: 10–37 mm	28	6–24 months	Epistaxis, crusting, whistling, obstruction	96%
Kazkayasi, M., Tuna, E., Kilic, C. (2010)	Local mucosal flap	Bullous middle turbinate flap	10–15 mm	1	18 months	Obstruction, crusting, and foreign body sensation	100%
Daneshi, A., Mohammadi, S., Javadi, M., Hassannia, F. (2010)	Alloplast	Titanium membrane	15–30 mm	10	10–15 months	Nasal obstruction, crusting, whistling	100%
Dhar, V., Watts, S. (2009)	Local mucosal flaps	Bilateral mucosal flaps crossing over	≤5 mm	Not mentioned	Not mentioned	Not mentioned	Not mentioned
Lee, H.R., Ahn, D.B., Park, J.H., Kim, Y.H., et al. (2008)	Local flap and interposition graft	Unilateral advancement mucosal flap and temporalis fascia interposition graft	Mean 15 mm	14	3–23 months	Not mentioned	85.7%
Islam, A., Celik, H., Felek, S.A., Demirci, M. (2009)	Local flaps and interposition graft	Superior flap from one side and inferior flap from other side with interposition graft	8–17 mm	10	5–26 months	Nasal obstruction, epistaxis, crusting, whistling	70%
Teymoortash, A., Werner, J.A. (2009)	Local mucosal flap	Unilateral inferior meatal flap	5–26 mm	13	2–7 months	Epistaxis, obstruction, crusting, whistling, pain	100%
De Gabory, L., Stoll, D. (2008)	Enlargement of perforation	Posterior enlargement of perforation	10 mm	10	16 months	Nasal block, epistaxis, headache, crusting—all improved, statistically significant	NA

Contd...

Contd...

Authors	*Technique*	*Surgery*	*Size of perforation*	*Number of patients*	*Follow-up*	*Symptom control*	*Success in closure*
Lee, K.C., Lee, N.H., Ban, J.H., Jin, S.M. (2008)	Local flaps and interposition graft	Bilateral local flaps with human dermal allograft	2–10 mm	11	Mean 15 months	Nasal obstruction, epistaxis, whistling, dryness, pain	91%
Barry, C., Eadie, P.A., Russell, J. (2008)	Free flap	Radial forearm free flap	Not mentioned	1	18 months	Not mentioned	100%
Riberio, J.S., da Silva, G.S. (2007)	Local mucosal flap and interposition	Bilateral superior and inferior flaps with cartilage and temporalis fascia	10–35 mm	258	Minimum 1 year	Obstruction, crusting, bleeding, whistling, headache—all improved	99.6%
Shikowitz, M.J. (2007)	Local flap	Vascularized mucoperiosteal pull through flap	17–29 mm	10	Not mentioned	Nasal obstruction, crusting, epistaxis, whistling	90%
Ceylan, A., Illeri, F., Celenk, F., Yilmaz, M., Uslu, S. (2007)	Local flap	Unilateral upper lateral cartilage mucoperichondrial flap	3–25 mm	24	28 months	Obstruction, bleeding, whistling, headache	79%
Kilty, S.J., Brownrigg, P.J., Safar, A. (2007)	Local flap	Anteriorly pedicled inferior turbinate flap	10–30 mm	20	Mean 7.6 months	Nasal obstruction, crusting, and epistaxis	80%
Andre, R.F., Lohuis, P.J., Vuyk, H.D. (2006)	Local flaps with interposition grafts	One side inferior advancement or rotation flap, and other side bipedicled from upper lateral, interposition with human dermal allograft, fascia, or cartilage	5–20 mm	43	3–138 months	Not mentioned	93%

Contd...

Contd...

Authors	*Technique*	*Surgery*	*Size of perforation*	*Number of patients*	*Follow-up*	*Symptom control*	*Success in closure*
Heller, J.B., Gabbay, J.S., Trussler, A., Heller, M.M., Bradley, J.P. (2005)	Local flap	Facial artery musculomucosal flap	20–40 mm	6	10–30 months	Crusting, epistaxis, dryness	100%
Friedman, M., Ibrahim, H., Ramakrishnan, V. (2003)	Local flap	Anteriorly based inferior turbinate flap	15–30 mm	10	18–36 months	Not mentioned	70%
Zhang, Q., Zhang, J., Li, S. (2003)	Local flap and free graft	One side single or double local mucosal flap and opposite side free graft	8–15 mm	8	Not mentioned	Not mentioned	100%
Newton, J.R., White, P.S., Lee, M.S. (1999)	Local flap	Unilateral local flap, bipedicled with septal bone or temporalis fascia	20 mm	11	Mean 10 months	Crusting, epistaxis, whistling	91%
Ayshford, C.A., Shykhon, M., Uppal, H.S., Wake, M. (2006)	Local flap and interposition grafts	Unilateral or bilateral anteriorly based inferior turbinate flap and human dermal allograft	10–25 mm	17	Not mentioned	Not mentioned	76%
Mobley, S.R., Boyd, J.B., Astor, F.C. (2001)	Free flap	Radial forearm free flap	30–40 mm	1	24 months	Crusting, epistaxis, and headache	100%
Eng, S.P., Nilssen, E.L., Ranta, M., White, P.S. (2001)	Enlargement of perforation	Posterior enlargement of perforation	15–50 mm	13	3–20 months	Obstruction, crusting, epistaxis, whistling, pain	NA
Woolford, T.J., Jones, N.S. (2001)	Local flap and composite graft	Unilateral posterior based local mucosal flap and composite conchal graft	10–40 mm	11	19.8 months	Not mentioned	73%
Foda, H.M. (1999)	Local flaps and interposition	Bilateral mucosal advancement/bipedicled flap with connective tissue interposition flap	10–40 mm	20	6–36 months	Crusting, nasal obstruction	90%

(NA: Not available).

the perforation. With longer horizontal dimension, the mucous membrane can be mobilized in the vertical direction to bring the edges of the perforation together. However, the suturing of the posterior extent of the septal perforation becomes technically difficult. Hence, it is the author's preference to use the open rhinoplasty approach in these patients. The nasal septum is accessed through the dorsal approach, bilateral mucoperichondrial septal flaps are raised off the septal cartilage when present, or the flaps are separated from each other by careful dissection of the scar tissue. The perforation margins are then separated to fashion two mucoperichondrial/mucoperiosteal flaps with a perforation in each flap (Fig. 19.2C). The upper lateral cartilages are then separated from the dorsal edge of the septal cartilage. The soft tissue flaps are further developed on either side by lifting them off the maxillary crest and vomer and then along the floor of the nasal cavity, inferior meatus, and the under surface of the inferior turbinate. The flap is left attached to the margin of the inferior turbinate (Fig. 19.2D). The mucous membrane remains tethered to the floor by the nasopalatine vessels entering the nose from the palate; these can be cut during the blunt dissection and the bleeding stops in a few minutes. This moves the inferior edge of the perforation superiorly. The mucoperichondrium/mucoperiosteum on the undersurface of the nasal bones and upper lateral cartilages is carefully raised (Fig. 19.2E). This is done for a sufficient length to bring the superior flap downward so as to move the superior edge of the perforation inferiorly. Both the superior and inferior flaps are moved as an advancement flap leaving the base attached widely. The perforation edges are then sutured with 4-0 polydioxanone sutures with a reverse cutting P3 needle in a vertical mattress suture (Fig. 19.2F). The flaps are mobilized enough before suturing to make sure that the closure is tension-free (Fig. 19.2G). A sheet of porcine collagen sheet is then placed between the flaps to keep the sutured sites separate (Fig. 19.2H). If nasal septal cartilage or bone is still available, it can be used instead of collagen sheet. Presence of a connective tissue layer between the repaired mucous membranes helps it heal better (Kridel, 1999; Metzinger, 2005; Stoor and Grenman, 2004;). When this is not available, the author prefers porcine collagen sheet because it is (a) easily available, (b) ready to use from the packet, (c) the architecture is very close to human tissue, (d) it is acellular and hence nonimmunogenic, (e) there is no additional donor site morbidity, and (f) it is resistant to collagenase enzymes. The upper lateral cartilages are then sutured back to the dorsal border of the septal cartilage. Silicone splints are placed in both nostrils and left in position for 1 week. If the septal support is weak, the septal framework is reconstructed using conchal or rib cartilage graft in the usual manner. If the perforation is large and the edges of the perforation are not coming together without tension after mobilizing the flaps, a reduction rhinoplasty is performed to reduce the height of the dorsum. This helps release more soft tissue for moving the flaps. Sometimes, the internal nasal valve angle may appear narrow after the flaps are sutured and the nasal cavity may appear smaller as the inferior flaps have been lifted off the floor of the nasal cavity. However, due to stretching of the nasal mucosa, the flaps are seen to line the nasal floor and the undersurface of upper lateral cart lages within 4–6 weeks after the procedure (Figs. 19.3A and B).

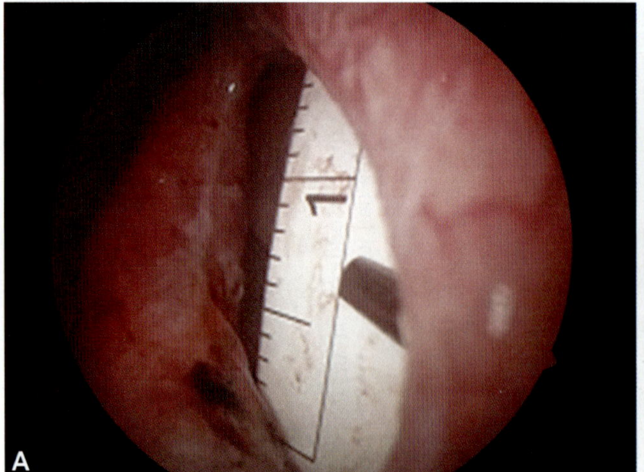

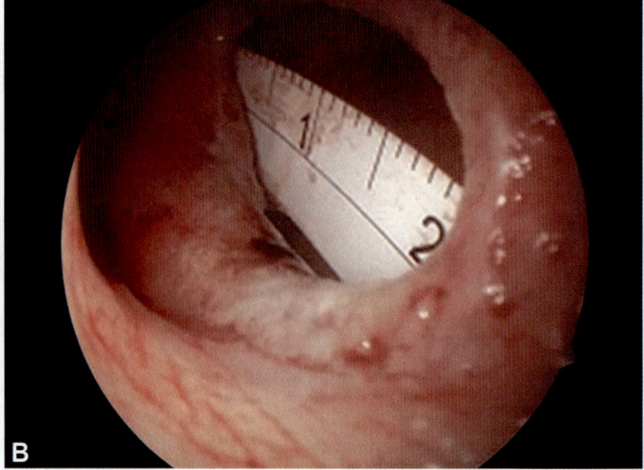

Figs. 19.2A and B: Author's surgical technique for repairing septal perforations. (A) Vertical measurement. (B) Horizontal measurement.

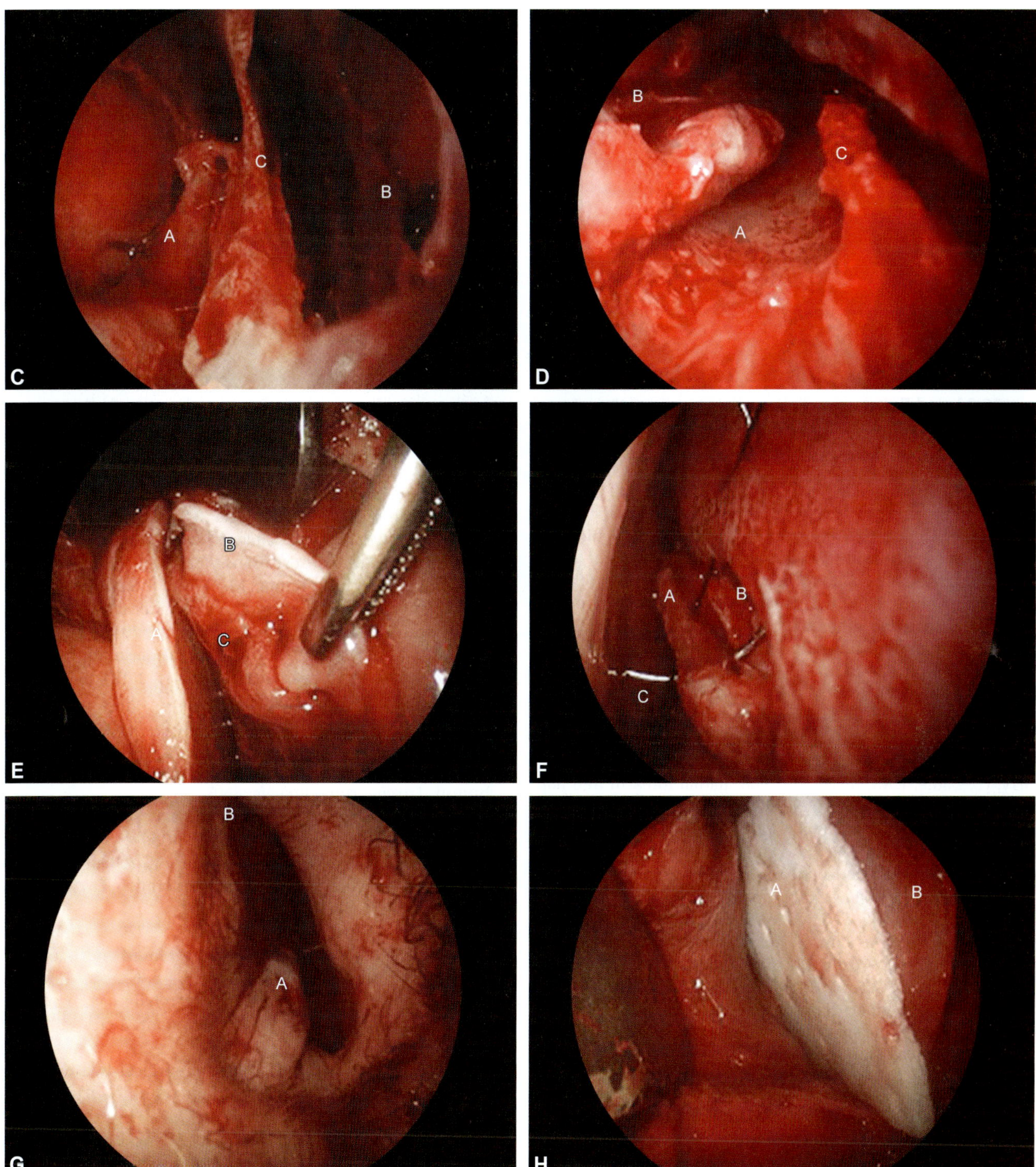

Figs. 19.2C to H: (C) Septal flaps raised. A—perforation margins of right flap, B—perforation margins of left flap, C—perforation margins of septal cartilage. (D) Inferior mucosal flap raised on right side. A—nasal floor, B—inferior mucosal flap raised form nasal floor, C—maxillary crest. (E) Left superior mucosal flap raised. A–dorsal edge of septum, B—superior edge of left upper lateral cartilage, C—superior mucosal flap raised from undersurface of left upper lateral cartilage. (F) Right mucosal margins being sutured. A—inferior margin of septal perforation, B—superior margin of septal perforation, C—reverse cutting needle during vertical mattress suture. (G) Left perforation margins sutured. A—sutured site, B—internal nasal valve angle. (H) Porcine collagen sheet between repaired mucosal sites. A—porcine collagen, B—septal cartilage.

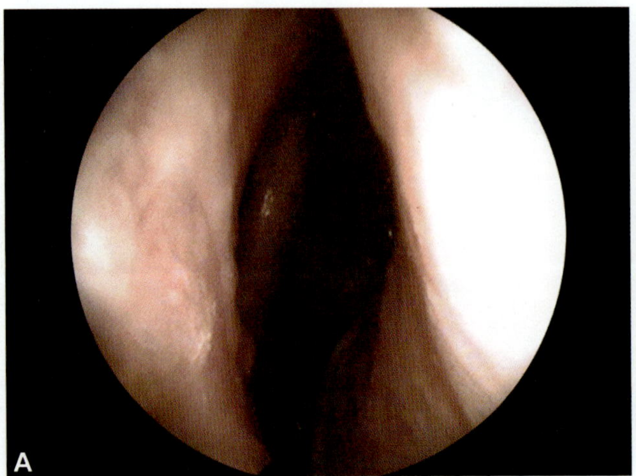

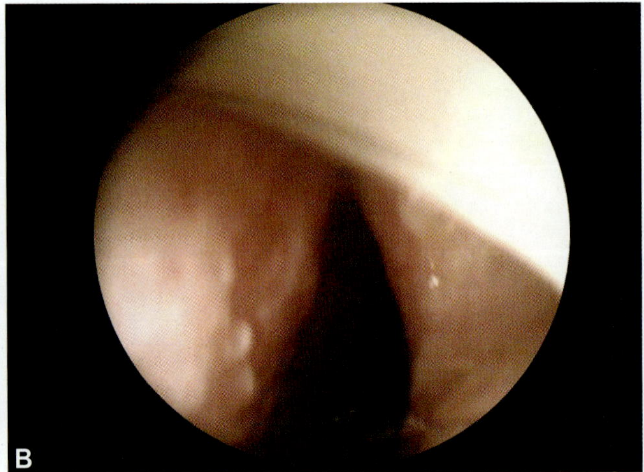

Figs. 19.3A and B: Before and after photographs of the internal nasal valve using the author's surgical technique. (A) Preoperative picture with septal perforation, (B) postoperative picture in the same patient with perforation closed.

REFERENCES

Al Kadah, B., Tengg, S., Deimann, J., Schneider, M., Schick, B., 2012. Experience with individual obturators to treat nasal septum perforation. *Laryngohinootologie*. 91(11), pp. 694-8.

André, R.F., Lohuis, P.J., Vuyk, H.D., 2006. Nasal septum perforation repair using differently designed, bilateral intranasal flaps, with nonopposing suture lines. *J Plast Reconstr Aesthet Surg*. 59(8), pp. 829-34.

Ayshford, C.A., Shykhon, M., Uppal, H.S., Wake, M., 2003. Endoscopic repair of nasal septal perforation with acellular human dermal allograft and an inferior turbinate flap. *Clin Otolaryngol Allied Sci*. 28(1), pp. 29-33.

Barry, C., Eadie, P.A., Russell, J., 2008. Radial forearm free flap for repair of a large nasal septal perforation: a report of a case in a child. *J Plast Reconstr Aesthet Surg*. 61(8), pp. 996-7.

Blind, A., Hulterstorm, A., Breggren, D., 2009. Treatment of nasal septal perforations with a custom made prosthesis. *Eur Arch Otorhinolaryngol*. 266(1), pp. 65-9.

Castelnuovo, P., Ferreli, F., Khodaei, I., Palma, P., 2011. Anterior ethmoidal artery septal flap for the management of septal perforation. *Arch Facial Plast Surg*. 13(6), pp. 411-4.

Ceylan, A., Ileri, F., Celenk, F., Yilmaz, M., Uslu, S., 2007. Upper lateral cartilage inner mucoperichondrial flap technique for the repair of nasal septal perforation. *ORL J Otorhinolaryngol Relat Spec*. 69(4), pp. 245-50.

Chen, F.H., Rui, X., Deng, J., Wen, Y.H., Xu, G., Shi, J.B., 2012. Endoscopic sandwich technique for moderate nasal septal perforations. *Laryngoscope*. 122(11), pp. 2367-72.

Chhabra, N., Houser, S.M., 2012. Endonasal repair of septal perforations using a rotational mucosal flap and acellular dermal interposition graft. *Int Forum Allergy Rhinol*. 2(5), pp. 392-6.

Daneshi, A., Mohammadi, S., Javadi, M., Hassannia, F., 2010. Repair of large nasal septal perforation with titanium membrane: report of 10 cases. *Am J Otolaryngol*. 31(5), pp. 387-9.

De, Gabory, L., Stoll, D., 2008. Treatment by enlargement of septal perforations. *Rev Laryngol Otol Rhinol (Bord)*. 129(1), pp. 43-8.

Deng, C., Li, R., Yang, J., Huang, Q., Xu, L., 2006. Repairing large perforation of nasal septum with titanium membrane and local pedicled mucoperiosteum flap. *Lin Chuang Er Bi Yan Hou Ke Za Zhi*. 20(8), pp. 358-9.

Dhar, V., Watts, S., 2009. Closure of nasal septum perforation: a novel technique. *Clin Otolaryngol*. 34(4), pp. 403-4.

Dosen, L.K., Haye, R., 2008. Silicone button in nasal septal perforation. Long term observations. *Rhinology*. 46(4), pp. 324-7.

Eng, S.P., Nilssen, E.L., Ranta, M., White P.S., 2001. Surgical management of septal perforation: an alternative to closure of perforation. *J Laryngol Otol*. 115(3), pp. 194-7.

Facer, G.W., Kern, E.B., 1979. Nasal septal perforations: use of Silastic button in 108 patients. *Rhinology*. 17(2), p. 1150120.

Fairbanks, D.N., 1994. Fairbanks GR Nasal septal perforation: 25 years experience with the flap and graft technique Am J Cosmetic Surg. 11, pp. 189-94.

Federspil, P.A., Schneider, M., 2006. The custom made septal button. *Laryngorhinootologie*. 85(5), pp. 323-5.

Foda, H.M., 1999. The one-stage rhinoplasty septal perforation repair. *J Laryngol Otol*. 113(8), pp. 728-33.

Friedman, M., Ibrahim, H., Ramakrishnan, V., 2003. Inferior turbinate flap for repair of nasal septal perforation. *Laryngoscope*. 113(8), pp. 1425-8

Giacomini, P.G., Ferraro, S., Di, Giarolamo, S., 2011. Ottaviano F large nasal septal perforation repair by closed endoscopically assisted approach. *Ann Plast Surg*. 66, pp. 633-6.

Goyal, M.K., Goyal, S., 2011. Prosthetic rehabilitation of large nasal septal defect with an intranasal stent: a clinical report. *Indian J Dent Res*. 22(5), pp. 719-22.

Goy, H.S., Husain, S.S., 2007. Different surgical treatments for nasal septal perforation and their outcomes. *J Laryngol Otol*. 121(5), pp. 419-26.

Grutzenmacher, S., Lang, C., Saadi, R., Mlynski, G., 2002. First findings about the nasal airflow in noses with septal perforation. *Laryngorhinootologie*. 81(4), pp. 276-9.

Heller, J.B., Gabbay, J.S., Trussler, A., Heller, M.M., Bradley, J.P., 2005. Repair of large nasal septal perforations using facial artery musculomucosal (FAMM) flap. *Ann Plast Surg*. 55(5), pp. 456-9.

Islam, A., Celik, H., Felek, S.A., Demirci, M., 2009. Repair of nasal septal perforation with "cross-stealing" technique. *Am J Rhinol Allergy*. 23(2), pp. 225-8.

Kazkayasi, M., Tuna, E., Kilic, C., 2010. Bullous middle turbinate flap for the repair of nasal septal perforation. *J Otolaryngol Head Neck Surg*. 39(2), pp. 203-6.

Kilty, S.J., Brownrigg, P.J., Safar, A., 2007. Nasal septal perforation repair using an inferior turbinate flap. *J Otolaryngol.* 36(1), pp. 38-42.

Kridel, R.W., 1999. Septal perforation repair. *Otolaryngol Clin North Am.* 32, pp. 695-724.

Kridel, R.W.H., Foda, H., Lunde K.C., 1998. Septal perforation repair with acellular human dermal allograft. *Arch Otolaryngol Head Neck Surg.* 123, pp. 73-8.

Lee, D.H., Yoon, T.M., Lee, J.K., Joo, Y.E., Kim, I.Y., Jang, W.Y., Moon, K.S., Jung, S., Lim, S.C., 2012. Clinical utility of the inferior turbinate flaps in the reconstruction of the nasal septum and skull base. *J Craniofac Surg.* 23(4):e322-6.

Lee, H.P., Garlapati, R.R., Chong, V.F., Wang, D.Y., 2010. Effects of septal perforation on nasal airflow: computer simulation study. *J Laryngol Otol.* 124(1), pp. 48-54.

Lee, H.R., Ahn, D.B., Park, J.H., Kim, Y.H., Sin, C.M., Youn, S.J., Kim, J.S., 2008. Endoscopic repairment of septal perforation with using a unilateral nasal mucosal flap. *Clin Exp Otorhinolaryngol.* 1(3), pp. 154-7.

Lee, K.C., Lee, N.H., Ban, J.H., Jin, S.M., 2008. Surgical treatment using an allograft dermal matrix for nasal septal perforation. *Yonsei Med J.* 30;49(2), pp. 244-8.

Li, F., Liu, Q., Yu, H., Zhang, Z., 2011. Pedicled local mucosal flap and autogenous graft for the closure of nasoseptal perforations. *Acta Otolaryngol.* 131(9), pp. 983-8.

Lindemann, J., Kuhnemann, S., Stehmer, V., Leiacker, R., Rettinger, G., Keck, T., 2001. Temperature and humidity profile of the anterior nasal airways of patients with nasal septal perforation. *Rhinology.* 39(4), pp. 202-6.

Lindemann, J., Leiacker, R., Stehmer, V., Rettinger, G., Keck, T., 2001. Intranasal temperature and humidity profile in patients with nasal septal perforations before and after surgical closure. *Clin Otolaryngol Allied Sci.* 26(5), pp. 433-7.

Mansour, H.A., 2011. Repair of nasal septal perforation using inferior turbinate graft. *J Laryngol Otol.* 125(5), pp. 474-8.

Ma, Y.X., Tao, A.Z., Lu, C., Tian, H., Dong, B.C., 2011. Endoscopic repair of nasal septal perforation with acellular dermal matrix and pedicled mucoperichondrial flap. *Zhonghua Er Bi Yan Hou Tou Jing Wai Ke Za Zhi.* 46(6), pp. 455-8.

Metzinger, S.E., 2005. Diagnosing and treating nasal septal perforations. *Aesthet Surg J.* 25, pp. 524-9.

Meyer, R., 1994. Nasal eptal perforations must and can be closed. *Aesthetic Plast Surg.* 18, pp. 345-55.

Mobley, S.R., Boyd, J.B., Astor, F.C., 2001. Repair of a large septal perforation with a radial forearm free flap: brief report of a case. *Ear Nose Throat J.* 80(8):512.

Moon, I.J., Kim, S.W., Han, D.H., Kim, S.T., Min, Y.G., Lee, C.H., Rhee, C.S., 2011. Predictive factors for the outcome of nasal septal perforation repair. *Auris Nasus Larynx.* 38(1), pp. 52-7.

Mullace, M., Gorini, E., Sbrocca, M., Artesi, L., Mevio, N., 2006. Management of nasal septal perforation using silicone nasal septal button. *Arch Otorhinolaryngol Ital.* 26(4), pp. 216-8.

Murray, A., McGarry, G.W., 2000. The clinical value of septal perforation biopsy. *Clin Otolaryngol Allied Sci.* 25(2), pp. 107-9.

Neumann, A., Morales-Minovi, C.A., Schultz-Coulon, H.J., 2011. Closure of nasal septum perforations by bridge flaps. *Acta Otorrinolaringol Esp.* 62(1), pp. 31-9.

Newton, J.R., White, P.S., Lee, M.S.W., 2003. Nasal septal perforation repair using open septoplasty and unilateral bipedicled flaps. *J Laryngol Otol.* 117, pp. 52-5.

Osma, U., Cureoglu, S., Akbulut, N., Meric, F., Topcu, I., 1999. The results of septal button insertion in the management of nasal septal perforation. *J Laryngol Otol.* 113(9), pp. 823-4.

Park, J.H., Kim, D.W., Jin, H.R., 2013. Nasal septal perforation repair using intranasal rotation and advancement flaps. *Am J Rhinol Allergy.* 27(2), pp. 42-7.

Pedroza, F., Patrocinio, L.C., Arevalo, O., 2007. A review of 25-Year Experience of Nasal Septal Perforation Repair. *Arch Facial Plastic Surgery.* 9, pp. 1-7.

Pless, D., Keck, T., Wiesmiller, K.M., Lamche, R., Aschoff, A.J., Lindemann, J., 2004. Numerical simulation of airflow patterns and air temperature distribution during inspiration in a nose model with septal perforation. *Am J Rhinol.* 18(6), pp. 357-62.

Purna, S.C.R., Annapurna, A.P.D., Ahmed, S.B., Vurla, S., et al., 2013. Two piece nasal septum prosthesis for a large nasal septum perforation: a clinical report. *J Prosthodont.* 22(2), pp. 143-7.

Raol, N., Olson, K., 2012. A novel technique to repair moderate-sized nasoseptal perforations. *Arch Otolaryngol Head Neck Surg.* 138(8), pp. 714-6.

Ribeiro, J.S., da, Silva, G.S., 2007. Technical advances in the correction of septal perforation associated with closed rhinoplasty. *Arch Facial Plast Surg.* 9(5), pp. 321-7.

Rokkjær, M.S., Barrett, T.Q., Petersen, C.G., 2010. Good results after endonasal cartilage closure of nasal septal perforations. *Dan Med Bull.* 57(10), p. A4196.

Romo, T 3rd., Sclafani, A.P., Falk, A.N., Toffel, P.H., 1999. A graduated approach to the repair of nasal septal perforations. *Plast Reconstr Surg.* 103(1), p. 66-75.

Shikowitz, M.J., 2007. Vascularized mucoperiosteal pull through flap for closure of large septal perforation: a new technique. *Laryngoscope.* 117(4), pp. 750-5.

Stoor, P., Grenman, R., 2004. Bioactive glass and turbinate flaps in the repair of nasal septal perforations. *Ann Otol Rhinol Laryngol.* 113, pp. 655-61.

Tardy, M.E, Jr., 1976. Alternatives in nasal reconstruction (five flaps and a graft). *Laryngoscope.* 86, pp. 1824-7.

Taskin, U., Yigit, O., Sisman, S.A., 2011. Septal perforation repairing with combination of mucosal flaps and auricular interpositional grafts in revision patients. *Otolaryngol Head Neck Surg.* 145(5), pp. 828-32.

Tastan, E., Aydogan, F., Aydin, E., Can, I.H., Demirci, M., Uzunkulaoglu, H., Unlu, I., 2012. Inferior turbinate composite graft for repair of nasal septal perforation. *Am J Rhinol Allergy.* 26(3), pp. 237-42.

Teschner, M., Willenborg, K., Lenarz, T., 2012. Preliminary results of the new individual made magnet based nasal septal button. *Eur Arch Otorhinolaryngol.* 269(3), pp. 861-5.

Teymoortash, A., Hoch, S., Eivazi, B., Werner, J.A., 2011. Experiences with a new surgical technique for closure of large perforations of the nasal septum in 55 patients. *Am J Rhinol Allergy.* 25(3), pp. 193-7.

Teymoortash, A., Werner, J.A., 2009. Repair of nasal septal perforation using a simple unilateral inferior meatal mucosal flap. *J Plast Reconstr Aesthet Surg.* 62(10), pp. 1261-4.

Wong, S., Raghavan, U., 2010. Outcome of surgical closure of nasal septal perforation. *J Laryngol Otol.* 124(8), pp. 868-74.

Woolford, T.J., Jones, N.S., 2001. Repair of nasal septal perforations using local mucosal flaps and a composite cartilage graft. *J Laryngol Otol January.* 115, pp. 22-5.

Yenigun, A., Meric, A., Verim, A., Ozucer, B., Yasar, H., Ozkul, MH., 2012. Septal perforation repair: mucosal regeneration technique. *Eur Arch Otorhinolaryngol.* 269(12), pp. 2505-10.

Zhang, Q., Zhang, J., Li, S., 2003. Endoscope-assisted repair of large nasal septal perforation using a complex mucoperichondrial flap and free tissue graft. *Chin Med J (Engl).* 116(1), pp. 157-8.

Facial Plastics

Section 2

Chapters Outline

Analysis of Aging Face 20

KV Vishwas, Ullas Raghavan

Chapter Overview

Pearls and Pitfalls

Pearls

- Meticulous analysis of facial features helps to understand age related changes in various tissue layers. Only after completing this thorough analysis can a surgeon formulate an appropriate treatment plan to suit the patient's unique anatomy and desires.
- The surgeon must appreciate the aesthetic flaw that concerns the patient before offering a management plan.

Pitfalls

- Asymmetries of the face are common. Make the patients aware of these asymmetries and the consequent limitations they impose on achieving desirable results preoperatively.
- Spend time with patients to understand their motivation and timing of surgery thoroughly. Patients seeking aesthetic treatments to satisfy external motivations are poor candidates for aesthetic treatments.

20.1 INTRODUCTION

In humans, the process of physical aging is believed to be due to a decrease in the restorative capacity of the tissue stem cells (Sharpless and DePinho, 2004). Even though these changes affect the whole body, they leave their mark on the face, which is the most exposed and noticed part of the body, more evidently than elsewhere in the body.

The attitude of our society has changed over the last few decades, gradually accepting "youth" as the desired outlook. Social stigma and reluctance associated with aesthetic surgery has virtually disappeared and surgery to look younger has become much more acceptable. Management of aging has also evolved over the years by incorporating both surgical and nonsurgical options with equal footing. Addressing the causes and consequences of aging has been the focus of many surgeons' and researchers' attention over the decades (Giampapa, Campo and Ramirez, 2003).

Aging of the face is known to affect every constituent part of the facial structure. It is much more complex than a simple ptosis of the skin and soft tissues. The behavior of skin, fat, muscles, salivary glands, and the underlying bony skeleton with aging involve both anatomic and physiological dynamics. An aesthetic facial plastic surgeon has to address changes affecting each layer of the facial tissues to achieve a long-lasting and natural appearing result.

20.2 AGE-RELATED CHANGES IN FACIAL STRUCTURES

Skin

- Reduction of thickness
- Reduction of elasticity and elastic recoil
- *Pigmentation* and coarse *wrinkles*

Skin is influenced by intrinsic as well as extrinsic factors. Some of the important external influences contributing to skin aging include excessive exposure to sun or other sources of *ultraviolet radiation*, toxins such as smoking, hormonal changes (Leung and Harvey, 2002), and sleeping position (Sarifakioglu, et al., 2004). Damage to collagen and elastic fibers as well as the reduction in cross-links between collagen fibers causes reduced skin thickness along with low elasticity and skin recoil. This causes sagging of the skin, apparent excess of skin, and wrinkling. Static and dynamic rhytids develop in the forehead, glabella, lateral (Crow's feet) and infraorbital region, upper and lower lips. Patients may present seeking correction of these or prominent melolabial fold and groove, marionette lines, or tear trough deformities. Aging is accompanied by appearance of *age spots* and an increase in the size of skin pores (Zimbler, Kokoska and Thomas, 2001).

Fat and Muscles

- Loss of subcutaneous fat
- Loss of volume of fat pads
- Accumulation of fat in areas such as submental and submandibular regions
- Loss of muscle tone
- Loss of muscle mass
- Dynamic wrinkles

Many of the changes in the facial architecture are secondary to changes in the superficial musculoaponeurotic system (SMAS). A loss of tone and bulk brings about gross variation in the profile that is accentuated by the appearance of rhytids. The activity of muscles of expression leads to the development of dynamic rhytids, which later becomes static rhytids.

With age there is loss of subcutaneous fat, reduction in volume of fat pads, and redistribution of fat. Lipoatrophy contributes to a loss of the normal convex facial contour (Ascher, et al., 2006) seen in youth. In addition, it causes increased hollowness of periorbital area, brow, forehead, cheek, mental, perioral, and temple areas. The osseocutaneous ligaments holding the fat pads in their normal position become attenuated with age leading to soft tissue ptosis. Bony margins such as the orbital margins become prominent due to a change in fat orientation. Fat accumulation occurs in submental, nasolabial, and jowl areas. All these changes lead to ill-defined jawline and cervicomental angle, prominent melolabial folds, and deep melolabial grooves. These changes lead to gradual change in shape of the young "V" shaped face to an inverted "V" configuration seen later in life.

There may be retro-orbicularis oculi fat ptosis, laxity of orbicularis oculi muscle, and laxity of upper lid skin leading to brow ptosis and dermatochalasis. Involution of the levator aponeurosis may lead to ptosis of the upper lid. Pseudoherniation of orbital fat leads to prominent medial and central fat pads in the upper lid. Similarly eye bags may form in the low lid area due to pseudoherniation of medial, central, and lateral fat pads. At the same time, tear trough deformity is caused by descent of suborbicularis oculi fat (SOOF), which leads to the inferior orbital rim being exposed.

Jowls are created by the downward pull and ptosis of facial portion of platysma (Zimbler, Kokoska and Thomas, 2001). Other contributing factors include ptosis of midface soft tissues, laxity of mandibular cutaneous and masseteric cutaneous ligaments, and loss of definition of chin and jawline.

Facial Bones

- Loss of volume
- Remodeling

The facial skeleton undergoes significant changes primarily due to loss of volume and remodeling of bone. A reduction in height and overall size of the facial skeleton fails to support the overlying soft tissue envelope, giving the appearance of sagging and drooping. The floor of the orbits sinks resulting in lateral bowing of the lower lid and increased scleral show. The periorbital soft tissues of youth are shallow in a narrow orbit, described as being an unbroken convex line from the lower eyelid to the cheek (Hamra, 1996). With progressive aging, those dimensions become wider and deeper as skeletonization of the orbit occurs, beginning in the fourth decade. Resorption of mandible and maxilla along with loss of dentition causes a loss of support to the labial and mental tissues, producing an appearance of excess soft tissue and wrinkles. The areas of muscle attachment start appearing more pronounced. Position of the eyebrow steadily descends from well above the supraorbital rim to a point at or below it. Loss of eyebrow volume is partly a result of bony absorption in the supraorbital region.

Exocrine Glands

- Subluxation
- Secretory changes

The exocrine glands in the face such as submandibular salivary glands and the lacrimal glands undergo significant anatomic changes along with an altered secretory capacity. The submandibular glands subluxate, causing swelling in the submandibular region, which sometimes persists even after a facelift procedure. Subluxation of the lacrimal glands adds fullness to the lateral part of the upper eyelids.

20.3 CONSULTATION

Consultation provides an opportunity for the surgeon to develop a rapport with the patient to assess their aesthetic concern, motivation, and expectation from intervention. As in any aesthetic surgery, patients considering surgical treatment of the aging face should be scrutinized thoroughly to identify the appropriate candidate. The surgeon must understand the aesthetic flaw that concerns the patient before offering a management plan.

Motivation of the patient must be assessed, seeking to know if it is internal motivation or external motivation driving him/her toward the treatment. The essential questions to pose during the interview include the reason for contemplating treatment, the timing behind the decision, and any prior attempts at therapy. Not being satisfied with previous results and going for revision to correct minor or perceived anomalies may be due to a body dysmorphic disorder. Spending time listening to the patient and reaching an understanding on the expectations and the final outcomes, go a long way in avoiding patient and surgeon dissatisfaction, legal hassles, and expensive suits.

A consultation in front of a three-way full-face mirror helps the patient to point out the anomaly that is of concern to them and serves as a platform for discussion regarding patient's perspective and concerns. It also helps the surgeon to educate the patient on normal anatomy, facial aesthetics, and enhancements that are possible given his or her unique facial characteristics. During the consultation, the patient faces the mirror and the surgeon stands behind the patient with his left hand on the left side of the patient's face and the right hand on the right half of the face. The senior author uses this module in all his consultations.

The expectations of the patient are assessed and a picture of what is realistically achievable by the surgeon is conveyed to the patient. With the advent of "no win no fee" legal practice, it might be worthwhile spending a small amount of time on documenting (either on paper or through video documentation) patient's expectations and achievable targets with due consent. At the end of consultation, if the surgeon has any doubts about the expectations of the patient, he or she must be referred for a psychological assessment.

A full medical history must be obtained. Most patients requesting rhytidectomy are in their fourth to sixth decade and may have multiple medical problems, and taking various medications. History of smoking is significant as this is one of the commonest causes of postoperative skin necrosis. Uncontrolled diabetes mellitus and previous radiotherapy to the face can also affect tissue vascularity. Psychosocial history is important to identify clinically depressed patients who seek aesthetic surgery. These patients may not be suitable candidates for surgery. Photo documentation and informed consent is essential prior to surgery.

A DSLR camera with low f-number (1–1.8) and 18–105 mm lens is ideal for portrait photographs in frontal, profile, 45° oblique, basal, and helicopter views. It is essential to set up a photographic lab in the clinic for uniformity and ease of serial documentation.

With the advent of increased international travel and medical tourism, the likelihood of a facial plastic surgeon encountering patients from different ethnic backgrounds is high. It is essential to know the interethnic variations in facial morphology in order to provide tailor-made surgical plans for the consulting patient. Forehead height, interocular distance, and nasal width show much variation among various ethnic groups. The least amount of variability is found in the ear height and upper, middle, and lower facial widths (Fang, Clapham and Chung, 2011). Delayed midface aging has been noticed among Asian and Afro-Caribbean races as well as delay in aging among Caucasians with prominent cheek bones (Hamra, 1996).

20.4 FACIAL ASYMMETRY

Facial asymmetry is not uncommon and should be identified and pointed to the patient prior to surgery. Facial asymmetry, such as hemifacial atrophy, may become more noticeable with age. Clinically visual inspection of the entire face, palpation to differentiate soft tissue from bony defects, comparison of the dental midline with the facial midline, and dentomandibular variations are noted. It is important to note that the fat pad density around the cheek on the hemiatrophic side needs to be altered to allow for appropriate correction of the underlying mandibulomaxillary deformities (Zufferey, 2005; Cheong and Lo, 2011). In such cases, a thorough clinical assessment followed by photo documentation, cephalometric assessment, and three-dimensional reconstructed computed tomography scan are obtained as needed (Figs. 20.1A and B).

20.5 CLINICAL EXAMINATION

The skin quality and rhytids must be assessed using Fitzpatrick's and Glogau's classifications (Glogau, 1996; Ho and Brissett, 2006) (Tables 20.1 and 20.2). The neck laxity is assessed using Dedo's classification (Lam and Williams, 2003a). Fitzpatrick's classification helps the surgeon in deciding on the benefit of skin pretreatment and resurfacing. Scars and pigmentary changes should be noted and the patient informed accordingly. Any suspected lesions should be biopsied and treated. Hairline and hair loss should be assessed and documented.

The wrinkle units may also be measured by objective profilometric ratios for better standardization in reviewing the results (Hatzis, 2004). The thickness and elasticity of the facial skin are crucial factors in achieving satisfactory results when surgical options are being considered.

The face is divided into the classical "Horizontal thirds" from menton to subnasale (lower third), subnasale to glabella (midface), and glabella to trichion (upper face) (Fig. 20.2).

Upper Third of Face

The most prominent parameters to assess in the upper third of the face are the height of the forehead, position of the hairline, and glabellar and forehead rhytids. The vertical rhytids in the glabella are secondary to the corrugator supercilii over action, while the horizontal rhytids are due to procerus muscle activity. The horizontal rhytids on the forehead are due to the action of frontalis muscle (Fig. 20.3). It is important to assess whether the rhytids are hyperfunctional lines noticeable only on muscle contraction (dynamic) or present at rest secondary to actinic changes (static). Palpation of the forehead lightly with patient alternately contracting and relaxing his/her forehead musculature helps delineate the frontalis distribution.

Midface

The shape and position of the brow varies with sex and age. Brow position and shape is well appreciated on standard photography and allows objective comparison of pre- and postoperative results. Understanding the brow lid relation is crucial for proper planning of surgical procedures. The male brow is situated at or below the level of the supraorbital ridge, with the lateral and the medial ends being situated at the same horizontal level (Lam and Williams, 2003b). In a young female, the eyebrow is situated at or above the level of the supraorbital ridge, with the peak at the level of the lateral limbus or lateral to it. As age advances, the lateral brow tends to become ptotic leading to lateral hooding of the upper eyelid. Studies

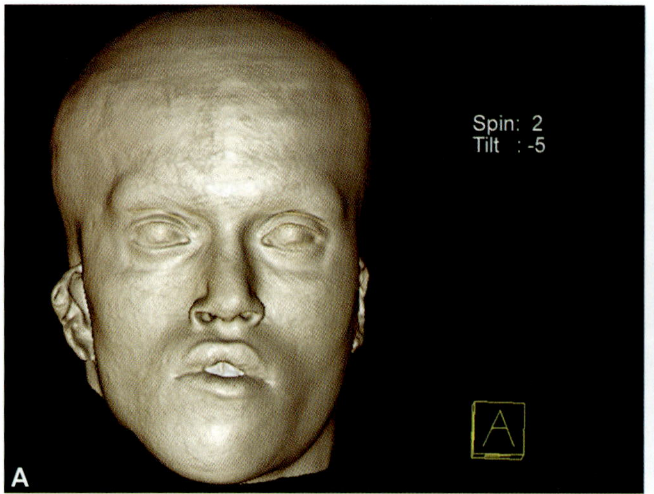

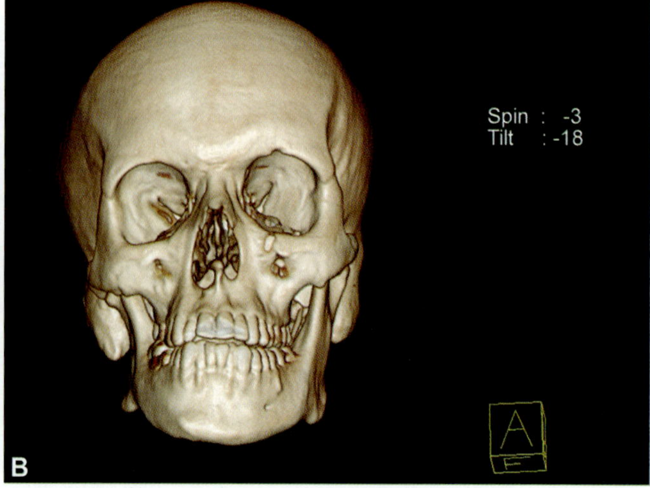

Figs. 20.1A and B: Three-dimensional soft tissue (A) and bony reconstruction (B) of a patient with hemifacial microsomia.

Table 20.1: Fitzpatrick's classification of skin types.

Type	*Skin color and features*	*Tanning ability*
I	White skin, blue eyes, blonde/red hair	Always burn, does not tan
II	White skin blue eyes	Easily burns, does not tan
III	Darker white skin	Mild burn, average tan
IV	Brown skin	Occasionally burns, tans easily
V	Dark brown skin	Rarely burns, tans very easily
VI	Black skin	No burns, dark tan

Table 20.2: Glogau's classification.

Type	*Severity*	*Age range*	*Characteristics*
I	Mild	20–30	Little wrinkling, no keratosis, requires little or no make up
II	Moderate	30–40	Early wrinkling with facial motion, early actinic keratosis
III	Advanced	50+	Persistent wrinkling, discoloration with telangiectasias, visible actinic keratosis
IV	Severe	60–70	Generalized wrinkling, actinic keratosis with or without malignancy

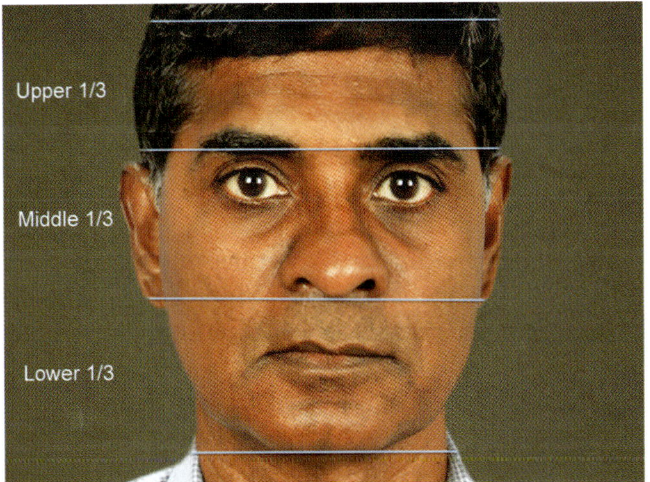

Fig. 20.2: Horizontal thirds of the face.

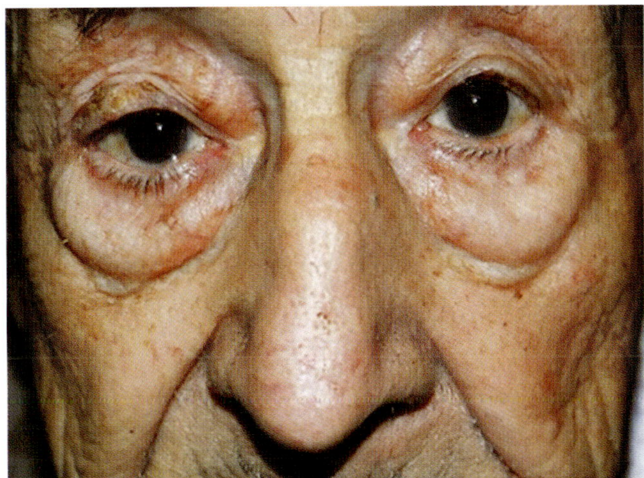

Fig. 20.4: Changes in the mid-third of face with age. Periorbital soft tissue ptosis, herniation of orbital fat in the upper and lower lids, deepened nasojugal folds, ptotic nasal tip, midface ptosis, and prominent melolabial folds can be seen.

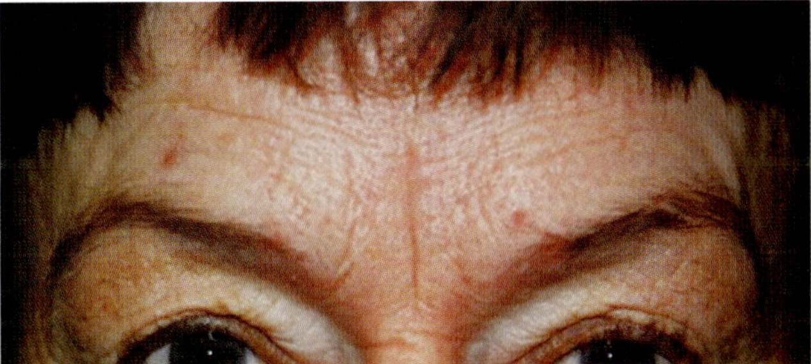

Fig. 20.3: Changes in upper third of the face with aging. Skin surface changes, vertical and oblique glabellar rhytids, and horizontal forehead rhytids can be seen.

have shown that the medial brow tends to get elevated in approximately half the patients with age.

In addition to changes in brow position, there is an excess of upper lid skin (*dermatochalasis*) and fat protuberance from medial and central fat pads. Possibility of upper lid ptosis must be kept in mind and if present it should be recorded. The lower eyelids may show excess skin, thickening of the orbicularis oculi, or fat protrusion from lateral, central, and medial fat pads (Fig. 20.4). The tone of the lower lid may reduce causing malposition of the lower lid margin, which can range from increased scleral show to frank ectropion. The distance between brow and upper lid margin, *mean reflex distance* 1 (MRD1) between upper lid margin and mid-pupil, and MRD2 distance between lower lid margin and mid-pupil must be recorded and compared to the expected normal level (Lam and Williams, 2003b).

The nose also shows alterations with age. The ligaments supporting the tip of the nose weaken and lengthen. This causes the tip to become ptotic making the nose look longer. The alar support reduces, contributing to alar collapse and resulting in nasal blockage (Sajjadian and Guyuron, 2009).

The malar prominence, produced in part by malar fat pad position, changes with age due to its inferior and medial movement. This in turn increases the depth of the nasolabial groove and leads to development of a nasojugal fold. The lower orbital margin becomes exposed leaving a tear trough deformity. The subcutaneous malar fat pad and the SOOF should be assessed individually in their contribution to a ptotic cheek segment. The position of eyeball to the cheek prominence must be assessed in the profile. If the anterior part of cornea and the infraorbital rim are in the same line, it is called neutral vector. If the cornea is behind the infraorbital rim, it is a positive vector, and if it is in front, it is a negative vector (Lam and Williams, 2003b). The surgeon should proceed very carefully with lower lid surgery in patients with a negative vector because of a high risk of lid malposition in the postoperative period. The orbital rim definition, lid position, the vector, and scleral show are important parameters to consider before embarking on any surgical interventions in the periorbital and midface area.

Lower Face

Soft tissue changes are responsible for an aged look (Fig. 20.5). The underlying bony changes in the lower part of the face make the soft tissue changes appear worse. Perioral lip lines, marionette lines, chin dimpling, jowls, and loss of jawline add years to the face and need a trained eye to discern the necessary corrections to be done. With advancing age, there is loss of height of mandible, particularly in edentulous patients. The decrease in height has the dramatic effect of reducing the facial height and leaving excess soft tissue. Loss of teeth contributes to change in the facial profile. The lips move posteriorly due to lack of dental support. Labiomandibular folds (marionette lines) and nasolabial folds become more noticeable with age. Jowls may be considered as the lower part of labiomandibular folds. The upper part of marionette lines is visible at rest and can be corrected with soft tissue augmentation. However, the lower part, which forms the jowl, is made more noticeable on smiling. Neck and lower face lift is ideal for correcting the appearance of the jowls. Surgery for correcting marionette lines and nasolabial folds can give suboptimal results unless deep plane lift or sub-SMAS techniques are used (Ivy, Lorenc and Aston, 1996).

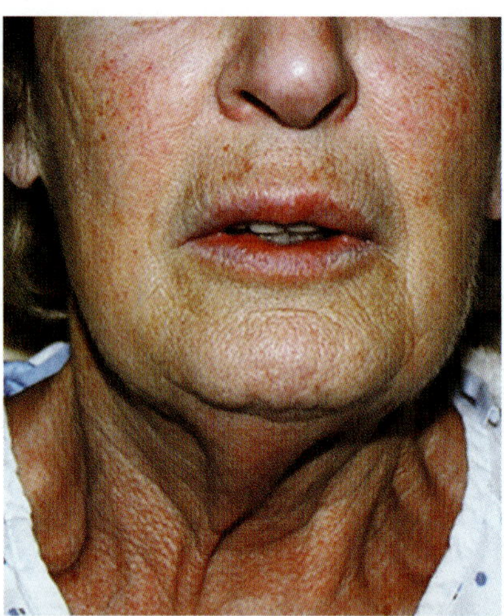

Fig. 20.5: Midface, lower face, and neck changes with age—note the platysmal bands, jowls, marionette lines, perioral rhytids, and nasolabial folds along with pigmentary changes.

Neck

The submental area needs detailed evaluation in order to provide improved aesthetic outcomes. Palpation is done to assess pliability of the neck skin, position of hyoid bone, chin, submandibular glands, and presence of isolated fat masses. The cervicomental angle becomes obtuse with aging and in some cases disappears completely. Some people, with anteriorly placed cervical structures do not have a well-developed cervicomental angle even in their youth. The submandibular salivary glands also become lax because of the loss of ligament support with advancing age. This laxity may persist despite a facelift unless it is identified preoperatively and specific corrective measures are undertaken during surgery. The anterior edge of the platysmal muscle sheet separates in the midline and presents as neckbands. The submental fat may protrude between the separated muscles and contribute to fullness in the submental region.

Neck also changes with age. Dedo (1980) has classified appearance of the neck. Certain anatomic configuration can result in limited success in surgery. The treatment for neck rejuvenation can be tailored according to the Dedo's classification (Table 20.3). A more detailed description of aging neck and double chin can be found in Chapter 25, volume 2.

SUMMARY

A patient seeking rejuvenation of aging face should be carefully assessed. It is essential that the right patient with appropriate expectations and insight be selected for surgical or nonsurgical intervention. The aesthetic changes secondary to aging should be assessed appropriately.

Table 20.3: Dedo's classification of neck laxity.

Type	*Laxity*	*Possible technique*
I	Youthful neck line	None
II	Skin laxity	Submental liposuction
III	Excess adipose tissue	Lower face and neck lift
IV	Platysmal banding	Platysmaplasty and face/neck lift
V	Microgenia or retrognathia	Chin implant with face/neck lift
VI	Low hyoid bone	Can never achieve a good cervicomental angle

This assessment will help in tailoring the surgery to the patient's unique facial characteristics. Using the right techniques for the right patient will result in a satisfied patient and surgeon.

REFERENCES

Ascher, B., Coleman, S., Alster, T., Bauer, U., Burgess, C., Butterwick, K., Donofrio, L., Engelhard, P., Goldman, M.P., Katz, P. and Vleggaar, D., 2006. Full scope of effect of facial lipoatrophy: a framework of disease understanding. *Dermatologic Surgery*, 32, pp. 1058-69.

Cheong, Y.W. and Lo, L.J., 2011. Facial asymmetry: etiology, evaluation, and management. *Chang Gung Medical Journal*, 34(4), pp. 341-51.

Dedo, D.D., 1980. "How I do it"—plastic surgery. Practical suggestions on facial plastic surgery. A preoperative classification of the neck for cervicofacial rhytidectomy. *Laryngoscope*, 90, pp. 1894-6.

Fang, F., Clapham, P.J. and Chung, K.C., 2011. A systematic review of inter-ethnic variability in facial dimension. *Plastic and Reconstructive Surgery*, 127(2), pp. 874-81.

Giampapa, V.C., Campo, A.F. and Ramirez, O.M., 2003. Anti-aging medicine and the aesthetic surgeon: a new perspective for our speciality. *Aesthetic Plastic Surgery*, 27, pp. 493-501.

Glogau, R.G.,1996. Aesthetic and anatomic analysis of the aging skin. *Seminars in Cutaneous Medicine and Surgery*, 15, pp. 134-8.

Hamra, S.T., 1996. The role of orbital fat preservation in facial aesthetic surgery. *Clinics in Plastic Surgery*, 23, p. 17.

Hatzis, J., 2004. The wrinkle and its measurement: a skin surface profilometric method. *Micron*, 35(3), pp. 201-19.

Ho, T. and Brissett, A.E., 2006. Preoperative assessment of the aging patient. *Facial Plastic Surgery*, 22, pp. 85-90.

Ivy, E.J., Lorenc, Z.P. and Aston, S.J., 1996. Is there a difference? A prospective study comparing lateral and standard SMAS facelifts with extended SMAS and composite rhytidectomies. *Plastic and Reconstructive Surgery*, 98, pp. 1135-43.

Lam, S.M. and Williams, E.F., 2003a. Lower facial rejuvenation. In: S.M. Lam and E.F. Williams, eds. *Comprehensive facial rejuvenation: a practical and systematic guide to surgical management of the aging face*. Lippincott and Wilkins. pp. 105-51.

Lam, S.M. and Williams, E.F., 2003b. Upper and midfacial facial rejuvenation. *Comprehensive facial rejuvenation: a practical and systematic guide to surgical management of the aging face*. Lippincott and Wilkins. pp. 54-104.

Leung, W.C. and Harvey, I., 2002. Is skin aging in the elderly caused by sun exposure or smoking. *British Journal of Dermatology*, 147, pp. 1187-91.

Sajjadian, A. and Guyuron, B., 2009. An algorithm for treatment of the drooping nose. *Aesthetic Surgery Journal*, 29(3), pp. 199-206.

Sarifakioglu, N., Terzioglu, A., Ates, L. and Aslan, G., 2004. A new phenomenon: 'sleep lines' on the face. *Scandinavian Journal of Plastic and Reconstructive Surgery and Hand Surgery*, 38(4), pp. 244-7.

Sharpless N.E. and DePinho R.A, 2004. Telomeres, stem cells, senescence, and cancer. *Journal of Clinical Investigation*, 113, pp. 160-8.

Zimbler, M.S., Kokoska, M.S. and Thomas, J.R., 2001. Anatomy and pathophysiology of facial aging. *Facial Plastic Surgery Clinics of North America*, 9(2), pp. 179-88.

Zufferey, J.A., 2005. Cheekbone: dynamic and anti-aging structure of the midface. *European Journal of Plastic Surgery*, 27, p. 359.

21 Facial Aging and Role of Botulinum Toxin in Aging Face

Frederick Wong, Gordon Soo

Chapter Overview

Pearls and Pitfalls

Pearls

- Respect the fact that Botox and filler injections are medical procedures.
- Follow all medical protocols for preparing patients for treatment.
- Patients undergoing Botox injection should be warned not to massage the injection site to prevent unintended dispersal and paralysis of neighboring muscles.
- Use filler material judiciously; always look for signs of potential ischemia such as blanching.
- Using blunt tipped cannulas for filler injection reduces the risk of injuring blood vessels and consequent bruising and intravascular injection.
- An "Injection First-aid Kit" consisting of a nitroglycerine ointment, aspirin tablet, sterile hyaluronidase injection, and hot packs should be available in every clinic performing filler injections.

Pitfalls

- Do not take Botox and filler injections too lightly. It is a mistake to think that they are "just a procedure" with little or no risk to the patient.
- Being caught unprepared for complications that can, and do, happen.
- Failure to keep good and clear documentation of the following:
  - Dosages
  - Sites of injection
  - Preoperative discussion with your patients.

21.1 INTRODUCTION

Facial plastic surgery is a unique discipline of otorhinolaryngology, as most of the patients present with very direct "symptoms". Very often, patients walk into our clinic and say, "Doctor, I would like to have my forehead wrinkles removed", or "Doctor, I would like to look younger". While the history taking seems a lot more straightforward, there are often hidden agendas or social implications that have to be discussed before jumping to a diagnosis, and incising (or needling) the patient.

Facial rejuvenation is in evergrowing demand, as people now live longer and are generally healthier than before. With a healthier and more energetic body, they strive to have an appearance that matches their biological but not their chronological age. In some industries, e.g. the entertainment and hospitality industries, the competitive marketplace almost demands youth as a prerequisite for gainful employment and success. Methods of rejuvenation can be classified into invasive (surgical), minimally invasive, or noninvasive. Minimally invasive methods such as *fillers* and *botulinum toxin* (BTX) have gained popularity due to their almost immediate effect, lower risk, and shorter downtime.

21.2 INITIAL ASSESSMENT OF PATIENTS

The surgeon should ascertain the patient's present concern(s), the duration, and any associated social or emotional impact on him/her. Previous plastic surgery procedures that the patient has undergone and the patient's own perception of his/her results are important to elucidate. This helps the surgeon to gauge patient's expectation of any intended treatment.

While true *body dysmorphic disorder* (BDD) is uncommon, anxiety and depression are sometimes seen in patients seeking facial rejuvenation (Clarke, et al., 2012). In fact, they are quite common in the general population. While these conditions do not preclude plastic procedures, they certainly need to be addressed. Involving a psychiatrist as part of the routine assessment of such a patient is sound clinical practice as he/she can guide the surgeon regarding the suitability of a patient to undergo any rejuvenation procedure. Extra time may be needed to explore the expectation of these patients. While having an in-house psychologist is a luxury that most practices cannot afford, it is helpful to ask patients to complete a screening questionnaire at the outset. For patients who demonstrate BDD traits, or are suspected of an undiagnosed/untreated psychiatric condition, a further psychiatric consultation should be initiated.

21.3 CLINICAL EXAMINATION—LOOK FOR SIGNS OF AGING

Physiological changes in *aging* may occur due to intrinsic or extrinsic causes. When we age, our skin gradually loses its turgor and thickness. Cellular changes include reduction in size of keratinocytes and fibroblasts, and increase in activity of melanocytes. Soft tissue changes include dermal elastin fiber alteration and the loss of hyaluronic acid in a connective tissue matrix. As a result, our skin becomes thinner, more friable, drier, more wrinkled, and takes longer to heal after injury. Extrinsic factors, such as sun exposure and tobacco smoking, cause similar skin aging, but the cumulative effect is to accelerate the whole process leading to signs of premature aging.

Wrinkles can generally be classified into dynamic and static types. *Dynamic wrinkles* appear in younger people, around the age of 30–40. They are caused by facial muscle contractions and form in a plane perpendicular to the direction of contraction of the underlying muscle. Generally speaking, they respond well to BTX treatment with the pharmacological relaxation of the facial muscles. *Static wrinkles*, on the other hand, are due to fibrosis over the subcutaneous layer, which is again due to aging and repeated muscle contraction. They behave more like subcutaneous scars and are refractory to BTX treatment. Surgical methods such as subcision and filler injection are required to correct this problem.

21.4 PATIENT COUNSELLING—CHOOSE YOUR WEAPONS WISELY AND CORRECTLY

After a thorough history taking and examination, the surgeon has to generate a treatment plan for the patient. At this point in consultation, the surgeon should have an understanding of the expectation and risk acceptance level of the patient. Although most, if not all, patients desire for "the most effective procedure with minimal risk and zero down time", such a procedure does not exist. Usually, the effectiveness level of any surgery or procedure corresponds directly to its risk profile and invasiveness. Therefore, the surgeon has to decide whether the patient is a candidate for a surgical procedure or a noninvasive intervention, or someone not suitable for either of these options. The first two categories are not mutually exclusive, as patients who have undergone plastic surgery in the past may be happy to undergo some maintenance procedures from time to time.

In the past, some surgeons focused mainly on lifting for facial rejuvenation. While it is important to lift the sagging tissues, overlifting can often lead to an "operated" and unnatural look. In recent years, *volumization* is gaining popularity as either a standalone treatment modality or a complimentary adjuvant procedure to achieve a more natural look together with face lifting.

Surgical volumization involves lipotransfer and is usually done under general anesthesia or sedation. For patients who prefer a less-invasive procedure under local anesthesia, filler injections offer a good alternative. When performed correctly, some of the fillers can also give a partial lifting effect. In addition, BTX can also be injected into selected antagonistic muscle areas to create a lifting effect by paralyzing the downward pulling muscles, in contrast to its most popular use for relaxing the uplifting muscles.

Discussion regarding photographic documentation and image simulation are beyond the scope of this chapter; its importance in preoperative counseling and medicolegal use cannot be emphasized enough.

Finally, a detailed explanation of risks of the procedure and proper consenting is a definite must. For example, while it is an extremely rare complication, filler injection(s) can lead to skin necrosis and blindness. Patients need to be made aware of this, instead, of thinking that they are just having "touchups" to make them look good for an upcoming social event.

21.5 BOTULINUM TOXIN

What Is It?

Botulinum toxin is an exotoxin produced by the bacterium *Clostridia botulinum*. It is the toxin-causing botulism, a potentially fatal paralytic condition. Since the 1970s, the serotype A of BTX (BTX-A) has been used clinically for treating hyperfunctional muscular disorders. Botulinum toxin works by the inhibition of acetylcholine release from the nerve terminals at the neuromuscular junction.

The chemical structure of BTX consists of a heavy chain and a light chain (Aoki and Guyer, 2011). The BTX heavy chain binds to the receptors on the membranes of cholinergic neurons, leading to endocytosis of the molecule; thereafter, the BTX light chain cleaves the intracellular proteins that are involved in neurotransmitter exocytosis, hence inhibiting their release. Without the release of the acetylcholine neurotransmitter, muscle contraction cannot be effected.

There are seven serotypes of BTX (types A–G) found in nature, and they target different intracellular proteins in the nerve terminal (Table 21.1). The commonest serotypes used clinically are serotype A and serotype B (Table 21.2).

Table 21.1: Serotypes of botulinum toxin.

Serotype	*Targeted intracellular protein*
A	SNAP-25
B	VAMP/Synaptobrevin
C1	SNAP-25 and Syntaxin
D	VAMP/Synaptobrevin
E	SNAP-25
F	VAMP/Synaptobrevin
G	VAMP/Synaptobrevin

(SNAP-25: Synptosomal-associated protein 25 kDa; VAMP: Vesicle-associated membrane protein).

Storage and Reconstitution

Botulinum toxin is supplied in powder form and requires reconstitution with normal saline before injection. It can be stored in a medical refrigerator at 4°C before reconstitution. Each vial of Allergan Botox contains 100 units; one *unit* of Allergan Botox corresponds to the calculated median intraperitoneal lethal dose (LD50) in mice, i.e. the unit dose that would lethally kill 50% of a sample of mice. If another brand of BTX is used, then the dosage may need to be adjusted. For example, Dysport is less concentrated than Botox, and the effect of every unit of Botox corresponds to about 2.5–3 units of Dysport. The dosage mentioned in this chapter will be based on the use of Allergan Botox.

With a 5 mL syringe and an 18-gauge needle, sterile normal saline can be injected into the Botox vial for reconstitution. Depending on the concentration required, usually 1 mL, 2 mL, 4 mL, or 5 mL of normal saline is injected into the vial for reconstitution. For cosmetic indications, the authors usually dilute 100 units of Botox with 2 mL of normal saline. A less concentrated solution would cause more diffusion of the BTX due to excessive fluid volume, which could lead to unwanted and unacceptable paralysis of the adjacent muscles. On the other hand, if too high a concentrated solution is used (1 mL saline to the 100 units of Botox, making up BTX 100 units/mL), it may be difficult to achieve precise dosage, especially in areas where only one unit is needed.

Botulinum toxin loses its effect gradually after reconstitution. The manufacturer recommends using Botox

Table 21.2: Examples of botulinum toxins.

Commonest serotypes	*Examples*
Type A	Botox (USA)
	Reloxin/Dysport (USA)
	Siax (Korea)
Type B	Myobloc (USA)

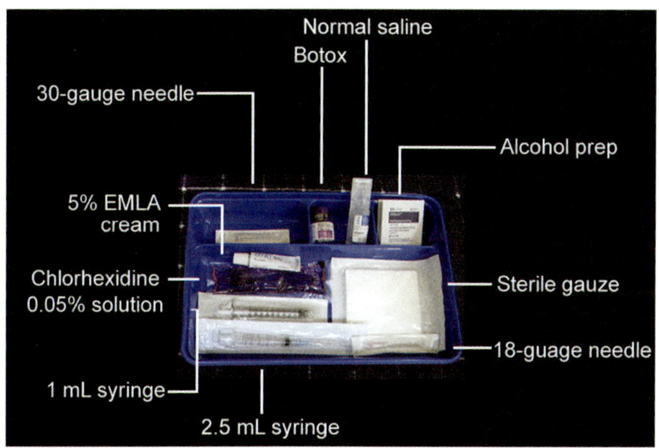

Fig. 21.1: Equipment needed for botulinum toxin injection. (EMLA: Eutectic mixture of local anesthetics).

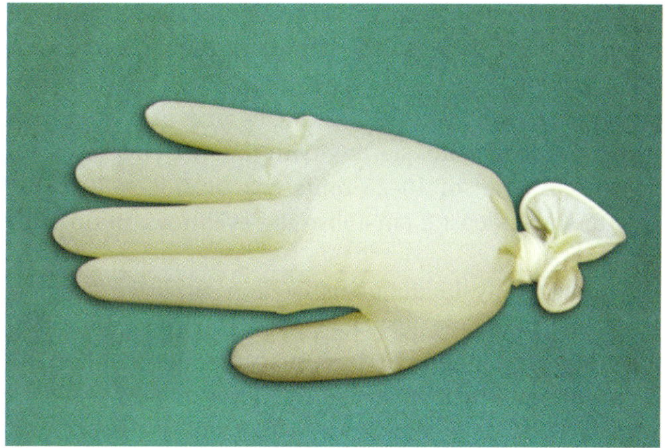

Fig. 21.2: Cheap and easy technique to assemble an ice pack with sterile glove, ice, and water to decrease bruising after injection of botulinum toxin and fillers.

within 24 hours of reconstitution. But in clinical practice, there is no universal consensus on the shelf time after dilution and most doctors use it up to 1-2 weeks after reconstitution. Some authors have suggested using normal saline preserved with 0.9% benzyl alcohol for reconstitution to prolong the effective duration for which reconstituted BTX may be used (Meyer and Blitzer, 2009).

More recently, it has been noted in a study that an oral intake of a zinc supplement and the enzyme *phytase*, 4 days before the injection of BTX, could improve its duration and effect by 30% (Koshy, et al., 2012). A tablet containing both zinc and phytase ingredients is commercially available for this purpose (Zytaze, USA).

Technique of Botulinum Toxin Injection (Fig. 21.1)

Before injection, a topical anesthetic, e.g. 5% eutectic mixture of local anesthetics (EMLA) cream can be applied onto the skin surface for 30–60 minutes, under an occlusive dressing, e.g. a piece of cling film or Tegaderm (3M) for this purpose. Ice packs can achieve further pain control together with vasoconstrictive effects, and can be prepared with large sterile gloves (size 8 or above) with ice cubes and water sealed within (Fig. 21.2).

After reconstitution with normal saline, BTX is drawn up into 1 mL syringes with an 18-gauge drawing needle (Small, 2012a). It is a good practice to mark the sites of intended injection and even take a photograph for future reference. Betadine or chlorhexidine solution can be used for the *sterilization* of the skin, and ice packs can also be placed on any pending injection sites for a few seconds. These ice packs create vasoconstriction and reduce the risk of vascular puncture. In addition, they provide a further anesthetic effect.

The patient is then asked to contract the muscles of facial expressions to exaggerate the wrinkles (Fig 21.3). With this maneuver, the responsible muscles become more visible and palpable for a more precise injection. The needle is inserted perpendicularly to the muscle in maximal contraction and the required dosage is injected.

After injection, gentle pressure is applied on the injection site to minimize bleeding and ecchymosis (Small, 2012a). After applying pressure for 1 minute, ice packs can be applied to the injection site again for another half a minute. It is important to watch the site of the ice pack application to avoid cold damage. Massaging the site is contraindicated to avoid any unintended dispersion of BTX. The common sites of BTX treatment are listed in Table 21.3. Specific precautions and techniques are as follows.

It is important to note that, in general, Asian patients have weaker musculature than Caucasian patients, and the dosage of BTX required will be less (Table 21.3). For example, according to the authors' experience, 1 unit of BTX is usually adequate to paralyze the procerus muscle, whereas in some Western textbook up to 2.5 units may be recommended. It will be more judicious to start with a low dose in Asian patients, with the option of repeat injections if the effect is inadequate.

Frontalis Muscle

The frontalis muscle is responsible for horizontal wrinkles over the forehead. It is one of the commonest sites for BTX treatment.

The patient is asked to raise his/her brows to make the frontalis muscle prominent. Mark the sites of intended injection, which should be *at least 1 cm* apart (Meyer and Blitzer, 2009; Small, 2012a). One unit of BTX is then injected to each site, starting with the one closest to the hairline. A total of 10–25 units can be injected, taking care to stay at least 2 cm above the eyebrows, in order to avoid ptosis.

Occasionally, inadequate injection can leave a persistent rhytid, usually just above the eyebrow. A second injection can be done in 2 weeks, carefully observing the 2-cm margin from the eyebrow. Half a unit BTX can be used instead of one unit per injection site, as the frontalis muscle is already weakened.

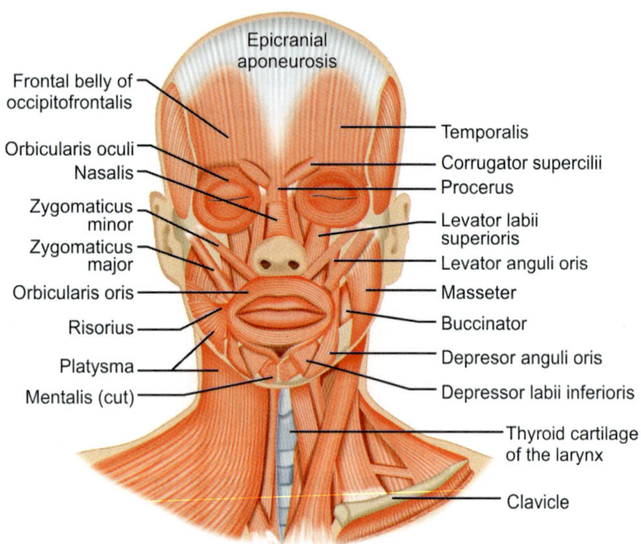

Fig. 21.3: Anatomy of facial musculature.

Corrugator Muscles

The patient is asked to frown, so that the two heads of corrugator supercilii are visible and palpable just medial to each eyebrow. Locate the main bulk of the muscle, and inject one unit into each site. Avoid going too lateral above the eyebrow.

Procerus Muscle

Located right at the center of the glabella, the procerus muscle is usually treated together with the two corrugator supercilii muscles. Usually, 3–4 units are enough to correct the horizontal rhytids over the nasion.

Orbicularis Oculi

The orbicularis oculi is a flat and superficial sphincteric muscle surrounding the orbit. It is responsible for closure of the eyes as we blink and sleep. Its contraction is also the cause of periorbital wrinkles; especially the lateral periorbital wrinkling, which is commonly described as *Crow's feet*. The patient is asked to squint so that Crow's feet and the contracted orbicularis oculi muscle are easily visible. One unit can be given for each injection point, at each strand of contracted muscle. A total of up to 5–7 units may be injected into each side. Subdermal injections should be given; therefore, a wheal should be visible at each injection point (Small, 2012a). It is important to avoid injection within the orbital rim by targeting the lateral part of the muscle (Meyer and Blitzer, 2009). Intraorbital injection is likely to lead to diplopia due to the paralysis of extraocular muscles.

Table 21.3: Common botulinum toxin treatment areas and dosage.

Muscles dosage	*Signs*	*Dosage per site [unit(s)]*	*Maximum dosage (whole area)*
Frontalis	Forehead horizontal wrinkles	1–2	10–25 units
Corrugator	Glabellar lines (vertical)	1–2	2–5 units per side
Procerus	Transverse nasal lines	1–2	5 units
Orbicularis oculi (lateral part)	Crow's feet	1	10 units per side
Transverse nasalis	Bunny lines	1	2.5 units per side
LLSAN	Gummy smile	1	5 units per side
Orbicularis oris	Smoker's lines	0.5–1	2.5 units
Depressor anguli oris	Downturned corners of mouth	1	2–5 units per side
Platysma	Platysmal band	2	20 units
Masseter	Square jaw	5	30 units per side

(LLSAN: Levator labii superioris alaeque nasi muscle).

Transverse Nasalis

Bunny lines are formed when the patients squeeze their noses. Two units of BTX can be injected directly to the muscle at each injection site, taking care not to go too deep to avoid a periosteal injection. Avoid the lateral margin of the nasal dorsum where the angular artery is located. A total of five units are usually used for both sides.

Levator Labii Superioris Alaeque Nasi Muscle

Excessive activity of this muscle leads to exaggerated upper lip retraction during smiling, also known as *gummy smile*. In order to avoid this undesirable look, the levator labii superioris alaeque nasi muscle (LLSAN) muscle can be injected, resulting in less upper lip retraction and more covering of upper gum during smiling. The upper attachment of the muscle is injected, right above the point where nasolabial fold joins the alar rim. You can feel the muscle by putting a finger on the spot and ask the patient to smile. Start with one to two units but sometimes as much as five units per side is needed.

Depressor Angular Oris

This muscle is responsible for a downturned angle of mouth, and to some extent, the *marionette lines*. The patient is asked to clench his/her teeth, and the muscle can be palpated just posterior to the marionette line. Avoid the depressor labii inferioris muscle, which lies more medially. A distance of at least 1 cm from the lip commissure is needed, to avoid causing lip asymmetry. Around 2–5 units can be injected into each side.

Orbicularis Oris

It is a sphincteric muscle surrounding the oral orifice. The patient is requested to whistle in order to have a better view of the contracted part of muscle. Very small amount of injection should be done each time to avoid oral incompetence and drooling. Avoid the lateral 1 cm from the lip commissure for upper lip, and 2 cm from the lip commissure for the lower lip, in order to avoid changing the shape of the lip. Injection should be given within 0.5 cm from the vermillion border. Inject 0.5–1 units subcutaneously into each point, with a maximum dosage of 1–2 units for each side of the upper and lower lips, respectively.

Platysma

The *platysma* muscle can create banding in the neck in older patients. Ask the patient to strain the two platysmal bands by grimacing and the bands will become more visible. Palpate the muscle and inject two units of BTX into each point, with a total of 3–4 injection points along the muscle band. A total of 20 units can be injected for the whole neck. The areas to avoid are within 2 cm from the jaw line and within 4 cm above the clavicle.

Masseter

Masseter injections are very popular in Asia, where a slim facial profile is desired. First, ask you patient to clench his/her teeth and bite firmly. Draw a line between the earlobe and nasal alae, and then delineate the anterior and posterior borders of masseter by palpation. All of the injection points should be between these three lines as mentioned above. Five units can be injected into each point, with a maximum dosage of 30 units on each side. If there is pre-existing asymmetry between the two masseters, which is often seen, the dosage can be adjusted accordingly.

Postinjection Care

The patient is advised against facial massage or lying prone on the bed for 24 hours. Ice packs can be applied intermittently to promote vasoconstriction and to minimize the risk of bruising. The patient is informed that at least 3 days are needed before he/she experiences the beginning of the BTX effect. This may also vary between individuals. If there is any sign of allergy, they should contact the surgeon immediately.

The authors usually examine the patient on the day following the injection. Though the effect of BTX is usually not evident by then, any minor complications, e.g. bruising and headache, should have manifested. Bruising can be managed with warm treatment and antibruising ointment, e.g. heparinoid ointment, and headaches can usually be controlled with analgesics.

The next follow-up will usually be 2 weeks later, when the full effect of BTX would have taken place. For any incomplete effect, further BTX can be injected at this time.

Complications

General

General complications include bruising, infection, asymmetry, undercorrection, and overcorrection. Antibody-induced therapy failure is rare (<1%) with the current formulation, but when it happens, repeated injection can become ineffective (Dressler and Hallett, 2006).

Fortunately, most of the complications from BTX are shortlived and can be managed.

1. Bruising should be avoided as much as possible by ice treatment and manual pressure after injection.
2. Infection can be minimized with sterile injection technique.
3. Asymmetry due to undercorrection can be treated with additional injection, 2 weeks later.
4. For overcorrection, patients need to be reassured, as they always get better with time.

To avoid development of antibodies, the smallest effective dose should be injected each time. Should the effect of BTX diminish with repeated injection, another brand or serotype of BTX can be tried.

Specific

Ptosis: For frontalis injection, ptosis can result if the injection is done too low (<1–2 cm of the brow). If that happens, then 0.5% of apraclonidine eyedrops can be used to relieve the condition temporarily. It stimulates the Muller's muscle, which is sympathetically controlled, and helps reduce ptosis by 1–2 mm. However, the patient will need to apply the eyedrops repeatedly 2–3 times per day, until the effect of BTX wears off. Usually, the improvement is noticeable as the effect of BTX weakens; this happens before the full effect of BTX (3–6 months) wears off.

Diplopia: It results from inadvertent injection of extraocular muscles during treatment of Crow's feet or BTX migration into those muscles. Although these are usually temporary, they can be very disturbing to the patients. Ophthalmological consultation with possible eye patching can be considered.

Lip and Cheek Ptosis

This is an often-neglected complication, which can happen when BTX is inadvertently injected into the zygomaticus major muscle, over the inferior lateral deep surface of orbicularis oculi. Smile asymmetry and oral incompetence can result.

Drooling and Oral Incompetence

This is usually due to overinjection of the orbicularis oculi, and sometimes seen with injection of the LLSAN. It is a very disabling problem for the patients. However, with time, all patients improve, as the effect of BTX is temporary.

Masseter Weakness

For masseter injections, the patient should be forewarned of this complication. It usually manifests as problem with chewing hard foods such as steak. Repeated injection increases the likelihood of this complication, as the muscle undergoes some atrophy. In order to minimize this complication, a combination of other facial contouring procedures can be offered to the patient, such as thread lift, radiofrequency, or even surgery. These adjuvant procedures help in decreasing the need for repeated injection of masseter muscles.

21.6 FILLERS INJECTION

What are Fillers?

Fillers are materials used to fill up spaces in the body. Facial fillers are materials that can be injected into the face, aiming to rejuvenate and enhance facial features.

What are the Types of Fillers?

Fillers may be classified in different ways based on the following: by the depth of injection, by the longevity of the products, or by origin of the materials. The latter classification is most commonly used for a comprehensive review of fillers, and is shown in Table 21.4 (Maas, et al., 2009).

However, clinically it is more practical to classify fillers according to their longevity, as most patients are obviously more concerned with the duration of effect rather than their origin. A classification of common fillers, according to their longevity, is shown in Table 21.5 (Small, 2012b).

Preparation (Fig. 21.4)

For anxious patients, a premedication with 2 mg oral diazepam can be given 15 minutes before the procedure, provided there is no contraindication. However, this is usually not required.

The authors suggest using blunt tip side ported facial aesthetic *cannulas* for all types of injections in order to reduce the risk of inadvertent intravascular injection, which can lead to serious complications. Commercially packed hyaluronic acid can either be aspirated into a syringe with Luer Lock and cannula, or a cannula can simply be attached to the syringe provided by the manufacturer. A 26G cannula can be used for most types of fillers.

Table 21.4: Classification of fillers according to origin.

Origin	*Product*	*Allergy test (skin) required*
Autologous	Fat*	No
	Fascia*	No
Allogenic (human)	Collagen (Cosmoderm, Cosmoplast)	No
	Dermal matrix (Cymetra)	No
	Fascia (Facian, Tutoplast)	No
Xenogenic	Bovine collagen (Zyderm, Zyplast)	Yes
	Porcine (Evolence)	No
	Avian hyaluronic acid (Hylaform)	No
Cross-species	Hyaluronic acid* (Restylane, Juvederm)	No
Alloplastic	Calcium hydroxyapatite* (Radiesse)	No
	Poly-L-lactic Acid* (Sculptra)	No
	Polymethymethacrylate—PMMA (Artecoll)	No
	Polyacrylamide (Aquamid)	No
	Silicone (Silkon)	No

The more commonly used products in practice nowadays are marked with an asterisk.

Table 21. 5: Classification of commonly used fillers according to their longevity.

Classification	*Duration of action*	*Type of filler*	*Mechanism of action*
Short term	3 months to 1 year	Hyaluronic acid	Volume restoration
Medium term	Up to 2 years	Calcium hydroxyapatite	Volume restoration
			Fibroblast ingrowth framework
		Poly-L-lactic acid	Collagen stimulation
Long term	10 years or more	PMMA	Microgranuloma formation
		Polyacrylamide	Tissue integration
		Silicone	Fibroblast stimulation

(PMMA: Polymethymethacrylate).

Nowadays, commercially available hyaluronic acid with added lignocaine mixtures is available. The author recommends using these preparations to minimize pain and discomfort for the patients.

Topical anesthetic cream, such as 5% EMLA, can be applied to the injection sites 45 minutes before the procedure. Occlusive dressing such as Tegaderm (3M) or cling film can be used to allow better absorption. Ice packs can be prepared with sterile gloves filled with ice and cold water (Fig. 21.2).

Specific Preparations for Poly-L-lactic Acid (Fig. 21.5)

The preparatory work for poly-L-lactic acid takes place well before the actual injection. The medication comes in powder form, and needs to be reconstituted with sterile water 24–72 hours before injection. The authors would, however, recommend that an even earlier reconstitution (as early as 5 days before injection) to allow better dissolution of the powder in the liquid medium prior to the procedure is optimal. Usually, 5–6 mL of water can be added. Right before injection, the reconstituted medication needs to be shaken well, and an additional 1 mL of 2% lignocaine can be added for anesthetic effect. The 2.5-mL or 5-mL syringes with Luer-Lock are used for injection and account for easier handling. The reconstituted medication is aspirated into the syringes and connected to a cannula.

For poly-L-lactic acid, a cannula of a larger gauge, such as 22G, should be used instead of the 26G cannula used for other fillers. This is because some undissolved

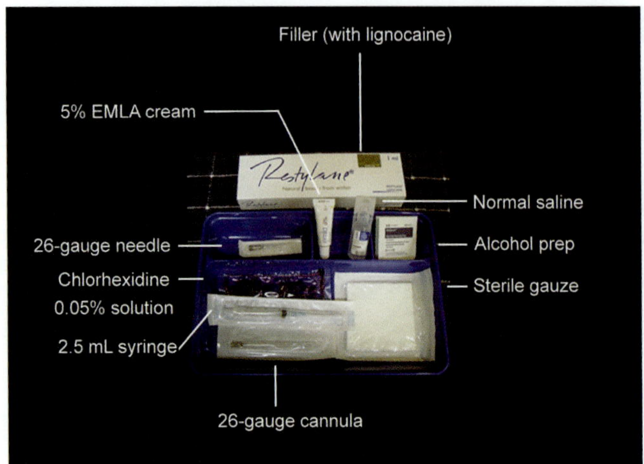

Fig. 21.4: Equipment needed for hyaluronic acid filler injection. (EMLA: Eutectic mixture of local anesthetics).

Fig. 21.5: Equipment needed for poly-L-lactic acid filler injection. (EMLA: Eutectic mixture of local anesthetics).

medications will persist in powder form, clogging up the lumen of the cannula if it is too small. A needle of the same size is also needed for skin puncturing.

Technique of Filler Injection

Following the application of topical local anesthetic cream, the area is sterilized with betadine or chlorhexidine solution. Sterile ice packs can be applied for a further 30 seconds to achieve vasoconstriction and an additional anesthetic effect. The needle, either used alone or connected to a 2.5-mL syringe, is used to puncture the skin, taking care to go only through the dermis and not further forward. This helps to minimize the risk of vascular puncture. If it happens, the surgeon needs to apply manual pressure on the site for 1 minute to prevent bruising, and choose an adjacent site for puncture instead.

The syringe containing filler with cannula is then inserted through the same puncture site, dissecting under the skin to the desired depth and area. With the cannula, a blunt dissection of soft tissue can be achieved and any blood vessels can be either avoided or pushed aside without puncturing. Filler is then injected on the way out.

There have been a few techniques described including linear thread, fanning, cross-hatching, layering, and depot. Each one of them gives a different filling pattern and should be chosen according to the injection site and desired effect (Small, 2012b; Maas, et al., 2009).

Linear Threading (Fig. 21.6)

Insert the needle or cannula along a linear area of planned filler injection. Inject the filler upon withdrawal of the needle, taking care not to inject while coming through the skin. This technique is suitable for a linear area of filling, such as the nasolabial fold.

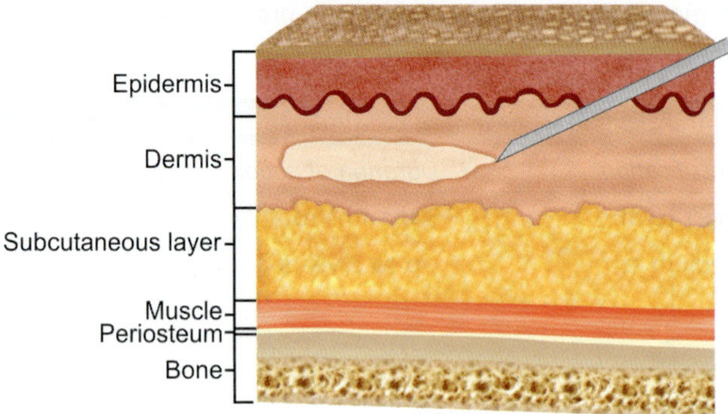

Fig. 21.6: Linear threading technique for injection of dermal fillers.

Fanning (Fig. 21.7)

Insert the needle or cannula into a single puncture point, and cover a fan-shaped area by repeated injections at different angles. Areas such as the chin are suitable to be treated with this technique.

Cross-hatching (Fig. 21.8)

Multiple puncture points are needed for injection in a square grid pattern. This is especially good for volumization, such as malar augmentation.

Layering

The filler is injected into layers of different depth. For example, the deep dermis is treated first, followed by

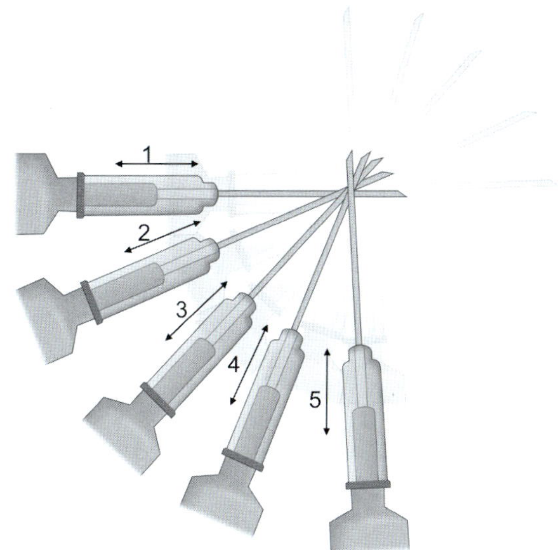

Fig. 21.7: Fanning technique for injection of dermal fillers.

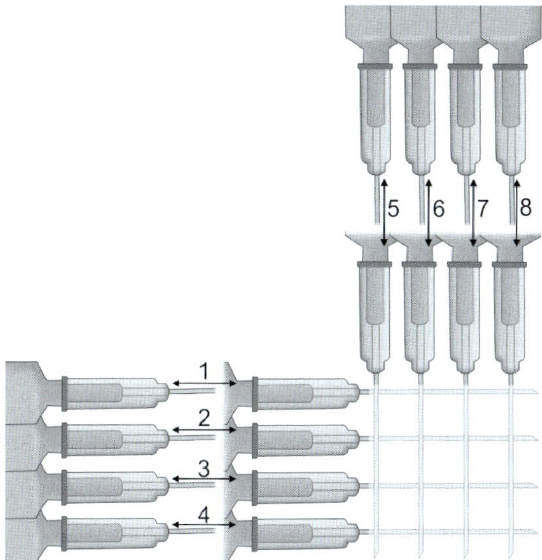

Fig. 21.8: Cross-hatching technique for injection of dermal fillers.

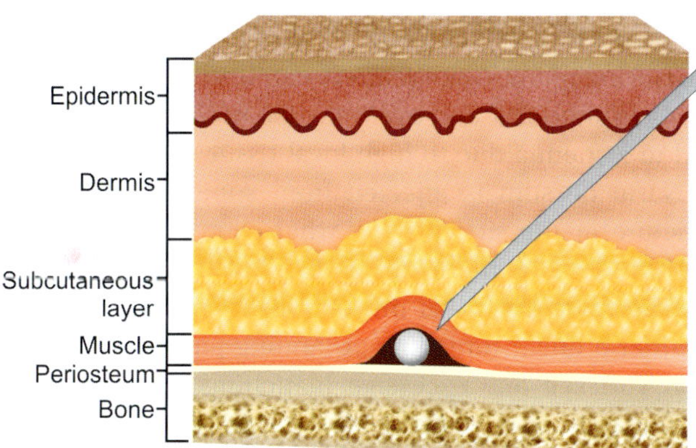

Fig. 21.9: Supraperiosteal depot injection of dermal filler.

another injection into superficial dermis. Areas requiring firm structural support can be treated with this method.

Depot (Fig. 21.9)

This technique is commonly used for longer-term filler such as poly-L-lactic acid. The depth of injection for poly-L-lactic acid differs from the usual recommendation, as palpable or visible nodule formation is a complication. Usually, a deeper level of injection is recommended to minimize this complication.

The cannula is inserted into the desired area, usually below the muscle, and a depot of medication is injected. It can give an overall rejuvenated appearance, and minimize the problem of visible nodules as there is a thick layer of soft tissue covering the medication.

The common areas that need filling on the face include the forehead, temple, tear trough, cheek, nasolabial folds, marionette lines, chin, and the nose. They are summarized in Table 21.6 (Small, 2012b).

Forehead

The material more commonly used for forehead filling is poly-L-lactic acid. A puncture site is made over the temple, and the syringe with cannula is inserted under the deep temporal fascia. When the conjoint tendon is reached, go deep under the *frontalis muscle*. The medication can then be injected either as linear threads or fanning, depending on the area for rejuvenation. Common forehead problems include horizontal rhytids and suprabrow depression. Patients need to be forewarned that if the supraorbital nerve is encountered, there will be a "lightning" sensation radiating up to the scalp. With the use of the blunt tip cannula, no actual harm will be done.

Temple

Puncture site and depth are similar to forehead injection; however, depot of medication is injected under the deep temporal fascia. There have been case reports of superficial temporal vessels puncture and intravascular injection with the use of needles. This complication has become minimal since the introduction of blunt tip cannulas.

Table 21.6: Common facial areas for filler injection.

Anatomical sites	*Entry point*	*Plane of injection*
Forehead	Temple area	Deep to frontalis muscle
Temple	Temple	Deep to deep temporal fascia
Tear trough	Underneath maxilla	Subcutaneous/deep to orbicularis oculi
Nasolabial fold	Angle of mouth	Subcutaneous/deep to orbicularis oris
Marionette line	Lowest point of line	Subcutaneous
Chin	Lowest point of chin	Just above the periosteum
Nose	Sites to be augmented	Deep to nasal muscles

Tear Trough

The medical term for this is the *nasojugal groove*, which is a demarcating line between the medial part of lower eyelid and the cheek. With aging it becomes deeper as the orbital septum loosens and the infraorbital fat herniates downward. The puncture point is over the lateral aspect of maxilla with the cannula pointing 45° upward and medially. Hyaluronic acid can be injected subcutaneously, while care must be taken to ensure that poly-L-lactic acid is injected more deeply underneath the orbicularis oculi muscle.

Nasolabial Fold

Puncture the skin over the lower end of the *nasolabial fold*. Advance the cannula along the fold, with a linear thread of filler injected, usually during withdrawal. In the past, cases of buccal mucosal puncture have been reported with the use of needle. Nowadays it seldom happens, but the patient needs to be forewarned that they may feel the cannula poking against their oral cavity.

Marionette Line

It is medically termed the *melomental fold*. The puncture site is over the chin line, at the lower end of the marionette line. Advance the cannula just underneath the skin, and inject only a minimal amount. This is a very thin area, and overinjection can lead to visible nodules or lumps. Massage vigorously if that happens.

Chin

Chin augmentation is quite safe in general, due to the thick layer of tissues covering this region. Puncture at the tip of the chin and advance the cannula until the deep periosteum is met. Inject the filler in a fanning pattern.

Nose

The nose is a dangerous area to be injected due to the rich vascular supply and thin and tight soft tissue envelope. Yet it is one of the most commonly augmented areas in Asian patients. The areas to take extra precaution include the lateral nasal groove, where the angular artery is situated, the adherent nasal tip skin, and the edge of the nostril, which is the end point of nasal blood supply. Puncturing of the angular artery can lead to skin necrosis due to thrombosis, and overinjection of nasal tip can also lead to ischemia due to high local tissue pressure.

Nasal dorsum is injected from superior to inferior. Puncture at the site of radix where you would like the higher end of augmentation to be, and advance the cannula between the nasal muscles and periosteum. Inject in either a linear threading or fanning pattern.

If you see any excessive blanching, stop injection immediately and squeeze the excess fillers out from the puncture hole. Refer to the section "Complications and Their Management" if there are signs of impending necrosis.

After Injection

With hyaluronic acid, manual molding is needed to achieve the final shape. With poly-L-lactic acid injection, a postinjection massage is needed for 5 minutes, taking care to squeeze evenly the area where a "nodule" is felt. The "nodule" is a concentrated nidus of the medication, which can potentially lead to overstimulation of collagen and longer-term nodule formation.

The patient should rest in the recovery area after injection. A review of the injection site(s) should be performed after 30 minutes. Any problems such as erythema, swelling, or ischemia should be managed accordingly. The patient is instructed to massage the area for 5 minutes, 5 times a day for 5 days to prevent nodule formation.

Pitfalls and Precautions

Serious complications such as blindness and skin necrosis occured with the use of needles in the past (Lazzeri, et al., 2012). This was due to accidental intravascular injection of the filler obstructing the blood vessels. Even without a direct puncture and intravascular injection, blood supply may be compromised due to excessive extravascular injection leading to vascular compression and reduced or absent tissue perfusion. That is especially common in areas where the blood supply depends on small caliber vessels, e.g. the nasal tip.

It is thus important that the surgeon injects filler material judiciously, always looking for important telltale signs of potential ischemia such as blanching of the nasal tip. If that happens, then all further injections need to be stopped, and excessive filler squeezed out from the puncture site. Observe for a few minutes. If the condition does not improve after this, consider the following "first-aid" measures.

An "*Injection First-aid Kit*" should be available in your clinic if you perform filler injections. It consists of a *nitroglycerine* ointment, aspirin tablet, sterile *hyaluronidase*, and hot packs (Small, 2012b).

If you choose to use a needle for injection, make sure that you aspirate each time before injecting to reduce the chance of an intravascular injection. However, a better way to prevent this complication is by employing blunt-tip cannulas. Some surgeons prefer to use hyaluronic acid fillers exclusively for all areas of the face because it can be neutralized with an injection of hyaluronidase in case of vascular compromise or if the patient is dissatisfied with the result of the filler injection.

Although poly-L-lactic acid is considered safer than other fillers with regard to intravascular injection, there are pitfalls associated with it. Due to its collagen-stimulating ability, it is not recommended for use in thin-skinned area, including the nasal dorsum and periorbital regions. Cases of visible and palpable nodule formation have been reported in the past. In order to avoid this from happening, it should not be injected into the aforementioned areas, and the patients should perform vigorous massage for 5 days after the injection. That helps the surgeon to spread out the medication evenly and ensure a more even stimulation of collagen formation.

Follow-up Visits and Repeated Injections

Patient should return for a follow visit on the day following the injection to look for signs of complications, including skin mottling, bruising, infection, etc. Undertake remedial action with the first-aid kit as mentioned above, if there is any doubt about the perfusion of the injected area. Infection usually manifests as erythema, warmth, and tenderness. Systemic antibiotics should be given if that happens.

The effect of the filler will wear off after a certain period depending on the longevity of the filler. While repeated injections are possible, the authors, in general, do not recommend this practice for areas with thinner skin, e.g. the dorsum of nose. With repeated injections subcutaneous scarring can get worse and eventually the vascular supply of the skin may be jeopardized. If the patient is satisfied with the effect of the filler and would like a permanent result, then a formal rhinoplasty should be offered as a long-term solution.

Complications and their Management

Bruising

This is one of the commonest complications. It is usually due to inadvertent vascular puncture. Ice pack application and manual pressure in case of vascular damage can minimize the incidence. Should it happen, topical medication such as a heparinoid can be used together with warm treatment to promote vasodilation and dissolution of the bruise.

Blindness

This is an extremely rare but terrifying complication. It is due to retrograde flow of filler causing central retinal artery embolism. If this complication happens, treatment will need to be initiated quickly, preferable within 90 minutes. Treatments mentioned in the literature include intravenous acetazolamide, oral steroids, and topical steroids, with variable effects (Lazzeri, et al., 2012).

Skin Necrosis

The aforementioned "first-aid kit" can be used in patients with impending skin necrosis/skin mottling. Apply the hot packs to the affected area first to facilitate vasodilatation. About 600 mg of chewable aspirin is given to the patient for an anticoagulation effect, and nitroglycerine ointment or patch is then applied onto the area for further stimulated vasodilatation. Note that monitoring of the vital signs is needed with the use of nitroglycerine. Hyaluronidase can then be injected to the area to dissolve the hyaluronic acid. Usually 30–50 units of hyaluronidase are needed. The patient should be admitted to hospital for further monitoring.

Infection

It can present as erythema or nodules, which are due to bacterial infection. Observing a strict aseptic technique for injections can minimize this risk. Should this complication happen, treatment with systemic antibiotics is needed. If there is a collection of hyaluronic acid with infection, hyaluronidase can be injected to dissolve the filler.

Formation of Nodules

Poly-L-lactic acid injection is associated with a very specific type of complication, which is nodule formation. The nodules formed are nidus of the medications, surrounded by the fibers and collagen. If it is only palpable and not visible, then most patients will choose to ignore it, waiting for it to subside in 1-2 years of time. Visible nodules can be treated with repeated injection of normal saline and aspiration.

Asymmetry/Undercorrection/Overcorrection

Facial asymmetry due to hyaluronic acid filler over injection can be treated with hyaluronidase. Undercorrection can be easily treated with another session of filler injection. However, it is prudent to wait for a few days for the initial swelling to subside before a final assessment can be made.

When using poly-L-lactic acid fillers the surgeon should impress upon the patient that the improvement achieved immediately after injection will disappear after 1-2 days. It can then take 6-12 weeks for the final results to become apparent, since the mechanism of action of this filler is stimulation of collagen formation by the body. Therefore, patience is needed before scheduling another session for the patient.

CONCLUSION

Neurotoxin and fillers injections are the bread and butter of facial plastic surgery. The techniques are easy to acquire with a short learning curve. However, sound knowledge of facial anatomy and a thorough analysis of facial deformity using well-established principles of facial aesthetics are key skills that the surgeon must possess before practicing this art form. It is a common pitfall to ignore and/or forget the associated serious potential complications associated with these treatments. These can be negated and/or minimized with appropriate precautions.

REFERENCES

Aoki, K.R. and Guyer, B., 2011. Botulinum toxin type A and other botulinum toxin serotypes: a comparative review of biochemical and pharmacological actions. *European Journal of Neurology*, 8(Suppl. 5), pp. 21-9.

Clarke, A., et al., 2012. Low priority? A cross sectional study of appearance anxiety in 500 consecutive referrals for cosmetic surgery. *Psychology, Health and Medicine*, 17(4), pp. 440-6.

Dressler, D. and Hallett, M., 2006. Immunological aspects of Botox, Dysport, and Myobloc/NeuroBloc. *European Journal of Neurology*, 13(Suppl. 1), pp. 11-5.

Koshy, J.C., et al., 2012. Effect of dietary zinc and phytase supplementation on botulinum toxin treatments. *Journal of Drugs in Dermatology*, 11(4), pp. 507-12.

Lazzeri, D., et al., 2012. Blindness following cosmetic injections of the face. *Plastic and Reconstructive Surgery*, 129(4), pp. 995-1012.

Maas, C.S., et al., 2009. Neuromodulators and injectable soft tissue substitutes. In: I. Papel, ed. *Facial plastic and reconstructive surgery*. New York, NY: Thieme. Chapter 28, pp. 337-53.

Meyer, T.K. and Blitzer, A. 2009. Botulinum toxin for facial wrinkles. In: I. Papel, ed. Facial plastic and reconstructive surgery New York, NY: Thieme. Chapter 30, pp. 369-77.

Small, R., 2012a. A practical guide to botulinum toxin procedures. Philadelphia, PA: Lippincott Williams.

Small, R., 2012b. A practical guide to dermal filler procedures. Philadelphia, PA: Lippincott Williams.

22 Lasers and IPL in Facial Plastics

PP Cheang, A D'Souza

Chapter Overview

Pearls and Pitfalls

Pearls

- Be familiar with the chromophore that is targeted, in order to select the appropriate laser.
- Take a detailed skin and tanning history, as appearances sometimes can be deceiving.
- Perform a test patch in a non-conspicuous area to ascertain the appropriate laser parameters.
- Consider antiviral prophylaxis in ablative and fractional ablative laser treatment.

Pitfalls

- Beware of dark skin tones, use lower fluence and longer wavelengths.
- PIH is common in Fitzpatrick 3 and above.
- Aggressive treatment with laser will produce long-lasting erythema, resulting in PIH.
- Postoperative sun exposure can lead to severe hyperpigmentation.

22.1 INTRODUCTION

Ever since the emergence of the first laser in 1960, there has been a significant explosion in laser technology. The choice of devices now can encompass the entire electromagnetic spectrum. Currently, lasers, light-based treatment such as intense pulsed light (IPL) plus an array of other heat technologies form a myriad of choices for the modern facial plastic surgeon in the treatment of skin aging. Improvement in light and laser-based technology has allowed the physician to treat not only signs of aging, such as rhytids, pigmentations, and lentigines, but also for addressing vascular lesions, scars, skin texture irregularities, and skin laxity.

22.2 ESSENTIAL CONCEPTS

Laser

Laser stands for **L**ight **A**mplification by **S**timulated **E**mission of **R**adiation. They are an intense build-up of a photon cascade created when photons are dropped down from a metastable state to the ground state. The metastable state is an in-between, long-lived energy state acquired when photos are first excited by electrical energy, chemical energy, and radio frequency waves or light.

There are three characteristics that define laser:

1. Monochromatic (same wavelength)
2. Coherent (same temporal and spatial phase)
3. Collimated (parallel)

The use of laser in the face is based on the concept of *selective photothermolysis*, proposed by R Anderson and JA Parrish in 1983. There are three main principles associated with this:

1. The wavelength of light is preferentially absorbed by the desired target structure (*chromophore*) and can penetrate the tissue sufficiently to reach that structure.
2. Pulse duration or exposure time is less than or equal to the time necessary for cooling of the target structures.
3. Sufficient *fluence* (energy density) is used to reach an irreversibly damaging temperature within the target structure.

Once the laser beam reaches the skin surface, four outcomes can occur:

1. Absorption
   In the therapeutic sense, the aim is for the laser light to be absorbed by the target tissue. Absorption of this laser energy leads to the controlled destruction of the target, without significant damage to the surrounding tissues. These specific light-absorbing targets are known as chromophores. The three main chromophores in the body are *melanin*, (oxy) hemoglobin, and water. The amount of light that gets absorbed depends on the wavelength of the laser used and the absorption spectrum of the specific targeted chromophore (Fig. 22.1).
   Light that is not absorbed is reflected, scattered, or transmitted—none of these have any biological effect.
2. Reflection
   Reflection occurs when light hits the skin at an angle. Approximately 5% of the laser beam will be reflected from the stratum corneum, particularly if the skin is dry and scaly. This is the reason why protective eye shields are required when working with lasers. To minimize reflection, light beam should be directed perpendicularly to the skin. Clear gel or oil can be applied to dry skin. There should be no reflective surfaces nearby.
3. Scattering
   Once laser has passed the stratum corneum, light can scatter within the tissue matter. Scattering defocuses the light, resulting in spreading of the beam and causing irradiation of a larger area. Scattering occurs predominantly within the dermis and happens more with shorter wavelength. Longer wavelength penetrates deeper into the skin, causes less scattering, and therefore less thermal damage. Consequently, the choice of a specific laser will depend on the depth of the desired tissue target.
4. Transmission
   Light energy not absorbed, reflected, or scattered will be transmitted to deeper structures such as the subcutaneous layer. This happens predominantly in longer

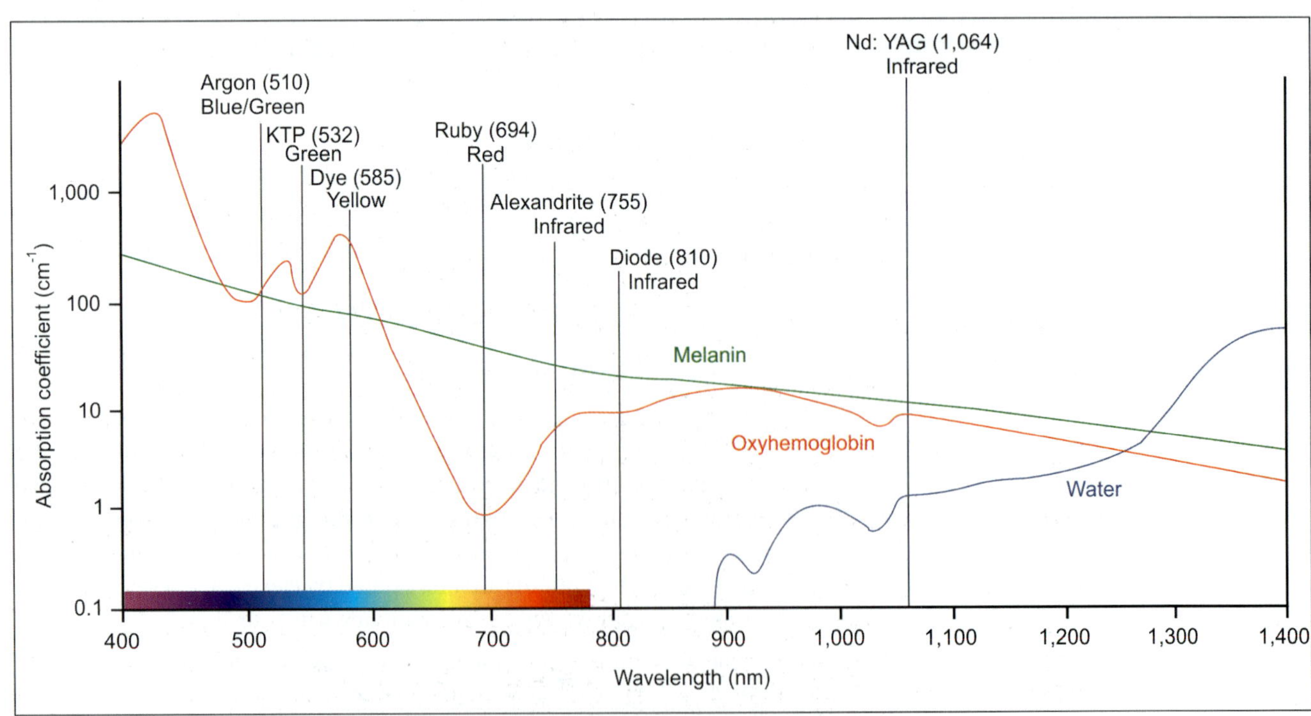

Fig. 22.1: Absorption spectra of the three main skin chromophores.

wavelength, as shorter wavelengths of 300–400 nm will already have been scattered. Depth of penetration of the laser light increases with increasing wavelength. However, at high water absorption wavelengths (2940 nm), penetration is decreased as light is trapped in the upper layers of the skin where water is most abundant.

The concept of selective thermolysis depends on the following laser parameters:

1. Wavelength
   As mentioned above, the wavelength of the laser chosen needs to correspond to the absorption maximum, or lie within the absorption spectrum of the intended target chromophore (Fig. 22.1).
   Melanin has a decreasing absorption spectrum from 400 nm to 750 nm. The absorption spectrum of hemoglobin is from 400 nm to 600 nm, with absorption peaks of oxyhemoglobin at 418, 548, and 577 nm. Water shows increasing absorption at mid- to far-infrared portion of the spectrum.
2. Pulse duration
   Pulse duration, also known as 'pulse width' of the laser beam, is the time needed for energy to go from zero intensity to maximum intensity and back to zero. Clinically, the pulse duration used is related to the *thermal relaxation time* (TRT) of the target chromophore. The TRT is the time needed for the chromophore to disseminate 63% of its peak temperature. Or in other words, in a heated region of tissue, TRT is the time required for the peak temperature to decrease to 37% of the total rise.
   Smaller targets have shorter TRTs. The TRTs of some common chromophores are listed in Table 22.1. The laser pulse duration must be shorter or equal to the TRT of the target chromophore to allow for selective damage (Allemann and Kaufman, 2011).
   The laser light can be delivered either in a continuous wave or in a pulsed wave. The continuous wave light is emitted over an uninterrupted period of time. Truly pulsed lasers are high powered, emitting ultrashort single pulses with extremely high energies. Measurements are from nanoseconds to milliseconds. This is different to the manipulated continuous beams where mechanically shutters serve to produce interrupted beams. These shorter emission times are of the duration between 1 ms and 1 s. The concept of selective photothermolysis only applies to pulsed lasers as continuous laser light leads to bulk heating and nonselective tissue damage.

Table 22.1: Thermal relaxation times (TRTs) of common laser targets.

	Size (μm)	*TRT (approximate)*
Tattoo ink particle	0.5–4	10 ns
Melanosome	0.5–1	1 μs
Erythrocyte	7	2 μs
Blood vessel	50	1 ms
Blood vessel	100	5 ms
Blood vessel	200	20 ms
Hair follicle	200	10–100 ms

3. Fluence
   Energy density or fluence is defined as the energy applied per unit area (J/cm^2).
   Fluence (J/cm^2) = Power density × time, where
   Power density = $W/\pi\ r^2$ (power applied to per unit area) and
   Energy (J) = Power (W) × Time (s)
   The fluence delivered by the laser beam must be high enough to actually destroy the target chromophore within the defined pulse width.
4. Spot size
   This is the diameter of the laser beam, measured in millimeters. Spot size influences the fluence as well as the depth of penetration and the scattering of the laser beam. Power density = $W/\pi\ r^2$ (power applied to per unit area). Thus, the fluence is inversely proportional to the square of the radius of the spot size.
   Decreasing the spot size by half will increase the fluence by a power of 4. Furthermore, smaller spot size has less penetration and therefore scatters more. To maintain the same energy density with a smaller spot size, the fluence would have to be reduced by a factor of 4.
   Based on these concepts, the wavelength, pulse duration, fluence, and spot size must all be tailored to the properties of the target chromophore and clinical indication to achieve a satisfactory outcome and reduce complications. In most cases, the clinical target and the target chromophore are the same. The only exception is in laser hair removal, which is discussed below in its relevant section.

Ablative versus Nonablative Lasers

In skin resurfacing, lasers used are broadly categorized into ablative and nonablative lasers. Ablative lasers remove the outer layers of aged or photo-damaged skin.

Dermal heating results in denaturation and modification of collagen structure, stimulating neocollagenesis thus improving the appearance of fine rhytids and skin that had begun to lose its elasticity. Ablative lasers like CO_2 and erbium-doped yttrium aluminum garnet (Er:YAG) continue to be the gold standard for treating fine facial rhytids and photoaging.

Nonablative skin rejuvenation refers to the techniques of achieving dermal heating indirectly through an intact epidermis. Nonablative systems can utilize light (IPL), thermal energy (lasers, radio frequency), or ultrasound. Each differs in its derived energy field, but the resultant energy-tissue interaction is similar. Tissue penetration and thermal injury are to the level of dermis and subcutaneous layer, without producing burns to the epidermis. Dermal neocollagenesis induced this way thus serves to limit adverse effects and reduces the recovery period significantly.

Light-based nonablative systems can be divided into three main categories: visible lasers such as the pulsed-dye laser (PDL), mid-infrared lasers, and IPL.

The PDL was used primarily as a vascular laser. When it was noticed that hypertrophic and acne scars showed clinical improvement with collagen changes histologically (Alexiades-Armenakas, Dover and Arndt, 2008), its role in the treatment of photo-damaged skin was suggested. The PDL at 585 nm and 595 nm was used to treat rhytids, but the results have been modest compared to the ablative systems. Since it is predominantly vascular targeting, it has only superficial penetration to the papillary dermis.

Infrared lasers such as the neodymium-doped yttrium aluminum garnet (Nd:YAG) at 1064 and 1320 nm were the prototype of nonablative rejuvenation. The majority of the studies using these two lasers showed mild but reproducible improvement in perioral and periorbital rhytids. Histology analysis after treatment from the 1450 nm diode laser and 1540 nm erbium-doped phosphate glass laser also demonstrated increase in dermal thickness, correlating with increase in dermal collagen following laser rejuvenation using infrared wavelengths (Alexiades-Armenakas, Dover and Arndt, 2008).

Intense Pulsed Light

Intense pulsed light systems are high intensity light sources emitting noncoherent light with a broad wavelength (515–1200 nm). They are not lasers but are similarly based on the principle of selective photothermolysis. The core technology involves the use of polychromatic broadband flash lamps equipped with optical filters. As multiple wavelengths are delivered, multiple chromophores can be targeted with the same light exposure—melanin, hemoglobin, water, and collagen. Theoretically, they can be used to treat vascular lesions, pigmentations, and dermal atrophy in the same setting. However in practice, there is the complexity in selecting cutoff filters to be more specific in treating the intended target and also to prevent shorter wavelength from leaking through and causing epidermal damage.

The IPL is mainly used in treating vascular lesions and pigmentations, as well as skin rejuvenation in some cases. Rhytid improvement with IPL devices is modest. However, as IPL is able to target both melanin and hemoglobin, there is global improvement in dyspigmentation and vascularity. This serves to increase the patients' perception of improvement, as improvement in pigmentation and vascularity is more easily detectable than mild changes in rhytids (Ciocon, Boket and Goldberg, 2009).

Other Heat Technologies

This group includes technologies that deliver low-level heat to the deep dermis layer for collagen shrinkage and skin tightening effect. These can be radio frequency systems (Thermage, Pelleve) delivering electrical energy, pulsed infrared light (Titan), or ultrasound (Ulthera). They can be used in combination with infrared lasers or IPL concomitantly.

22.3 REGION: FACE

Anatomy of the Skin

Covering the entire body, the skin is our principal barrier to the external world. There are two layers of the skin: the epidermis and the dermis. The epidermis is further separated into five strata from superficial to deep: corneum, lucidum, granulosum, spinosum, and basale. Thickness of the epidermis varies by individual and body location, with the thinnest skin on the eyelid and the thickest on the palm and sole. The dermis consists of a superficial papillary and a deeper reticular part. The adnexal structures (hair follicles, eccrine sweat glands, and apocrine sweat glands) contain epithelial stem cells that are essential for healing.

Important components of the skin include collagen, elastin, glycosaminoglycans (GAGs), and dermal water. Collagen is the main determinant of skin tensile strength, with type I collagen the most abundant. Elastic fibers are responsible for skin elasticity. The GAGs are the major

Table 22.2: Fitzpatrick skin type.

Fitzpatrick skin type	*Response to sun exposure*	*Examples*
I	Always sunburn Do not tan	Fair-skinned, freckled Blue-eyed Celts
II	Always sunburn Tan minimally	Fair-skinned, blonde-haired Blue-eyed Scandinavians
III	Sometimes burn Tan moderately	Fair-skinned, brown hair Brown-eyed Unexposed skin is white
IV	Seldom burn Tan easily	Light brown skin, dark brown hair Brown-eyed Unexposed skin is tan Mediterranean, Hispanic
V	Rarely burn Tan profusely	Brown skinned Darker Mediterranean Orientals, Eastern Indians
VI	Never sunburn Deeply pigmented	Africans

components of the dermal ground substance, binding to water molecules extensively. They are the major determinant of dermal hydration. Dermal water is essential for the proper structural configuration and function of proteins and is extensively bound in younger skins.

Fitzpatrick Skin Types

Fitzpatrick devised a classification of skin types (Papel, 2009), taking into account the skin color and reaction to sun exposure (Table 22.2). Those with lighter skin are more likely to develop postoperative erythema, whereas those with darker skin type are more at risk of postinflammatory hyperpigmentation or hypopigmentation.

22.4 PRESENTATION: RHYTIDS

Aging Process

Like all organs, the skin undergoes a natural, chronological aging process. This process is influenced by both intrinsic and extrinsic factors. Extrinsic factors of aging include sun exposure, which has a cumulative effect, and lifestyle factors such as smoking. Nicotine causes vasoconstriction of the dermal plexus, increases carboxyhemoglobin, and results in elastosis and telangiectasia as both collagen and elastin in the dermis are reduced.

Intrinsic factors that affect aging are mainly our genetic makeup, ethnicity, and hormonal changes. Pigmented skin confers more protection against ultraviolet light and may contribute to more resistance in aging. The degree of aging varies in different races due to differences in skin characteristics, e.g. wrinkling in Orientals has been documented to occur later and with less severity than in Caucasians (Farage, et al., 2008). A reduction in estrogen in postmenopausal women causes reduced synthesis of collagen and elastin.

As we age, the skin becomes thinner. This thinning is predominantly in the dermis alongside a decrease in subcutaneous fat. The size and metabolic rate of fibroblasts are reduced, bringing about a reduction in collagen synthesis. The collagen fibers produced are also more fragmented, thickened, and loosely woven. The ratio of collagen III to collagen I increases by 30% after 65 years. This results in a reduced potential for stretching.

Chronic *photodamage* also causes the synthesis of structurally and functionally abnormal elastic fibers, which degrade slower, accounting for the decrease in skin elasticity. The GAGs are increased but clumped together, abnormally localized to the superficial band of elastic material, resulting in inefficient water binding. Total dermal water is increased in photo-damaged skin, but in its unbound form, it is unable to interact with other dermal structural components.

The above process results in skin appearance that is dry and wrinkly, with a yellowish hue. The decrease in dermal matrix and elasticity of dermal blood vessels can cause easy bruising and senile purpura. Pigmentary irregularities are also common, be it hyperpigmentation (melanin) or hypopigmentation (scarring). Together with *actinic keratoses*, *telangiectasia*, and wrinkles, they form the hallmark of aging.

Classification of Rhytids

Wrinkles, or rhytids, are what bothers most patients when they age. *Rhytids* may be static (present at rest) or dynamic (dependent on muscle movement). The commonest rhytidosis scale used is the *Glogau classification* (Glogau, 1996):

1. Mild — Little or no wrinkles
2. Moderate — Early wrinkling (dynamic wrinkles)
3. Advanced — Persistent wrinkling (static wrinkles)
4. Severe — Severe wrinkling, gravitational, and dynamic forces affecting the skin

Laser treatment is indicated for static and not dynamic wrinkles.

Treatment Options

Ablative Laser Skin Resurfacing

Laser skin resurfacing is extremely effective in treating photoaging, improving the appearance of periorbital and perioral rhytids, dyspigmentation, vascularity, and elastosis. The chromophore in skin is water; hence, these lasers act by targeting intracellular water, in the process ablating a layer of photo-damaged skin in a precise fashion. To control the depth of thermal damage that occurs in tissue, the pulse duration needs to be <1 ms. Sufficient energy must be delivered within this time to achieve tissue vaporization.

The CO_2 laser operates at a wavelength of 10600 nm, which is in the near-infrared region. Early low power systems (<1000 W) required longer on-times, with the potential of causing deeper thermal damage and resulting in scarring frequently. Since the early 1990s, newer, high-energy CO_2 laser can be used in extremely short pulses (<1 ms), resulting in more precise vaporization. It has been calculated that the necessary fluence to achieve pulsed-laser ablation of skin tissue is 5 J/cm^2. The result is little heat damage to deeper structures and char-free tissue removal.

Each pulse of the CO_2 laser removes 100 microns (±40 microns) of tissue. One pass may be enough for mild rhytids or sun damage, but three passes are needed to effectively reduce wrinkles and scars in moderate-to-severe cases. The only exception is in the eyelids where no more than two passes should be used. Gentle wiping of the desiccated debris in between passes is important, as any water remaining on the skin may absorb laser energy and block it targeting the dermal tissue. Clinical end point is reached when yellow chamois-looking skin is seen, signifying reticular dermis.

Re-epithelialization starts from the undamaged epithelial cells lining the adnexal structures of the skin. In the following 7–10 days, new collagen and elastic fibers reform in the upper dermis, further tightening the skin. Complete recovery may require 1 month. Thus, the patient downtime is significant in a fully ablative CO_2 laser. A multitude of CO_2 laser systems are available on the market. Most reports have shown significant improvement in photoaged skin regardless of the system used. Most patients with wrinkles attain a 50–90% improvement (Alexiades-Armenakas, Dover and Arndt, 2008).

The next ablative laser developed for skin resurfacing was the *Er:YAG laser*. Emitting a wavelength of 2940 nm, it is near the largest absorption peak by the water molecule and has a higher affinity for water. This makes it more capable of removing extremely thin layer of tissue, with scant thermal damage. However, as there is smaller depth of penetration, less collagen shortening is stimulated. A single pulse of the Er:YAG laser at 5 J/cm^2 will ablate 20–25 microns of tissue.

Compared to the CO_2 laser, the Er:YAG laser promised more rapid healing, less discomfort, and less redness. However, the results are superficial, with limited success in removing deep winkles (Kauvar and Hruza, 2005). It also has poorer hemostasis, as penetration is not deep enough for blood vessel coagulation. Bleeding increases with successive passes with the Er:YAG laser, where it is virtually bloodless with CO_2 laser. The overall efficacy of the Er:YAG laser is comparable to the CO_2 laser, but the CO_2 laser is still the more superior system in most comparative studies.

Complications of Ablative Lasers

- Erythema and edema
  Erythema occurs during the healing phase when skin starts to re-epithelialize. It lasts for at least 1 month but can be as long as 6 months. The Er:YAG has a shorter duration of erythema and edema than the CO_2 laser, typically lasting 2–4 weeks.
- Pruritus
  This can happen in 90% of patients. Oral antihistamine can be prescribed if there is no evidence of fungal colonization.
- Infection
  Patients may develop bacterial (*Staphylococcus aureus, Pseudomonas*), fungal (*Candida*), or viral (herpes simplex) infection. Most infections are temporary and can be managed by appropriate topical or systemic treatment.
- Dyschromia
  Transient hyperpigmentation is common. It happens overall in 36% of all skin types but 100% in skin type IV and above patients. Post inflammatory hyperpigmentation starts 30 days after laser ablation. Hypopigmentation occurs late, 6–12 months post-treatment, and mostly in those with skin types I and II and in cases with prolonged erythema.
- Permanent scarring
  Mainly occurs as a result of infection, or when the depth of ablation is too deep. This happens in <1% of cases. Scarring can be treated with topical/intralesional steroids. Special caution with a reduced number of passes or reduced fluence should be used in the treatment of specific areas like the eyes or the neck.

Nonablative Lasers

As mentioned earlier, nonablative systems include vascular lasers, midinfrared lasers, and IPL. The advantage of nonablative methods is the ease of postoperative care. Post-treatment erythema and edema are minimal, resolve within hours, with the patients able to return to normal daily activities immediately. The drawback is that it induces dermal changes only, with limited benefit for those who have both epidermal and dermal changes secondary to photoaging. The improvement is mild and nonspecific, with multiple treatments required to provide minimal incremental improvement.

Fractional Resurfacing

Fractional photothermolysis is the latest technology in laser skin resurfacing. The concept behind this approach is to thermally alter a fraction of the skin, leaving intervening areas of normal skin. The areas of thermal damage are in the forms of arrays of columns, known as microscopic thermal zones (MTZs). The MTZs comprise approximately 15–25% of the skin surface area per treatment session. The uninjured tissue that surrounds these columns then serves to repopulate the ablated columns by fibroblast activity and neocollagenesis as in ablative laser resurfacing.

The advantages of fractional laser lie in the fact that it causes lower epidermal and dermal thermal damage. There is preservation of the overlying stratum corneum, with coagulation of dermal blood vessels. Erythema and edema resolves within a few days. However, the improvement in rhytids and photodamage is not as significant as with ablative resurfacing, and multiple sessions spaced at 1- to 4-week intervals maybe needed.

22.5 PRESENTATION: VASCULAR LESIONS

Port Wine Stains

Port wine stains (PWS) are capillary vascular malformations. They are present in 0.3% of neonates and present at birth as cutaneous patches on the head and neck. With increasing age, the lesions grow with the child, and change their color from pink to purple. They also become thickened, darker, and nodular. Spontaneous bleeding or hemorrhage can occur by fifth decade.

Differentiation between PWS and other vascular malformations is essential in determining long-term prognosis and implementing appropriate therapy (Table 22.2). The PWS are usually isolated lesions but may be associated with serious syndromes such as *Sturge-Weber syndrome* (large facial PWS, ipsilateral leptomeningial vascular malformations, ipsilateral choroidal vascular malformations, and glaucoma) and *Klippel-Trenaunay syndrome* (capillary venous vascular malformation and hypertrophy of affected limb).

Treatment Options

Pulsed-Dye Laser

Using the principles of selective photothermolysis, the main chromophore in vascular lesions is oxyhemoglobin. Hemoglobin has absorption peaks at 418, 542, and 577 nm for oxy-, deoxy-, and methemoglobin, respectively. The strongest peak is at 418 nm (blue), but strong absorption by melanin and its limited penetration depth preclude the use of this wavelength. *Argon laser* (blue-green light 488 and 514 nm) is preferentially absorbed by oxyhemoglobin in the ectatic dermal vessels, but the long exposure time means heat can diffuse and cause injury to surrounding structures. Clinically, this produces a high incidence of scarring, atrophy, and hypopigmentation (Kauvar and Hruza, 2005).

Pulsed dye laser has a wavelength of 577 or 585 nm, providing increased depth of clearance. The treatment produces intravascular thrombosis without epidermal or dermal damage. The exposure time or pulse duration must be chosen to match the diameter of the blood vessel being treated. For most target tissues, the TRT can be approximated in seconds as the square of the target dimension in millimeters. A 0.1-mm PWS vessel should therefore cool in approximately 10^{-2} s or 10 ms. The PDL selectively damages vascular tissue with no inconsequential absorption by melanin in fair-skinned individuals.

The laser can be safely used in skin types I–IV when there is no suntan present. It cannot be used to treat skin types V and VI, because the higher density of melanin results in decreased vascular absorption and the possibility of epidermal damage.

The heterogeneity of the size and depth of blood vessels in PWS makes them difficult to treat. Range of improvement reported following PDL in children has been from 50% lightening in 87% of patients to nearly 100% clearance. In adult patients, four laser treatments resulted in >75% lightening in 36–44% of patients, with at least 50% lightening in 75% of patients.

Complications of PDL

- Reticulation
  Reticulated erythema is common when smaller spot sizes (3–5 mm) are used at high fluence, producing "footprinting" of the laser spots. The reticulation resolves after the second or third treatment. Using a larger spot size (10 mm) alleviates the problem.
- Immediate skin whitening
  This occurs as a consequence of epidermal damage due to overly aggressive laser parameters or poor skin-cooling techniques. Test sites should be carried out to determine the appropriate parameters. When graying or whitening occurs, the skin should be cooled immediately, with topical antibiotic ointment used to prevent crusting.
- Hyperpigmentation
  This is common when treating lesions on extremities or type III or IV skin. Judicious use of sunscreen and active skin-cooling techniques can decrease the incidence of hyperpigmentation.
- Hypopigmentation
  This indicates the use of aggressive laser parameters, improper skin cooling, or treatment of sun-tanned skin. Hypopigmentation is almost always transient, but it can last up to 3 months.
- Atrophic and hypertrophic scars
  Scarring rarely occurs following PDL treatment to PWS. Skin cooling is important to avoid this complication.

Intense Pulsed Light

The chromophores targeted by IPL in vascular lesions include oxyhemoglobin (predominantly found in clinically red lesions), deoxyhemoglobin (predominantly in blue lesions), and methemoglobin and therefore are suitable to treat the different kind of vascular lesions.

In the treatment of PWS, it is found that the 585 nm PDL deposits more of its energy in the superficial vessels, with less amount of light available to target the deeper vessels, limiting treatment efficacy. The IPL in contrast has variable pulse duration, and the multiple split light pulses cause additive heating, leading to coagulation of vessels of different diameters of both superficial and deep components of PWS. Hence, IPL can be used in PDL-resistant PWS cases. In a side-by-side study, both PDL and IPL were found to lighten PWS, but the PDL seemed to have better efficacy (Faurschou, et al., 2009).

Hemangioma

Hemangiomas are common benign vascular lesions of childhood. Typically, they undergo a period of rapidly enlargement by cellular proliferation, followed by involution after the first year of life. As involution is not always complete, 50% of the patients may be left with telangiectasia, epidermal atrophy, and redundant fibrofatty tissue. There is some evidence to suggest that lesions that involute slowly are more likely to leave a residuum, whereas those that involute rapidly are likely to achieve complete involution.

Treatment Options

Pulsed-Dye Laser

The PDL have become the widely used modality for treating superficial component of hemangiomas since 1989. Treatment is normally carried out during the proliferative phase of superficial hemangioma, where the laser can minimize or even halt the superficial growth. It is also useful in treating complications such as ulcers associated with superficial hemangiomas.

Laser therapy can also be used to treat residual telangiectasia and atrophic scarring, which can happen after involution of a hemangioma. The shorter exposure time and the larger spot size of a PDL are ideal for the treatment of vascular matting.

Proliferating hemangioma can cause destruction to the papillary dermis, leading to atrophy. Skin resurfacing should only be carried out after all the residual telangiectasias have been adequately treated with a PDL.

Intense Pulsed Light

The IPL systems have been used effectively to treat hemangiomas, capillary malformations, and telangiectasia. The wavelength used is of 500–670 nm for vascular lesions.

Interstitial Laser

Given the limited depth of penetration of light at 585 nm, PDL has no effect on compound or deep hemangiomas. Interstitial laser therapy, originally developed for treating malignant tumors, has since been adapted for treating deep vascular lesions. Quartz fiber coupled to a near-infrared laser (Nd: YAG) can be introduce percutaneously or transmucosally into the substance of a hemangioma, under ultrasound guidance. The epidermis and papillary dermis can be protected from thermal damage by active skin cooling.

Telangiectasia

Telangiectasia is a dilated venule, capillary or arteriole visible to the human eye, and measuring 0.1–1 mm in diameter. On the face, telangiectasia develops secondary to genetic predisposition, chronic actinic damage, collagen vascular disorders, or vascular regulation disorder such as acne rosacea. Its presentation is mainly cosmetic disfigurement.

Treatment Options

For telangiectasia in the lower extremities, sclerotherapy remains the gold standard. However, this is not effective for facial telangiectasia. The PDL and IPL are the treatment of choice, with virtually no scarring due to their vascular specificity (Figs. 22.2A and B). Erythema, flushing, and telangiectasia associated with rosacea can also be effectively treated with IPL. It is at least as effective as PDL in reducing the signs and symptoms (Table 22.3).

22.6 PRESENTATION: UNWANTED FACIAL HAIR

Since the mid-1990s, laser hair removal has become a widely accepted treatment modality for long-term hair reduction. This approach has come to rival electrolysis in successful treatment of small hair-bearing areas. To be successful in treating unwanted facial hair with lasers, one must understand the mechanism of hair growth and how lasers work to target the hair follicle.

Classification of Patients with Excess Hair

Unwanted hair can be divided into four main categories:

- Hypertrichosis
  This is excess body hair in a nonandrogen-dependent fashion. It can affect both males and females and can be further subdivided into congenital and acquired, as well as localized and generalized forms. The commonest cause is genetic and ethnicity. Other causes include metabolic conditions (porphyrias, internal malignancies), medications (minoxidil, cyclosporine, and phenytoin), and rarely tumors or malformations.
- Hirsutism
  By contrast, hirsutism is excess hair in women in androgen-dependent locations, primarily in the face. It can be either idiopathic or due to excess androgens. Excess androgens can be endogenous (polycystic ovarian syndrome, congenital adrenal hyperplasia, or adrenal tumors) or from exogenous sources.
- Unwanted facial hair
  This is by far the commonest reason for patients seeking hair removal. The acceptable amount of facial and body hair is very dependent on culture and society. Excess hair on the face or certain body parts such as the forearms and legs can be distressing to some people. It is important to understand the patient's specific concerns and expectations.
- Medical reasons
  Hair-bearing flaps for reconstruction may contain unwanted hair, which may interfere with normal function. Treatment to the donor site is therefore indicated before surgery.

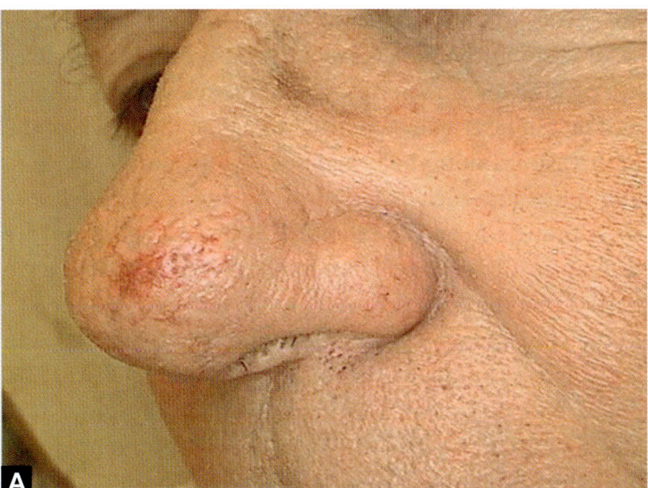

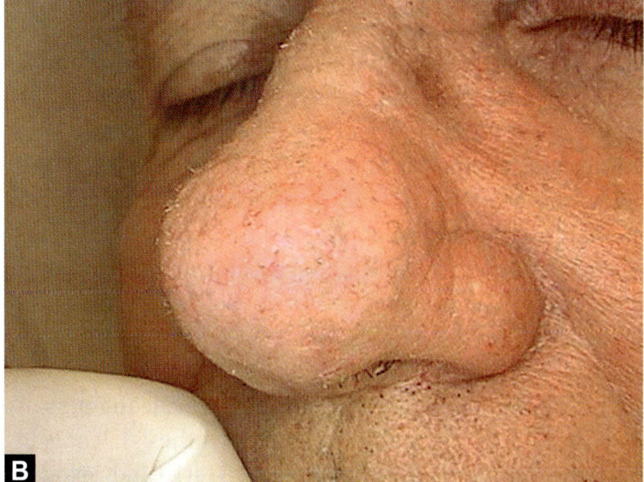

Figs. 22.2A and B: Treatment of telangiectasia by pulsed-dye laser (PDL). (A) Patient with nasal telangiectasia before and (B) after treatment with PDL.

Table 22.3: Comparison between hemangioma and vascular malformations.

Hemangioma	*Vascular malformation*
Benign vascular tumor	Malformation of blood vessels
Histology: endothelial proliferation	Ectatic dilatation of vessels in papillary dermis
Appears after birth But manifest by 6 months	Appears at birth
Proliferates in 1st year (8–18 months)	Grows with child
Involutes 2–9 years of age 75% involute by 7 years Involution may not be complete Residual telangiectasia, redundant fibrofatty tissue and epidermal hypertrophy	Does not involute
Fifty percent of capillary hemangioma in head and neck region	Associates with intracranial vascular malformation
Types: • Superficial hemangioma – Cutaneous component, bright red vascular papule • Deep Hemangioma – Subcutaneous component only – Bluish-colored nodule within the skin – No superficial red plaque • Compound hemangioma – Have both a superficial and deep component	Types: • Capillary telangiectasia – (Port wine stain) – Abnormally enlarged capillaries – Low pressure • Venous – Clusters of enlarged veins, no feeding arteries – Low pressure • Cavernous – Abnormal cluster of enlarged capillaries – No significant feeding vessels – Low pressure • Lymphatic (macro, microcystic) • AV malformation – Arteries shunt directly to veins, no capillaries, multiple feeding arteries, high pressure

Hair Biology

Anatomically, a terminal hair follicle can be divided into three sections from superior to inferior: infundibulum, isthmus, and the inferior segment. The infundibulum is the hair follicle orifice on the skin surface to the entrance of the sebaceous duct. The isthmus is the short middle section from the entrance of the sebaceous duct to where the arrector pili muscle attaches. The inferior segment lies below the arrector pili muscle attachment and includes the hair bulb and dermal papilla. The hair bulb contains germinative matrix cells and melanocytes. Melanin is produced by melanocytes within the bulb and transferred to matrix cells. The hair shaft is a cornified structure that protrudes above the surface of the skin.

Hair growth is asynchronous and cyclical. The phases of hair follicle are anagen (active synthesis), catagen (intermediary regression), telogen (rest), and exogen (shedding). Hair shaft growth and pigmentation only takes place during anagen, the duration of which is dependent on body location: anagen in the scalp lasts for 4–6 years, the upper lip 2–5 months, arms and legs 1–3 months and 4–6 months, respectively (Ross 1999). Each follicle has its own cycle, independent of adjacent follicles. During transition from anagen to catagen, there is cessation of melanin production and apoptosis of melanocytes, an important fact in laser hair removal. Moreover, the depth of the bulb varies among hair stages, 2–7 mm during anagen, and more superficially (1.5 mm) during late telogen.

Although *laser hair removal* is based again on the principles of selective photothermolysis, the difference here is that the target chromophore (melanin) is different to the clinical target (hair matrix and the stem cells). The hair matrix contains melanin, but the stem cells do not. These follicular stem cells are located in the outer root sheet, in an area called the bulge, near the attachment of the arrector pili muscle, approximately 1.5 mm below the epidermis. This means it is in close vicinity to the bulb of a terminal hair follicle during late telogen/early anagen phase. Because the depth and pigmentation of the bulb are dependent on the stage of the hair cycle, it is possible that the cycle influences the susceptibility to laser injury. Follicles should be most easily inactivated during early anagen (Goldberg, 2008).

Treatment Options

Melanin has an absorption spectrum of 600–1,100 nm. Lasers or light sources that operate in the red or near-infrared region (Ruby laser 694 nm, Alexandrite laser 755 nm, and Nd:YAG laser 1064 nm) and noncoherent light sources with cutoff filters are suitable. However, there is a caveat: melanin in the epidermis presents a competing site for absorption of the light energy, causing epidermal injury. This can be avoided by cooling the epidermis. Fortunately, follicular melanin is about 2–6 times denser than the epidermal melanin, with the highest concentration in the hair bulb.

To destroy the nonpigmented stem cells, heat must diffuse from the pigmented area (hair) to the target. Thus, the clinical target is destroyed by heat diffusion rather than by direct heating, a theory different to selective thermolysis. Melanin absorbs photons of light, becomes activated, and then releases the extra energy in the form of heat to the target tissue, in this case the hair follicle. The pulse duration therefore has to be shorter than the TRT of the hair follicle (20–30 ms), but longer than that of the hair shaft (3–5 ms), to prevent the hair shaft from vaporization and subsequent loss of chromophore.

Color contrast between epidermis and the hair shaft (and bulb) are paramount in determining the optimal wavelength. For high contrast (fair skin and dark hair), shorter wavelengths such as the Ruby laser 694 nm and Alexandrite laser 755 nm can be used. For darker skin with lighter hair, longer wavelengths should be used, such as the Nd:YAG 1064 nm (Figs. 22.3A to D).

Nonlaser light sources such as IPL devices have also been shown to be effective in hair removal. Cutoff filters can be used to achieve certain wavelengths, and thus can be altered based on the patients' skin color and hair color, and the desired depth of penetration.

Laser does not destroy hair in the resting stage of the cycle; therefore, repeated sessions are required for maximum treatment efficacy. Treatments are usually spaced 4–6 weeks apart. Even in the best candidates with dark hair and fair skin, permanent hair removal is not possible. However, the bulb damage results in induction of catagen and telogen, with subsequent hair growth becoming lighter and finer. In the majority of patients, permanent hair reduction is achieved, with only one or two sessions being required annually for maintenance.

22.7 PRESENTATION: FACIAL DYSCHROMIA

Different types of pigmentations can occur in the face, causing patients to seek advice and treatment. The common pigmentations seen include solar lentigos (age spots), ephelides (freckles), seborrheic keratoses, pigmented nevi, melasma, and birth marks. Care must be taken to evaluate these and differentiate them from a malignant process.

Treatment Options

The IPL has been reported to be one of the most effective light-based methods for the treatment of melanocytic hyperpigmentation. The primary advantage of light-based treatments is that most hyperpigmented lesions can be removed completely in one or two treatments. Darker lesions and lesions in the deeper layer of the dermis would require more number of treatments.

The localization of the pigment target is a key determinant for the selection of the appropriate therapeutic wavelength. The PDL has less penetration than IPL, making it more appropriate for pigmented epidermal lesions. With the use of different filters, the IPL device is capable of emitting wavelength spectra in the ranges 870–1400 nm for pigmented lesions. The immediate end point from IPL treatment of dyschromia should be visible darkening of the treated brown spots. These typically crust over 24 to 48 hours and peel off within 7 days.

For junctional or dermal lesions, Q-switched lasers (Ruby, Alexandrite, and Nd:YAG) are more effective. In Q-switched lasers, energy is stored in the laser medium during its off interval. This enables the delivery of pulses with extremely high-peak power in nanoseconds, resulting in deeper dermal penetration. It is particularly useful in treating melasma and lentigines.

22.8 PRESENTATION: HYPERTROPHIC SCARS

Although there is a role for laser in the treatment of scars, the mechanism remains unclear. It is thought that laser helps to remove pigment within the scar by inducing capillary destruction. The chromophore in this case is hemoglobin. Fibroblast modulation subsequently occurs,

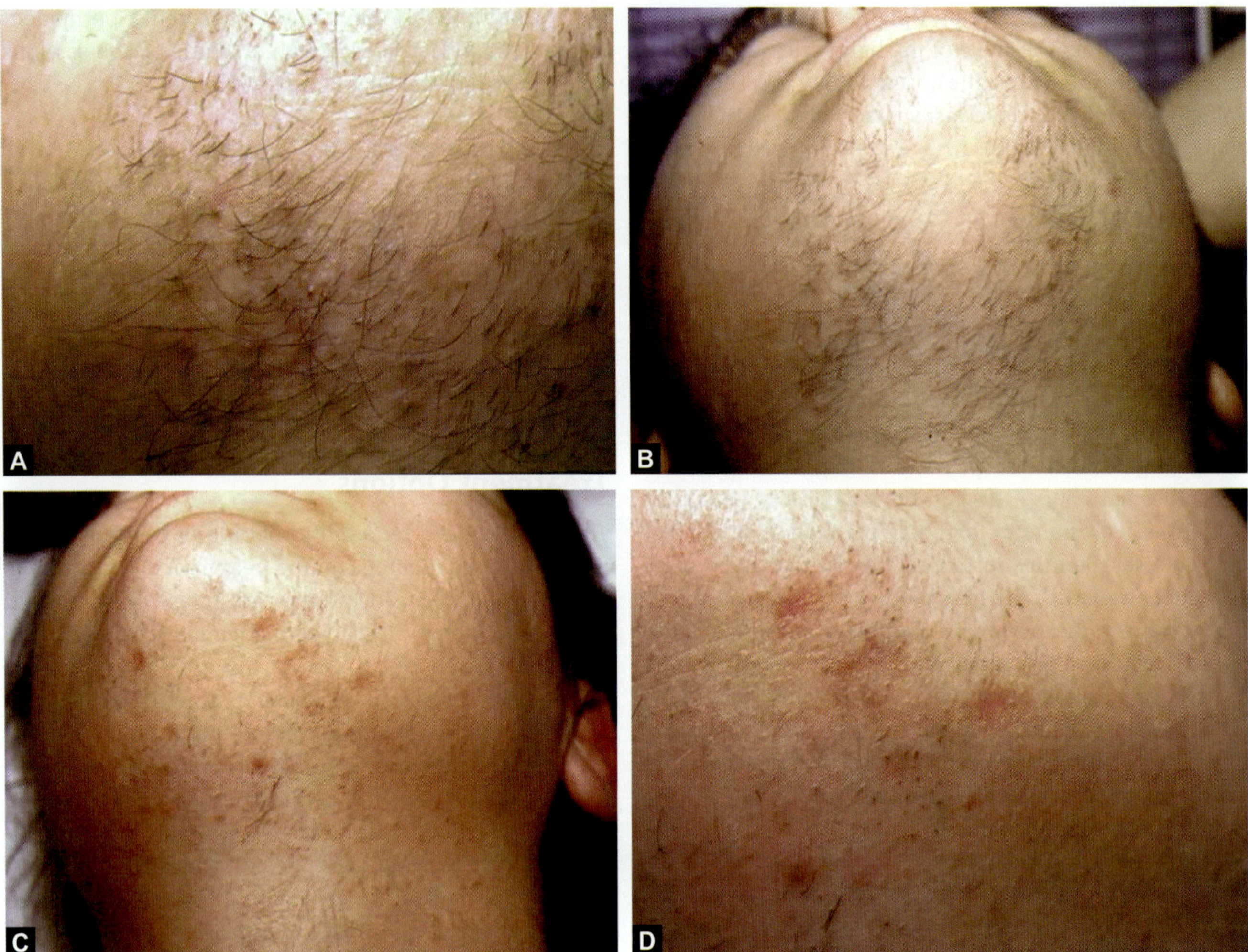

Figs. 22.3A to D: Laser hair removal before (A and B) and after six treatments (C and D). For Fitzpatrick type I–III, 755-nm Alexandrite is recommended. If the patient is a Fitzpatrick type IV–VI, the first choice would be the 1064 Nd:YAG. (Nd:YAG: Neodymium-doped yttrium aluminum garnet).

resulting in remodeling of collagen and ultimately scar improvement (DiBernarnardo and Pozner, 2009).

Treatment Options

The PDL is the treatment of choice for scar revision. Two to six treatment sessions are necessary, with improvement seen in scar color, height, texture, and pliability. Side effects are minimal, with purpura the most common complication. This can last for 7–14 days. Depending on the energy density employed, vesicles and crusting could also occur. Hyperpigmentation is a risk in darker skin types. The 1064 nm Nd:YAG has also been utilized. Its penetration depth is greater than PDL, but its efficacy reduces with thicker scars. Also in terms of improving the fresh, highly vascularized appearance of scars, PDL is still the recommended choice. Intralesional steroid can be used in conjunction with laser treatment.

22.9 FUTURE TRENDS

Laser technology is advancing at a remarkable rate in the field of aesthetic surgery. The future trend sees us marching toward less invasive technologies and using combining treatments. Fractional resurfacing is gaining more popularity due to its remarkably short recovery time. Research is also being carried out on combining fractional laser with photodynamic therapy, as the ablative columns created by fractional resurfacing facilitate the delivery of phototherapy agent.

There will always be a strong patient demand for the nonablative rejuvenation, with minimum downtime associated. The results produced from current nonablative systems are still modest compared to what can be achieved in ablative laser resurfacing. With time, it is hoped that a truly effective noninvasive methods can be found.

REFERENCES

Alexiades-Armenakas, M.R., Dover, J.S. and Arndt, K.A., 2008. The spectrum of laser skin resurfacing: nonablative, fractional and ablative laser resurfacing. *Journal of American Academy of Dermatology*, 58(5), pp. 719-37.

Allemann, I.B. and Kaufman, J., 2011. Laser principles. *Current Problems in Dermatology*, 42, pp. 7-23.

Ciocon, D.H., Boker, A. and Goldberg, D.J., 2009. Intense pulsed light: what works, what's new, what's next. *Facial Plastic Surgery*, 25(5), pp. 290-300.

DiBernarnardo, B.E. and Pozner, J.N., 2009. *Lasers and nonsurgical rejuvenation*. Spain: Elsevier.

Farage, M.A., Miller, K.W., Elsner, P. and Malbach, H.I., 2008. Intrinsic and extrinsic factors in skin ageing: a review. *International Journal of Cosmetic Science*, 30, pp. 87-95.

Faurschou, A., Togsverd-Bo, K., Zachariae, C. and Haedersdal, M., 2009. Pulsed dye laser vs. intense pulsed light for port-wine stains: a randomised side-by-side trial with blinded response evaluation. *British Journal of Dermatology*, 160, pp. 359-64.

Glogau, R.G., 1996. Aesthetic and anatomic analysis of the aging skin. *Seminars in Cutaneous Medicine and Surgery*, 15(3), pp. 134-8.

Goldberg, D.J., 2008. *Laser dermatology pearls and problems*, Oxford: Blackwell Publishing.

Kauvar, A.N.B. and Hruza, G.J., 2005. *Principles and practices in cutaneous laser surgery*. Florida: Taylor & Francis Group.

Papel, I., 2009. *Facial plastic and reconstructive surgery*. 3rd ed. New York: Thieme Medical Publishers.

Ross, E.V., Ladin, Z., Kernel, M. and Derrick, C., 1999. Theoretical considerations in laser hair removal. *Dermatologic Clinics*, 17(2), pp. 333-56.

Brow Ptosis and Its Management

23

Sandeep Uppal

Chapter Overview

Pearls and Pitfalls

Pearls

- Long-term success rate in brow lift is reduced in patients with developmental low brows and/or exceptionally high foreheads in whom concealed incisions have to be placed remote from the brow.
- Longevity of brow lift is improved when permanent cranial fixation of inferior forehead flap periosteum is performed to unicortical bony tunnels with a braided polyester suture.
- Only bipolar diathermy should be used near the hair follicles, and that too discreetly, to prevent irreversible hair follicle damage and postoperative alopecia.
- Avoid midforehead and direct brow lift incisions in patients with thick sebaceous skin as these patients are more prone to unsightly scars.
- Remove the Rainey clips only with special clip removers, and definitely not by pulling them off the scalp, to minimize bleeding at the time of closure.
- The results of corrugator myotomy during transblepharoplasty brow lift can be made more durable by placing an interposition fat graft between the cut ends of the muscle.
- It is difficult to correct asymmetrical brows because of asymmetrical development of the bony orbits. The right brow and/or orbit are lower in 85% of patients, and the left in 7% of patients.

Pitfalls

- Performing blepharoplasty in the presence of pseudodermatochalasis leading to upper lid fullness worsens brow ptosis. Thorough preoperative assessment of the entire forehead, brows, and eyes should be performed to differentiate dermatochalasis from pseudodermatochalasis.
- Aggressive resection of brow depressors can produce noticeable irregularities in the skin on redraping; hence it should be avoided.

23.1 INTRODUCTION

The periorbital area plays an important role in conveying an impression of a person's vitality, age, expression, and mood. The eyebrows form an aesthetic unit within this broad region and frame this area superiorly. The upper one third of the face is the first area in which the earliest signs of aging become apparent. Patient's often present with droopy eyelids and/or visual problems secondary to brow ptosis with or without excessive upper eyelid skin. Slight improvements in this area can translate into excellent aesthetic results. However, even minor imperfections are perceptible and aesthetically unpleasing.

23.2 SURGICAL ANATOMY OF THE FOREHEAD, BROW, AND EYE

Layers of Scalp

The scalp is composed of five layers from the superficial to deep plane. These are as follows:

1. **S**kin
2. **C**onnective tissue (dense): subcutaneous tissue
3. **A**poneurosis: galea aponeurotica
4. **L**oose areolar tissue (connective tissue)
5. **P**ericranium (periosteum)

Although both the subgaleal and subpericranial planes are avascular and easy to dissect, subperiosteal plane is relatively more difficult to dissect because of two reasons: (1) the periosteum is firmly attached to the underlying scalp bones; (2) the subgaleal plane is distensible, whereas the periosteum is robust and less pliable.

Galea aponeurotica is a continuation of the superficial musculoaponeurotic system (SMAS) layer in the neck and face. SMAS is substantial over the parotid and neck but becomes very thin over the zygomatic arch. In the temporal area SMAS is represented by the temporoparietal fascia (TPF), which lies superficial to the superficial layer of deep temporal fascia (DTF) and directly underneath the skin and subcutaneous tissue. The SMAS then continues as galea in the scalp, which splits to ensheathe the frontalis, occipitalis, and periauricular muscles. The transition between the TPF and galea occurs at the temporal fusion line.

The periosteum over the frontal bones fuses to form the arcus marginalis at the supraorbital rim and then becomes continuous with the periorbita and orbital septum. It is essential that these decussating fibers of arcus marginalis be released for satisfactory and durable brow lift results.

The DTF fuses with the periosteum at the temporal ridge. At about 2 cm superior to the zygomatic arch, the DTF splits into the superficial and deep layers. The intermediate fat pad lies deep to the superficial layer of DTF, whereas the deep temporal fat pad lies deep to the deep layer. It is important that the surgeon does not violate the deep layer of DTF; otherwise, atrophy of the deep temporal fat pad and resultant temporal wasting may ensue.

Neurovascular Bundles

Temporal Branch of the Facial Nerve

The temporal branch of the facial nerve (Fig. 23.1A), which innervates the frontalis muscle, lies within the TPF. The temporal branch emerges from the substance of the parotid gland and travels beneath the parotid-masseteric fascia, and then crosses the zygomatic arch at a deep plane overlying the periosteum (Fig. 23.1B). As it crosses the zygoma, the nerve divides into multiple distinct branches, which anastomose with one another as they course superiorly (Sabini, Wayne and Quatela, 2003). Over the zygomatic arch, the posterior ramus of the temporal branch lies at a distance of roughly 1.7 cm anterior to the porion and the anterior ramus 1.2 cm posterior to the zygomaticofrontal suture line and 2.54 cm lateral to the lateral canthus (Fig. 23.1A) (Davies, et al., 2012).

Above the zygomatic arch the parotid-masseteric fascia merges into the innominate fascia within the area of adhesion between the TPF and superficial layer of DTF. The temporal branches course through the innominate fascia to reach the undersurface of the TPF to its entrance to the frontalis muscle, which it supplies through its undersurface. The nerve is located within 2 mm of the various vessels that cross from the subcutaneous plane, through the TPF to DTF in the temporal region (Sabini, Wayne and Quatela, 2003). Sentinel vein (Fig. 23.2), which is one of the larger of these vessels, is encountered during endoscopic brow lift and midface lift procedures, and is a surgical landmark for the temporal branch of the facial nerve. Sentinel vein is encountered in the region of superolateral orbital rim, near the tail of the non-ptotic brow.

The inferior temporal septum (ITS) extends from the lateral corner of the temporal ligamentous adhesion (TLA) toward the external acoustic meatus. The potential space between the ITS and the superior temporal septum (STS) does not contain any major branches of the temporal branch of facial nerve. Hence, this area may be dissected without direct visualization. The ITS forms the superior border of a triangular compartment between the superficial temporal fascia and the underlying DTF and contains some branches of the zygomaticotemporal nerve, the sentinel vein, and the temporal branches of the facial nerve within a fatty layer. The DTF divides itself into superficial and deep components above the level of the ITS (Fig. 23.1B).

To avoid injury to the temporal branch of facial nerve, the surgeon must choose a plane of dissection, which is either deep or superficial to TPF. For the bitemporal or

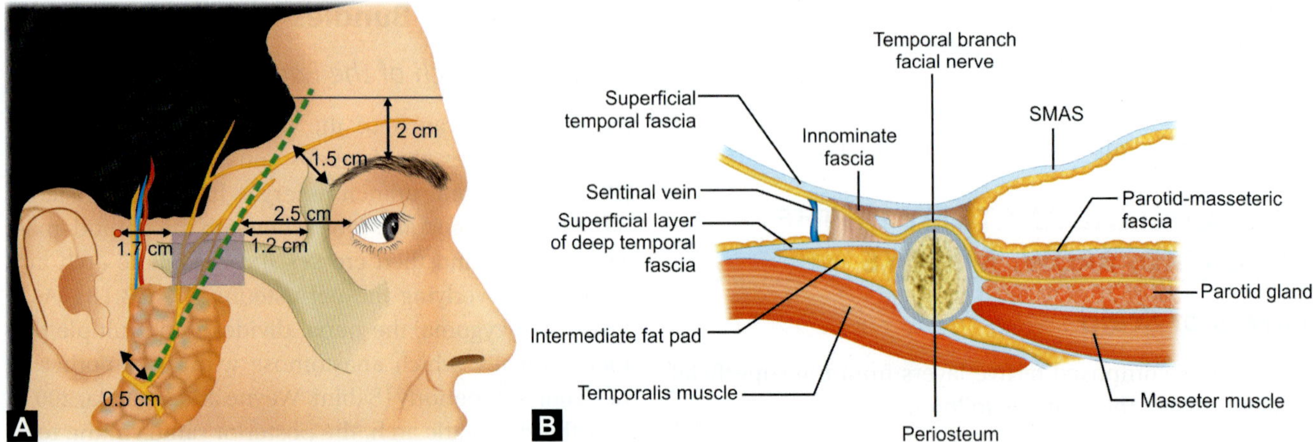

Figs. 23.1A and B: (A) Topography of the temporal branch of the facial nerve and its relationship to the helical root, lateral orbital rim, zygomatic arch, and eyebrow. A rough surface landmark for the facial nerve is Pitanguy's line which is drawn between a point 0.5 cm inferior to the tragus to a point 1.5 cm superior and lateral to the eyebrow (dotted green line). (B) Note the relationship between the facial nerve, temporoparietal fascia, deep temporal fascia, and sentinel vein. (SMAS: Superficial musculoaponeurotic system).

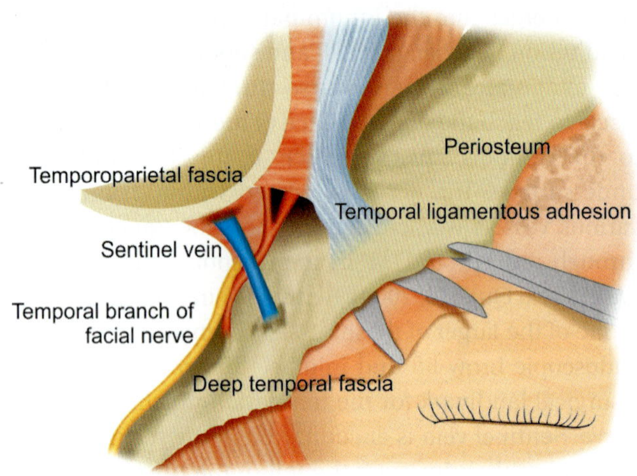

Fig. 23.2: Relationship between the facial nerve, deep temporal fascia, sentinel vein, temporoparietal fascia, temporal ligamentous adhesion, and periosteum in the region of the temporal fusion line. *Source*: Modified from Henderson, J.L., Larrabee, W.F., 2007. Analysis of the upper face and selection of rejuvenation techniques. *Otolaryngol Clin N Am*, 40, pp. 255–65.

endoscopic brow lift approach, a subgaleal or subperiosteal plane of dissection is chosen medial to the temporal line of fusion. In the temporal area, injury to facial nerve is avoided by staying superficial to the superficial layer of DTF in the superior temporal area and deep to the superficial layer of DTF and superficial to the intermediate fat pad in the inferior temporal and zygomatic arch region. The surgeon should avoid aggressive flap elevation and traction in the region of the tail of brow. Inadvertent injury to the temporal branch of the facial nerve by entering a superficial plane of dissection is also avoided by dissecting superficial to the DTF in the temporal area and then penetrating the temporal line of fusion from lateral to medial to enter the subperiosteal plane medial to the line of fusion.

Sensory Innervation of the Forehead

The sensory innervation of the forehead is by the supraorbital and supratrochlear nerves, which are branches of the first division of the trigeminal nerve. The supraorbital notch/foramen can be palpated at the midpupil about 2.4–3.2 cm from the midline. The supratrochlear foramen is located over the medial aspect of the supraorbital rim, 1.7–2.2 cm lateral to the midline.

The supraorbital nerve divides into a superficial and a deep branch. Like the supratrochlear nerve, the superficial division of the supraorbital nerve initially runs in a subgaleal plane, then pierces the frontalis muscle, and finally supplies the skin of the forehead and anterior hairline region. The deep branch frequently exits at the supraorbital notch but it may also exit from a foramen located up to approximately 1–1.5 cm superior to the orbital rim in approximately 10% of patients. The deep division of the supraorbital nerve runs between the deep layer of the galea and the underlying periosteum and pierces the galea approximately 0.5–1.5 cm medial to the superior temporal line (STL) at the level of the coronal suture to innervate the frontoparietal scalp (Knize, 1995).

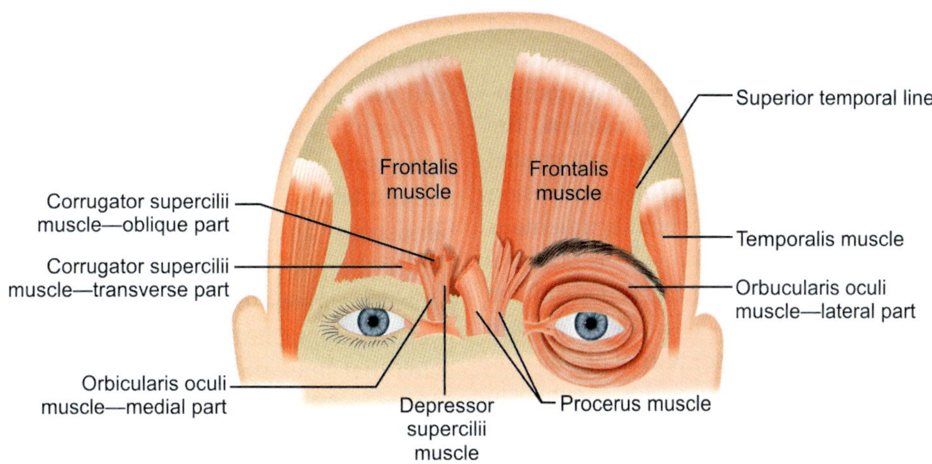

Fig. 23.3: Illustration showing brow elevator and depressors.
Source: Modified from Fitzgerald, R., 2013. Contemporary concepts in brow and eyelid aging. *Clin Plastic Surg,* 40, pp. 21–42.

Brow Elevator and Depressors

The three-dimensional position of an individual's brow is determined by the relative contribution of brow elevator versus brow depressors (Fig. 23.3). The frontalis muscle is the only elevator of the brow and forehead. Its contraction leads to horizontal forehead rhytids. The galea divides into anterior and posterior layers in the forehead. The anterior galea inserts into the dermis above the orbital rim. Frontalis muscle arises within the galea at the level of the anterior hairline and inserts into the skin of the eyebrow. It is often a bifid muscle with an area of deficiency between the right and left halves in the middle of the forehead. The depressors of the brow include the orbicularis oculi, corrugator supercilii, depressor supercilii and procerus muscles, all of which are innervated by the facial nerve.

Knize (1996) has shown through his anatomical studies that the lateral margin of frontalis muscle almost always ends or becomes noticeably tempered along or just lateral to the temporal fusion line and its continuation as the STL. The frontalis muscle stops short of the tail of the brow making the lateral brow more prone to loss of elevation with aging. Relaxation of the frontalis muscle causes the brow and orbicularis muscle to fall leading to obliteration of upper lid sulcus and prominence of upper eyelid skin fold. Such patients benefit from a temporal forehead lift or brow lift, which repositions the brow and orbicularis muscle at the rim. With aging, along with brow ptosis, there is also dermatochalasis, i.e. excessive accumulation of skin in the upper lid. This may need to be addressed along with brow ptosis in patients presenting with restriction in field of vision.

Orbicularis oculi is a concentric muscle, which originates at the medial orbital bone, and interdigitates with the frontalis muscle superiorly and medially. The orbicularis oculi is functionally divided into three parts: preseptal, pretarsal, and orbital. Its orbital portion is responsible for squinting and dynamic rhytids, including Crow's feet. It is also responsible for medial and lateral brow ptosis.

The corrugator supercilii is the largest of the depressor muscles. It has a transverse and an oblique head, originates at the medial orbital bone and bony glabella, and spreads superolaterally to join the frontalis and orbicularis muscles in the region of the midbrow. Contraction of the corrugators draws the eyebrows medially and depresses their medial aspect to create vertical or oblique glabellar rhytids.

The depressor supercilii are relatively small depressors that run approximately vertically between the medial orbital bone and the medial head of the brow.

The procerus is often a bifid muscle. It originates from the nasal bones and fans superiorly to meet the frontalis and orbicularis muscles and inserts into the skin. It draws the medial brows inferiorly and is responsible for the horizontal glabellar and dorsal nasal rhytids.

Ellis and Masri (1989) studied 60 patients and divided them into three groups according to their dominant animation pattern: brow lifters, frowners, and squinters. They established that brow ptosis was more prominent laterally in the squinters and medially in frowners. Uniform displacement of the eyebrows was noted in the brow lifter group.

Orbital Retaining Ligaments

The STS separates the frontal periosteum medially from the DTF laterally and continues inferiorly as the TLA at the boundary between of the periorbita, forehead, and temporal area (Fig. 23.4). Temporal ligamentous adhesion is formed by the confluence of the superficial temporal fascia with galea aponeurotica and periosteum. The lateral part of frontalis muscle usually becomes attenuated along the STS and TLA. Temporal ligamentous adhesion is continuous medially with the supraorbital ligamentous adhesion, which maintains the medial brow in its position. Orbicularis retaining ligament (ORL) is a fascia beneath the orbicularis oculi muscle that inserts into the periosteum around the superior, lateral and inferior part of orbital rim. In these areas, the overlying soft tissues are attached to periosteum and fixed to bone, which helps in attaching the muscle and stabilize it into position. All these attachments are present within 3 cm from the edge of the orbit. These structures also restrain brow elevation and must be comprehensively released during brow lift surgery.

Brow Anatomy

As the galea approaches the upper forehead, it splits into the superficial galea and deep galea planes to envelop the frontalis muscle (Fig. 23.5). The deep galea plane splits again to envelop the galea fat pad, which contains the transverse head of the corrugator supercilii muscle. This eyebrow fat pad allows the movement of the frontalis muscle in the lower forehead and is continuous inferiorly with the suborbicularis space in the eyelid.

Deep to the galea fat pad is the subgalea fat pad glide plane space. The floor of the glide plane space is the deepest layer of the deep galea plane, which is fused with periosteum and is fixed to the underlying frontal bone. Under the glide plane space, the subgalea fascia plane, which separates the deep galea plane from periosteum over the upper forehead, is obliterated. A layer of deep galea that lines the undersurface of galea fat pad forms the roof of this space. Corrugator supercilii muscle rests on the medial roof of this space as it passes through the galea fat pad before inserting into the dermis.

The multiple layers of the deep galea plane then come together and fuse to the orbital rim before they enter the orbit to form the suborbicularis oculi muscle fascia and the orbital septum. The superficial galea plane that covers the surface of the frontalis muscle continues over the surface of the orbicularis oculi muscle (Knize, 2007).

The lateral eyebrow position is more stable in individuals where the layers of the galea completely envelop the galea fat pad and fuse again along the entire superior orbital rim. Lateral eyebrow ptosis is likely to appear

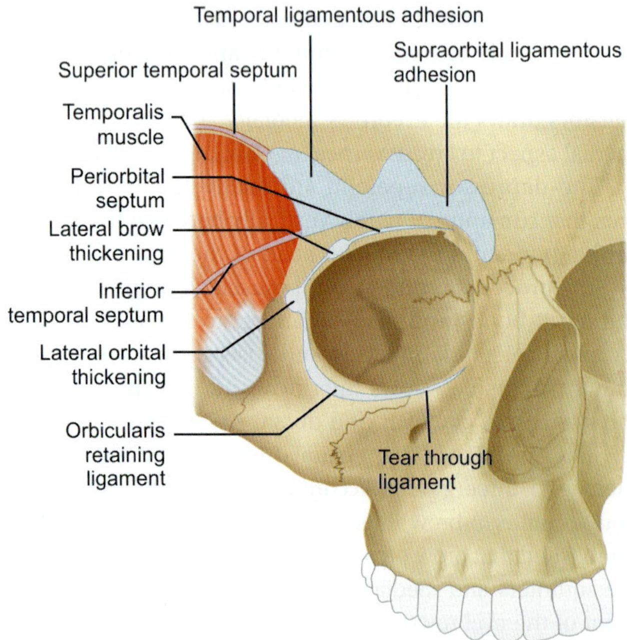

Fig. 23.4: Ligamentous adhesions, tissue thickenings, and retaining ligament that help maintain the brow position.
Source: Modified from Moss, C.J., Mendelson, B.C., Taylor, G.I., 2000. Surgical anatomy of the ligamentous attachments in the temple and periorbital regions. *Plast Reconstr Surg*, 105, pp. 1475-90.

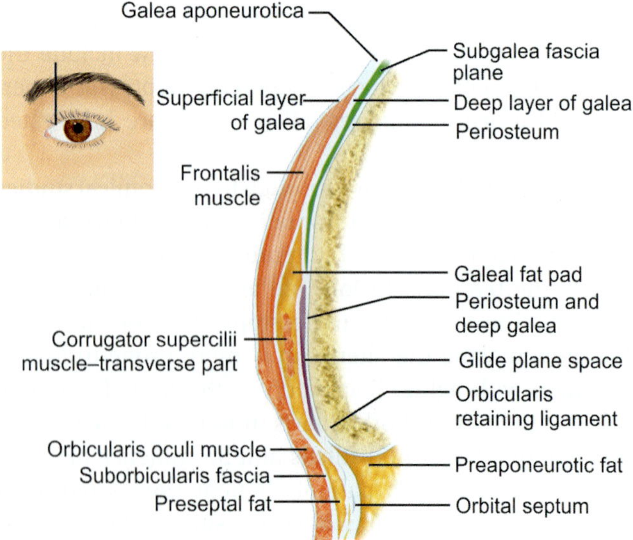

Fig. 23.5: Sagittal cross-sectional anatomy of the forehead, brow, and upper lid in the lower forehead.
Source: Modified from Fitzgerald, R., 2013. Contemporary concepts in brow and eyelid aging. *Clin Plastic Surg*, 40, pp. 21–42.

earlier in patients where the envelope around the galea fat pad is incomplete laterally, which allows the fat pads to slide down over the orbital rim.

23.3 BROW AESTHETICS

Due to the very important interrelationship between the eyes, brows, and forehead, it is important that the surgeon assesses these areas not only individually but also appreciates the delicate and extremely significant interrelationships between them before proceeding with treatment. Individual patient anatomy, their ethnic background, age, body habitus, facial shape, degree of functional and aesthetic deformity, underlying pathology leading to brow ptosis, and patients expectations from surgery influence the surgeons decision regarding the treatment plan to achieve a natural-looking result.

It is important to realize that there is no ideal brow shape. Descriptions of an "ideal brow" have changed over the years, depending on many factors, including the age of the subject or the observer, culture, race, gender, shape of the face, and current aesthetic trends. Differences in the brow shape exist between males and females, and should be considered during assessment and planning to obtain gender appropriate results.

Ideal Male Brow

Men have a more prominent supraorbital ridge than women, which is responsible for a more masculine and angular appearance to the brow. The male forehead is more sloping than the female forehead, and the anterior male hairline is more posteriorly placed than the female hairline.

The male brow should sit at or just below the supraorbital rim. It is heavier and flatter than the female brow and should taper only marginally from medial to lateral extent. Although the brow may be slightly elevated in the region of the lateral limbus, it should not arch as much as the female brow. An excessively thin and arching brow that has been positioned above the supraorbital rim imparts a feminized appearance in a male patient and should be avoided at any cost, lest it should be done for male to female gender realignment. The surgeon should aim to individualize the brow position to achieve facial harmony based on the position of the hairline, height of the forehead, and characteristics of the glabellar complex.

Coventionally eyebrow ptosis is said to exist when the distance from the midpupil to the top of the brow is <2.5 cm. This figure is totally arbitrary and may not be relevant in all patients. The distance between the inferior border of the eyebrow and the upper lid margin is equal to the vertical height of the eye from palpebral fissure to palpebral fissure.

Female Brow

According to Westmore's principles of periorbital aesthetic ideals in women, the brow should lie just above the superior orbital rim and the highest arch of the brow should lie at the lateral limbus. The medial border of the brow should lie on a vertical line with the alar-facial crease. The lateral end of the brow should lie on a line drawn from the alar-facial crease tangent to the lateral canthus. The lateral brow should lie at the same horizontal level as the medial brow.

However, public opinion of eyebrow aesthetics, as per the survey performed by Schreiber, Singh and Klatsky (2005), suggests that the public prefers the overall position of the eyebrow to be lower, the arch to be more lateral in relation to its position over the lateral limbus, and the lateral eyebrow to be higher than the medial eyebrow. The current trend for an aesthetically pleasing brow peak is in the region of the lateral canthus than the lateral limbus. This position prevents a more startled and angular look to the brow. The brow should be fuller in its medial aspect and then taper elegantly toward its lateral part. The lateral brow should end in a line extending from the nasal ala to the lateral canthus, and should begin on a vertical line extending from the nasal ala or from the medial canthus. By convention brow is considered ptotic if it is <26–28 mm above the midpupil (Fig. 23.6).

The average height of the female forehead (eyebrow to hairline) should be between 5 and 6 cm (Fig. 23.6). For forehead heights of 7 cm and more, techniques to shorten the forehead should be considered.

23.4 AGE-RELATED CHANGES IN BROW'S SHAPE AND POSITION

In a teenager, the brow is full and well supported, and the upper eyelid sulcus is well defined. In middle age, there is mild brow ptosis and some fullness of the sulcus. There is age-related progressive deflation along with temporal brow ptosis and hooding, obliteration of the superior eyelid sulcus, and prominence of upper eyelid fold.

Matros, et al. (2009) have demonstrated through their study of 70 women that medial and midbrow is elevated

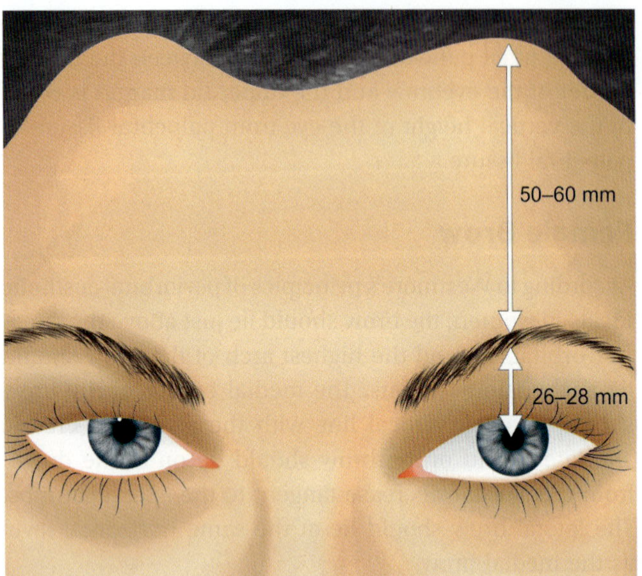

Fig. 23.6: In females the height of the brow from midpupil is 26–28 mm, and the height of the anterior hairline from the brow is 50–60 mm.

in older as compared to younger women (Matros, Garcia and Yaremchuk, 2009). It has been suggested that this may be attributable to hyperactive frontalis muscle compensating for obstruction of the visual field due to upper lid dermatochalasis and age-related lid ptosis. Studies comparing longitudinal photographs of individuals have shown that brows descend in 29% of patients, remain stable in 30% of patients, and elevate in the remaining patients. It is important to assess the position of the brow in each individual patient and the surgeon should ask the patient to bring facial photographs of his/her youth. This is important to avoid excessive elevation of brows, which creates a surprised look and may exacerbate an aged appearance.

The position of eyebrows is maintained by the opposing action of elevator, depressor muscles, and the support offered by periorbital ligamentous adhesions and retaining ligaments (Figs. 23.3 and 23.4). There is a gradual disruption of these supporting structures and the balance between the pull of elevator and depressors with age leading to brow ptosis, especially in its lateral part.

Facial aging involves both soft tissue descent and loss of volume. When this involves the eyebrows, brow ptosis develops, which affects the balance and aesthetic appearance of the face. Aging causes descent and loss of volume of galeal and preseptal fat pads. There is a lack of frontalis muscle support to suspend the eyebrows lateral to the temporal fusion line. The more medially the plane of temporal line is placed in relation to the eyebrow, the less the frontalis muscle resting tone there is for suspensory support for the lateral eyebrow. Moreover, instability of superficial temporal fascia plane lateral to the zone of adhesion facilitates lateral brow ptosis over time causing temporal hooding. As skin elasticity decreases, the forehead, temple, and glabellar skin descend. If brow ptosis is severe, a visual deficit may develop in the superior and temporal quadrants.

The supratarsal crease disappears, and Crow's feet and deep forehead creases appear due to the repetitive action of the orbicularis oculi and the frontalis muscles. Brow ptosis imparts an appearance of tiredness, sadness, and anger. It commonly represents only a cosmetic concern.

Brow ptosis is often unrecognized by the patient. More commonly, the patient may complain about excessive upper eyelid skin with hooding, not recognizing the contribution of ptotic brow position as a major contributing factor to the resultant appearance of upper lid redundancy. It is thus important for a facial plastic surgeon to educate the patient about the important role of brow position in upper lid redundancy and stress the importance of brow repositioning before any intervention of the upper lid skin. In fact, in a large proportion of patients, brow repositioning alone may help the surgeon to meet the patients' aesthetic and functional goals entirely.

In patients with marked brow ptosis, the eyelid skin above the supratarsal fold descends over the eyelid crease decreasing the visibility of the pretarsal skin segment. Reduced visibility of pretarsal skin is particularly common in the oriental races. When one brow is more ptotic than the other, eyelid asymmetry may be secondary to asymmetric brow ptosis, with it being worse on the more ptotic side (Fig. 23.7A). The surgeon has to be particularly vigilant to pick up lid asymmetry resulting from brow asymmetry and tailor the surgical correction accordingly. If symmetric skin only or skin muscle blepharoplasty is performed in these patients without addressing the brow asymmetry, it will be converted to a much more significant eyelid asymmetry postoperatively. In these patients, asymmetry is corrected by performing a greater temporal scalp excision on the more ptotic side, providing more support to the brow using a temporal crest anchoring suture through a bone tunnel or by using a superiorly based temporal periosteal flap. Additionally, more supratarsal crease eyelid skin and muscle may be removed on the more ptotic side.

Hairline and Scalp

The surgeon has to consider various parameters related to a male patient's hair pattern while deciding on the surgical approach to employ for brow lifting. These include patients favored hairstyle, current hair pattern, degree and type of male hair loss pattern and thinning, predicted future hair pattern based on family history of hair loss, current hair density, and height of the frontal and temporal hairline. The surgeon should deliberate and choose a surgical approach that is discreet at the time of surgical procedure and will remain so in the years to come. Endoscopic brow lift procedures can prove to be challenging in patients with a high forehead and frontal bossing due to the limited access afforded by straight endoscopes and limited angulation of instruments. The degree of mobility of scalp skin should be assessed.

The coronal approach is the gold standard approach for brow lifting and allows the surgeon to address not only brow ptosis but also forehead and glabellar rhytids, and a low-lying anterior hairline.

Patients with a high but stable hairline and those who have forehead hair growing inferiorly are candidates for the pretrichophytic and trichophytic approaches. Female patients with high forehead who desire a lower frontal hairline are also good candidates for this approach (Figs. 23.8A and B).

Patients with receding hairlines and prominent forehead rhytids are good candidates for the midforehead approach with incision placement around a rhytid. Patients with a low and stable hairline are suitable for the endoscopic brow lift approach.

In younger patients, early lateral hooding can be treated with an isolated temporal lift with the incision hidden in the temporal tuft of hair. It is often possible to do this without disrupting the temporal fusion line.

Eyebrows

When determining which brow lifting procedure to perform, the surgeon should assess the position, shape, symmetry, and mobility of the eyebrows (Figs. 23.9A to C). Patient's assessment must be performed when the patient is in the sitting position, and the brow elevator and depressors in the relaxed position (Fig. 23.9B). Patients with ptotic eyebrows have a tendency to involuntarily elevate the brow with frontalis muscle contraction (Fig. 23.9A). The surgeon can help the patients to achieve relaxation of the frontalis muscle by asking them to close their eyes. The position of the eyebrows is noted while the patient's eyes are closed. The patient is then asked to open his/her eyes slowly without contracting the frontalis muscle, while the surgeon maintains the brows in the relaxed position manually (Fig. 23.9B). Patient is photographed with brows in repose, initially with eyes closed and then with eyes open in neutral position without contracting the frontalis muscle. The surgeon can then manually elevate the brows to demonstrate the aesthetic and functional benefit of brow lifting (Fig. 23.7B). Manually, lifting the brow helps the surgeon to identify concealed lid margin and upper lid crease. A surgical plan regarding the degree of brow lifting and position of brows is then developed taking into account the aesthetic desires and functional needs of the patient.

The quality, density, and direction of the eyebrow hair are also assessed. Patients with thick eyebrows with hair growing in a superior direction are suitable candidates for direct brow lifting procedures as the nature of the eyebrow helps the surgeon to hide the surgical scar. At the same time, the surgeon should note the degree of prominence of supraorbital ridge and superior orbital rim as well as the volume of the eyebrows. Female patients with prominent supraorbital ridge or superior orbital rim appear more masculine and can benefit from reduction of these structures to give a more balanced appearance to the face (Figs. 23.8A to F). In these patients, a blepharoplasty or coronal approach is more appropriate. Patients with volume loss in the brows will benefit from filler injections or fat grafting. This gives a more youthful appearance to the brow and also helps the surgeon to elevate the brow to a small degree.

On average, the distance from the top of the brow to the forehead is about 5 cm and from midpupil to the central brow about 2.6–2.8 cm. If the later distance is <2.5 cm, one should not lift the central brow.

Eyes

It is important to obtain a history of dry eyes or previous ophthalmic procedures like laser-assisted in situ keratomileusis surgery (LASIK), which can lead to temporary denervation of portions of cornea and predispose the patient to corneal injury in the postoperative period. In patients with these risk factors, an ophthalmic consultation for slit-lamp examination of the ocular surface is arranged.

It is important to assess the TPS, BFS, and MRD1 in patients under consideration for upper face and periorbital rejuvenation (Fig. 23.10). In young female patients,

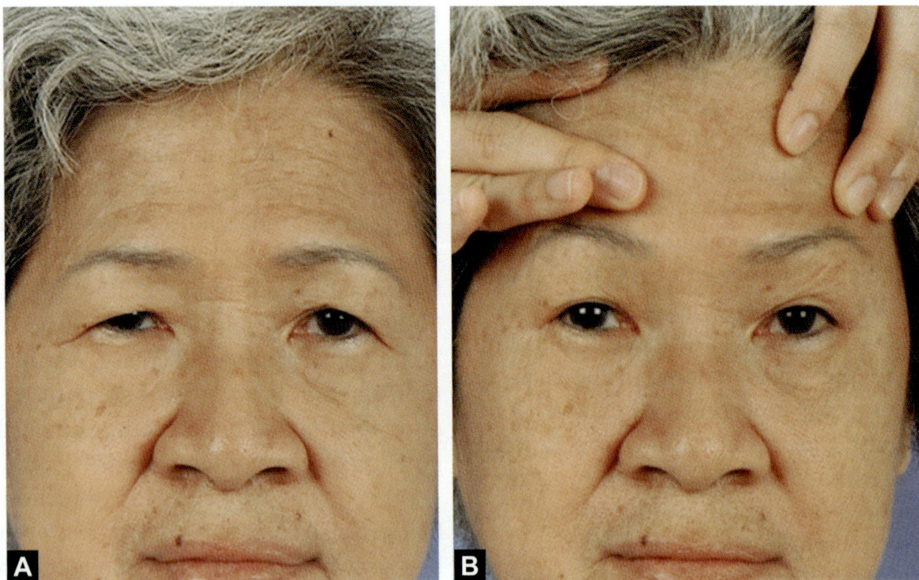

Figs. 23.7A and B: Patient with right brow ptosis secondary to facial nerve paralysis: (A) Forehead in repose. Right brow is more ptotic and there is more pseudodermatochalasis on that side compared to the left. This leads to an impression of upper lid ptosis on the right side. (B) Elevation of the brow helps identify any hidden upper lid ptosis by measuring MRD 1 accurately. This patient does not have any overt upper lid ptosis. (MRD: Marginal reflex distance).

PTS:PSS ratio is roughly 1.0:1.5 in the medial brow and 1.0:3.0 in the lateral part as it arches superiorly in the region of lateral limbus and lateral canthus (Fig. 23.11A).

The youthful eye is long and full, with a parallel lid margin and crease. The aging process changes this relationship depending on the type of volume loss and dermatochalasia (Fig. 23.11B). The PTS:PSS ratio may be used to assess patients for upper lid volume loss with a purpose of volume replacement using fillers or fat grafting (Fig. 23.11B). It has been suggested that the symmetry of TPS may be more important than symmetry of marginal reflex distance (MRD)-1 in the perception of facial appearance.

It is important to determine if there is an underlying unilateral or bilateral eyelid ptosis (Figs. 23.7A and B) by measuring the MRD-1 (distance between pupillary light reflex and the margin of the upper lid in primary gaze), a distance of 3.5–5 mm is normal. The MRD-2 (distance between the pupillary light reflex and lower lid margin in primary gaze) is also measured; a distance of >5 mm is adequate.

Prominence of the eyelid sulcus and the degree of asymmetry between the two sides is noted. Pre-existing lagophthalmos is also noted. The contribution of brow ptosis to appearance of the upper eyelid region should be recognized and factored into the degree of resection of upper eyelid skin if concomitant upper lid blepharoplasty is planned. In this situation, and also in patients who have undergone previous blepharoplasty, ptosis surgery, or brow lift, a conservative resection of upper lid skin is required to prevent iatrogenic lagophthalmos.

The surgeon should assess the eyes to identify unilateral or bilateral upper lid ptosis, and whether it is discovered only after raising the brow, or conversely whether it disappears on raising the brow. If ptosis is present, an appropriate ptosis repair procedure is incorporated in the surgical plan.

Levator excursion is recorded while holding the brow in repose (annulling the effect of the frontalis muscle contraction) and requesting the patient to first look down and then up. The difference in upper eyelid margin excursion between maximum down gaze and up gaze is the levator excursion. A difference of <4 mm between the eyelid position looking downward and then upward is deemed as poor levator function: a movement of 5–7 mm is fair; 8–15 mm is good; and >15 mm is normal. In patients with severe brow ptosis, the brow must be elevated before the eyelid margin can be visualized to assess levator function.

The presence of upper eye lid scars, herniation of fat pads, lid tone, lid position at rest, shape, size and symmetry of palpebral aperture, position of lateral canthus, lid

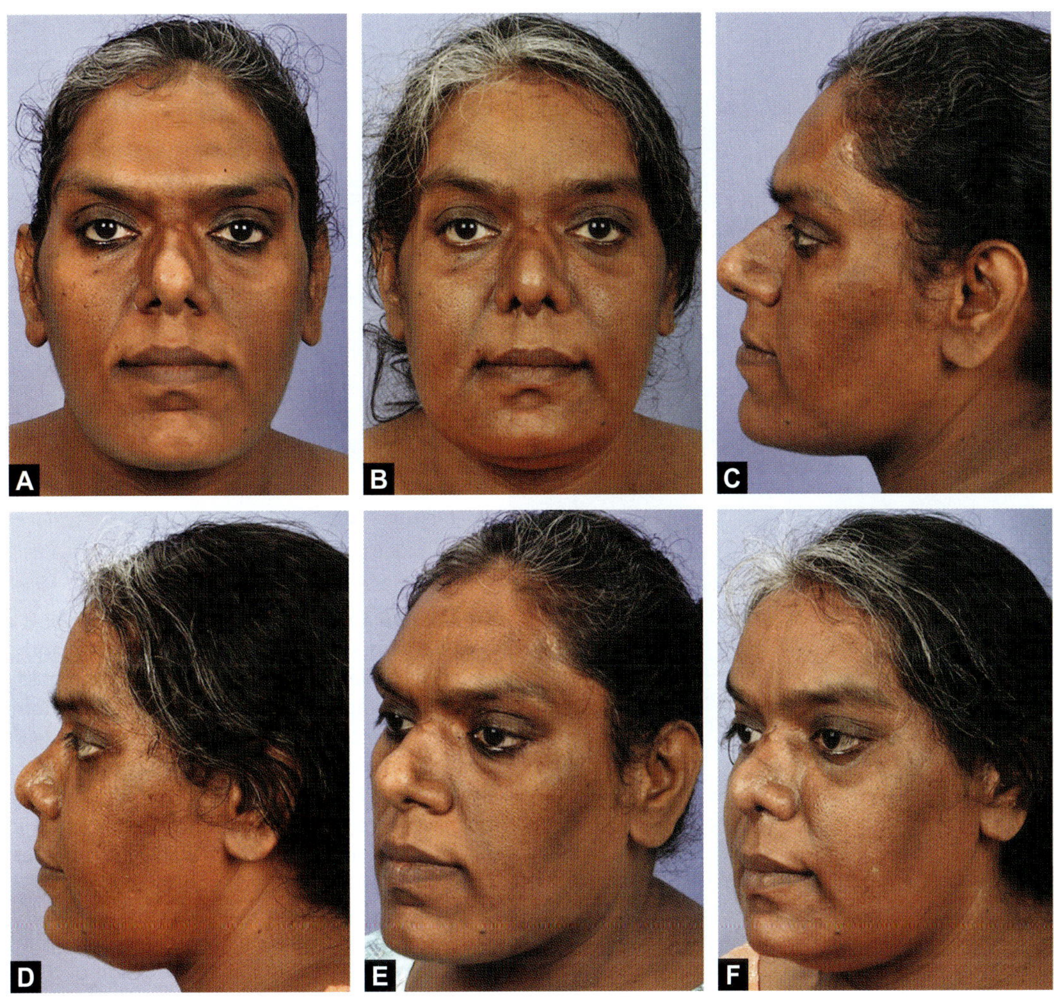

Figs. 23.8A to F: (A, C, and E) Preoperative photographs of a patient with acromegaly. Patient has a high and sloping forehead, prominent supraorbital ridges, large nose, prominent malar eminences, prominent angles of mandible and chin, which gives a very masculine appearance to her face. (B, D, and F) 3-month postoperative photographs of the patient after reduction rhinoplasty, trichial forehead lift approach for forehead contouring with 8 mL hydroxyapatite bone cement and reduction of supraorbital rims and ridges. She also underwent malar, chin and angle of mandible reduction.

retraction, exophthalmos, enophthalmos, scleral show, and lower lid negative vector should be noted. The surgeon assesses the degree of brow elevation that can be safely performed to prevent postoperative lagophthalmos (Fig. 23.12). This is important to prevent lagophthalmos and the risk of corneal injury in the postoperative period. The presence of Bell's phenomenon is documented.

23.5 MANAGEMENT

Nonsurgical Rejuvenation of Brow and Forehead

The aim of nonsurgical rejuvenation of the brow and forehead is many fold—restoring the lost brow volume, restoring volume to the upper eyelid sulcus, brow elevation to a more natural and aesthetically pleasing position, and effacement of forehead, glabellar, and periorbital rhytids.

Volumizing the eyebrows helps the surgeon to improve skin redundancy caused by ptosis and atrophy of the brow fat and may help him/her to elevate the brow to a certain degree. This process should not be considered as the principal tool for brow elevation. Brow elevation is primarily achieved through chemodenervation (botulinum toxin injection) of brow depressors or through surgical means.

If a patient has a full brow, e.g. a young patient, lifting using chemodenervation gives a pleasing result. On the

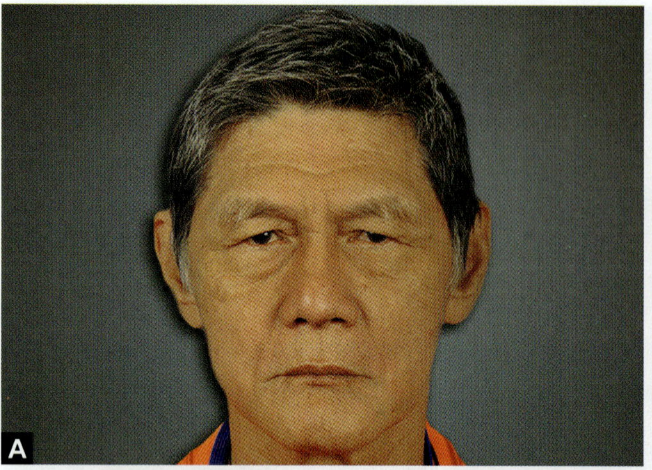

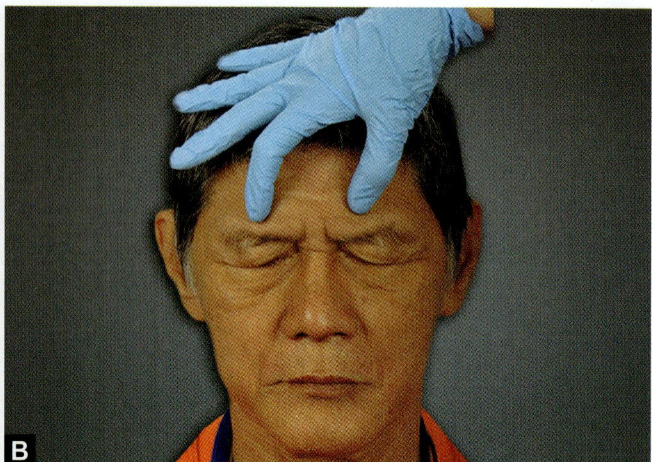

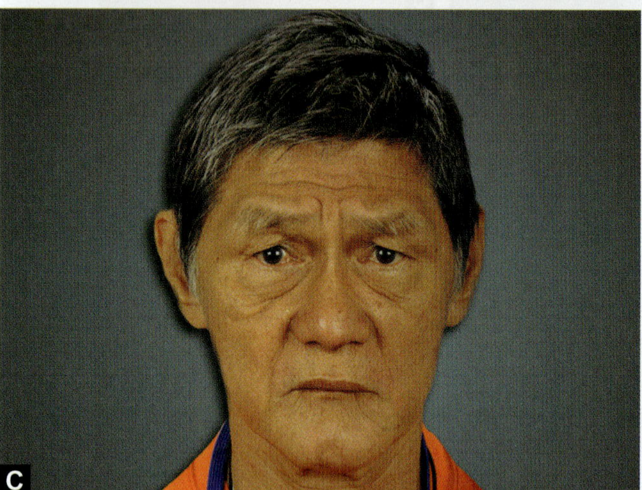

Figs. 23.9A to C: (A) Preoperative photograph of a patient presenting with severe reduction in temporal and superior fields of vision secondary to severe brow ptosis and mild dermatochalasis. This photograph was taken in the patient's normal configuration where he keeps the frontalis muscle contracted to keep the eyes open. Prominent forehead rhytids due to persistent contraction of the frontalis muscle are seen. Note the forehead rhytids, which point to the artificially raised brow. Hence, it is important to take photograph of the patient's with the frontalis muscle relaxed to appreciate the true position of the brow. (B) The patient was unable to open his/her eyes when frontalis muscle is maintained in relaxed position manually. (C) Temporal hooding is apparent despite maximum voluntary contraction of the frontalis muscle.

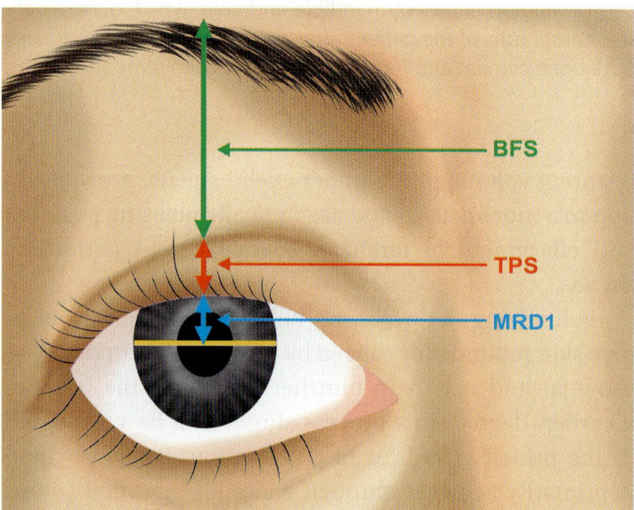

Fig. 23.10: Illustration showing the parameters that are measured when brow and periorbital rejuvenation is being considered. (BFS: Brow fat span; TPS: Tarsal platform show, MRD1: Marginal reflex distance-1).

other hand, both nonsurgical and surgical elevations of a deflated brow may reveal a skeletonized looking orbit and are aesthetically undesirable.

Further details of nonsurgical rejuvenation of the upper face and periorbital area have been discussed elsewhere in the book and will not be covered here any further.

Surgical Rejuvenation of Brow and Forehead

The goals associated with rejuvenation surgery of upper third of the face include the following:

- Elevation of ptotic eyebrows including lateral hooding
- Correction of eyebrow asymmetry
- Reduction of rhytids (transverse forehead; vertical, oblique, and transverse glabellar; Crow's feet)
- Excision of redundant upper eyelid skin
- Elevation of lateral canthus (if needed).

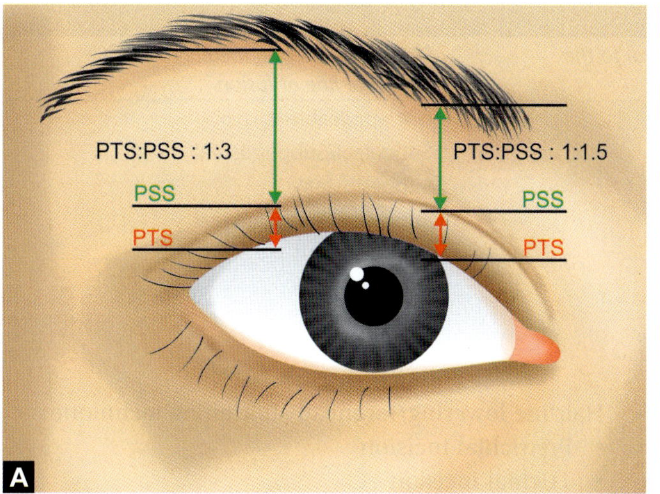

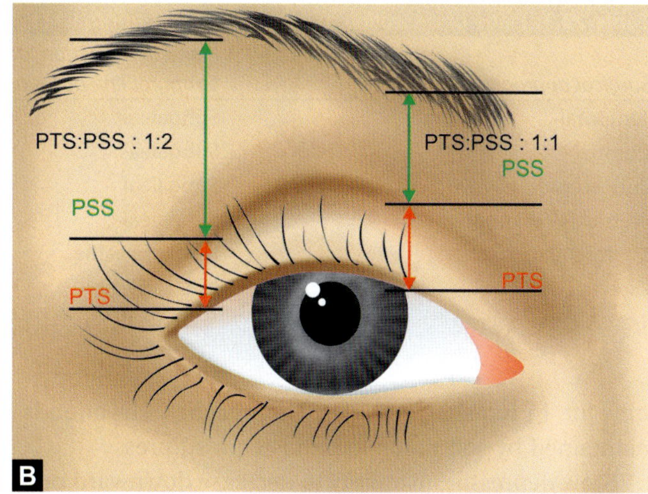

Figs. 23.11A and B: Illustrations showing the PTS and PSS in the medial and lateral part of the upper lid. (A) In young female patients, pre-tarsal show (PTS): pre-septal show (PSS) ratio is roughly 1.0:1.5 in the medial part and 1.0:3.0 in the lateral part as the brow arches superiorly in the region of lateral limbus and lateral canthus. (B) This illustration demonstrates a change in PTS:PSS ratio to 1:1 in the medial part and 1:2 in lateral part due to aging related brow ptosis and upper lid volume loss.

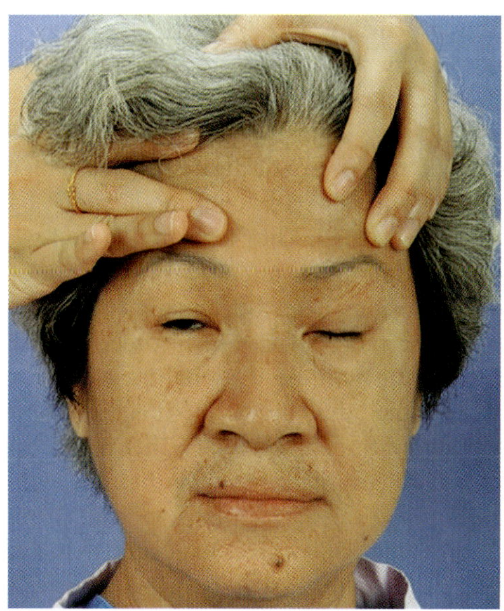

Fig. 23.12: Assessment of brow elevation that can be performed safely in a patient without causing lagophthalmos. On the right excessive brow elevation has been performed, which is causing lagophthalmos. On the left side just enough brow elevation has been performed to prevent lagophthalmos.

Younger patients initially develop heaviness and ptosis of lateral brow leading to pseudodermatochalasis of the upper eyelid and may benefit more from brow and forehead procedures rather than upper eyelid blepharoplasty. Surgical correction of temporal ptosis helps the surgeon to efface Crow's feet to a certain degree. As signs of upper face and periorbital aging develop further with advancing age, many patients are likely to benefit from combined brow lift and upper eyelid blepharoplasty.

Surgical Management

A range of surgical procedures for brow elevation and forehead rejuvenation are available and will be described briefly in the following section (Table 23.1). In endoscopic and non-endoscopic closed procedures, the degree of brow elevation is dependent on the amount of flap release. On the other hand, the amount of skin excision determines the degree of brow elevation in open approaches. Intraoperative brow asymmetries and inadequate brow elevation require release of the tissues in the periorbital area and cannot be dealt with solely by applying suspension sutures, which will not lead to a stable long-term result.

The vertical vector of elevation of forehead flap leads to the best biomechanical effect in elevating the brow. The surgeon should not depend upon lateral vector of displacement for effacement of glabellar rhytids but instead on corrugator myotomy.

In brow lift procedures with a temporal lift component (coronal, endoscopic, and temporal brow lift), a stable elevation is obtained by the fascia-to-fascia (galea to DTF) suture approximation and ultimately tissue fibrosis. In the medial part of the forehead, elevation is obtained by skin-to-soft tissue sutures and fibrosis in direct and midforehead lift and skin to bone fixation in endoscopic

Table 23.1: Plane of dissection in various brow lift approaches.

Surgical approach	*Plane of dissection lateral to the temporal line of fusion*	*Plane of dissection medial to the temporal line of fusion*
Temporal	Subgaleal	Not applicable
Coronal	Subgaleal	Subgaleal/Subperiosteal
Endoscopic	Subgaleal	Subperiosteal
Pretrichial/Trichophytic	Subgaleal	Subgaleal/Subperiosteal
Midforehead	Not applicable	Subcutaneous
Direct	Not applicable	Subcutaneous
Transblepharoplasty	Subgaleal	Subperiosteal

brow lift. In transblepharoplasty approaches, elevation is maintained by soft tissue to periosteum sutures.

Brow depressor myoplasty to decrease downward pull on the brow helps the surgeon to secure the elevated brow position in transblepharoplasty, endoscopic, and coronal forehead lift. When the corrugator is modified through the eyelid incision, the periosteum in the lower central forehead and the glabellar retaining ligaments remain intact and are not disrupted. Medial brow elevation can thus be minimized or avoided.

Percutaneous Suspension Antiptosis (APTOS) Suture Lifting

Suture materials with unidirectional barbs and fixed to long needles are available for brow lifting (Fig. 23.13). The suture material is introduced through small temporal incisions in a subcutaneous plane to pull the brow up and anchor it to the temporal fascia. The thread is fixed to subcutaneous tissues due to the anchoring effect of unidirectional barbs, which engage the subcutaneous fat, pulling it together and distributing it evenly along the whole length. These techniques are more suitable for temporal brow ptosis. They have the advantage of very short down time and can be performed under local anesthesia. They lead only to a shortlived lift and are not preferred in the author's practice. Hence, they will not be discussed further.

Surgical Approaches

The following general categories (Fig. 23.14) of upper face rejuvenation surgical procedures are available:

- Coronal incision
- Limited incision, non-endoscopic
- Limited incision, endoscopic
- Midforehead incision
- Direct brow lift incision
- Blepharoplasty incision
- Hairline lowering/forehead shortening technique
  - Pretrichial incision
  - Trichial incision

The procedure of choice for a particular patient is dictated by the following criteria:

- Hairline position
- Density of hair
- Pattern of hair loss
- Stability of hair line
- Family history of hair loss
- Laxity of scalp tissues
- Degree of aging deformity: functional and aesthetic
- Amount of improvement desired by the patient.

Unless there are specific contraindications based on the above criteria, the author feels that closed short scar endoscopic technique is suitable for most patients.

Hairline incisions help the surgeon to remove excess forehead skin in patients with high forehead and can be used to lower the hairline. Coronal incision is the gold standard incision, and allows for the most amount of lift that is stable and predictable. This is the approach of choice in patients with very low hairline who desire the hairline to be raised to improve facial proportions. The incision offers the widest exposure that allows for contouring of the forehead. This incision as well as the blepharoplasty incision allows for contouring of the supraorbital ridge and superior orbital rim as well as suspension of the ptotic lacrimal gland. Ablation of brow depressors may be performed with coronal, endoscopic, pretrichial and trichophytic brow lift approaches.

Temporal Lift

Temporal lift is suitable for patients with isolated lateral brow ptosis and good medial brow position, and female patients with relatively straight brows who desire more peaked lateral brow. In this approach, access is achieved through a 5–6 cm incision made 2–3 cm posterior to the

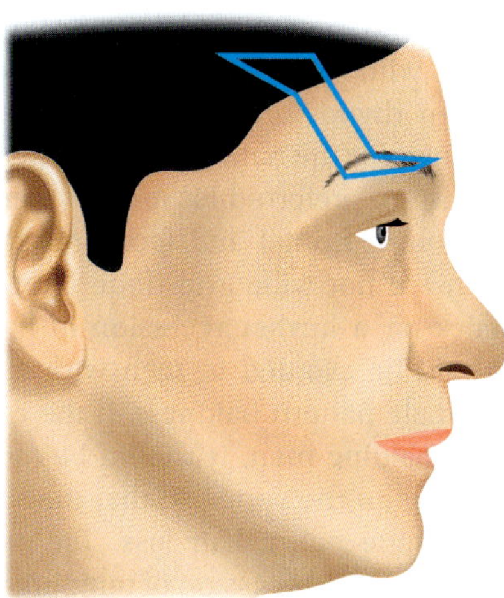

Fig. 23.13: Antiptosis (APTOS) suture for lateral brow lift.

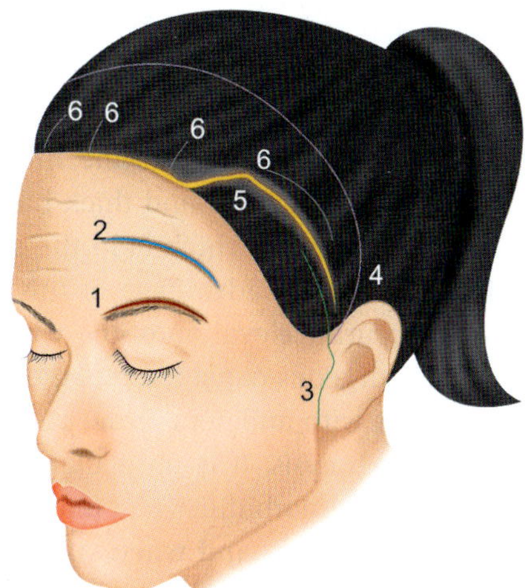

Fig. 23.14: Incisions used for brow lift and forehead rejuvenation: (1) Direct brow lift incision. (2) Midforehead lift incision. (3) Temporal extension of face lift incision. (4) Coronal incision. (5) Pretrichial/Trichial incision. (6) Endoscopic brow lift incisions. *Source*: Modified from Henderson, J.L., Larrabee, W.F., 2007. Analysis of the upper face and selection of rejuvenation techniques. *Otolaryngol Clin N Am*, 40, pp. 255–65.

temporal hairline; skin flap is raised in a plane superficial to the DTF through blunt dissection till 2 cm above the orbital rim. According to the author's practice, adequate lift is then achieved by release of lateral temporal ligamentous adhesions and lateral brow thickening under endoscopic control while identifying and preserving the sentinel vein. Once free, the temporal brow is secured into position by placing a deep suture from DTF to TPF. Some surgeons prefer to raise the skin in the subcutaneous plane instead of the subgaleal plane.

Temporal Extension of Rhytidectomy Incision

In patients who are undergoing a facelift at the same sitting as a brow lift the preauricular component of the facelift incision can be extended superiorly into the temporal region. The temporal component of the incision and the subsequent plane of dissection are similar to temporal lift.

Transblepharoplasty Browpexy

Under local or general anesthesia, the transblepharoplasty browpexy procedure is performed through an upper lid supratarsal crease incision. Then a preseptal suborbicularis plane of dissection is followed all the way to the orbital rim. Ptotic galeal fat is identified superior to the arcus marginalis. Forehead periosteum is then elevated in between the temporal crests from the orbital rim to the hairline, except for a small triangle based along the orbital rim between the supraorbital notches. If upper lid skin excision or preaponeurotic fat excision is required as a part of simultaneous blepharoplasty, it is best left till the end of the procedure. Forehead flap fixation is achieved either with a 3.5-mm Endotine implant or sutures passed through monocortically drilled bone tunnels.

If medial brow elevation or effacement of glabellar rhytids is desired, the preseptal plane can be followed medially to divide the corrugator and procerus muscles. Transpalpebral corrugator myectomy avoids disrupting the supraorbital ligamentous adhesions that hold the medial brow in place, and this prevents unnecessary elevation of medial brow. The corrugator can be divided between the supraorbital and supratrochlear nerves and an interposition fat graft positioned between the cut ends of the muscle for longer-lasting results.

Paresthesias and dysesthesias of the forehead that result from dissection of the supratrochlear nerves in open or endoscopic brow lift procedures are reduced with the transpalpebral approach. Hyperinfiltration of the medial brow with 0.5% lidocaine reduces the bleeding during corrugator resection.

The incisions are hidden within a natural skin crease in the transblepharoplasty approach. The amount of tissue dissection is limited with the benefit of causing less bruising and postoperative edema. However, the amount of brow elevation that can be achieved is limited.

Direct Brow Lift

This approach involves making an incision, preferably zigzag, just superior to the brow and raising a subcutaneous skin flap to excise skin with the aim of elevating the brow. It allows for precise elevation of whole or part of brow while preserving the sensation to the forehead. It is particularly suitable for men with high hairline, minimal forehead rhytids, extensive hair loss, and thick bushy brows with superiorly directed hair, which help the surgeon to hide the incision. The main advantage of this approach is that it leads to accurate elevation of the whole or part of the brow. Many surgeons consider it as the procedure of choice for patients with unilateral brow ptosis secondary to facial nerve paralysis. It is particularly suited for patients with significant morbidities that make them unfit for a more extensive surgery and when surgery is being performed for functional rather than aesthetic improvement. In a proportion of patients with thick sebaceous skin, the scar may be perceptible requiring scar revision and dermabrasion. Traumatic alopecia and decreased sensation to the forehead are other risks associated with this approach.

Midforehead Lift

In this approach, the incision is placed around a horizontal midforehead rhytid, which is completely excised. The incision is broken in the midline or paramedian positions. The skin incision is beveled away from the center to allow eversion during closure. This incision tends to conceal the scar better than the incision made directly above the brow. A subcutaneous skin flap is elevated from the midforehead to the level of the supraorbital rims. Once the orbicularis oculi is identified it is suspended to the periosteum with 3–4 mattress sutures. The redundant skin is excised and the incision is closed accurately in layers.

It is suitable for men with thin non-oily skin in whom the postoperative scar is more acceptable. However, the patient should be warned against an expected scar that is perceptible for many months after surgery. This approach is particularly useful in patients in whom static forehead reanimation is planned for paralyzed forehead, and in those who have deep forehead rhytids, a receding hairline, and eyebrows which are unlikely to conceal a direct brow lift scar. The approach offers excellent symmetry and durability, and is suitable for patients with significant brow ptosis.

Coronal Forehead Lift

This gold standard approach offers real decrease in scalp and forehead skin redundancy, which allows for better brow elevation, and secure and long-lasting improvement. Patients with low hairlines, generalized brow ptosis, and deep rhytids are particularly suited for this approach. It allows for the hairline to be raised by 1–2 cm. This approach is not preferred for men as there is a thinning or recession of frontal and temporal hairline with age. Most men are not willing to trade improvement in brow aesthetics for a further recession of hairline. This approach should be avoided in men with a family history of severe male pattern baldness. If the coronal incision is used in balding men, it should be modified and placed posteriorly on the vertex so that the scar remains camouflaged despite future hair loss. The incision may be modified to decrease recession of temporal hairline by placing it pretrichially in the temporal area and excising the forehead skin anterior to it. Since skin has a tendency to stretch, more skin needs to be excised if an incision is made further away from the brow. For coronal lift, the ratio of excised skin to the final degree of brow elevation is 2:1.

The dissection is carried out in the subperiosteal plane medial to the STL and subgaleally lateral to the line, till the orbital rim is exposed. If needed, corrugator and procerus myotomy may be performed under direct visualization after releasing the arcus marginalis, lateral orbital thickening, STS and conjoint tendon. After obtaining the desired forehead lift, the flap periosteum is suspended with 3–4 horizontal mattress suspension sutures to cortical bony tunnels and DTF with 3–5 mm of overcorrection to allow for some postoperative tissue relaxation. After redraping the scalp with the brow in the elevated position, excess skin is excised along the coronal incision. A drain is inserted and skin is closed with staples. Galea is not repaired as it increases the risk of alopecia and postoperative pain. Pressure bandage is applied to the forehead for 24 hours and staples are removed after 10 days.

Endoscopic Brow Lift

The endoscopic brow lift is particularly suited for a patient with normal forehead height without severe brow ptosis. Patients with thick inelastic scalp skin, high frontal hairline, and a very sloping forehead or frontal bossing are not good candidates for this approach (Figs. 23.8A, C, and E). This approach is particularly popular with patients because of small incisions and well hidden scars, short down time, and decreased risk of postoperative complications like alopecia and sensory loss. The anterior hairline is altered minimally with the endoscopic approach;

hence this technique is preferred in women (Figs. 23.15A, B, C, D, G, and H). The steep learning curve with the use of endoscopic instruments and the cost of equipment is a distinct disadvantage of this technique. Corrugator, procerus, and frontalis myoplasty is also more technically challenging.

Endoscopic brow lift is usually performed through one 1.5-cm sagittal, two 1.5-cm parasagittal, and two 3–4 cm temporal incisions made parallel to the hair shafts. The sagittal and parasagittal incisions are placed radially 1.5 cm behind the hairline whereas the incisions in the temporal areas are placed tangentially. The temporal incisions are made within the temporal tuft of hair 2 cm behind the frontotemporal hairline. The medial extent of the temporal incision is placed lateral to the temporal line and the incision is made parallel to the lateral brow. This orientation of the temporal incision helps the surgeon to elevate the tail and lateral part of brow in a superolateral vector. The parasagittal incision is made in line with the proposed peak of the brow near the junction of the frontal and frontotemporal hairlines. In patients with temporal hair loss, the parasagittal incisions can be placed more laterally along the anterior margin of the temporal hairline.

Aging-related brow ptosis results from scalp skin and brow fat sagging relative to the periosteum. Thus, elevating the skin in the subgaleal plane makes intuitive sense. However, there is a debate in the literature regarding the best plane for dissection, subperiosteal, or subgaleal. Cadaveric studies have shown that the difference in elevation achieved between the two techniques is not statistically significant. However, there is more tension in the flap in subperiosteal dissection than in subgaleal dissection. However, there is some evidence to suggest that subperiosteal lifts result in more permanent fixation because the periosteum adheres to bone more than galea.

The skin flap is raised in a subperiosteal plane medial to the temporal line through the sagittal and parasagittal incisions, and superficial to the DTF through blunt dissection via the temporal incisions. Alternatively, the dissection may be performed in the subgaleal plane medial to the temporal line but transition to the subperiosteal plane 2 cm above the supraorbital rim or when the neurovascular bundle is visualized. The lateral incision in the temporal scalp is used to divide the temporal line of fusion and conjoint tendon between the central subperiosteal dissection and the lateral subgaleal dissection.

Subperiosteal dissection is preferred as it offers protection to deep branch of the supraorbital nerve. The dissection is then carried all the way to the rim preserving the supraorbital and supratrochlear neurovascular bundles. Total release of conjoint tendon, supraorbital ligamentous adhesion, TLA, lateral brow thickening, lateral orbital thickening and ORL, and arcus marginalis are essential to obtain a successful result from endoscopic brow lift. Flap liberation around the orbital margins is performed till orbital fat is visible through thinned tissues.

The posterior scalp skin is also undermined for a few centimeters to accommodate flap advancement. The forehead skin is then elevated by pulling on the superior incisions till the desired eyebrow position, shape and brow peak are achieved. In patients with thick and immobile scalp skin and heavy brows, some lateral overcorrection is advisable.

Next, a suction drain is placed across the forehead and secured to the skin. Care must be taken not to tighten the drain-securing suture too tightly to the skin as this may lead to alopecia. After the desired brow elevation has been achieved, an ellipse of skin is usually excised along the temporal incision. The galea of the temporal skin flap is secured to the DTF with two 2-0 polydioxanone (PDS) horizontal mattress sutures while the brow is lifted laterally and overcorrected.

Once symmetric release of the forehead flap has been achieved, the flap is elevated and the edges of the parasagittal and sagittal incisions are retracted and the site of flap suspension is marked on the forehead. The periosteum of the flap is secured in an elevated position with 2-0 PDS suture to monocortical bony tunnels drilled into the skull. The incisions are closed with surgical staples. Healing time of periosteum to bone has been documented and ranges from 7 days to 12 weeks leading to a stable result.

Pretrichophytic and Trichophytic Approach

In the pretrichial approach, the incision is placed along the anterior hairline, between the junction of the hairline and the cephalic margin of the forehead, and thus allows for the hairline to be lowered by excision of the cephalic forehead skin. In contrast, the trichophytic incision (Figs. 23.15E and F) is made 2 mm posterior to the frontal hairline centrally and within the temporal hair laterally. Care is taken to bevel the incision parallel to the direction of the hair follicles to preserve them. This allows the hair to grow through the incision and helps to camouflage it. The pretrichial lift can be performed in either the subcutaneous, subgaleal, or subperiosteal plane.

Since a high forehead gives a masculine unattractive appearance to the female face, this technique is particularly

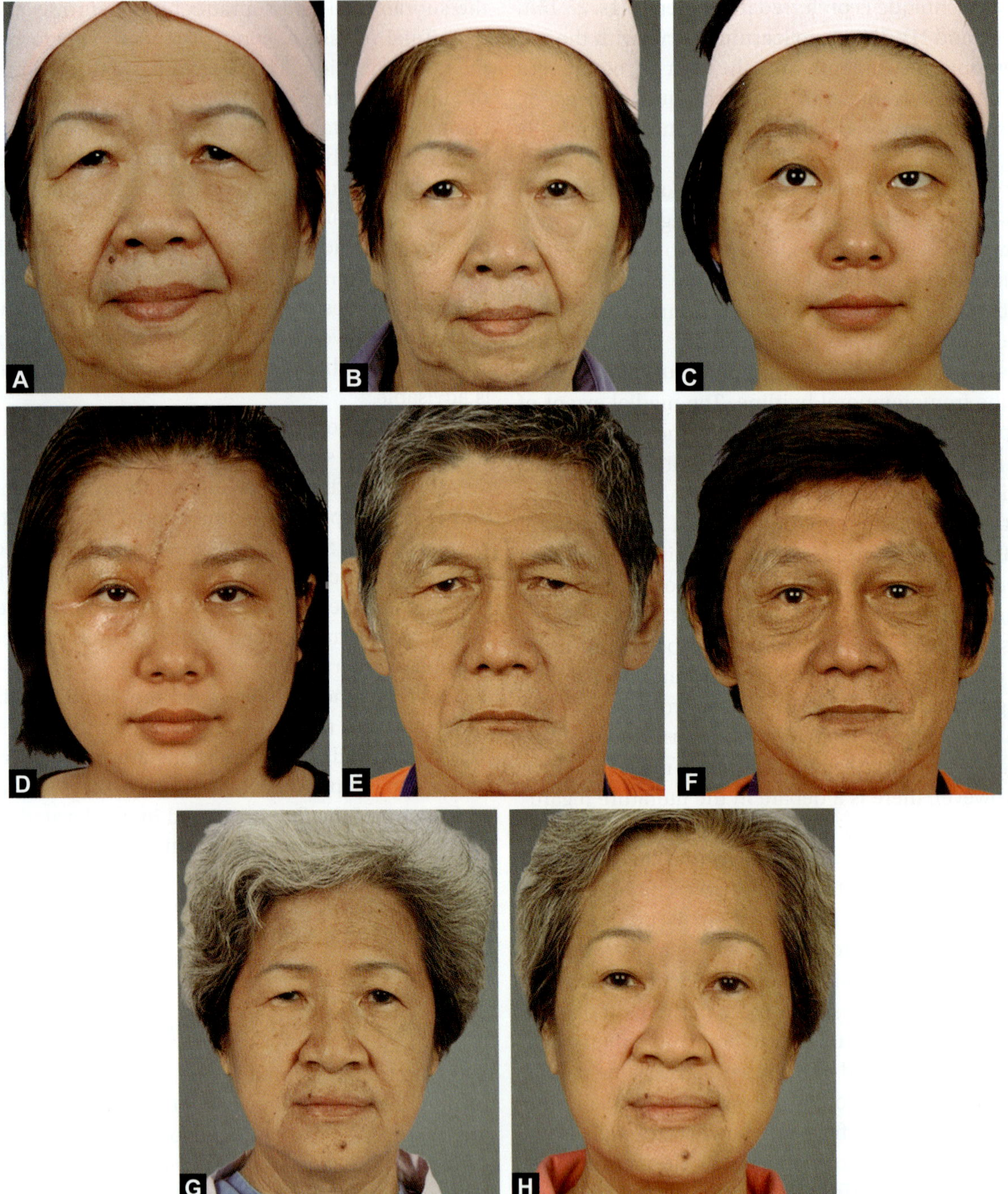

Figs. 23.15A to H: (A) Preoperative frontal view of a patient with restriction of superior lateral field of vision due to brow ptosis and dermatochalasis. (B) 9-month postoperative frontal view of the same patient after endoscopic brow lift and bilateral upper lid blepharoplasty. (C) Preoperative frontal view of a patient with right brow elevation and right upper lid scar following road traffic accident and suturing of laceration in a neighboring country. Notice that there is also asymmetry in the appearance of upper lid crease with development of right double eyelid after repair of lid laceration. Patient had right orbital floor fracture repair in our institution 1 week after the trauma. (D) 2-week postoperative view of the patient after interval left brow lift, right upper lid and forehead scar revision, and bilateral upper lid blepharoplasty. Notice the more symmetrical position of brows and eyelid creases. (E) Preoperative frontal view of a patient with brow ptosis and dermatochalasis restricting superior lateral field of vision. (F) 5-month postoperative frontal view of the patient after trichophytic brow lift and upper lid blepharoplasty. (G) Preoperative frontal view of a patient with brow ptosis restricting superior lateral field of vision. (H) 5-month postoperative frontal view of the patient after endoscopic brow lift. Notice the improvement in brow position and unmasking of the upper lid crease.

suitable for patients who wish their high forehead to be lowered (Figs. 23.8A to F). Patients with a receding hairline can also benefit from lowering of the hairline. These patients would not be suitable for coronal or endoscopic brow lift approaches, which will raise the hairline even further.

The supratrochlear and supraorbital nerve branches are transected if the subgaleal and subperiosteal planes are chosen, resulting in a loss of skin sensation. However, these planes are easy to raise and allow the periorbital thickenings and arcus marginalis to be released, and the corrugator and procerus muscles to be transected. On the other hand, the subcutaneous plane is more difficult to dissect and requires a more meticulous surgical technique using sharp dissection. Although dissection in this plane causes more bleeding, it allows the surgeon to release dermal attachments, which leads to better effacement of heavy forehead wrinkles.

The subgaleal and subperiosteal planes are similar to the coronal and endoscopic lift procedures. If subcutaneous plane of dissection is chosen, it starts at the hairline and continues inferiorly all the way to the level of superior orbital rims and laterally to the temporal line of fusion. The dissection should be kept superficial to the plane of TPF to protect the temporal branch of facial nerve. Removal of subgaleal areolar tissue in the temporal area helps the surgeon to cause scar fixation of the lateral brow in an elevated position and leads to a more long-lasting lateral brow elevation. If required, the corrugator and procerus muscles are transected under direct vision. Any redundant forehead skin is excised. The galea of the temporal flap is anchored to the DTF with 2-0 PDS, and skin is closed with staples. Excess temporal skin is excised (the author prefers to excise skin posterior to the temporal incision so that the incision remains within the temporal tuft of hair). For each 5-mm excess skin that is excised, approximately 1 mm of long-term elevation in lateral brow is expected. This happens because the posterior flap slides anteriorly and decreases the effectiveness of lateral lift. If there is brow asymmetry, maximal correction is achieved on the more ptotic side first. The excision of redundant skin flap on the less ptotic side is reduced by roughly five times the extent of required difference in correction between the two sides. For medial brow asymmetry, twice the millimeters of desired brow correction is excised on the lower side. After brow symmetry has been achieved, the central incision is sutured in two layers with a few 4-0 PDS sutures for the galeal or periosteal layer and 6-0 running locking nonabsorbable monofilament suture or 6-0 Vicryl rapide for the skin.

23.6 POSTOPERATIVE CARE

Antibiotic ointment is applied liberally to the incisions every 2-3 hours for 5-7 days, when the sutures are removed. Staples are removed in 2 weeks. Patients are advised to apply iced compresses to their eyes for 10 minutes every hour for the first 24 hours when they are awake. The hair can be shampooed after 48 hours and drain is usually removed on the first or second postoperative day. The patient is instructed to maintain a head-up position when resting for 3 days and refrain from heavy exercises for 3 weeks.

23.7 COMPLICATIONS

Headaches

Patients may experience headaches and nausea/vomiting for the first few days after surgery. Regular oral analgesics and antiemetic medication is prescribed.

Loss of Forehead and Scalp Sensation

This is commonly a sequel of pretrichial, trichophytic or coronal approaches where subgaleal or subperiosteal plane of dissection is chosen for dissection. Sensation usually returns, beginning around the brow and spreading toward the vertex, but it may take up to 1 year for this to happen. Patients are instructed that they should not shower with hot water or use hair dryers on high heat settings to avoid burns to the scalp.

Hematoma

Usually, the result of injury to the superficial temporal, supratrochlear, supraorbital or zygomaticotemporal arteries, this complication is more commonly encountered during coronal brow lift. Meticulous dissection and attention to hemostasis helps the surgeon to avoid the complication. Small hematomas can be managed conservatively with pressure bandage, whereas larger hematomas need to be evacuated.

Alopecia

Damage to the hair follicles from poorly executed nonbeveled incisions, excessive use of diathermy near the hair follicles, too superficial subcutaneous dissection, and excessive wound closure tension predispose to alopecia.

Facial Nerve Paralysis

The temporal branch of the facial nerve may be injured while raising the flap in the temporal area. Excessive traction on the flap during endoscopic dissection in the lateral orbital and temporal area predisposes to this complication. The surgeon should also exercise caution while using diathermy in the vicinity of sentinel vein since the temporal branch is located within 2 mm of this structure in the majority of patients.

Brow Asymmetry

Inadequate release of arcus marginalis and periorbital ligaments predisposes to poor brow elevation and brow asymmetry.

Lagophthalmos

Concurrent or prior blepharoplasty increases the risk for lagophthalmos. Mild lagophthalmos usually resolves with massaging the upper lids and squinting exercises. Measures for protection of cornea from exposure keratitis like artificial tears and taping the eye are instituted during the initial postoperative period. Patients are instructed to use preservative-free ophthalmic ointment at night and artificial tears during the day for the first few weeks postoperatively or until all signs of corneal irritation have waned.

SUMMARY

The surgeon should assess the whole of the upper face from the hairline to forehead skin, forehead and glabellar rhytids, brow shape and position, the upper eyelid and the periorbital area as a single unit while planning rejuvenation surgery to this area. It is a common misconception among patients that droopy eyelids are caused by excess upper eyelid skin. Patients need to be educated regarding the contribution of brow ptosis to their symptoms. There are specific differences in brow aesthetics between men and women, which need to be kept in mind while contemplating brow surgery to achieve aesthetically pleasing results for our patients.

REFERENCES

Davies, J.C., Fattah, A., Ravichandiran, M. and Agur, A.M., 2012. Clinically relevant landmarks of the frontotemporal branch of the facial nerve: a three-dimensional study. *Clinical Anatomy,* 25, pp. 858-65.

Ellis, D.A. and Masri, H., 1989. The effect of facial animation on the aging upper half of the face. *Archives of Otolaryngology—Head and Neck Surgery,* 115, pp. 710-3.

Knize, D.M., 1995. A study of the supraorbital nerve. *Plastic and Reconstructive Surgery,* 96, pp. 564-9.

Knize, D.M., 1996. An anatomically based study of the mechanism of eyebrow ptosis. *Plastic and Reconstructive Surgery,* 97, pp. 1321-33.

Knize, D.M., 2007. The importance of the retaining ligamentous attachments of the forehead for selective eyebrow reshaping and forehead rejuvenation. *Plastic and Reconstructive Surgery,* 119, pp. 1119-20.

Matros, E., Garcia, J.A. and Yaremchuk, M.J., 2009. Changes in eyebrow position and shape with aging. *Plastic and Reconstructive Surgery,* 124, pp. 1296-301.

Sabini, P., Wayne, I. and Quatela, V.C., 2003. Anatomical guides to precisely localize the frontal branch of the facial nerve. *Archives of Facial Plastic Surgery,* 5, pp. 150-2.

Schreiber, J.E., Singh, N.K. and Klatsky, S.A., 2005. Beauty lies in the "eyebrow" of the beholder: a public survey of eyebrow aesthetics. *Aesthetic Surgery Journal,* 25, pp. 348-52.

Mid-Face Lift 24

Sandeep Uppal, Nadia Ashraf, Ullas Raghavan

Chapter Overview

Pearls and Pitfalls

Pearls

- Make every effort to understand the patient's aims and expectations from surgery, timing of surgery, as well as their emotional and financial situation.
- Surgery should only be undertaken in those who have realistic expectations of outcome and are likely to be compliant with preoperative and postoperative instructions.
- "One-size-fits-all" approach is doomed to failure in facial rejuvenation surgery. Customize facelift surgery according to the patient's unique facial features and aging-related changes.
- Patients should be able to commit to the downtime associated with the proposed procedure; otherwise they will be dissatisfied postoperatively.
- All the important landmarks and surgical incisions should be marked preoperatively with the patient in sitting position to simulate the effect of gravity.
- Thread lift procedures do not lead to predictable or long lasting results and should only be offered to patients unwilling to undergo surgery.

Pitfalls

- Electrocautery close to the sentinel vein puts the temporal branch of facial nerve at risk as it lies within 2 mm of this vein in most patients.
- Dissection in a subplatysmal plane in the neck risks injuring the marginal mandibular nerve.
- Devil ear deformity is likely to result if care is not taken in placement of incision around the ear lobule.

24.1 INTRODUCTION

Ever since the dawn of civilization humans have aspired to look younger than their chronological age. With an increase in average life expectancy and general health over the last few decades' patients often perceive a mismatch between their aged facial appearance and how young they feel physically. It is well documented in literature that beauty and youth bestow advantages in social interactions, job prospects, and social mobility to an individual. As a result, the acceptance of cosmetic surgery has become increasingly more acceptable in certain sections of society. The aim of facelift surgery is to remove visible signs of facial aging. Patients now present to facial plastic

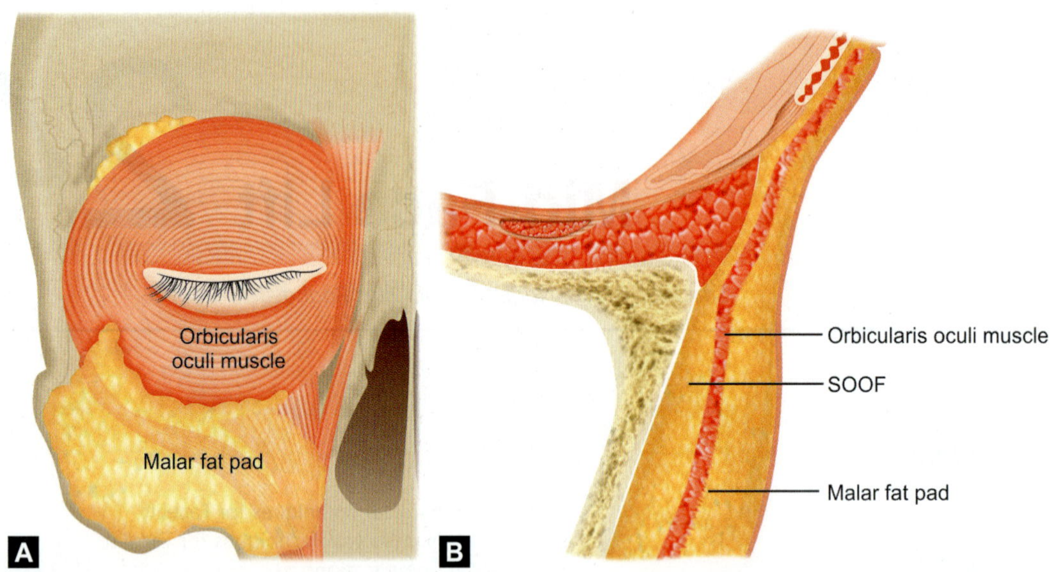

Figs. 24.1A and B: Illustration showing the relationship between the orbicularis oculi muscle, suborbicularis oculi fat pad (SOOF), and malar fat pad.

surgeons at an earlier age for facelift, often with an aim of correcting early and minimal signs of facial aging. Facial plastic surgeons now have a variety of facelift procedures in their armamentarium that can be customized to the needs of an individual patient. This chapter aims to provide an overview of the relevant facial anatomy, facial aging, patient assessment, various facelift techniques, and possible complications of these procedures. A detailed description of the technical aspects of each procedure is beyond the scope of this chapter.

24.2 SURGICAL ANATOMY

The midface is the area between the bicanthal plane (horizontal plane transecting the medial and lateral canthi) and the oral commissure. The layers of midface in superior part differ from layers in inferior aspect. In the superior part, the layers from deep to superficial include bone, periosteum, preperiosteal fat, suborbicularis oculi fat pad (SOOF), facial musculature (orbicularis oculi, zygomaticus major and minor, levator labii superioris alaeque nasi, and levator anguli oris), subcutaneous fat, and skin. It is important to realize that SOOF is separate from the orbital fat, which lies deep to the orbital septum (Figs. 24.1 to 24.3).

In the lower midface, the layers from deep to superficial include bone, periosteum, facial musculature (zygomaticus major and minor, levator labii superioris alaeque nasi, and levator anguli oris), malar fat pad, and skin.

The subcutaneous fat in midface is divided into various compartments (Fig. 24.4). The nasolabial fat compartment is the most medial of the major cheek fat compartments. The orbicularis retaining ligament is its superior boundary, SOOF is a lateral and deep boundary, and zygomaticus major muscle is its inferior border. Lateral to the nasolabial fat compartment is the malar fat that is composed of three compartments: the medial, middle, and lateral temporal-cheek. The orbicularis oculi muscle separates the superficially placed malar fat pad from the SOOF that is located deep to it (Figs. 24.1A and B). Suborbicularis oculi fat pad is intimately related to the periosteum of the lateral infraorbital rim, maxilla, as well as the origin of the zygomaticus major and minor muscles. The medial fat lies lateral to the nasolabial fat. Its superior boundary is the orbicularis retaining ligament and the lateral boundary is the middle cheek septum. The middle cheek fat compartment lies between medial and lateral temporal-cheek fat. It is bounded superiorly by the superior cheek septum and laterally by lateral cheek septum. A point of fixation is present at its junction with medial compartment and inferior orbital compartment. The lateral boundary is the lateral cheek septum. The lateral temporal-cheek fat, which is the most lateral of all the cheek fat compartments, extends from the forehead to the cervical region. It is bounded medially by the lateral cheek septum, whereas the superior and inferior temporal septa represent the superior boundaries. The

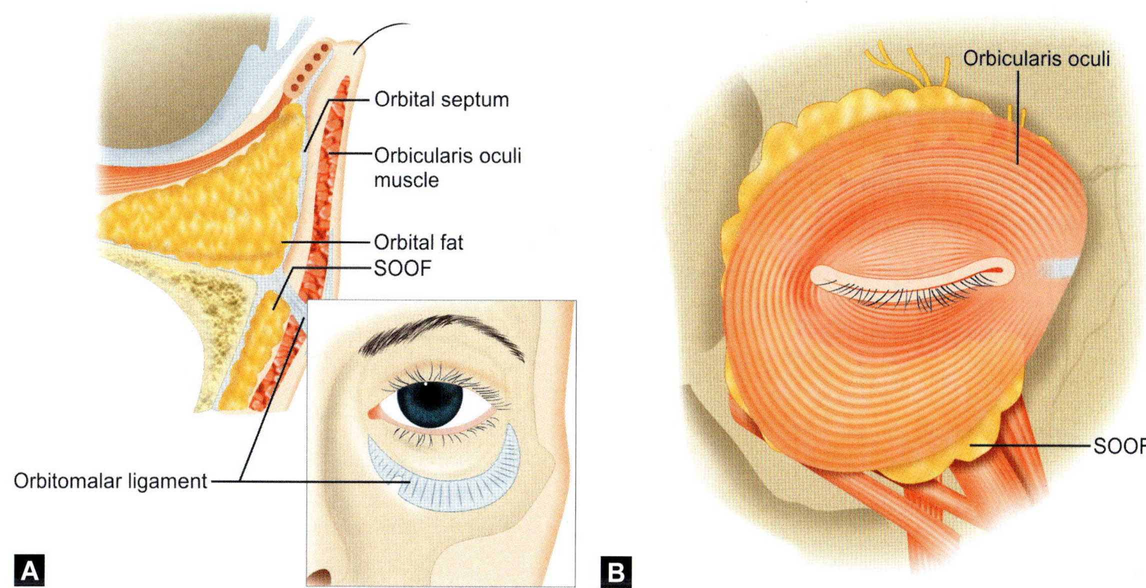

Figs. 24.2A and B: Suborbicularis oculi fat pad (SOOF) is separate from the orbital fat, which lies deep to the orbital septum. The two fat compartments are separated by orbitomalar ligament.

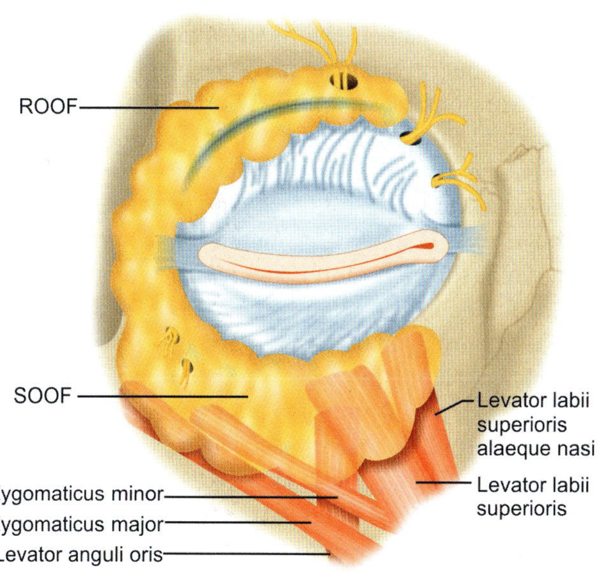

Fig. 24.3: In this illustration, the orbicularis oculi muscle has been removed to demonstrate the relationship between suborbicularis oculi fat pad (SOOF) and muscles of the upper midface. (ROOF: Retro orbicularis oculi fat pad).

other subcutaneous fat compartment in the midface is the infraorbital fat compartment, which is bordered superiorly by the orbicularis retaining ligament.

Superficial musculoaponeurotic system (SMAS), which is a continuous fibrous sheath of variable thickness, extends all the way from the scalp to the neck. It surrounds and interconnects the muscles of facial expression and extends to the cheek and nose. Superficial musculoaponeurotic system divides the subcutaneous fat into a superficial layer and deep layer. The superficial layer has fibrous septae that extend from the SMAS to the dermis and help disperse the force of contraction of facial muscles to the skin leading to facial expression. The deeper layer of fat is free of septae.

Motor nerves enter the deep surface of the muscles in the midface except the levator anguli oris and buccinator muscles, which are innervated through their superficial surface. Sensory nerves and vessels originate deep to the fascia but their terminal branches run within it or superficial to it. In the temporal area, SMAS is located immediately beneath the skin and subcutaneous tissue, overlying the superficial layer of deep temporal fascia. Superficial musculoaponeurotic system becomes a thin layer over the zygomatic arch but again becomes substantial over the parotid and neck. Superficial musculoaponeurotic system layer in cheek contains the parotid masseteric fascia. Superficial musculoaponeurotic system is tenuous over the anterior cheeks, lips, and nose.

The temporal branch of the facial nerve (Fig. 24.5) crosses the middle third of the zygomatic arch, midway between the lateral canthus and the tragus. It is thus safest to dissect the anterior and posterior thirds of the zygomatic arch before the middle third. In midface lift, the subperiosteal dissection over the zygomatic arch is

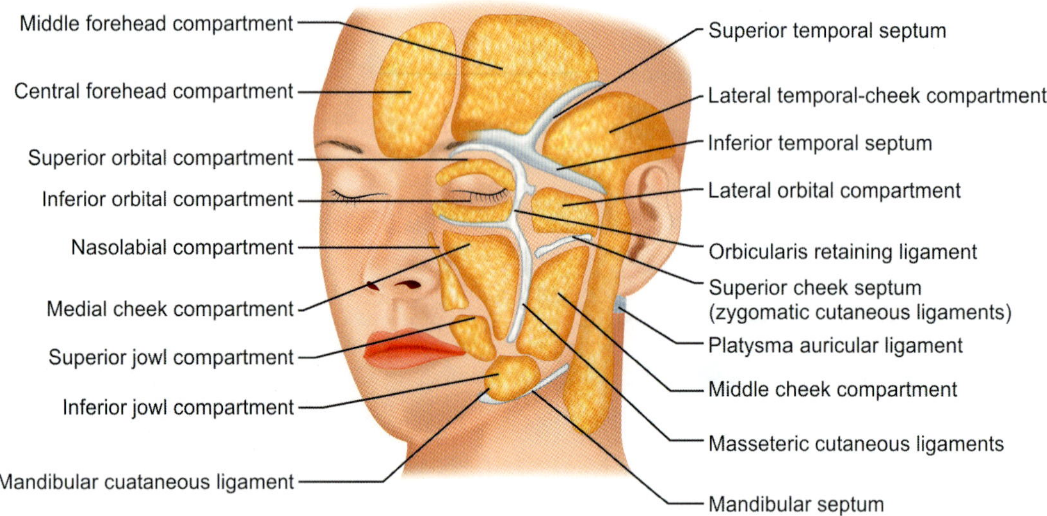

Fig. 24.4: Illustration showing the superficial fat compartments and cutaneous ligaments of the face.

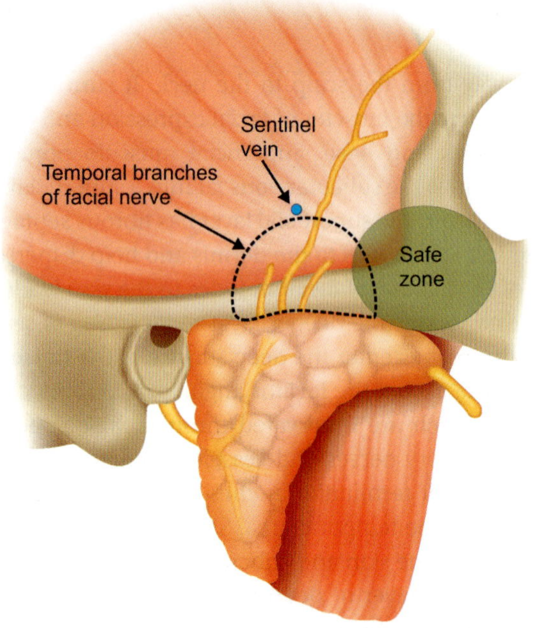

Fig. 24.5: Illustration showing the temporal branches of facial nerve over the zygomatic arch and the safe zone to start the subperiosteal dissection in midface lift surgery.

begun anteriorly first, this area is devoid of any temporal branches of the facial nerve, which helps enter a safe plane of dissection.

The zygomaticotemporal branch of the facial nerve lies posteroinferior to the lateral canthus adjacent to one of three temporal veins. The zygomatic branch exits the parotid gland deep to the parotid masseteric fascia about 1 cm under the zygomatic arch and travels forward into the buccal space beneath the origin of the zygomatic major. Some branches of the facial nerve supplying orbicularis oculi pass superficial to the attachment of these muscles. The buccal branches leave the mid-parotid gland deep to the parotid masseteric fascia, running just inferior to the parotid duct. They perforate this fascia and enter the buccal fat compartment between the fibers of the masseteric-retaining ligaments of the cheek. Facial nerve branches become superficial medial to an arch drawn 2 cm lateral to the oral commissure and are at risk if excessive subcutaneous dissection is carried out medial to this area. It is important to note that there are no branches of the facial nerve along the zygomatic prominence or infraorbital rim and this is therefore a safe area for access to and suturing of the malar fat pad. Figure 24.6 shows the danger zones of facial nerve. Figures 24.4 and 24.7 show the retaining ligaments of the face. Figure 24.8 shows the relationship of facial nerve to these retaining ligaments.

There are a number of fascial thickenings and osseocutaneous ligaments, which help maintain the position of the midface structures. These include the lateral orbital thickening, tear trough ligament, and the orbicularis-retaining ligament. Other ligaments include the zygomatic cutaneous (also called McGregor's patch) and masseteric-cutaneous ligaments. A true osseocutaneous ligament, the tear trough ligament, has recently been described on the maxilla (Wong, Hsieh and Mendelson, 2012). Cephalad to this ligament is the palpebral part of orbicularis oculi, and caudal to the ligament is the

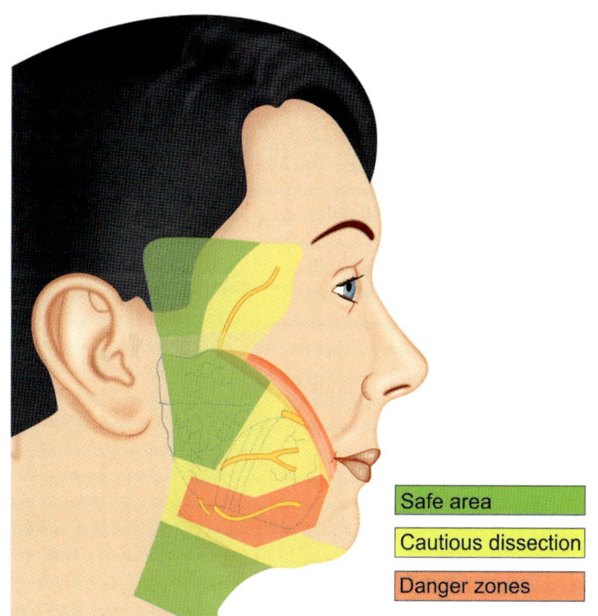

Fig. 24.6: Illustration showing the safe zones, danger zones, and areas where the surgeon needs to be cautious during facelift surgery to prevent injury to facial nerve.

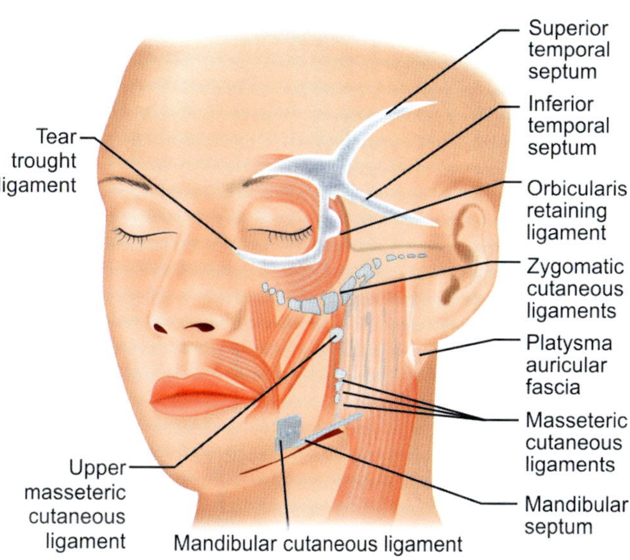

Fig. 24.7: Illustration demonstrating the retaining ligaments that support the soft tissues of the face. These need to be released to obtain an effective facelift.

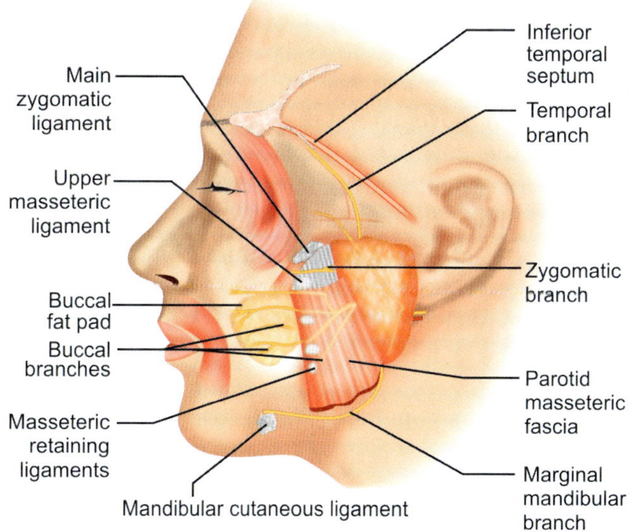

Fig. 24.8: Illustration showing the relationship of the facial nerve branches to the retaining ligaments of the face.

orbital part of this muscle, with the ligament sandwiched between the two parts. It begins medially, at the level of the insertion of the medial canthal tendon, just inferior to the anterior lacrimal crest, and extends approximately to the medial-pupil line, where it continues laterally as the bilayered orbicularis retaining ligament. The prominence of the tear trough is due to the tear trough ligament. This ligament should be released in midface lift procedures and during filler injection and fat grafting to the tear trough area. Other ligaments need to be released effectively to obtain a satisfactory lift during facelift surgery (Figs. 24.4 and 24.7).

The deep fat pad in the midface, which is deep to the facial muscles, is the buccal fat pad, which consists of anterior, intermediate, and posterior lobes. The Bichat fat pad is placed underneath the masseter and it spreads medially and superiorly. Fine branches of facial nerve pass through this fat.

The soft tissue layers of the midface attenuate and fuse inferomedially to form the melolabial fold. The levator labii superioris alaeque nasi muscle lies under the upper third of the melolabial fold and the orbicularis oris muscle under the lower third. There exists a soft tissue gap between these muscles in the middle third of the fold.

Midfacial Aging

Facial aging is a multifactorial process. It is contributed to by loss of volume of fat and bone, skin surface changes, facial descent, and line formation (Beer and Beer, 2009).

Skin changes include irregular pigmentation and the development of actinic keratoses and telangiectasia.

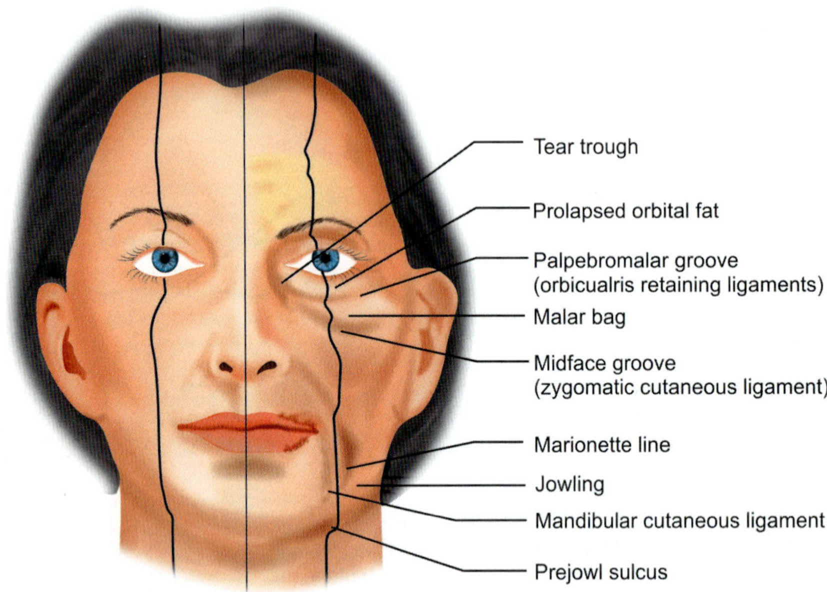

Fig. 24.9: Illustration showing changes on the face with aging.

Actinic keratoses in particular scatter light unevenly and change light reflection from the skin. In addition, there are changes in the skin thickness and elasticity, which in turn cause wrinkles.

The midface is a key area for volume loss with age and inferior migration of malar fat pad (Fig. 24.9). Loss of volume is caused by a combination of thinning of collagen and elastic fibers, fat atrophy, and bone resorption. In a young individual, there is a smooth transition from the lower eyelid margin to the cheek. With aging, the orbital fat prolapses forward and the midface descends to transform the single convex surface of the eyelid and cheek into a double convexity.

Reduced eyelid tone results from skin and muscle laxity. Laxity of the orbital septum in the upper and lower eyelids leads to pseudoherniation of fat through the orbital septum. A sling-like structure consisting of orbicularis oculi muscle and the tarsoligamentous system supports the lower eyelid. Aging leads to lengthening of these structures leading to lower eyelid laxity and involutional ectropion. Additionally there may be rounding of the lateral canthus, excessive scleral show, and malposition of the lower canaliculus and epiphora. Treatment of involutional ectropion is by lower eyelid tightening procedures.

Decrease in tone of the orbicularis oculi muscle leads to an increase in the height of the lower eyelid. There is formation of tear trough deformity, malar crescents, and festoons. The vertical length of the lower eyelid increases, which causes the infraorbital rim to be made visible through the thin lower eyelid skin. This gives a hollowed-out appearance to the infraorbital area and results in formation of a tear trough deformity medially.

Along with this, there is laxity of the orbicularis-retaining ligaments and zygomatic cutaneous ligaments. This results in movement of the eyelid-cheek unit downward and the downward displacement of the junction between the eyelid and midface. With age, descent of SOOF and malar fat pad causes the bony orbital rim to become exposed, which gives the infraorbital area a hollow appearance.

The bony skeleton of the face loses volume with age, which in the midface, leads to a wider orbital aperture and reduced anterior projection of the cheek. There is resorption of mandibular and maxillary bones leading to a reduction in vertical height of the midface and decreased chin projection. This, in turn, reduces support for the overlying soft tissues.

The midfacial fat pads around the zygoma and periorbital areas, which form the malar prominence, descend and atrophy with age. The fat pads that descent with age include the malar pad (Fig. 24.10), which is held up by true ligaments to the malar eminence; buccal fat pad, which is held up by false ligaments; and SOOF fat pad, which forms part of the malar crescent and is bound to the periosteum.

Malar fat pad descent causes the nasolabial crease to become more prominent. It also exposes the lateral

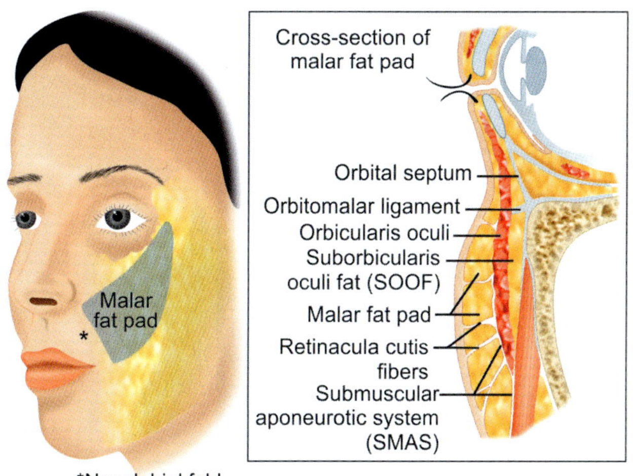

Fig. 24.10: Illustration showing the location of malar fat pad and its relationship to other structures of the midface.

orbital rim and deepens the nasojugal (tear trough) crease. Furthermore, as the malar fat pad descends, it separates from the SOOF, producing a faint diagonal groove in the infraorbital area parallel to the nasolabial crease. This happens due to reduced ligamentous support, the effect of gravity, and reduced malar bone support. This tends to occur around the early 30s and can lead to the appearance of dark circles beneath the eyes. Patients who have poor bone support or midface retrusion may undergo these changes earlier.

Key areas of the face to analyze preoperatively include position of the lateral canthi, projection of the cheek, and depth of the nasolabial creases (Figs. 24.11A to D). Areas of the midface with loss of volume should be assessed, with a plan for how to reposition fat pads medially, laterally, or in the submalar region to improve the deficiency.

The "smile test" can be used to assess whether there is a need for volume augmentation. If the malar fat pad ascends when the patient smiles, then an increase in volume is not needed and malar fat pad lift will be successful. If volume is lacking when the patient smiles, then it is likely that a filler or implant will be needed (Keller, et al., 2014).

Global volume loss transforms a youthful oval face in the frontal view to a flat and deflated face in old age. Volume loss is particularly prominent in the cheek area. Skin flaccidity and loss of volume of the subcutaneous tissue and fat modify the facial contour along several vectors created by the different fascia attachments.

Lifting the cheeks using SOOF lift or midface lift techniques can be used for midface rejuvenation. This indirectly improves the nasolabial crease, tear trough deformity, and jowling. Volume restoration to the midface and infraorbital area along with lower eyelid blepharoplasty restores a youthful appearance in such patients.

Aging of the Lower Face and Neck

Descent and laxity of soft tissues and masseteric cutaneous and mandibular cutaneous ligaments lead to development of jowls with aging. Along with this, there is resorption of mandible, which leads to development of sulcus in the prejowl and postjowl area.

In a youthful looking neck, the mandibular projection is adequate, the inferior border of the mandible is well defined, and the cervicomental angle is between 105° and 120°. A superiorly and posteriorly based hyoid located at C2 and C3 levels gives rise to an aesthetically pleasing neck with well-defined cervicomental angle. Such patients are more likely to achieve superior aesthetic results following lower face and neck rejuvenation procedures. On the other hand, an anteriorly and low placed hyoid at the levels of C4 and C5 leads to vertically orientated neck muscles with poorly defined neck lines, these anatomical variants are poor prognostic indicators for neck rejuvenation procedures.

Chin projection is also crucial to neck aesthetics. Retrognathia gives the appearance of an apparently short neck and blunting of cervicomental angle. With age, there is resorption of the mandibular height, which highlights skin changes resulting from SMAS laxity. These patients are likely to benefit from mandibular augmentation. A ptotic submandibular gland, lateral projection of deep cervical fat into the submental area, and prominent anterior belly of digastric muscles can also contribute to an ill-defined jaw and neckline and may need to be addressed (Stuzin, et al., 2002; Marten, et al., 2005).

In the neck skin laxity, platysmal diastasis and banding are seen with advancing age and may require platysmaplasty or nonsurgical procedures like botulinum toxin injection for aesthetic improvement.

There is drooping of the angle of the mouth and development of marionette lines due to relaxation and sagging of ligaments around the mouth and chin. Later in life patients develop perioral rhytids and a prominent chin crease. These can be minimized with facial fillers and facelift techniques that lift cheek tissue away from the area of the mouth. Perioral rhytids are best addressed with dermabrasion or laser resurfacing, these techniques are more suited for patients with Fitzpatrick skin types I and II.

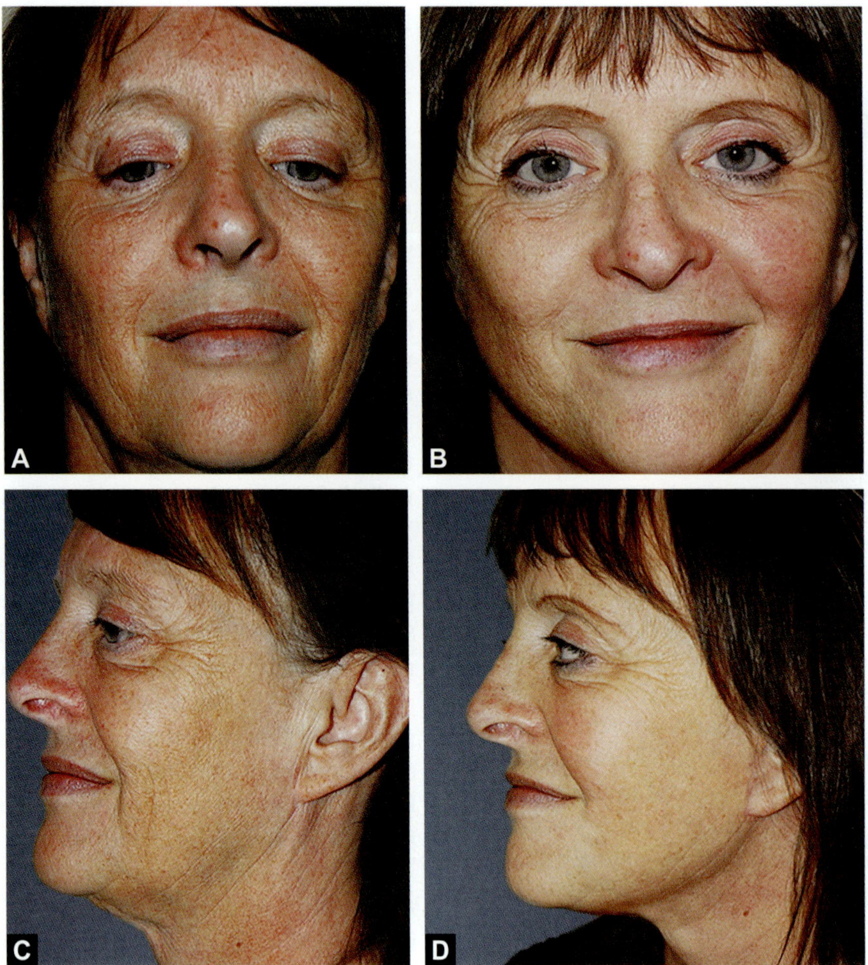

Figs. 24.11A to D: (A and C) Preoperative photographs demonstrating deep nasolabial fold, tear trough, nasojugal fold, prejowl sulcus, jowl, and platysmal banding. (B and D) Postoperative photograph after facelift with reduced nasolabial fold, tear trough, and nasojugal folds. Reduced jowls and more defined neck and jawline are also evident.

24.3 PREOPERATIVE ASSESSMENT

In today's competitive environment, it is essential that every facial plastic surgery clinic present a pleasant and welcoming environment to the patient. The staff must be warm, friendly, and well informed. The staff should be happy to pamper the patients presenting for elective aesthetic surgery. Basic courtesies like keeping to scheduled appointments and spending enough time with the patient must be observed. The surgeon and his/her staff should make every effort to understand the patient's aims and expectations from surgery, timing of surgery, as well as their emotional and financial situation. Each patient is asked to complete a detailed questionnaire to determine the goal of surgery, past medical history including previous surgeries, drug allergy, current medications, and any contraindication to surgery like smoking. Surgery should only be undertaken in those who have realistic expectations of outcome and are likely to be compliant with pre- and postoperative instructions. Any comorbidity that may compromise the operative result must be addressed before committing to surgery. A detailed explanation of the surgical and nonsurgical options along with possible risks and complications of each procedure is given to the patient. The position of each incision that will be utilized at the time of surgery is explained and documented. It is emphasized to the patient that although every effort will be made to camouflage the incisions, the resultant scars may still be visible. Brochures detailing the surgical procedure, care required in the perioperative period, and what to expect at each stage of patient's journey are made available to the patient.

Standard preoperative photographs are arranged. Standard views include full-face frontal, full-face right and left lateral and oblique views, close up of each ear without jewelry and with hair pulled back, and close up of perioral area and submental neck.

All the signs of aging detailed in the previous section are looked for and documented. Presence of midface ptosis, prominent melolabial folds, jowl, platysmal bands, and ill-defined jawline are indications for facelift surgery. Patient is asked to sit in front of a three-way mirror and the surgeon takes note of their specific concerns. Repositioning the facial soft tissues along the proposed vectors of pull is performed to simulate the proposed improvements.

Patients with moderately thick and elastic skin with minimal sun damage, prominent cheek bones, strong jaw, and high hyoid bone are good candidates for facelift and vice versa. Patients who are overweight and have thick skin, heavy cheeks and prominent jowls are unlikely to get fantastic or long lasting results from surgery. It is important to have a frank discussion with patient regarding what is realistically achievable to prevent disappointment for the patient and surgeon alike in the postoperative period. The surgeon uses morphing software like the Mirror suite to indicate the likely improvements in the neck and jawline.

24.4 MIDFACIAL REJUVENATION

The midface has traditionally been the hardest region of the face to rejuvenate. Standard cervicofacial rhytidectomy does not specifically address the midface. Facial rejuvenation options for the midface include open or endoscopic midface lift, deep plane rhytidectomy, and composite facelift. These procedures may be combined with volume restoration using fillers or autologous fat transfer.

Injectable Fillers

Injectable fillers have come a long way since the first use of bovine collagen in the 1980s (Pontius, Chaiet and Williams, 2013). This product did not last long once injected and there were concerns about immunological response to it. Hence this material is not favored nowadays. Current injectable fillers include hyaluronic acid, calcium hydroxyapatite, and poly-L-lactic (PLLA) acid. Hyaluronic acid fillers tend to last for 9–18 months and are mostly used for effacement of melolabial crease, marionette lines, and tear trough deformity.

Injectable fillers that can be used in the deeper layers of the skin include Sculptra (PLLA) and Radiesse (calcium hydroxyapatite). These fillers are longer lasting than hyaluronic acid. Radiesse is particularly useful for filling prominent nasolabial folds when injected into the deep dermis or subdermis. Sculptra is predominantly useful for large volume substitution in the midface and has the added advantage of results lasting for 5 years and longer. Usually 2–3 injections of Sculptra 3–6 months apart are required depending on the amount of collagen production and volume restoration desired. The carrier material resorbs after injection and the active product within (PLLA) subsequently produces a low-grade inflammatory response resulting in production of new collagen. This process takes 3–4 months and the patients should be advised accordingly.

Fillers for facial rejuvenation have been described in detail in Chapter 21, Volume 2 and will not be discussed further in this chapter.

Fat Transfer

One more option for volume replacement in the midface is autologous fat transfer. Fat is harvested from the abdomen or thighs using fat harvesting cannulas. Since fat is autologous material, it is associated with less risk of foreign body reaction and granuloma formation as compared to fillers. Up to 50% of fat resorbs after transfer, the surgeon has to compensate for this loss by over-injecting at the time of fat transfer. Patient is counseled that they may require more than one session spaced 3–6 months apart to achieve optimal results.

Midface Lift Operative Techniques

There are various approaches that may be used for midface lift like endoscopic, nonendoscopic short scar, deep plane facelift, and composite facelift. The location of the incision dictates the plane of dissection and the method of fixation. Incisions include temporal, orbital, and oral.

Temporal Approach

A high temporal incision hidden behind the hairline is a popular approach with many surgeons, due to good scar cosmesis and the superolateral vector of pull (Keller, et al., 2014). This approach decreases the risk of eyclid malposition that may result from transorbital approaches. As well as the midface, it allows for lifting of the temples, lateral brow, and lower eyelids as a single unit.

Ramirez (1994) developed the endoscopic approach for full facelift. The procedure is performed under general anesthesia. After local anesthesia infiltration, two incisions

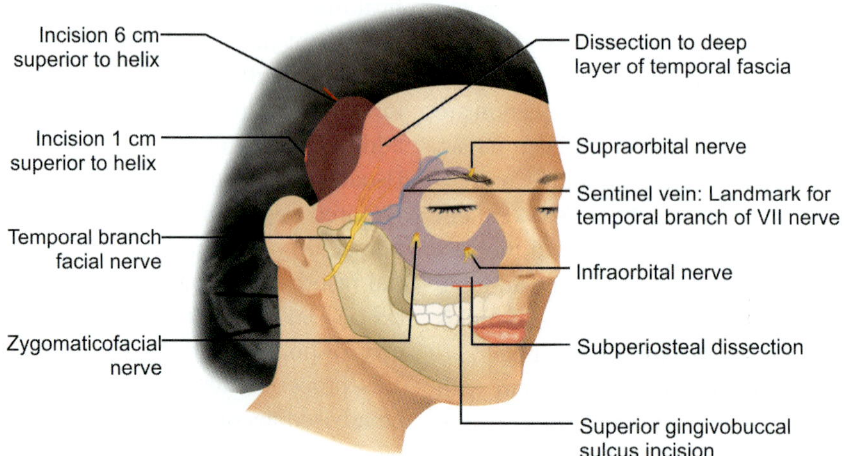

Fig. 24.12: Illustration to demonstrate the extent of dissection carried out in endoscopic midface lift procedures.

are placed 1.5 cm posterior to the anterior hairline (Fig. 24.12). The incisions are beveled in the direction of hair follicles to prevent injury and postoperative alopecia. One 2.5–3 cm incision is placed in the temporal area parallel to the lateral brow and is used for temporal access. The second 1.5 cm vertical incision is placed medial to the superior temporal septum. The dissection in the forehead is in the subperiosteal plane, whereas the dissection in the temporal area is subgaleal (deep to superficial temporal fascia and superficial to the deep temporal fascia), similar to endoscopic brow lift procedure. Two centimeter above the zygomatic arch, the dissection is carried to a plane deep to the intermediate fat pad all the way to the zygomatic arch, where the dissection is again carried out in a subperiosteal plane. This helps prevent injury to the temporal branches of facial nerve. Sentinel vein (Fig. 24.5) is a landmark for the temporal branch of the facial nerve, which travels in the superficial temporal fascia. Care must be taken not to damage the deep temporal fat pad otherwise temporal wasting may occur. This does not seem to happen if there is damage to the intermediate fat pad.

The conjoint tendon is released by sharp dissection under endoscopic control from lateral-to-medial to join the temporal and central pockets. The supraorbital and lateral temporal adhesions and arcus marginalis are released while preserving the supraorbital neurovascular bundle. The dissection is then carried down to the midface in a subperiosteal plane over the zygoma. The lateral orbital thickening is released while preserving 1 cm cuff of tissue around the lateral canthus to prevent it getting distorted. Zygomatic cutaneous, orbicularis retaining, and tear trough ligaments are released and the dissection is then carried out in a subperiosteal plane to the infraorbital area over the anterior face of the maxilla. The dissection extends all the way to the nasal bones, pyriform aperture, and the superior gingival buccal sulcus. An alternative is to make an incision in the upper gingivobuccal sulcus or along the pyriform aperture intranasally to raise a subperiosteal flap over the anterior face of maxilla. With either approach, the surgeon has to take care not to damage the infraorbital nerve and orbital contents. This is achieved by placing a finger over the infraorbital nerve and the orbital rim while performing the dissection.

A 2-0 polydioxanone periosteal suture (PDS) is used to suspend the SOOF and midface from the deep temporal fascia. A second suture is placed between the skin flap (posterior to the facial nerve) and the deep temporal fascia. The excess skin in the temporal area is distributed posteriorly and smoothened by suturing techniques. A single drain is inserted and skin closed with vertical mattress sutures or staples making sure that there is no step-off at the skin edges. Midface lift leads to bunching of excess skin in the lower eyelid, which is excised using skin pinch technique. Midface lift leads to tightening of the lower eyelid. This makes it difficult to perform a lower eyelid transconjunctival blepharoplasty after midface lift. If lower eyelid blepharoplasty is planned, it should be performed before midface lift. Patients are informed that they should expect to have marked edema of the face and distortion of the lateral canthus lasting for 8–12 weeks after midface lift.

Some surgeons prefer to address both ptosis of soft tissues and volume loss with a multimodal approach. Defatta and Williams (2011) advocate endoscopic midface lift in combination with lipotransfer, in order to address volume loss at the tear trough and infraorbital rim. Marten advocates lipotransfer with SMAS lift (Marten, 2008; Marten and Elyassnia, 2015). The advantages of using fat over a synthetic filler are that it is readily available, easy to harvest, biocompatible, and pliable. Implants can be used to compensate for atrophy of bone and fat. These can be used in the infraorbital region, malar bone, or anterior wall of maxilla (Terino and Edward, 2008).

Orbital Approach

The orbital approach involves a subciliary or transconjunctival incision (Albrecht, 2006). Dissection proceeds in the subperiosteal plane to elevate and then fix the midface soft tissues to the deep temporalis fascia posterior to the orbital rim at a level above the lateral canthus. This can cause bunching of tissue at the lateral orbital rim, which may be avoided if a transtemporal approach with concurrent temporal lift is used. The excess lower eyelid skin is excised and a canthoplasty or canthopexy is performed to create lower eyelid support. The key advantages with the orbital approach are the avoidance of risk to the facial nerve and a vertical vector of pull.

Deep Plane and Composite Facelift

The alternative preauricular incision involves a sub-SMAS deep plane rhytidectomy dissection. The dissection in this technique is continued deep to the malar fat pad but superficial to the zygomaticus major and minor muscles medially to avoid injury to facial nerve. The zygomatic cutaneous ligaments are released and anchored to deep temporal fascia in order to allow elevation of the malar fat pad. This approach gives a more posterolateral vector of pull. Ideally this vector should be parallel to the axis of the zygomaticus major muscle.

Rhytidectomy Techniques

Although transtemporal and orbital midface lift techniques help address midface aging-related changes, they do little to address lower face aging like jowls, prejowl sulcus, loss of definition of the jawline, and platysmal banding. A number of facelift techniques are available to address these issues. They differ from each other in the length of incision, extent and plane of soft tissue dissection, vector of lift, and time required for recovery. The surgeon decides on the most appropriate technique to use for an individual patient after careful history-taking and detailed physical examination.

Superficial plane of dissection-limited subcutaneous flaps: In an attempt to lift ptotic facial soft tissues, surgeons initially attempted raising limited subcutaneous flaps containing a thin layer of fat, pulling the skin posterosuperiorly, trimming the excess skin, and then suturing the skin edges together to obtain the desired lift. However, skin has a tendency to creep and stretch over time and consequently these techniques did not yield long lasting results. Any attempt to remove excess skin and close wounds under tension leads to an operated wind swept look and stretched scars, which are aesthetically unacceptable. Hence limited subcutaneous flap techniques are no longer favored for facelift surgery. Other planes of dissection like midcutaneous plane with a moderate amount of fat included in the skin flap, and supra-SMAS flaps where the flap is raised just above the SMAS layer have also been utilized but are not preferred.

Sub-SMAS plane of dissection: To overcome the problems associated with superficial skin flaps, Skoog (1974) described dissection in a deeper subfascial plane, which removes tension on the skin during closure and furthermore leads to improved results in the lower third of the face. Subsequent description of SMAS (Mitz and Peyronie, 1976) led to the advent of SMAS plication and imbrication techniques that led to improvement in the jawline. Pull on SMAS repositions and lifts the muscles it envelops, and skin it is attached to, without any tension on the skin edges.

In both SMAS plication and imbrication, a subcutaneous skin flap is raised in the preauricular and postauricular areas after making a classical facelift incision and SMAS is identified. In SMAS plication (Fig. 24.13), the anterior more mobile SMAS is sutured to the posterior immobile SMAS with 2-0 PDS leading to posterosuperior vector of pull on the attached structures. In SMAS imbrication, sub-SMAS dissection is carried out to dissect and excise a strip of SMAS and then the two edges of SMAS are sutured to each other to achieve the desired lift. In both techniques along with pull on the SMAS layer, the excess skin is excised in a way that the skin edges can be approximated without any tension on the wound.

Minimal Access Cranial Suspension Lift

The other contentious issue in facelift surgery is the vector of pull that should be utilized during surgery. The classical facelift techniques employ a posterosuperior vector of pull, whereas Tonnard and Verpaele (2007) and Verpaele, et al. (2007) feel that the vector of pull should be vertical since the descent of soft tissues due to gra-vity is in a

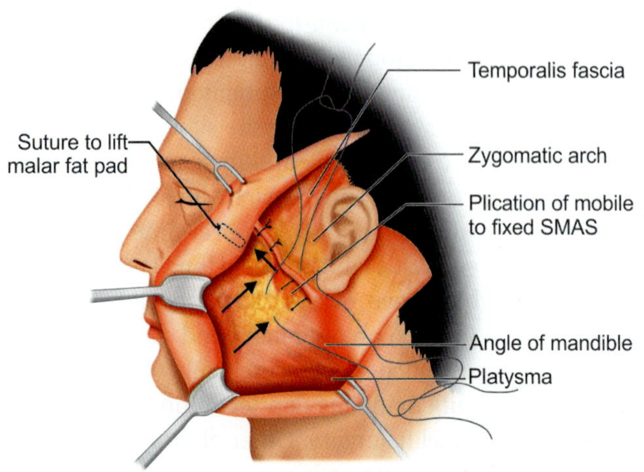

Fig. 24.13: Illustration showing superficial musculoaponeurotic system (SMAS) plication facelift procedure.

vertical direction. They are also proponents of short scar rhytidectomy employed in their minimal access cranial suspension (MACS) lift procedure (Figs. 24.14A to C), as the downtime associated with this procedure is 2 weeks compared to the longer recovery period in more aggressive facelift techniques.

Minimal access cranial suspension lift is a variation of the SMAS plication technique. In simple MACS lift (S-MACS), two PDS 2-0 purse string sutures are used to pull the SMAS in a vertical direction to correct jowling, marionette grooves, and cervicomental angle. The incision is limited to the preauricular portion of the classical facelift incision from the earlobe to the temporal area and then follows the temporal hairline along the sideburn to the level of the lateral canthus. Skin is undermined in a subcutaneous plane for 5 cm anteriorly and up to the mandibular angle inferiorly. In extended MACS lift, the incision is similar to S-MACS lift but it is extended for 1–2 cm along the anterior temporal line to the level of the tail of the eyebrow. In addition to the skin undermining carried out in S-MACS lift, an area of skin over the malar fat pad is also undermined. A U-shaped third purse string suture is used to anchor the malar fat pad and suspend it to the deep temporal fascia just superior lateral to the zygomatic frontal suture to correct nasolabial groove, midface descent, and shorten the height of the lower eyelid.

Deep Plane and Composite Rhytidectomy Approach

Hamra (1992a, 1992b) introduced the deep plane (Figs. 24.15A and B) and subsequently the composite facelift (Figs. 24.16A to C) procedure for rejuvenation of the mid and lower face in the 1990s. Both approaches (Figs. 24.17A and B) involved sub-SMAS dissection of the malar fat pad but the compo-site facelift incorporated a lower blepharoplasty approach with facelift dissection. It involved repositioning a composite flap of orbicularis oculi, cheek fat, and platysma muscle as one unit, so as to maintain the relationship of each structure to the other and also to the skin.

Hamra (1990) through his more aggressive sub-SMAS deep plane and composite facelift techniques (Hamra, 1992a, 1992b) demonstrated improved results in the middle third of face. Although his techniques improved results, they were challenged because of the associated prolonged postoperative recovery period and greater risk of complications like injury to facial nerve, prolonged edema, and risk of eyelid malposition and ectropion.

There is still debate in the literature regarding the facelift procedure that gives the best and most durable results. Becker and Bassichis (2004) evaluated deep plane facelift versus SMAS plication facelift in correcting the melolabial fold, jowl, and cheek areas of the face in short-term follow-up. In their study, deep-plane facelift did not seem to offer superior results over SMAS plication facelift in patients <70 years of age. On the other hand, Kamer and Frankel (1998) have shown through their retrospective study that the tuck rate following SMAS rhytidectomy was 11.4%, and that following deep plane rhytidectomy was 3.3% in their series, which suggests that deep plane rhytidectomy gives more desirable results. This debate is unlikely to be resolved because of the innumerable variables that dictate the choice of surgery for a patient. There is a suggestion that high SMAS deep plane facelift with other open procedures for neck rejuvenation offers satisfactory and durable rejuvenation to the midface, lower face, and neck (Marten, 1997; 2008). The facial plastic surgeon can choose from a plethora of surgical techniques and adopt them to the needs of each individual patient. In doing so the surgeon has to consider their unique anatomical characteristics, degree of aging, their goals, and aspirations as well as the downtime they are willing to commit toward achieving their goals.

24.5 SURGICAL TECHNIQUES FOR FACELIFT

The zygomatic arch, malar eminence, McGregor's patch, angle and inferior border of mandible, jowls, platysmal bands, melolabial folds, an arch 2 cm lateral to the oral commissure, Pitanguy line, and the extent of infiltration and dissection are all marked with the patient in the

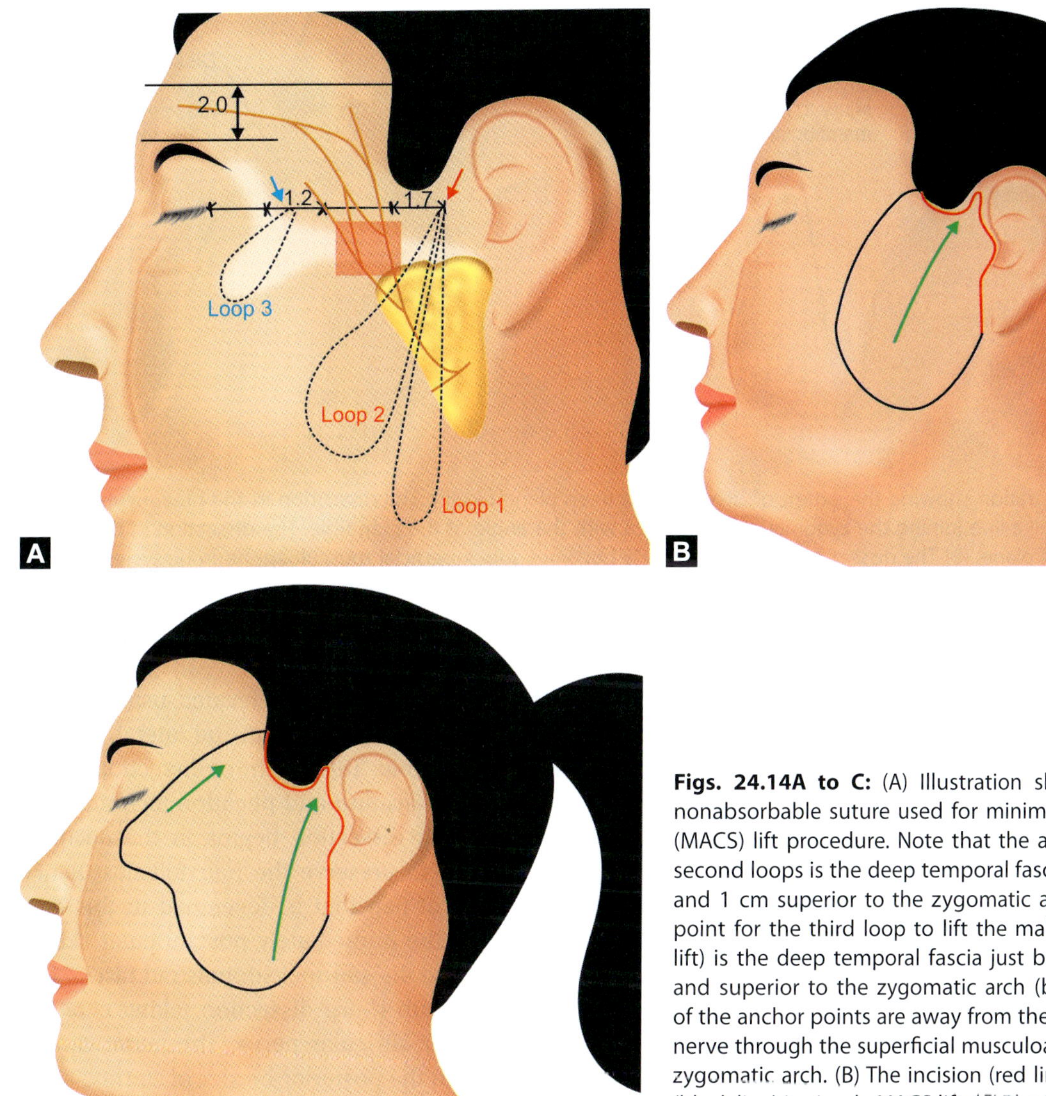

Figs. 24.14A to C: (A) Illustration showing the three loops of nonabsorbable suture used for minimal access cranial suspension (MACS) lift procedure. Note that the anchor point of the first and second loops is the deep temporal fascia 1 cm anterior to the helix and 1 cm superior to the zygomatic arch (red arrow). The anchor point for the third loop to lift the malar fat pad (extended MACS lift) is the deep temporal fascia just behind the lateral orbital rim and superior to the zygomatic arch (blue arrow). These positions of the anchor points are away from the temporal branches of facial nerve through the superficial musculoaponeurotic system over the zygomatic arch. (B) The incision (red line) and extent of dissection (black line) in simple MACS lift. (C) The incision (red line) and extent of dissection (black line) in Extended MACS lift.

sitting position in the waiting area before the start of the procedure. The procedure is carried out under intravenous sedation or general anesthesia with 1% lignocaine with 1:200,000 epinephrine infiltration.

It is of utmost importance that the surgeon plans and places facelift incisions and executes them meticulously so that scars are invisible and there is no distortion of hairline (temporal tuft of hair in women and sideburn in men) and ear lobule. If the sideburn hairline is 1–2 cm inferior to the level of the insertion of the superior portion of helical root, the surgeon can design an incision that extends into the temporal hairline. This will allow the hairline to be lifted in a posterosuperior direction to some degree. However, if the preauricular tuft of hair is at the level of helical insertion before surgery, there is a danger that it may be lifted above this level leading to a cosmetic deformity. This may be prevented by making a beveled zigzag trichial incision at the inferior aspect of the temporal tuft of hair. The incision is beveled in the direction of the hair shafts so that hair growth through the incision camouflages the scar. Avoid making the incision along the anterior aspect of temporal hairline. It is difficult to camouflage scars in this region as the hair are very fine, low density, and posteriorly directed.

The incision follows the natural curvature of the helical insertion. It is then hidden 2–3 mm behind the tragus and is then placed in a natural skin crease in the preauricular area. However in men, and in patients who wear a

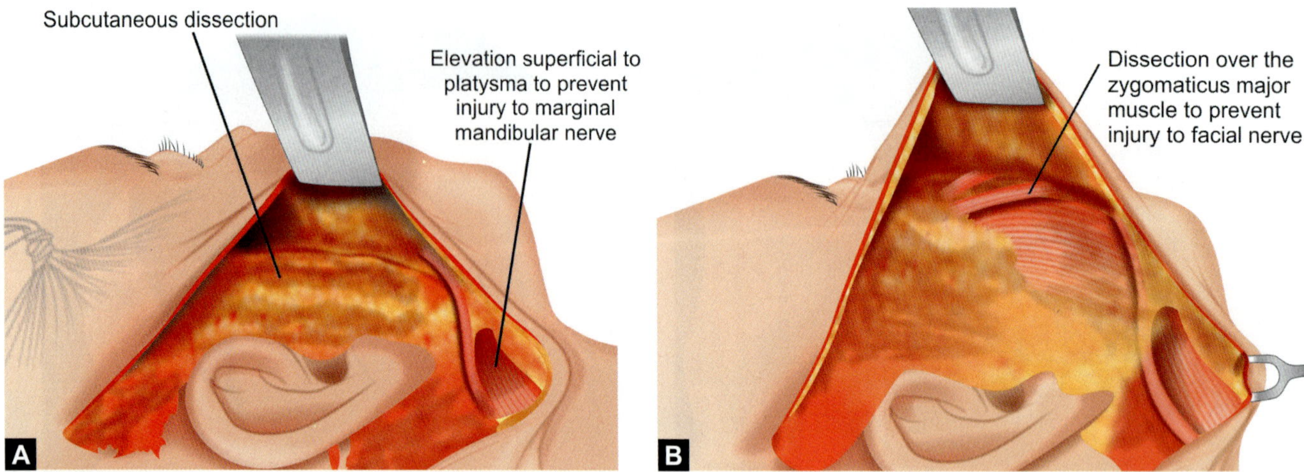

Figs. 24.15A and B: (A) Illustration showing the extent of dissection in deep plane facelift. The dissection in the preauricular area is in the subcutaneous plane till a line joining the zygomatic prominence with the angle of the mandible. The dissection in the neck is performed in a preplatysmal plane. (B) The dissection further anteriorly becomes sub-superficial musculoaponeurotic system (SMAS) but stays superficial to the zygomaticus major muscle to avoid injury to the facial nerve that supplies the muscle through its deep surface. Malar fat pad is lifted with the sub SMAS flap.

hearing aid, a gently curved incision is made in a natural preauricular skin crease from the superior attachment of pinna to the ear lobe to preserve a reasonable width of non-hair bearing skin in the preauricular area. This helps prevent the hair bearing bearded skin from being pulled posterosuperiorly on to the ear.

In both men and women, the incision is then carried around the ear lobule leaving a 3 mm cuff of skin attached to the ear lobule to prevent its distortion. The incision is then continued on to the posterior aspect of the pinna 7–10 mm anterior to the postauricular sulcus. Scar contraction in the postoperative period leads to the postauricular incision settling into the postauricular groove and prevents a visible scar in the postauricular area. The incision is then carried backward toward the hairline in a "lazy S" fashion at a level where most amount of the postauricular skin is covered by the pinna. Next the incision is carried posteriorly and inferiorly into the occipital hair. If there is marked laxity of the neck skin that needs to be addressed by a posterosuperior pull, the incision is carried along the postauricular hairline for a distance before being turned posteriorly. The authors prefers to place the incision 1–1.5 cm behind and parallel to the hairline along its entire length so that it is hidden within the hairline. The salient features to consider in planning a facelift incision are detailed in Figure 24.18.

The extent of elevation of subcutaneous skin flap and the plane of dissection varies from one facelift technique to other and is dictated by the redundancy of facial and neck tissues and the vector of pull. After making the incision, the preauricular skin is elevated using a knife for 2–3 cm up to a line drawn from the lateral canthus to the angle of mandible. This extent of dissection is sufficient for SMAS imbrication and plication techniques.

The postauricular dissection begins in the occipital area. Care is taken to preserve the hair follicles; hence the initial portion of flap that is developed in this area is relatively thick. The immediately postauricular skin is thin and adherent to the sternocleidomastoid fascia. It is elevated carefully with sharp dissection taking care not to injure the greater auricular nerve. The nerve can be seen emerging from the posterior border of sternocleidomastoid muscle (6.5 cm below the tragus) and should be identified and preserved. In the neck, dissection is carried out in a subcutaneous plane superficial to the platysma to prevent injury to the marginal mandibular nerve.

The extent of SMAS dissection depends on the degree of midface ptosis, jowl formation, and platysmal banding. In plication techniques, the SMAS is folded over itself and sutured. If SMAS imbrication is planned, an incision is placed in the SMAS 1 cm anterior and parallel to the preauricular skin incision from just below the zygomatic arch to just below the angle of mandible. Superficial musculoaponeurotic system is elevated for a distance of 1–2 cm from the parotid fascia. A 1–2 cm strip of SMAS is excised and the cut ends are sutured to each other. An alternative technique is to develop an inferiorly based SMAS flap attached below the level of ear lobule. This is then sutured to the mastoid periosteum and leads to better definition

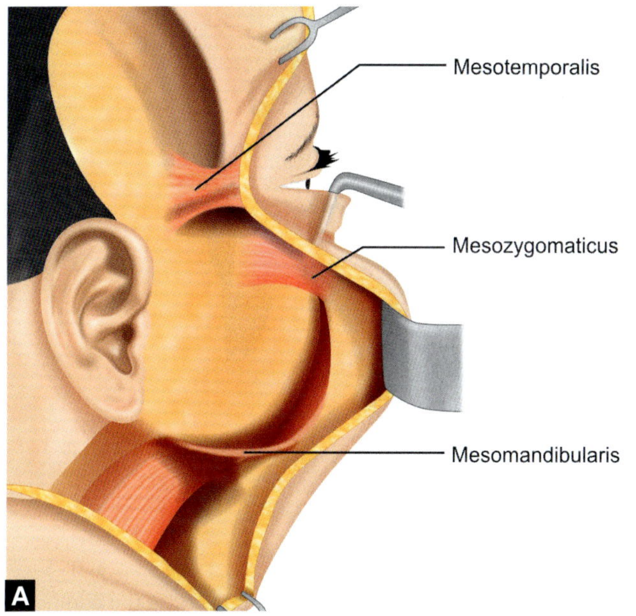

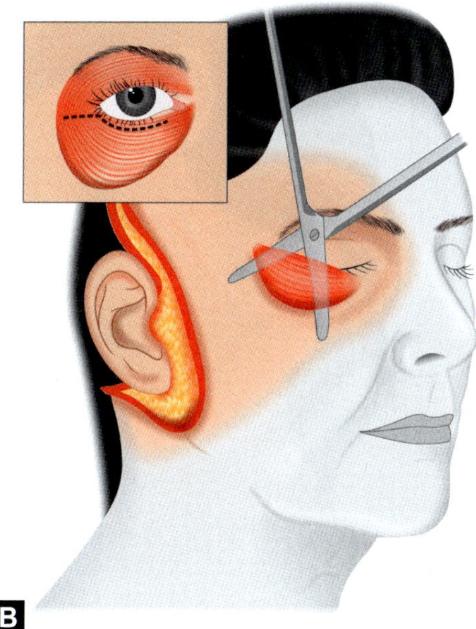

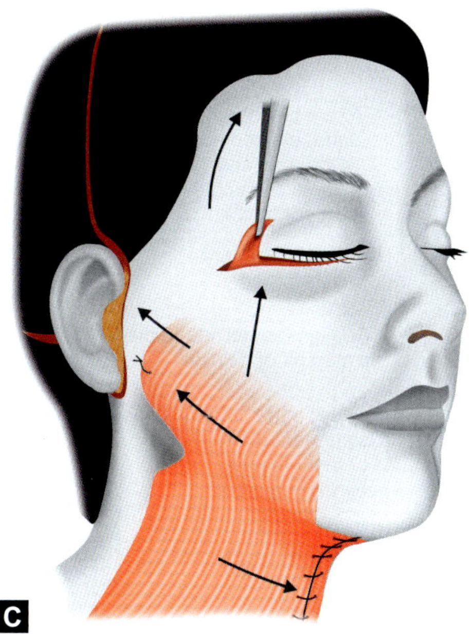

Figs. 24.16A to C: (A) Illustration showing the extent of dissection carried out in a composite facelift. Composite facelift involves even more extensive dissection than the deep plane facelift. The dissection in the neck and preauricular area is similar to deep plane facelift. In the temporal area, the dissection is in a plane that is superficial to the superficial layer of deep temporal fascia. This creates three mesenteries, mesotemporalis containing the temporal branch, mesozygomaticus containing the zygomatic branch, and mesomandibularis containing the mandibular branch of facial nerve. (B) Through a subciliary incision, the surgeon releases the orbicularis oculi muscle from its deep attachments from 5'o clock to 9'o clock (on the right side) and this plane is then joined to the suprazygomaticus major dissection carried out in a deep plane lift. (C) The released muscle is then suspended along with the malar fat pad and midface structures to the deep temporal fascia with sutures. Any redundant orbicularis oculi muscle is excised.

of the jawline due to the resultant pull on the platysma. The superior cut edges of SMAS are then approximated to each other with horizontal mattress sutures and suspended from the deep temporal fascia.

If deep plane facelift is planned, the surgeon elevates a sub-SMAS flap anterior to the line drawn from the lateral canthus to the angle of mandible. The dissection in the neck is supraplatysmal. An uninterrupted bridge of SMAS (mesomandibularis) is maintained between the two planes as it contains the marginal mandibular nerve. The dissection is then carried over the zygomaticus major muscle to elevate the malar fat pad attached to the skin flap. The zygomatic cutaneous and masseteric cutaneous ligaments are released, which helps in lifting the tissues. If composite facelift is planned, the orbicularis oculi muscle is released from its deep attachments through a subciliary incision (from 5'o clock to 9'o clock on the right side) and this plane is then joined to the suprazygomaticus major dissection carried out in a deep plane lift. The released muscle is then suspended along with the malar

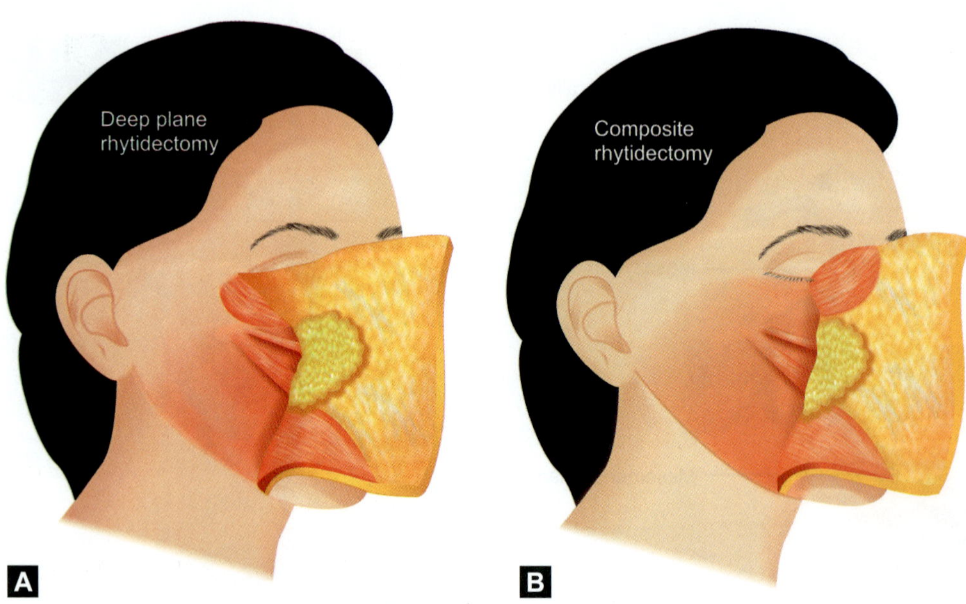

Figs. 24.17A and B: Illustration demonstrating the difference between deep plane and composite rhytidectomy. Note the additional release of orbicularis oculi muscle, which is then lifted along with the malar fat pad in composite facelift as compared to deep plane facelift.

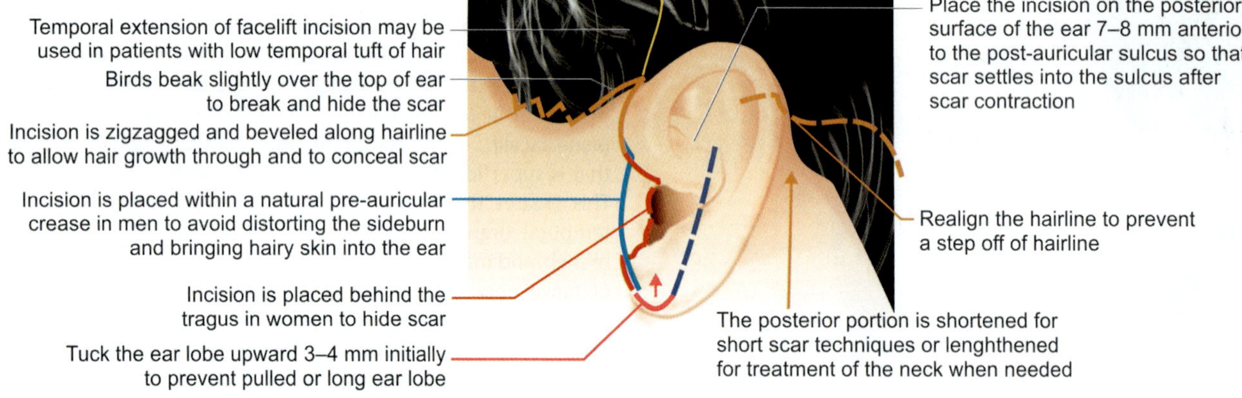

Fig. 24.18: Illustration showing the important factors to consider during facelift incision planning.

fat pad and midface structures to the deep temporal fascia with sutures. Any redundant orbicularis oculi muscle is excised.

Temporal extension of facelift incision is required in patients undergoing a simultaneous midface lift or composite facelift when repositioning of excessive tissue in the lateral brow and lateral orbital region is needed to prevent bunching after midface lift. The dissection is carried out in a subgaleal plane preserving a continuous bridge of SMAS (mesotemporalis) that contains the temporal branches of facial nerve. This plane is then joined to the subperiosteal midface lift plane further inferiorly.

A 2–3 cm incision is made just anterior to a preexisting submental crease to facilitate platysmaplasty and excision of excess fat from the neck. Neck rejuvenation has been discussed in detail in Chapter 25, Volume 2 and will not be discussed further in this chapter.

24.6 NONSURGICAL TECHNIQUES FOR FACELIFT

Thread Lift

Sutures with barbs directed unilaterally have been used to create a high contour of the midface, brow, and for giving the jawline more definition. Barbed sutures like APTOS (Sulamanidze and Sulamanidze, 2009) suture are introduced subcutaneously by means of a guiding needle and without the need for incisions. When tightened the barbs in the sutures engage the subcutaneous soft tissues and help lift it toward the anchor point. Thread lift techniques have the advantage of low downtime and can be performed under local anesthesia. However, the lift achieved is very mild and only suitable for addressing mild manifestations of soft tissue descent. They are not suitable for patients with a heavy face. They should only be considered for patients who refuse surgery and are happy with mild lifting that is hardly visible to other people.

24.7 COMPLICATIONS

Midface Lift

Midface lift procedures are generally safe with adequate knowledge of surgical anatomy and experience (Albrecht, 2006; Jacono and Ransom, 2013). However, the following complications may result from surgery.

Nerve Injury

Facial nerve injury is rare, as is injury to the sensory supraorbital and infraorbital nerves. Temporal and marginal mandibular branches of the facial nerve are most commonly injured. Weakness of the temporal branch of facial nerve may occur due to stretch injury or due to overzealous electrocautery in the vicinity of the sentinel vein. Marginal mandibular nerve is in danger of injury if dissection is carried out in a subplatysmal plane in the neck. Transient numbness in the territory of supraorbital and infraorbital nerves may occur but usually resolves within 9–12 months.

Alopecia

Alopecia along skin incisions may occur from injury to the hair follicles or excessive tension on the wound and can be prevented by meticulous surgical technique.

Distortion of Eyelid and Lateral Canthus

Care should be taken not to transect the orbicularis oculi muscle, as this can lead to denervation of this muscle and eyelid retraction, especially if the pretarsal portion is affected. When subciliary approach is used, there is always a possibility of lower eyelid malposition. Lateral canthal distortion is expected for a few weeks and usually recovers with massage. Sometimes patients experience chemosis and eyelid edema for >6 weeks, but these resolve spontaneously.

Brow Asymmetry

There is a risk of brow distortion, this usually settles with local massage. Rarely revision surgery to release and reposition the tissues may be necessary.

Facelift

Hematoma

Hematoma formation is the commonest complication following facelift surgery and occurs in up to 15% of patients (Rees and Aston, 1978; Lawson and Naidu, 1993). Ingestion of antiplatelet drugs, anticoagulants, vitamin E containing products, ginger, and herbal medications predisposes to hematoma formation. These drugs must be discontinued 2 weeks prior to surgery. Males are at increased risk of hematoma formation due to increased vascularity of hair-bearing facial skin. Hypertension [2.6-fold risk (Straith, Raju and Hipps, 1977)] and coughing or retching during extubation predispose to hematoma formation. Use of fibrin glue (Zoumalan and Rizk, 2008) and drains decrease the incidence of hematoma formation. Aspiration and antibiotics (Pitanguy and Ceravolo, 1981) may be used to treat minor hematomas identified within the first week. Major hematomas are drained by opening the incision line adequately. The bleeding point is identified and ligated followed by pressure bandage to the site. If left untreated, fibrosis and skin irregularity and dimpling may occur. Should this happen, massage and serial triamcinolone injections at 4–6-week interval may be helpful.

Infection

Infection is not common after facelift surgery. Cellulitis usually responds to broad-spectrum antibiotics. Untreated or unrecognized hematomas predispose to abscess formation, which requires incision and drainage followed by intravenous antibiotics.

Flap Necrosis

Necrosis of skin flap is a dreaded complication. Predisposing factors include history of smoking (Adamson and Moran, 1993) (12.6-fold risk), anticoagulant therapy, extensive subcutaneous dissection with damage to subdermal plexus, diabetes mellitus, and connective tissue disorders.

Patients are advised to stop smoking for 2 weeks prior to surgery. In smokers, limited undermining of skin should be carried out to decrease the risk of flap necrosis (Webster, et al., 1986). If necrosis occurs, it is treated conservatively with daily dressings till the area heals by secondary intention. If the scar is unacceptable, scar revision may be carried out after a few months.

Sensory and Motor Nerve Injury

Greater auricular nerve is most commonly injured nerve in facelift surgery (1–7%) (McKinney and Katrana, 1980; Kamer, 1996). Injury to facial nerve occurs in 0.5–2.6% of patients (Rees and Aston, 1978; Liebman, et al., 1988) with the temporal and marginal mandibular nerves being the most commonly affected. If injury is recognized at the time of surgery, direct anastomoses under microscopic control should be attempted. Most injuries are due to neuropraxia and 85% of injuries recover with time (Baker and Conley, 1979). If recovery is not noticed after 1 year of reconstructive surgery in the form of brow elevation or upper eyelid, platinum implants may need to be considered.

Poor Scars and Alopecia

Poor planning of incisions may lead to stair step deformity in the postauricular hairline, loss of temporal tuft of hair, and standing cutaneous deformity formation. This may require revision surgery for correction. Excessive wound tension closure predisposes to wide and hypertrophic scars and alopecia and should be avoided. If alopecia or loss of temporal tuft of hair occurs, hair transplantation may be considered.

Distortion of Ear Lobe

Failure to tuck the earlobe properly predisposes to it being pulled inferiorly during the healing phase leading to devil's ear deformity, which is difficult to correct. V-Y plasty may be used to recreate the inferior lobe sulcus.

REFERENCES

Adamson, P. and Moran, M.L., 1993. Complications of cervicofacial rhytidectomy. *Facial Plastic Surgery Clinics of North America,* 112, pp. 257-70.

Albrecht, P., 2006. Trans-inferior orbital rim anchorage and fascia roll multi-loop temporal anchorage in midface rejuvenation. *Aesthetic Surgery Journal,* 26, pp. 404-12.

Baker, D.C. and Conley, J., 1979. Avoiding facial nerve injuries in rhytidectomy. Anatomical variations and pitfalls. *Plastic Reconstructive Surgery,* 64, pp. 781-95.

Becker, F.F. and Bassichis, B.A., 2004. Deep-plane face-lift vs superficial musculoaponeurotic system plication face-lift: a comparative study. *Archives of Facial Plastic Surgery,* 6, pp. 8-13.

Beer, K. and Beer, J., 2009. Overview of facial aging. *Facial Plastic Surgery,* 25, pp. 281-4.

Defatta, R.J. and Williams, E.F., 3rd, 2011. Midface lifting: current standards. *Facial Plastic Surgery,* 27, pp. 77-85.

Hamra, S.T., 1990. The deep-plane rhytidectomy. *Plastic and Reconstructive Surgery,* 86, pp. 53-61; discussion 62-3.

Hamra, S.T., 1992a. Composite rhytidectomy. *Plastic and Reconstructive Surgery,* 90, pp. 1-13.

Hamra, S.T., 1992b. Repositioning the orbicularis oculi muscle in the composite rhytidectomy. *Plastic and Reconstructive Surgery,* 90, pp. 14-22.

Jacono, A.A. and Ransom, E.R., 2013. Anatomic predictors of unsatisfactory outcomes in surgical rejuvenation of the midface. *JAMA Facial Plastic Surgery,* 15, pp. 101-9.

Kamer, F.M., 1996. One hundred consecutive deep plane face-lifts. *Archives of Otolaryngology—Head and Neck Surgery,* 122, pp. 17-22.

Kamer, F.M. and Frankel, A.S., 1998. SMAS rhytidectomy versus deep plane rhytidectomy: an objective comparison. *Plastic and Reconstructive Surgery,* 102, pp. 878-81.

Keller, G., Quatela, V.C., Antunes, M.B., Sykes, J.M., Magill, C.K. and Seth, R., 2014. Midface lift: panel discussion. *Facial Plastic Surgery Clinics in North America,* 22, pp. 119-37.

Lawson, W. and Naidu, R.K., 1993. The male facelift. An analysis of 115 cases. *Archives of Otolaryngology—Head and Neck Surgery,* 119, pp. 535-9; discussion 540-41.

Liebman, E.P., Webster, R.C., Gaul, J.R. and Griffin, T., 1988. The marginal mandibular nerve in rhytidectomy and liposuction surgery. *Archives of Otolaryngology—Head and Neck Surgery,* 114, pp. 179-81.

Marten, T.J., 1997. Facelift. Planning and technique. *Clinics in Plastic Surgery,* 24, pp. 269-308.

Marten, T.J., 2008. High SMAS facelift: combined single flap lifting of the jawline, cheek, and midface. *Clinics in Plastic Surgery,* 35, pp. 569-603, vi-vii.

Marten, T.J. and Elyassnia, D., 2015. Fat grafting in facial rejuvenation. *Clinics in Plastic Surgery,* 42, pp. 219-52.

Marten, T.J., Feldman, J.J., Connell, B.F. and Little, W.J., 2005. Treatment of the full obtuse neck. *Aesthetic Surgery Journal,* 25, pp. 387-97.

McKinney, P. and Katrana, D.J., 1980. Prevention of injury to the great auricular nerve during rhytidectomy. *Plastic and Reconstructive Surgery,* 66, pp. 675-9.

Mitz, V. and Peyronie, M., 1976. The superficial musculo-aponeurotic system (SMAS) in the parotid and cheek area. *Plastic and Reconstructive Surgery,* 58, pp. 80-88.

Pitanguy, I. and Ceravolo, M.P., 1981. Hematoma postrhytidectomy: how we treat it. *Plastic and Reconstructive Surgery,* 67, pp. 526-9.

Pontius, A.T., Chaiet, S.R. and Williams, E.F., 3rd, 2013. Midface injectable fillers: have they replaced midface surgery? *Facial Plastic Surgery Clinics in North America,* 21, pp. 229-39.

Ramirez, O.M., 1994. Endoscopic full facelift. *Aesthetic Plastic Surgery,* 18, pp. 363-71.

Rees, T.D. and Aston, S.J., 1978. Complications of rhytidectomy. *Clinics in Plastic Surgery,* 5, pp. 109-19.

Skoog, T., 1974. *Plastic surgery: new methods and refinements.* Philadelphia, Pa: WB Saunders Co.

Straith, R.E., Raju, D.R. and Hipps, C.J., 1977. The study of hematomas in 500 consecutive face lifts. *Plastic and Reconstructive Surgery,* 59, pp. 694-8.

Stuzin, J.M., Feldman, J.J., Baker, D.C. and Marten, T.J., 2002. Cervical contouring in face lift. *Aesthetic Surgery Journal,* 22, pp. 541-8.

Sulamanidze, M. and Sulamanidze, G., 2009. APTOS suture lifting methods: 10 years of experience. *Clinics in Plastic Surgery,* 36, pp. 281-306, viii.

Terino, E.O. and Edward, M., 2008. The magic of mid-face three-dimensional contour alterations combining alloplastic and soft tissue suspension technologies. *Clinics in Plastic Surgery,* 35, pp. 419-50; discussion 417.

Tonnard, P. and Verpaele, A., 2007. The MACS-lift short scar rhytidectomy. *Aesthetic Surgery Journal,* 27, pp. 188-98.

Verpaele, A., Tonnard, P., Gaia, S., Guerao, F.P. and Pirayesh, A., 2007. The third suture in MACS-lifting: making midface-lifting simple and safe. *Journal of Plastic and Reconstructive Aesthetic Surgery,* 60, pp. 1287-95.

Webster, R.C., Kazda, G., Hamdan, U.S., Fuleihan, N.S. and Smith, R.C., 1986. Cigarette smoking and face lift: conservative versus wide undermining. *Plastic and Reconstructive Surgery,* 77, pp. 596-604.

Wong, C.H., Hsieh, M.K. and Mendelson, B., 2012. The tear trough ligament: anatomical basis for the tear trough deformity. *Plastic and Reconstructive Surgery,* 129, pp. 1392-402.

Zoumalan, R. and Rizk, S.S., 2008. Hematoma rates in drainless deep-plane face-lift surgery with and without the use of fibrin glue. *Archives of Facial Plastic Surgery,* 10, pp. 103-7.

25 Aesthetic Surgery of the Neck and Submental Region

Jamil Asaria, Ashlin J Alexander

Chapter Overview

Pearls and Pitfalls

Pearls

- Careful consideration of body habitus and patient anatomy must be taken into account when determining the ideal procedure(s) for refinement of the submentum.
- Excess neck skin and elasticity cannot be overlooked and may need to be addressed by facelift/necklift.
- Augmentation of the mentum may be necessary (by genioplasty or alloplastic augmentation) to improve the cervicomental contour.
- Appropriate contouring of the submental and neck region can have a dramatic impact on facial balance, and therefore, it should be viewed as importantly as the upper two-thirds of the face.

Pitfalls

- Procedures undertaken without detailed knowledge of the anatomy of the submental region can lead to permanent vascular and nerve injury.
- Selecting an inadequate procedure, or an isolated procedure without accounting for multiple sources of pathology in the submentum, can lead to disappointing aesthetic results.

25.1 INTRODUCTION

In many cultures, the neck is the cornerstone of an individual's beauty. Indeed, when patients present for a *facelift* consultation, the lower third of the face and cervical region are the areas that they are most commonly dissatisfied with and most wish to have corrected (de Castro, et al., 2012). To that end, achieving a youthful neck contour is of critical importance in achieving success in *facial rejuvenation*.

25.2 RELATIONSHIP BETWEEN NECK CONFIGURATION AND AESTHETICS

- In both male and female patients, definition of the jawline and submentum contributes significantly to the ideal aesthetic balance of the lower face and neck. The youthful neck is characterized by thin soft tissue, an acute *mentocervical angle* (80°–95°) with the hyoid bone at the apex of the angle, absence of horizontal wrinkles and vertical *platysmal bands*, and lack of excess fat and sagging skin. Furthermore, a strong chin, defined *mandibular angle* and distinct mandibular line that separates itself from the neck by casting a shadow along its inferior border, serves to delineate the two aesthetic units.

- Factors contributing to a heavy and poorly defined submental region include the skeletal configuration of the neck, muscular support, adipose tissue, and skin tone. During the aging process, the lower third of the face and neck undergo significant changes. Fat and soft tissues descend along the mandibular body and obscure its definition and produce *jowling*; these are central stigmata of the aging face. Platysmal laxity in the midline leads to vertical bands, which extend from the mentum to the clavicle, and can be quite aesthetically unpleasing. *Platysmal dehiscence* allows for descent of the submandibular glands and ptosis of deep cervical fat into the submental region, creating unwanted neck fullness; coupled with skin sagging, excessive superficial and deep cervical fat, and prominence of the anterior bellies of the digastric muscles; these findings lead to the classic "double chin" phenomenon. Mandibular hypoplasia, microgenia, and chin ptosis can further exacerbate the above-described effects.

25.3 ANATOMY AND CLASSIFICATION

- In 1980, Dedo formalized these changes into a classification system of the aging neck based on anatomic layers (Table 25.1). Conceptualizing the changes of aging using separate layers—skin, fat, muscle, and bone—helps one to direct surgical planning. Several key points can be highlighted regarding the anatomy of the lower face and neck.
- Anatomically, the neck is separated into different triangles; the borders of these triangles are based on the sternocleidomastoid muscles (SCMs), the anterior and posterior digastric muscles and stylohyoid muscle, the mandibular and clavicular borders, and the midline. From the aesthetic viewpoint, the submental and submandibular triangles are most important.
- *Neck skin* must be evaluated both in terms of redundancy and elasticity. High elasticity may permit less skin resection to manage redundancy as this skin can redrape over the tightened underlying structures more readily. Skin with poor elasticity, on the other hand, will likely require resection and resuspension in the retroauricular/mastoid region to take up the excess redundancy that will result after defatting and tightening of the underlying neck structures.

Table 25.1: Dedo's classification of cervical abnormalities.

Class	*Description*
I	Younger patient with minimal cosmetic deformity of neck, essentially normal
II	Laxity of cervical skin without significant fat deposition or muscle pathology
III	Pathologic layer of subcutaneous fat, which is either genetic or acquired
IV	Pathologic platysma, evident as anterior platysmal banding in thin patients, diagnosed by voluntary facial grimacing preoperatively
V	Microgenia or retrognathia
VI	Abnormally low hyoid position

- *Supraplatysmal* (i.e. subcutaneous) *fat* prominence manifests mostly anteriorly, particularly in the submental region. It is distinct from the deep cervical fat in this region. Supraplatysmal fat can be removed by liposuction or open lipectomy.
- Understanding the *platysma muscle* is critical to aesthetic surgery of the neck. This thin, sheet-like muscle originates from the fascia of the pectoralis and deltoid regions and extends superiorly, inserting onto the anterior mandible, the skin of the cheek, the oral commissure, and the orbicularis oris muscle. In the cheek, the platysma can extend up to nearly 4 cm superiorly from the mandibular border (Shah and Rosenberg, 2009). The platysma is innervated by the cervical branch of the facial nerve, on its deep surface. Closer to the mandibular border, upper branches of the cervical branch intermingle with lower branches of the marginal mandibular branch of the facial nerve. Exercising extreme care around the marginal mandibular nerve (MMN) is a well-understood concept, but even injury to the cervical branch can have a detrimental effect on smiling in those patients whose platysma has a significant contribution to lower lip depression. This is the so-called "MMN pseudoparalysis" (Daane and Owsley, 2003); cervical branch injury can be distinguished from MMN injury by asking the patient to evert his or her lower lip, which will remain functional due to an innervated mentalis muscle.
- The *superficial layer of the deep cervical fascia* is an investing layer that envelopes the SCM and anterior strap muscles, as well as the submandibular gland.

The MMN branches run within this fascial layer, which is deep to the platysma.

- In the neck, *deep cervical fat* exists deep to the platysma, primarily in that triangle bounded by the anterior bellies of the digastric muscle and the hyoid bone. Typically, this fat can extend laterally over the top of the anterior bellies of the digastric muscles. This compartment contains lymph nodes and is thus well vascularized, requiring careful hemostasis during fat removal. In this submental region, the deep cervical fat separates the platysma from the mylohyoid. Overresection of this fat can lead to the muscular fibers of the platysma healing into the mylohyoid muscle, leaving a very noticeable depression in the submental region, the so-called "cobra neck deformity".
- The *anterior belly of the digastric muscle*, innervated by the mandibular division of the trigeminal nerve, originates from the inner surface of the lower border of the mandible and extends downward to become the intermediate tendon, which attaches to the hyoid bone. Some authors advocate tangential surgical debulking of this muscle when it is excessive (Ramirez, 2008).
- A detailed description of submandibular gland anatomy is beyond the scope of this chapter; the reader is referred to a comprehensive overview provided by Ramirez (2008). Ptotic or enlarged submandibular glands can obscure an otherwise excellent neck contour; although some surgeons suggest removal of the glands, the authors do not advocate this approach and simply educate the patient of this possibility prior to surgery.
- Stuzin, Baker and Gordon (1992) described two types of *retaining ligaments* in the face: (1) true osteocutaneous (zygomatic and mandibular) and (2) a coalescence between the superficial and deep facial fascias (parotidocutaneous and masseteric cutaneous). In particular, the mandibular ligaments arise in the parasymphyseal region and insert into the overlying skin. This retaining ligament serves as the anterior border of the *jowl* complex while the jowl is bordered posteriorly by the anterior border of the masseter. Therefore, attempts at reducing prominent jowling should focus on releasing the mandibular cutaneous ligaments and repositioning the ptotic soft tissue above the mandibular border.
- The MMN terminates in more than two branches in 84% of people (Batra, Mahajan and Gupta, 2010). When it is anterior to the facial artery, it always courses above the lower border of the mandible. When its course is posterior to the facial artery, a recent study found that it traverses along the lower border of the mandible 52% of the time, below in 32%, and above in 16% of cases. It travels 1.2 cm below the mandibular border, and 1.5 cm below the angle, on average. It is always superficial to the facial artery and vein and typically courses within the superficial layer of the deep cervical fascia. The MMN is at risk in cervical liposuction where it crosses the mandible at the antigonal notch (approximately 2 cm lateral to the oral commissure) because the nerve becomes more superficial here.
- The *great auricular nerve* originates from the second and third nerves of the cervical plexus, crosses the posterior border of the SCM at the junction of the upper third and lower two-thirds of the muscle (*Erb's point*), and ascends to give sensation to the lower pinna and postauricular region. It travels on top of the SCM, at the same depth as the platysma. Therefore, dissection in this region should remain just superficial to the fascia of the SCM to protect this nerve.

25.4 PATIENT EVALUATION

- The patient consultation should begin with a full medical history and focused physical examination. Pertinent information on history includes discerning the patient's motivations and expectations and ruling out any psychiatric conditions. Medical conditions that place the patient at increased anesthetic risk should be identified. Conditions that impair wound healing (e.g. diabetes, peripheral vascular disease, collagen vascular disease, autoimmune disorders, head and neck irradiation, smoking, Accutane, and oral steroids) or increase the risk of bleeding (e.g. bleeding disorders, anticoagulants, and herbal medications) must be carefully teased out.
- Physical examination follows a systematic and stepwise approach. First, the skin is evaluated for elasticity; those with good skin elasticity will achieve a better result.
- Mandible contour and chin position are then evaluated, as these structures play an important role in the eventual result. Chin position is evaluated by dropping a vertical line from the vermilion border of the lower lip; in men, the pogonion should be tangent to this line, and in women, it should be 2–3 mm posterior to this vertical line. Appropriate chin position is key in achieving a satisfactory neck contour and *cervicomental angle.*

- Furthermore, as described by Zide, Pfeifer and Longaker (1999), the chin-nose relationship significantly influences facial harmony. While men will rarely perceive an implant as too large, the surgeon should err toward undercorrection in women. If an overly large implant is to be removed, the surgeon should consider replacement with a smaller implant; otherwise, the prior implant pocket will contract down unpredictably and could produce disfigurement of the region.
- It is important to determine whether the patient has microgenia, micrognathia, or retrognathia. "Microgenia" describes a patient who has a small mandible but retains normal occlusion (Angle Class I). "Micrognathia" refers to a mandible that is underdeveloped but has Angle Class II occlusion (overbite). "Retrognathia" refers to an anatomical configuration where the mandible is normal in size but is retruded leading to Class II occlusion. Both micrognathia and retrognathia lead to functional problems that require correction with orthognathic surgery before chin augmentation is considered. Overaugmentation in these patients may place the *pogonion* at the correct position but will do so at the expense of the *labiomental angle*, which can lead to a protruding chin soft-tissue pad and deepened *labiomental fold* (Zide, Pfeifer and Langaker, 1999).
- *Mandibular hypoplasia* is acquired secondary to bony resorption of the mandible. As soft-tissue atrophy and bone reduction occur with aging, a groove develops between the chin and jowl, termed the "prejowl sulcus". Microgenia and mandibular hypoplasia can be addressed with an alloplastic implant or *genioplasty*, whereas micrognathia and retrognathia benefit most from a bony advancement technique (e.g. *bilateral sagittal-split osteotomy*).
- Prior to *chin advancement* or augmentation, careful consideration should also be given to the position and depth of the labiomental fold. Women who have a high or indistinct labiomental fold (i.e. closer to the lower lip) will have the appearance of a large chin soft-tissue pad. Augmentation in these patients risks making the entire lower face enlarged, which can be aesthetically very unpleasing. Conversely, women with a low labiomental crease have the appearance of a smaller chin pad, and augmentation in these patients will accentuate the chin only.
- Native hyoid bone position—ideally situated at the level of the fourth cervical vertebrae or above—is critical to achieving an acute cervicomental angle. If the hyoid is low, the patient should be advised that, even with surgical correction, the cervicomental angle will remain obtuse.
- Cervical fat is assessed for amount and distribution; liposuction or open lipectomy with scissors may need to be employed to achieve the desired contour.
- Management of the platysma muscle is compulsory to achieve a high-quality result in the lower face and neck; laxity and vertical platysmal bands are identified and treated with plication and resuspension. Identification of prominent ptotic submandibular glands and bulky anterior bellies of the digastric muscles is important; again, although some surgeons recommend removal of the glands and debulking of the muscles in this case, most surgeons would agree that the associated risks are too great and instead simply educate their patients that this prominence may become even more apparent following surgery (Table 25.2).

Table 25.2: Anatomic factors in the assessment of the aging neck.

Step	*Description*
I	Skin elasticity
II	Mandible contour and skin position
III	Hyoid position, cervicomental angle
IV	Cervical fat
V	Platysmal banding
VI	Submandibular gland ptosis
VII	Prominent anterior belly of digastric

25.5 AUGMENTATION OF THE MENTUM

Augmentation of the mentum is indicated for hypogenesis of the mandible associated with an obtuse cervicomental angle. Options for augmentation include *sliding genioplasty* and alloplastic implants. The authors of this chapter generally prefer an alloplastic technique due to the facility of the procedure and low incidence of complications. Implant choices include premanufactured silicone implants and porous polyethylene. Advantages of silicone implants include ease of insertion, as well as removal, should implant-related complications develop in the future.

Surgical Technique

Placement of an alloplastic chin implant can be performed via an intraoral or submental incision. The primary advantage of the intraoral incision is the avoidance of an external scar. The disadvantage, however, includes the need for a larger dissection pocket, which can result in cephalic migration of the implant and higher risk of seroma or hematoma formation. The mental nerves are also at slightly higher risk via the intraoral route. There is also a risk of implant contamination with oral flora. These risks are minimized with an external approach.

The submental incision is generally well hidden and is preferred by the authors of this chapter. It is placed just anterior to the submental crease so as not to exaggerate the crease and create a depression at the site of the scar. A 15-blade is used to make a 2.5-cm incision through skin, subcutaneous tissue, and muscle down to the level of the periosteum. Stevens scissors are used to elevate the mentalis muscle superiorly just above the level of periosteum and just high enough to accommodate the height of the implant. The midline is marked with a marking pen along the inferior aspect of the mentum. Bilateral paramedian incisions are made in the periosteum 1 cm lateral to the midline, and periosteal elevation is initiated in a subperiosteal plane with a Joseph periosteal elevator. Thus, a 2-cm central strip of periosteum remains attached to the mandible; this is said to reduce the risk of mandible resorbing secondary to pressure from the implant.

A blunt Freer elevator is placed in the pocket, and the periosteum is manually elevated, taking care not to dissect superiorly in the region of the mental nerve, nor to detach the periosteum off of the inferior border of the mandible. The left hand is used to palpate the location of the elevator, ensuring that it is precisely parallel to the inferior border of the mandible. Dissection proceeds laterally for approximately 5–6 cm, enough to accommodate the lateral portion of the implant. Care is taken to stay below the level of the mental foramen.

Following the development of the pockets, the site is irrigated with Bacitracin solution to reduce bacterial load and prevent infection of the implant. A 3-0 polydioxanone (PDS) suture is placed in vertical orientation through the intact central periosteal strip. The implant is then guided into the pocket with a straight clamp. The implant is then folded acutely and the contralateral phalange of the implant is guided into the contralateral pocket. The midline marking on the implant is aligned with the central marking along the mentum, and the 3-0 PDS suture is passed through the implant and tied inferiorly. A second stabilizing suture of 4-0 Surgipro or Nylon is used to secure the implant in the midline inferiorly along the inferior border of the mentum. The ideal position of the implant should correspond to the inferior border of the mandible. Careful dissection of the subperiosteal pockets will prevent cephalic migration.

The lateral aspects of the implant are palpated to ensure that the implant is not folded or curled upon itself, and the surgical site is again irrigated with Bacitracin solution. The mentalis muscle is then closed separately above the implant with interrupted, buried 4-0 PDS sutures ensuring complete coverage of the implant. Subcutaneous tissue and deep dermis are closed with interrupted 5-0 PDS, and the skin closed with a running 5-0 Surgipro or Nylon suture.

25.6 SUBMENTAL LIPOSUCTION

Submental adiposity can contribute to cervicomental angle blunting and the resultant appearance of a double chin. *Submental liposuction* is an effective procedure to address localized adipose collection and can be performed as an isolated procedure or combined with complementary surgery. Extraction of fatty deposits in this region, when performed on ideal candidates, can result in marked improvement in neck contour. Good candidates for submental liposuction include patients of normal general body habitus, with elastic skin, well-defined mandible, high and posterior hyoid position, and well-defined, localized collections of subcutaneous fat (Table 25.3).

Liposuction was developed in the 1970s with the use of rigid cannula and suction device. Illouz (1983) described a modification of the technique, which included the use of tumescence to expand the surgical plane and reduce bleeding. Over the years, refinements in technique and equipment have allowed for more accurate fat removal with a reduction in the incidence of complications.

The principle of surgical liposuction is based on contouring submental fatty deposits by precise reduction of adipocytes in the region. Following suction-assisted avulsion of fat cells, recontouring relies on redrapage of the overlying skin envelope and subdermal contraction.

Surgical Technique

Prior to the procedure, the patient is marked in the upright position. The anatomical landmarks of the SCM laterally and the thyroid notch inferiorly are marked as the boundaries of liposuction. The extent of the fatty accumulations is palpated with the fingers, and the borders of the maximal submental collection are marked. The majority of the

Table 25.3: Factors impacting submental liposuction.

Factor	*Good candidate*	*Poor candidate*
Body habitus	Normal	Large with excess generalized adipose tissue
Skeletal features	Anterior, strong mentum, and well-defined mandible	Posterior, weak chin position, and poorly defined mandible
Hyoid position	High and posterior	Low and anterior
Muscular features	Taut platysma	Lax platysma
Adipose tissue	Well-defined, localized collection	Diffuse distribution
Skin tone	Elastic	Lax

submental fat is localized centrally in the submental area, and thus, liposuction is generally focused in this region with feathering into the surrounding tissues to create a smooth transition. Access to the submental fat deposit is via a small submental incision, wide enough to allow for smooth passage of a cannula. Care should be taken to avoid a large incision to maintain adequate suction during the procedure. Conversely, an incision that is too small will restrict cannula motion and result in excessive friction and tissue trauma. When treatment of the jowls is indicated, the approach is via an infralobular incision. Fine cannulas must be used to avoid nerve injury and contour irregularity in this sensitive region.

Cervicofacial liposuction can be performed under local anesthesia, intravenous sedation, or general anesthesia. The authors use a partial tumescent technique, infiltrating the treatment region with a 1:1 mixture of 0.5% lidocaine and 0.25% Marcaine with 1:200,000 epinephrine. Approximately, 20 cc of solution is used. Excessive infiltration is avoided to preserve the anatomic landmarks and to prevent distortion of the preplanned treatment regions.

Following infiltration of the tumescent anesthetic solution, a 15-blade scalpel is used to make a 5–8 mm incision, just anterior to the submental crease. The incision is undermined for a distance of 1 cm with Stevens tenotomy scissors to develop a subdermal plane, which will allow for insertion of the cannula. If jowl liposuction is to be performed, similar incisions are made in the infralobular crease. Fine cannulas must be used for cervicofacial liposuction to prevent excessive removal of fat and to avoid injury to neurovascular structures. In general, the authors prefer to use a 3- or 4-mm cannula in the submental region and a 2- or 3-mm cannula in the jowl region.

Prior to applying suction, the cannulas are used to create tunnels in a deep subcutaneous plane. The ideal plane of fatty resection is above the platysma muscle and deep to the dermis with the goal of leaving 1–2 mm of fat on top of the muscle and below the dermis to avoid adhesions of the muscle and contour irregularities of the skin. Once pretunneling is completed, negative pressure suction is applied via a commercially available electric liposuction pump or manually with a handheld syringe. With the nondominant hand supporting (but not pinching) the fat accumulation externally, the dominant hand is used to aspirate the adipose tissue with long, radial passes of the cannula in a fan-shaped pattern. The aperture of the suction cannula is directed away from the skin flap to avoid dermal injury leading to contour irregularities, and care is taken to sculpt the region in a smooth and even manner.

Extraction volumes vary for each patient, but in general, the total volume of fat extracted ranges from 10 to 100 cc. The incision sites are closed with a buried 5-0 PDS intradermal suture, and the skin is closed with interrupted 5-0 Surgipro or Nylon sutures.

To prevent postoperative hematoma or seroma collection, a pressure dressing is applied to the submental region and removed on the second postoperative day. A pressure garment may be recommended for use at night for a further 2 weeks to aid in redraping of the skin envelope.

25.7 SUBMENTAL PLATYSMAPLASTY

Loss of elasticity and laxity of the jowls, skin, and platysma of the submental region is best addressed by a *necklift* (commonly in combination with a facelift procedure). Ideal candidates for the procedure have normal body habitus and strong skeletal structure with a well-defined mandible, anterior chin position, and high and posterior hyoid bone.

The facial musculature of the face and neck is enveloped by the superficial musculoaponeurotic system

(SMAS), first described by Mitz and Peyronnie (1976). This layer is contiguous with the platysma in the submental region, and modification of SMAS-platysma unit is of primary importance when addressing laxity of the neck. Anteriorly, dehiscence and laxity of the platysma present as vertical banding of the neck.

While facelift is covered elsewhere in this text, a description of platysmaplasty is outlined below.

For patients presenting with central neck skin and platysmal laxity, in addition to posterior tightening of the SMAS-platysma, midline submentoplasty should be performed.

Surgical Technique

The amount of submental adipose tissue is first assessed and treated via liposuction prior to platysmaplasty. Following liposuction, a 2.5 cm incision is made just anterior to the submental crease. Wide subcutaneous elevation of skin is performed over the platysma muscle spanning to the anterior border of the SCM laterally and down to the thyroid notch inferiorly. Any excess central adipose collection is excised directly between the medial borders of the platysma, taking care to avoid excessive fat resection, which can result in contour irregularities. The medial border of the platysma is then elevated for a distance of 2–3 cm on each side, and any redundant muscle is clamped with a Kelly clamp and excised. Meticulous hemostasis using bipolar cautery is vital to prevent postoperative hematoma. The two anterior borders of the muscle are then brought together in the midline with a central corset technique. Horizontal mattress 3-0 Vicryl sutures are used for this purpose to approximate the muscle borders in the midline creating a tight midline sling. Partial platysmal resection or platysmal transection at the level of the hyoid bone may need to be performed in a small proportion of patients.

For the majority of patients, the platysma will be further tightened laterally and redundant skin excised via a postauricular incision, which is commonly combined with a facelift procedure.

SUMMARY

With the goal of producing a sharp cervicomental angle and well-defined jawline, aesthetic refinement of the submental region may involve a variety of surgical techniques. Options include contouring localized adipose collections in the neck, augmenting the skeletal structure of the mandible, and tightening the muscular sling. Commonly, a combination of these procedures is necessary for comprehensive treatment of the lower neck region. Proper patient evaluation is paramount to produce an optimal result.

REFERENCES

Batra, A.P.S., Mahajan, A. and Gupta, K., 2010. Marginal mandibular branch of the facial nerve: An anatomical study. *Indian Journal of Plastic Surgery*, 43(1), pp. 60-4.

Daane, S.P., and Owsley, J.Q., 2003. Incidence of cervical branch injury with "marginal mandibular nerve pseudo-paralysis" in patients undergoing face lift. *Plastic and Reconstructive Surgery*, 111(7), pp. 2414-8.

de Castro, C.C., Aboudib, J.H., Jr. and Roxo, A.C., 2012. Updating the concepts on neck lift and lower third of the face. *Plastic and Reconstructive Surgery*, 130(1), pp. 199-205.

Dedo, D.D., 1980. "How I do it"—plastic surgery. Practical suggestions on facial plastic surgery. A preoperative classification of the neck for cervicofacial rhytidectomy. *Laryngoscope*, 90 (11 Pt 1), pp. 1894-6.

Illouz, Y.G., 1983. Body countouring by lipolysis: a 5-year experience with over 3000 cases. *Plastic and Reconstructive Surgery*, 72, pp. 610-9.

Mitz, V. and Peyronnie, M., 1976. The superficial musculoaponeurotic system (SMAS) in the parotid and cheek area. *Plastic and Reconstructive Surgery*, 58, p. 80.

Ramirez, O.M., 2008. Advanced considerations determining procedure selection in cervicoplasty; part one: anatomy and aesthetics. *Clinics in Plastic Surgery*, 35, pp. 679-90.

Shah, A.R. and Rosenberg, D., 2009. Defining the facial extent of the platysma muscle: a review of 71 consecutive face-lifts. *Archives of Facial Plastic Surgery*, 11(6), pp. 405-8.

Stuzin, J.M., Baker, T.J. and Gordon, H.L., 1992. The relationship of the superficial and deep facial fascias: relevance to rhytidectomy and aging. *Plastic and Reconstructive Surgery*, 89(3), pp. 441-9.

Zide, B.M., Pfeifer, T.M. and Longaker, M.T., 1999. Chin Surgery: I. Augmentation—the allures and the alerts. *Plastic and Reconstructive Surgery*, 104(6), pp. 1843-53.

Correction of Lids (Blepharoplasty) 26

Don Julian De Silva, Brett Kotlus

Chapter Overview

Pearls and Pitfalls

Pearls

- Important criteria for the eyelid evaluation before blepharoplasty include position of the eyebrow, margin reflex distance (MRD), presence and location of skin crease, periorbital fat atrophy, orbital fat prolapse, and lower eyelid laxity.
- The most common indications for blepharoplasty are involutional changes and facial aging, other causes of eyelid changes must be excluded before these diagnoses are made including thyroid eye disease and ptosis.
- An appropriate preoperative assessment and management plan reduce the risk of complications from blepharoplasty, including identification of patients who may be unsuitable for surgery due to marked dry eye, active thyroid orbitopathy, or unrealistic expectations.
- Upper blepharoplasty is a procedure that involves the excision of variable quantities of eyelid skin, orbicularis oculi muscle, and preaponeurotic fat.
- Lower blepharoplasty procedure may be performed by transcutaneous or transconjunctival methods. The traditional transcutaneous technique results in a scar in the skin and a higher risk of lower eyelid retraction. The more contemporary transconjunctival technique avoids a skin scar and has a lower risk of eyelid retraction.
- With lower blepharoplasty, caution must be taken to avoid injury to the inferior oblique muscle that can result in intractable diplopia.

Pitfalls

- Common sequelae from blepharoplasty include swelling and ecchymosis. Additional complications include scarring, asymmetry, dry eye, and failure to achieve patient's expectations.
- Potentially devastating blepharoplasty complications include retrobulbar hemorrhage, permanent damage to visual function, and blindness.
- Over-resection of fat can result in a "hollowed-out" appearance of the upper eyelid and a "sunken" appearance of the lower eyelid.
- Rare and serious complications from blepharoplasty include diplopia and lower eyelid retraction.

26.1 INTRODUCTION

Blepharoplasty is derived from the Greek words blepharon meaning eyelid and plasty meaning formed. Blepharoplasty is commonly used to describe a number of eyelid procedures including upper blepharoplasty, lower blepharoplasty, and Asian blepharoplasty. Cosmetic blepharoplasty is one of the most popular esthetic surgeries. The forehead, brows, midface, and cheek have intimate relationship with the eyelids and need to be considered in evaluation of the eyelids.

26.2 EYELID ANATOMY

Upper Eyelid Anatomy—Key Points

The upper eyelid is a mobile structure that protects the eye from injury and enables the even distribution of tears on blinking. The surface anatomy of the upper eyelid includes the eyebrow, the eyelid crease, and the eyelid itself; the space between the eyebrow and the eyelid crease is termed the eyelid sulcus. The eyelid consists of three principal layers: anterior lamellar (skin, subcutaneous tissue, and orbicularis oculi muscle), middle lamellar (orbital septum), and the posterior lamellar (tarsal plates, striated and smooth muscles, and conjunctiva). Posterior to the orbital septum lays the preaponeurotic fat pads.

- Upper eyelid skin (termed anterior lamellar) is one of the thinnest in the body; beneath skin is the loose subcutaneous tissue of the eyelids with increased elastic fibers and minimal fat. A common sign of facial aging is laxity in the upper eyelid skin that can droop over the upper eyelid (termed dermatochalasis). If marked, the soft tissue may reduce the superior or temporal visual field.
- Orbicularis oculi muscle is an elliptical sphincter muscle that surrounds the globe. It is divided into two principal parts: the innermost palpebral part that is present in the eyelids and an outer orbital part. The function of the orbicularis oculi is to close the eyelids like a purse string. The muscle is innervated by the facial nerve from temporal and zygomatic branches on the deep surface and is not denervated or injured by transcutaneous eyelid surgery. The orbicularis muscle is the antagonist to the levator aponeurosis (striated muscle) and Müller's muscle (smooth muscle) both of which open the upper eyelids.
- Orbital septum (termed middle lamellar) forms a fibrous divide between the skin and the orbital cavity, and is a continuation of the periosteum at the orbital rim. The septum lies posterior to the medial palpebral ligament and anterior to the lateral palpebral ligament, and blends with the levator aponeurosis above the superior tarsal border. The orbital septum provides an important functional barrier in the eyelid that protects the spread of infection from superficial skin tissues to the orbital cavity.
- Tarsal plates (termed posterior lamellar) are a dense fibrous tissue that give the eyelids a defined shape and structure. The tarsus in the Caucasian's upper eyelid measures approximately 10 mm in height and 20 mm in length and is attached medially via the medial palpebral ligament to the lacrimal crest and laterally to Whitnall's ligament. Attached at the superior edge of the upper tarsus are the smooth muscle fibers of the levator superior tarsal muscle (Müller's muscle) and the aponeurosis of the levator palpebral superioris.
- Frontalis muscle lifts the eyebrows and indirectly lifts the upper eyelid. The frontalis is a weak elevator of the upper eyelid; however, it has an important role in upper eyelid as the activity of the frontalis muscle impacts the shape of the eyebrow and eyelid sulcus.
- Preaponeurotic fat lies immediately behind the septum and with facial aging the fat may prolapse anteriorly resulting in a bulge in the upper eyelid. There are two components to the fat, medial fat that is pale in color and central fat that is darker yellow. Laterally in the eyelid is the lacrimal gland and caution must be observed in this area as surgical reduction of the gland can result in marked hemorrhage and dry eye. A branch of the palpebral artery lays posterior to the medial fat pad and caution is required to avoid injury to this vessel to avoid hemorrhage.
- Common facial aging in the upper eyelid includes excess skin, photoaging, and rhytidosis, fullness of the upper eyelid with fat prolapsing anteriorly, and atrophy of the sub-brow fat pad.

Eyelid Measurements

- There is marked variability in eyelid measurements depending on ethnicity, age, sex, and environmental factors such as sun exposure.
- Although the normal male eyebrow is considered at the superior orbital rim and the female brow above the orbital rim, there is considerable variability in the position of the eyebrow and many patients have low eyebrows in youth.
- The normal distance between the upper and lower eyelids (palpebral distance) is 9 mm (however this is not necessarily an accurate measurement of eyelid position as the measurement is reliant on the position of the lower eyelid).
- The position of the upper eyelid is most accurately defined quantitatively by the MRD measurement from the central corneal light reflex to the upper eyelid

margin. This distance is normally 4–5 mm. If the MRD is <2 mm, there may be a droopy eyelid (termed ptosis) that needs to be further evaluated. Ptosis can be graded in terms of severity, mild ptosis MRD is >1 mm and severe ptosis MRD is ≤0 mm (Scoppettuolo, 2008).

- The skin crease is the distance from the upper eyelid margin to the supratarsal crease. Normally it is 6–8 mm in men and 8–10 mm in women, but can vary ethnically.

Blood Supply and Lymphatic Drainage of the Upper Eyelids

- The eyelids have a profuse blood supply from the lateral and medial palpebral arteries that form a marginal and peripheral arterial arch in the upper and lower eyelids. The lateral palpebral arteries are derived from the lacrimal artery and the medial palpebral arteries from the ophthalmic artery. The venous drainage is to the superior orbital vein and the facial vein.
- The lymphatic drainage of the medial one-third of the upper eyelid is to the submandibular lymph nodes and from the lateral two-thirds to the superficial parotid (periauricular) lymph nodes (Nerad, 2010).

Lower Eyelid Anatomy—Key Points

- Lower eyelid skin is very thin and similar to the upper eyelid with loose subcutaneous tissue and minimal fat.
- Orbicularis oculi muscle is present immediately beneath the thin lower eyelid skin as a ring around the eye attaching to the periorbital skin. The skin and orbicularis oculi muscle comprise the outer or anterior lamellar of the eyelid.
- Orbital septum is a fibrous membrane that compartmentalizes the orbital fat, provides an important barrier for preventing infection from the superficial eyelids to the deeper orbit. The orbital septum makes the middle lamellar of the eyelid.
- Tarsus and conjunctiva make the posterior lamellar of the eyelid. The tarsus gives the lower eyelid tensile strength and is 3–4 mm in height and 30 mm in length; its inner lining is covered with conjunctiva that abuts the globe.
- Lower eyelid retractors, also called the capsulopalpebral fascia, are sympathetically driven and the equivalent to Müller's muscle in the upper eyelid.

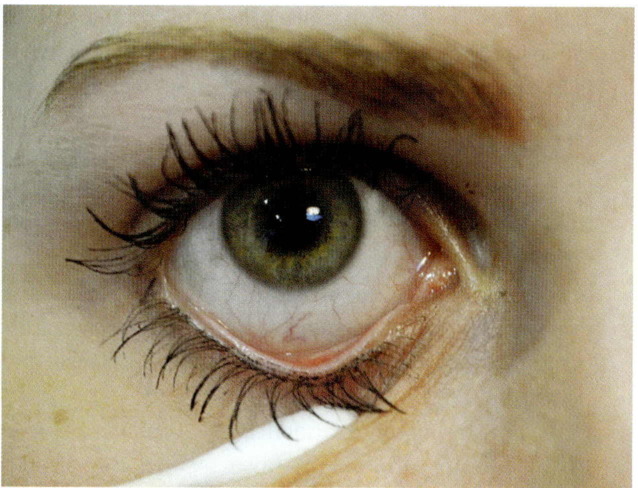

Fig. 26.1: Snap back test: laxity of the lower eyelid is assessed with the snap back test. The lower eyelid is pulled away from the globe (termed lower eyelid distraction), if the eyelid can be pulled ≥8 mm away from the globe this is defined as severe lower eyelid laxity. In evaluating the snap back test, the speed at which the lower eyelid returns to its normal position is also evaluated. Any patient who shows unilateral evidence of laxity should undergo evaluation to exclude VII nerve weakness; clinical signs of facial nerve paralysis including orbicularis oculi weakness should be discussed with the patient and fully evaluated before surgical treatment.

- Orbital fat in the lower eyelid is located in three compartments, medial, central, and lateral fat pads. The orbital fat is separated between the medial and central fat pads by the inferior oblique muscle and caution is required during surgery to avoid damage to this muscle (Harley, et al., 1986).
- Lower eyelid position usually rests 0–2 mm above the inferior border of the colored iris (termed corneal limbus). The lateral canthus is commonly positioned 1–2 mm superior to the medial canthus (i.e. up-sloping from medial to lateral); there is considerable variability in the natural position of the lateral canthus. If the lateral canthus is lower than the medial canthus, the lower eyelid should be evaluated for laxity.
- Lower eyelid laxity is evaluated with the snap-back test (Fig. 26.1) and eyelid distraction test. In the snap-back test, the lower eyelid is stretched away from the eye and time for the eyelid to return to its normal position is observed without blinking, laxity is defined by a slow return to the normal eyelid position. In the eyelid distraction test, the ability of the lower eyelid to be pulled away from the globe is measured, >6 mm is regarded as abnormal and implies lower eyelid laxity (Codner, McCord CD and Hester, 1998).

- The position of inferior orbital rim is of key importance in lower eyelid surgery and if the maxillary bone is relatively posterior (termed negative vector), there is an increased risk of lower eyelid retraction with lower blepharoplasty (Jelks and Jelks, 1993).
- Globe protrusion is the relative position of the globe to the orbital rim (>15 mm). There is considerable ethnic variability in relative globe protrusion; however, in patients with considerable globe protrusion, ophthalmology assessment is indicated to exclude orbital pathology including thyroid eye disease and neoplasia.
- Orbitomalar ligament attaches the orbicularis oculi to the inferior orbital rim (also termed the orbicularis-retaining ligament). In youth, there is a smooth continuity between the lower eyelid and cheek, with facial aging there can be distension of the ligament that gives rise to appearance of ring beneath the lower eyelid.
- Common facial aging of the lower eyelid includes fat prolapsing anteriorly that is seen as lower eyelid bags, loss of subcutaneous eyelid, and cheek fat that can accentuate the nasojugal hollows. Laxity and actinic changes of the lower eyelid skin can be seen as lines and wrinkles.
- Festoons or malar bags are lower eyelid changes that have fluid with associated redundancy due to folds of skin and orbicularis muscle.

Asian Eyelid Anatomy—Key Points

Asian blepharoplasty (also termed double-eyelid surgery) describes a procedure to place or define a pretarsal skin crease in Asian eyelid. Asian blepharoplasty results in the appearance of a more open eyelid, that can be a more sought after culturally defined aesthetic goal. The Asian eyelid has a different anatomy to the Caucasian eyelid with 50% of Asians having no upper eyelid crease. The key anatomical differences in comparison to a Caucasian eyelid are outlined below:

- Asian facial characteristics include relatively shallow orbits and minimally or noncantilevered supraorbital ridges that result in relatively greater soft tissues in the upper eyelid.
- The upper tarsal plate in Asian eyelids is relatively small 6.5–8.0 mm (compared to Caucasian eyelids 8.0–11.0 mm) (Chen and Khan, 2010). This is of key esthetic importance as a high crease in an Asian eyelid may not be aesthetically acceptable.
- In the Asian eyelid, there is lower insertion of the orbital septum on the levator aponeurosis, which results in a lower descent of the preaponeurotic fat, resulting in a fullness of the upper eyelid (pretarsal, preseptal, post-septal, or sub-brow fat). In addition, the inferior location of the fat blunts the insertion of the aponeurosis resulting in further blunting of the pretarsal skin crease (Lam, 2005).
- Commonly the Asian eyelid has a medial canthal (epicanthal) fold that can be modified with Asian blepharoplasty.
- The Asian eyelid crease tends to exhibit a medial taper as compared to a "Caucasian" crease that tends to follow a line parallel to the eyelid margin.
- Lash ptosis is described as a downward angulation of upper eyelid lashes as a result of redundant skin or lack of fibrous aponeurotic support immediately above the upper eyelid ciliary margin.

Salient features of upper and lower eyelid anatomy are shown in Figures 26.2A to F.

26.3 INDICATIONS FOR BLEPHAROPLASTY

Blepharoplasty (eyelid reshaping) may be indicated for various reasons.

Upper Blepharoplasty

- The most common indications for upper blepharoplasty are involutional changes and facial aging resulting in upper eyelid hooding and fullness. This may be due to excess upper eyelid skin, prolapse of orbital fat and/or lacrimal gland prolapse. This leads to changes in upper eyelid form that are deemed aesthetically unacceptable by patients. Initially there may be loss of superior (or temporal) visual field as a consequence of marked dermatochalasis. With severe dermatochalasis, there may be a loss of central vision.
- In addition to dermatochalasis, a proportion of patients develop age related brow ptosis that leads to the appearance of excess upper eyelid skin. This pseudodermatochalasis, must be recognized by the astute surgeon and brought to the attention of the patient as these patients require brow lifting to rejuvenate their upper eyelid appearance, although most patients will benefit from a combination of brow lift with blepharoplasty.

Lower Blepharoplasty

- There are two principal types of lower blepharoplasty, transcutaneous lower blepharoplasty (also termed lower subciliary blepharoplasty) and transconjunctival blepharoplasty. Lower blepharoplasty is always performed for aesthetic reasons. The most common indications for surgery are involutional changes and facial aging. Orbital fat that has prolapsed anteriorly in the lower eyelids is seen as lower eyelid bags. Lower eyelid skin laxity may be present with periorbital cutaneous rhytids. Festoons and malar crescents may also develop with age.
- Lower eyelid laxity requires eyelid tightening with canthopexy or canthoplasty.

Asian Blepharoplasty

- Upper eyelid fullness with absence or poor definition of upper eyelid crease is a common indication for Asian blepharoplasty.
- Minimal upper eyelid show and medial canthal (epicanthal) fold are other reasons for patients to seek blepharoplasty.

26.4 FEATURES IN CLINICAL HISTORY

Upper Blepharoplasty—Clinical Features

Upper blepharoplasty is one of the most common cosmetic surgical procedures of the face and is more common in

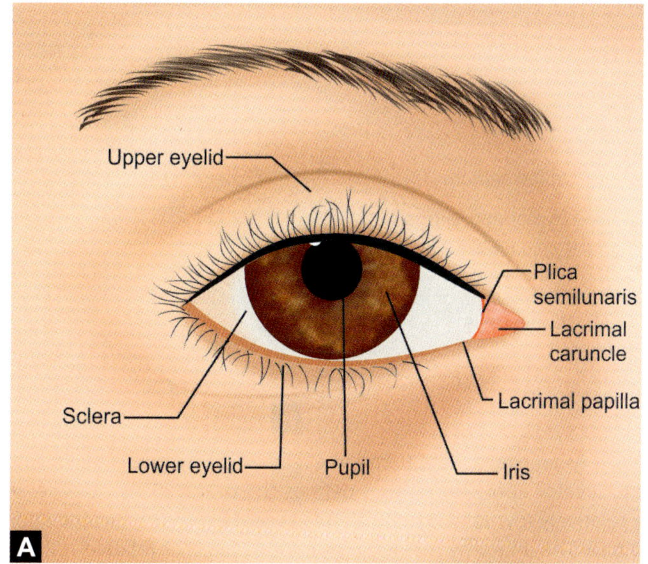

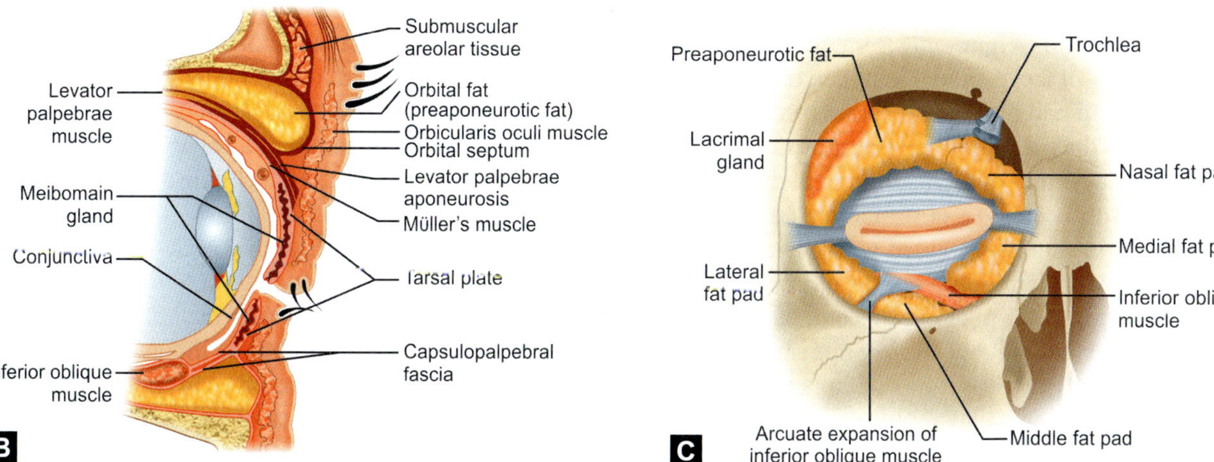

Figs. 26.2A to C: Eyelid anatomy: (A) Surface anatomy of Caucasian eyelid. The lower eyelid crosses through the lower part of the iris. (B) Caucasian upper eyelid—sagittal section. (C) Anatomy of right upper eyelid: coronal section.

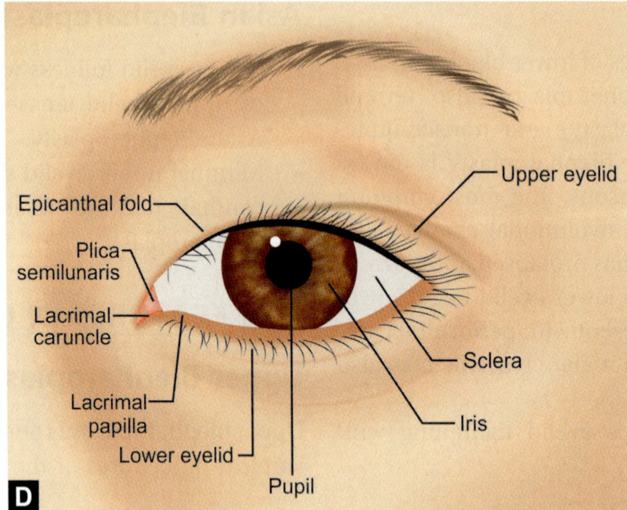

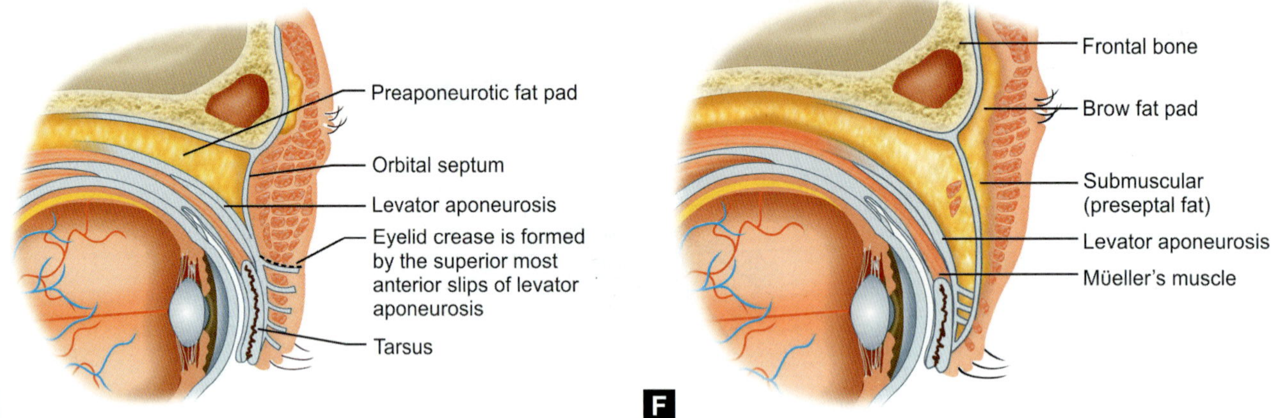

Figs. 26.2D to F: (D) Surface anatomy—Asian eyelid. (E) Caucasian eyelid anatomy in sagittal plane: in Caucasians, there is a relatively high attachment of orbital septum to levator aponeurosis that defines the pretarsal skin crease. (F) Asian eyelid anatomy in sagittal plane: in the Asian eyelid, there is a relatively low attachment of orbital septum to the levator aponeurosis, resulting in relatively low displacement of preaponeurotic fat pad. The anatomy results in the appearance of relative fullness in the upper eyelid and variable skin crease creation.

women than men, most commonly from 50 years of age. As a consequence of facial aging, there is a combination of degenerative and pathological processes resulting in an alteration in the skin and periorbital structures. There may be anterior displacement of orbital fat due to dehiscence of septal and muscle support of orbital fat. In addition, loss of elasticity of the skin coupled with environmental damage to the skin (commonly due to ultraviolet light) may result in redundant upper eyelid skin.

- Patients often complain of a droopy upper eyelid with fullness, women often describe difficulty putting cosmetics on the upper eyelids.
- Patients may complain of difficulty seeing as a consequence of the upper eyelid skin covering the superior and lateral field of vision.
- Patients with vocations or hobbies requiring frequent up gaze may have earlier functional impairment.
- Chronic medical conditions such as heart disease, hypertension, diabetes mellitus, hepatic disease, thyroid disease, glaucoma, and bleeding diatheses should be elicited.
- Patients with a history of dry eyes, previous laser refractive surgery, arthritic or autoimmune conditions require further evaluation including Schirmer's test (evaluation of the ability of the eye to produce tears after 5 min). Blepharoplasty in these patients is associated with a higher risk of postoperative dry eye and exposure keratopathy.
- The use of medications including herbal supplements with anticoagulant effects (e.g. aspirin, garlic, gingko

biloba, and vitamin E) should be ceased before surgery to reduce the incidence of postoperative bruising and hematoma formation.

Lower Blepharoplasty—Clinical Features

Lower blepharoplasty is a common cosmetic surgical procedure of the face and is more frequently encountered in women than men, from 50 years of age. With genetic factors, patients can have bags in the lower eyelids at a younger age.

As a consequence of degenerative and pathological processes, there is an alteration in the skin and periorbital structures resulting in anterior displacement of orbital fat due to dehiscence of septal and muscle support of the fat pads.

As indicated in the previous section, chronic medical conditions, previous surgery, and medication use should be elicited. Appropriate investigations should be performed and preoperative advice given to the patients to reduce the risk of postoperative complications.

Asian Blepharoplasty—Clinical Features

Asian blepharoplasty is a common surgical procedure worldwide; culturally the presence of a "double eyelid" is regarded as an attractive aesthetic for many Asians. In the Caucasian eyelid, the pretarsal skin crease is understood to represent the insertion of the levator aponeurosis into the dermis. The absence of a skin crease in some Asian eyelids is thought to result from a lower aponeurotic insertion point in the Asian eyelid with an increased amount of fat above the skin crease that inhibits folding. There has been a shift away from the principle of "Westernization" of Asian upper eyelids; modern Asian blepharoplasty maintains the inherent beauty and ethnicity of the Asian eyelid while lending more crease definition and a well-demarcated pretarsal shelf.

26.5 TYPICAL FINDINGS IN EXAMINATION

Basic ophthalmological assessment includes visual acuity, pupil size and response, visual fields, and extraocular movements. Any abnormal findings advocate referral for an ophthalmology assessment.

Upper Blepharoplasty—Examination Findings

- Upper eyelid skin excess.
- Bulging medial aspect of upper eyelid.
- Raised, asymmetrical, or multiple eyelid creases (>10 mm).
- Patient may have frontalis muscle overaction to elevate eyelid. This is particularly so in patients with pseudodermatochalasis.

Lower Blepharoplasty—Examination Findings

- Lower eyelid bags indicating orbital fat anterior prolapse (medial, central, and lateral fat compartments).
- Lower eyelid skin laxity.
- Lower eyelid assessed for canthal tendon laxity (snapback test and eyelid distraction test), requiring lid tightening techniques (canthopexy and canthoplasty).
- Hollowing below the lower eyelid between the junction of the eyelid and cheek may require volume augmentation (fat transfer, nonsurgical fillers, or facial implants).

Asian Blepharoplasty (Figs. 26.5A and B)—Examination Findings

- In 50% of Asian eyelids, there is an absence of a pretarsal skin crease.
- In 50% of Asian eyelids, there is a low skin crease.
- The nasal epicanthic fold can be referred to as an "inside" or "outside" fold. When the fold is set relatively high, the crease usually folds on the outside (Fig. 26.3).
- The configuration of the medial epicanthal fold can vary and the Flowers classification is based on the amount of visible caruncle. In type I, the caruncle is visible and resembles a Caucasian eyelid. In type II, the caruncle is partially obstructed, and in type III the fold is prominent and has an inversus component. Type IV resembles type I, except that the medial epicanthal fold is thick (Fig. 26.4). A medial epicanthoplasty is recommended for patients with type III or IV and is optional for patients with type II.

26.6 INVESTIGATIONS

- Photographic documentation of the eyelids in primary gaze, upward gaze, and down gaze.
- Consider blood investigations including clotting screen.
- Patients with systemic symptoms suggestive of thyroid eye disease need further biochemical investigations and referral to an endocrinologist.

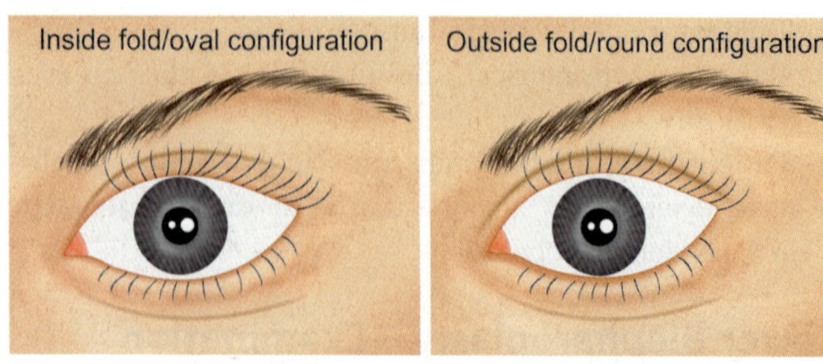

Fig. 26.3: Inside and outside epicanthal fold configuration.

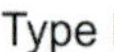

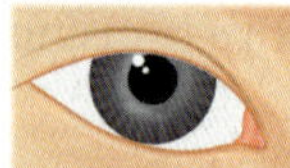

Type II

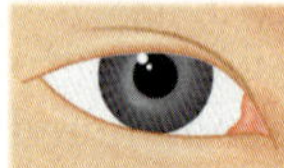

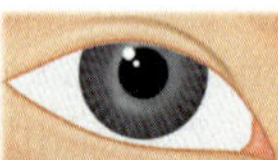

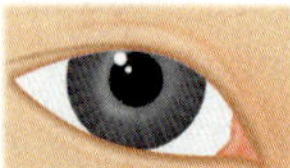

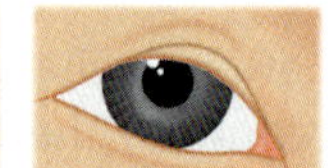

Type III

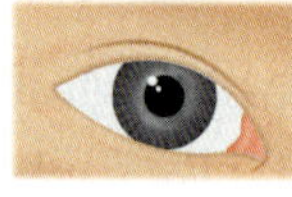

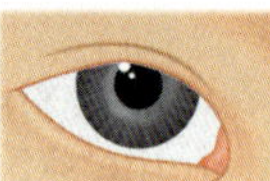

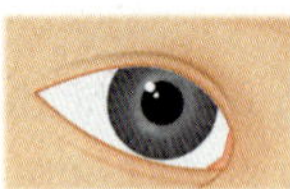

Type IV or pseudo Type I

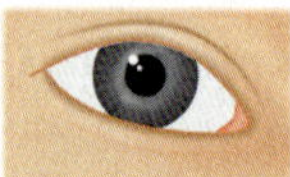

Fig. 26.4: Flowers classification of epicanthal folds.

- Exclude other causes of upper eyelid changes including oculomotor nerve palsy.

26.7 PREFERRED TREATMENT

Upper Blepharoplasty (Figs. 26.5A to B4)—Surgical Procedure

- The skin marking includes skin crease (men 6–8 mm, women 8–10 mm) and elliptical area for skin excision. There needs to be sufficient skin between the brow and the upper eyelid margin to allow complete eyelid closure, this amount is between 20 mm and 25 mm (25 mm is conservative and 20 mm is minimum when a more cosmetic procedure is required). Laterally the limit to skin excision is 1 cm lateral to the brow to avoid a visible scar; medially the limit is the lacrimal punctum to avoid webbing at the medial canthus. Markings can be performed with the patient sitting in upright or supine position (Fig. 26.5B1), although upright position is preferred by many to allow for the effect of gravity on brow position and upper eyelid skin.
- Once the excess skin is marked, performing a skin pinch test between the blepharoplasty markings is advised to ensure the patient is able to close their eyes, conservative surgery is advised to avoid functional dry eye and lagophthalmos after surgery.
- Local or sedative anesthesia is required for analgesia. The eyelid is infiltrated with local anesthetic with 1:100,000 epinephrine to reduce hemorrhage (Fig. 26.5B2).
- The use of ocular shields during blepharoplasty may prevent corneal or globe perforation.
- The skin is excised in accordance with the premarkings, a scalpel 15-blade or scissors is commonly used (Fig. 26.5B3). Alternatives are carbon dioxide (CO_2) laser, radiofrequency, or electrocautery device.
- In most patients, a strip of orbicularis oculi is excised to reduce fullness in the upper eyelid.
- The orbital septum is opened.
- In patients with anterior preaponeurotic fat prolapse, the fat pad (medial and/or central fat pad) is identified and reduced to give a deep superior sulcus between the eyelid and the brow. Fat excision should be conservative to avoid a "hollowed-out" appearance to the upper eyelid. Medial fat prolapse is common, and a pedicle of nasal fat can be created, cauterized, and excised. Meticulous hemostasis techniques are advocated to avoid orbital hemorrhage that has the potential to damage visual function.
- A more contemporary technique in the upper eyelid is fat preservation; the medial fat pad is transposed locally to an area of depression in the upper eyelid including an age-related depression over the superonasal orbital rim (Yoo, Peng and Massry, 2013).
- The skin is closed commonly with a continuous nonabsorbable suture (Fig. 26.5B4).
- Additional surgical technique may be required to provide an optimal aesthetic result including brow lifting, skin resurfacing, eyelid crease fixation, fat grafting, glabellar and lateral orbital chemodenervation (botulinum toxin).

Lower Blepharoplasty—Surgical Procedure

The treatment for lower eyelid facial aging includes transcutaneous lower blepharoplasty (also termed lower lid

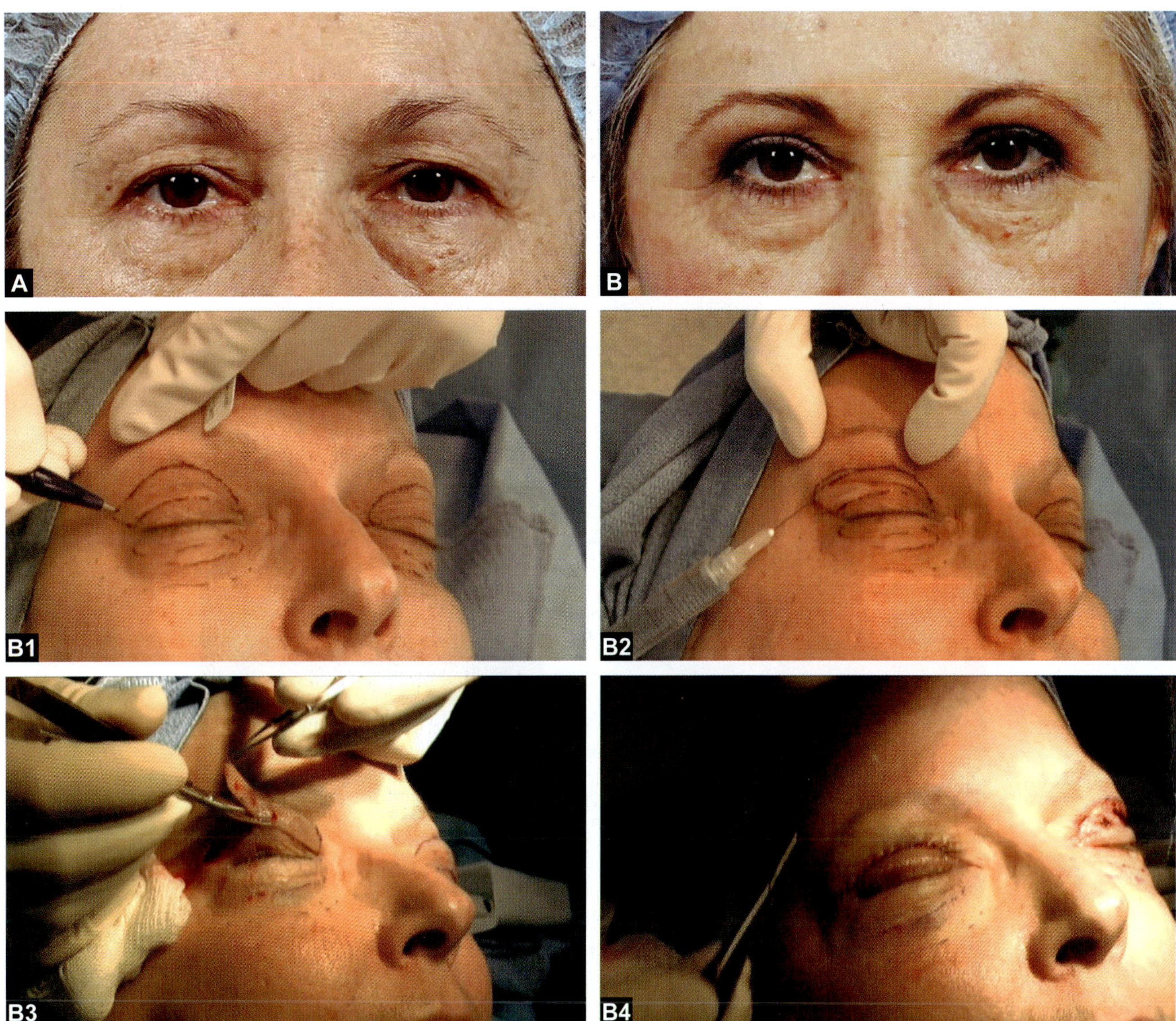

Figs. 26.5A to B4: Upper blepharoplasty. (A) Preoperative photograph of a patient. (B) Postoperative photograph of the patient after upper blepharoplasty. (B1 to B4) Intraoperative photographs. (B1) Upper blepharoplasty skin markings. (B2) Upper blepharoplasty local anesthetic infiltration. (B3) Upper blepharoplasty skin excision with scissors. (B4) Upper blepharoplasty skin closure with continuous suture.

subciliary blepharoplasty) and transconjunctival blepharoplasty (Hidalgo, 2011) (Figs. 26.6A to D3). Transcutaneous lower blepharoplasty is the more traditional technique for blepharoplasty, although more straightforward, it is associated with increased risk of complications including lower eyelid retraction, ectropion, and a rounded canthal angle (Neuhaus and Baylis, 1982).

- Transcutaneous lower blepharoplasty (also termed lower lid subciliary blepharoplasty)
  - Marking of the lower eyelid skin incision and orbital fat prolapse is done at the start of the procedure.
  - Local or sedative anesthesia is required for analgesia. The eyelid is infiltrated with local anesthetic with 1:100,000 epinephrine to reduce hemorrhage.
  - The use of ocular shields during blepharoplasty may prevent corneal or globe perforation.
  - The lower eyelid skin incision is 2–3 mm below the lower eyelid margin from the punctum to approximately 5 mm from the lateral canthus (Fig. 26.6C1).
  - The skin is excised in accordance with the premarkings, a scalpel 15-blade or scissors is commonly used, alternative procedures are skin tightening

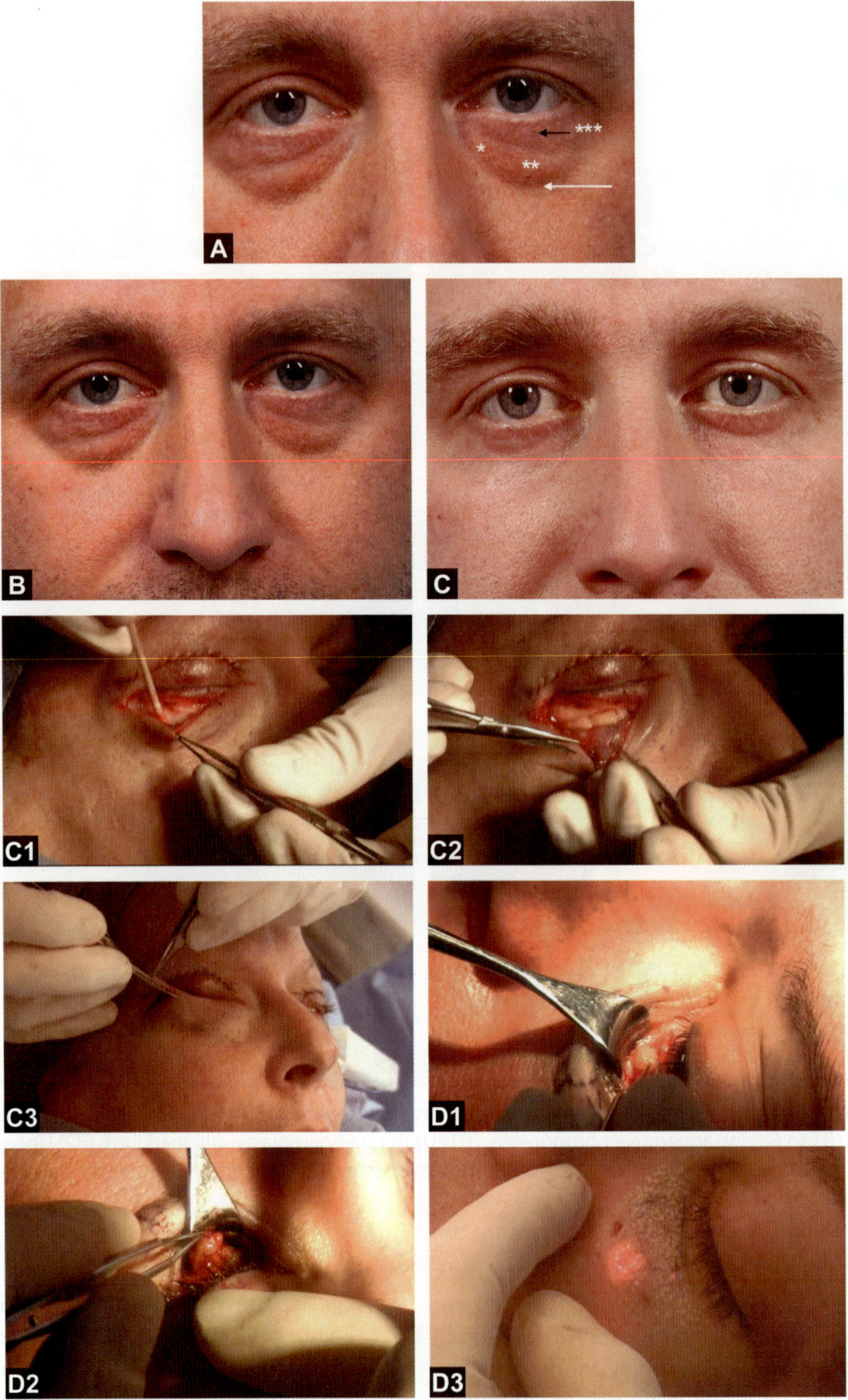

Figs. 26.6A to D3: Lower blepaharoplasty. (A) Facial aging of the lower eyelid: the black arrow marks the position of lower eyelid, the white arrow marks the lower eyelid-cheek junction, and white stars mark the orbital fat pads (one star, medial; two stars, central; three stars, lateral orbital fat pad). (B) Preoperative photograph of a patient. (C) Photograph of the patient after subciliary bilateral lower lid blepharoplasty. (C1 to C3) Lower blepharoplasty intraoperative photographs: subciliary approach. (C1) Subciliary incision and skin muscle flap formation. (C2) Identification of orbital fat through subciliary approach. (C3) Excess skin excision with scissors at the end of subciliary approach. (D1 to D3) Lower blepharoplasty intraoperative photographs: transconjunctival approach. (D1) Identification of prolapsing fat. (D2) Conservative fat pad excision. (D3) Blanching of skin during laser resurfacing to rejuvenate lower eyelid.

with a CO_2 laser or electrocautery device. Caution is required in the excision of lower eyelid skin as excessive skin removal can result in inability to close the eyelids and symptomatic dry eye and corneal exposure.
- An orbicularis oculi strip may be fashioned to support the lower eyelid.
- The orbital septum is opened (Fig. 26.6C2).
- Orbital fat prolapse is commonly excised. There are different surgical techniques to excise orbital fat that reduce orbital hemorrhage including: (1) clamping the fat, its excision and cautery before release of clamp, (2) electrocautery excision and hemostasis, (3) CO_2 laser excision and hemostasis. Between the nasal and central fat pads lies the inferior oblique muscle; caution is required to avoid damage to this muscle. Fat excision should be conservative to avoid a "hollowed-out" appearance to the lower eyelid. Meticulous hemostasis techniques are advocated to avoid orbital hemorrhage and rare complication of visual loss.
- Fat transposition is a more contemporary alternative to orbital fat excision in patients with a tear-trough depression. In this technique, the fat is not excised, instead it is moved in position to drape over the inferior orbital rim. The orbital fat is sutured in place over the orbital rim with absorbable sutures (Kawamoto, 2003).
- With lower eyelid laxity, a canthoplasty procedure is required to tighten the lower eyelid and avoid lower eyelid retraction in the postoperative period.
- The skin may be excised alone (skin pinch, Fig. 26.6C3) or advanced and excised with orbicularis muscle (skin muscle flap).
- The skin is closed commonly with a continuous nonabsorbable suture.
- Additional surgical technique may be required to provide an optimal aesthetic result including skin resurfacing, volume augmentation, and suborbicularis oculi fat lift.

- Transconjunctival blepharoplasty:
  - Marking of the lower eyelid orbital fat prolapse.
  - Local or sedative anesthesia is required for analgesia. The eyelid is infiltrated with local anesthetic with 1:100,000 epinephrine to reduce hemorrhage.
  - A traction suture retracts the lower eyelid inferiorly over an eyelid or Desmarres retractor.
  - The conjunctiva is incised at the inferior border of the tarsus from the punctum to approximately 5 mm from the lateral canthus. Anterior lamellar flap is then raised all the way to the inferior orbital rim. This approach is called the preseptal approach as the flap is anterior to the orbital septum, which must then be incised to access the orbital fat. Anatomy of the lower eyelid suggests that an incision made 5 mm inferior to the tarsus border, results in a postseptal plane of dissection that avoids traumatic dissection to the orbital septum and less risk of lower eyelid retraction.
  - Orbital fat prolapse is identified in three fat pads (medial, central, and lateral fat pads) and selectively excised or transposed (Figs. 26.6D1 and D2). There are different surgical techniques to excise orbital fat as discussed under upper blepharoplasty. Between the nasal and central fat pads likes the inferior oblique muscle, caution is required to avoid damage to this muscle.
  - The conjunctiva is not sutured closed.
  - With lower eyelid laxity, a canthopexy or canthoplasty procedure is required to tighten the lower eyelid and avoid lower eyelid retraction in the postoperative period.
  - Additional surgical technique may be required to provide an optimal aesthetic result including skin pinch excision, skin resurfacing (Fig. 26.6D3), and volume augmentation.
- *Fat-sparing lower blepharoplasty*: A more contemporary concept in lower blepharoplasty is preservation of the orbital fat. Traditional techniques favored excision of orbital fat; however, there is evidence that fat preservation with lower blepharoplasty results in more favorable long-term aesthetic results. The techniques are as above; however, the orbital fat is repositioned (termed fat transposition) over the inferior orbital rim in the tear-trough depression. The fat is secured over the orbital rim with an absorbable or nonabsorbable suture (Kawamoto, 2003).

Asian Blepharoplasty—Surgical Procedure

- *Skin incision method (also termed transcutaneous approach)*:

  This method of Asian blepharoplasty is most effective and gives durable long-term results (Fig. 26.7). It involves making a skin incision in the natural crease of the skin, which is usually invisible in a few months:

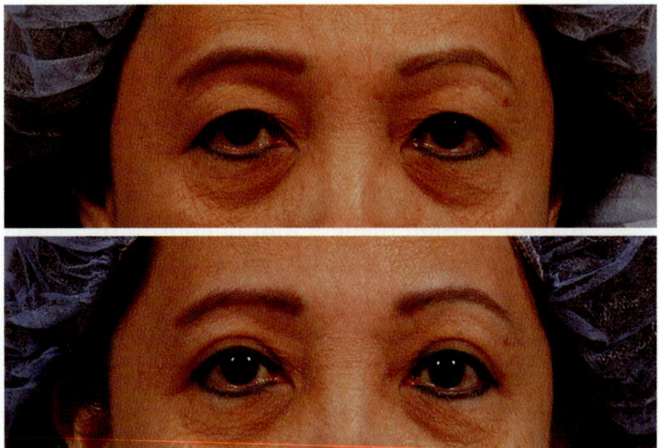

Fig. 26.7: Asian blepharoplasty: Asian blepharoplasty before and after photographs.

- The skin marking includes skin crease elliptical area for skin excision (approximately 3 mm).
- Local or sedative anesthesia with adrenaline is required for analgesia and to reduce hemorrhage.
- The skin is excised in accordance with the premarkings, a scalpel 15-blade is commonly used, and alternatives are CO_2 laser or electrocautery devise.
- A 3–5 mm strip of orbicularis oculi is excised.
- The orbital septum is incised.
- The anterior preaponeurotic fat is excised in accordance with the patients' objectives from surgery. Increased fat excision will result in a more open appearance to the eyelid and relatively higher skin crease. Fat excision should be conservative to avoid a "hollowed-out" appearance to the upper eyelid, particularly in the medial fat pad. Meticulous hemostasis techniques are advocated to avoid orbital hemorrhage and rare complication of visual loss.
- The pretarsal skin crease is recreated with three or more absorbable or nonabsorbable sutures between the skin, tarsus, and levator aponeurosis. The position of the skin crease can be raised with the sutures being placed higher through the levator aponeurosis.
- The skin is closed commonly with a continuous nonabsorbable suture.
- Additional surgical technique may be required to provide an optimal aesthetic result including medial canthoplasty.

- *Suture method (also termed transcutaneous approach)*: The suture or stitch method avoids any incisions in the skin, except for the passing of the stitches, and is very popular in the East, particularly Japan. The suture method is appealing as it avoids significant incisions in the skin. The stitches are buried underneath soft tissues and the recovery from surgery completes in a few days. The limitation with this method is that the sutures have relatively short effect compared to the other methods as the stitches weaken with time.
- *Partial-incision method*: The partial-incision method, with a small 1.5 cm incision, is a hybrid approach between the suture method and the full-incision method. Patients like this method as it has a relatively quick recovery of 1–2 weeks. The main disadvantage is that in some individuals there may be loss of skin crease in a few months to years. The results are however more long-lasting than the stitch technique alone.

26.8 COMPLICATIONS OF TREATMENT

Blepharoplasty Complications

- Surgical complications include persistent swelling, marked ecchymosis, dry eye, scarring, webbing, excess hollowing, undercorrection, and asymmetry.
- Corneal abrasion is inadvertent trauma to the corneal epithelium secondary to exposure, drying, chemical agents, or mechanical drying. Lubrication of the cornea with ointment or normal saline, or covering of the cornea during surgery is warranted to prevent this complication.
- The most serious complication from blepharoplasty is damage or loss of vision; this is understood to occur when bleeding tracks behind the eye compressing the optic nerve as a consequence of retrobulbar hemorrhage (termed orbital compartment syndrome). Immediate release of the pressure is indicated to prevent visual loss with a procedure to release the eyelid (termed lateral canthotomy and inferior cantholysis) (Lima, et al., 2009). The risk of retrobulbar hemorrhage after blepharoplasty is considered to be 0.05% and the risk associated with permanent vision loss 0.0045% (Hass, 2004).
- Globe perforation is a rare risk with any procedure around the eye. Caution must be observed when injecting local anesthetics and with needle techniques used around the eyes including traction sutures.
- Infection after blepharoplasty is rare.
- With cosmetic blepharoplasty, it is important that the patient has realistic expectations from the surgery to avoid disappointment from expectations of perfection.

Lower Blepharoplasty Complications

- With lower blepharoplasty, inadequate removal of the orbital fat can result in fat prolapse postsurgery, particularly the lateral fat pad can be under-resected. In addition over-resection of the fat pads can result in a hollowed-out appearance.
- Chemosis is defined as subconjunctival edema; increased risk factors include a low incision site, canthoplasty incision, and corneal exposure postoperatively.
- A subconjunctival hemorrhage is a red discoloration on the surface of the globe, although often alarming to a patient, it resolves spontaneously over a 2-week period.
- Damage to the inferior oblique muscle during lower eyelid surgery results in postoperative double vision (diplopia) (Harley, et al., 1986).
- Lower eyelid retraction occurs when scarring of the lower eyelid middle or posterior lamellar results in the eyelid being pulled inferiorly. In assessment of the eyelid before surgery, recognizing lower eyelid laxity and negative vector and supporting the lower eyelid reduces the risk of this complication. Lower eyelid supporting techniques include canthopexy and canthoplasty. In addition there is evidence that transconjunctival lower blepharoplasty technique preserves the orbital septum resulting in a reduced risk of eyelid retraction (Rohrich, Ghavami and Mojallal, 2011).
- Lower eyelid skin shortage caused by over-resection of skin can also result in an inferiorly displaced eyelid margin and ocular surface exposure.

Asian Blepharoplasty Complications

- The commonest complication requiring revision surgery is eyelid asymmetry.
- Medical canthoplasty techniques to alter the epicanthal folds can result in scarring.

REFERENCES

Anderson, R.L. and Dixon, R.S., 1979. Aponeurotic ptosis surgery. *Archives of Ophthalmology*, 97, pp. 1123-8.

Chen, W.P.D. and Khan, J.A., 2010. *Colour atlas of cosmetic oculofacial surgery*. 2nd ed. Saunders: Elsevier. p. 6.

Codner, M.A., McCord, C.D. and Hester, T.R., 1998. The lateral canthoplasty. *Operative Techniques in Plastic and Reconstructive Surgery*, 5, pp. 90-8.

Harley, R.D., Nelson, L.B., Flanagan, J.C. and Calhoun, J.H., 1986. Ocular motility disturbances following cosmetic blepharoplasty. *Archives of Ophthalmology*, 104, pp. 542-4.

Hass, A., 2004. Incidence of postblepharoplasty orbital hemorrhage and associated visual loss. *Ophthalmic Plastic and Reconstructive Surgery*, 20, pp. 426-32.

Hidalgo, D.A., 2011. An integrated approach to lower blepharoplasty. *Plastic and Reconstructive Surgery*, 127, pp. 386-95.

Jelks, G.W. and Jelks, E.B., 1993. Preoperative evaluation of the blepharoplasty patient. Bypassing the pitfalls. *Clinics in Plastic Surgery*, 20, pp. 213-23; discussion 224.

Kawamoto, H., 2003. The tear "TROUF" procedure: transconjunctival repositioning of orbital unipedicled fat. *Plastic and Reconstructive Surgery*, 112, pp. 1903-7; discussion 1908-9.

Lam, S., 2005. Esthetic facial surgery for the Asian male. *Facial Plast Surg.*, 21, pp. 317-23.

Lima, V., Burt, B., Leibovitch, I., Prabhakaran, V., Goldberg, R.A. and Selva, D., 2009. Orbital compartment syndrome: the ophthalmic surgical emergency. *Survey of Ophthalmology*, 54, pp. 441-9.

McCurdy, J.A. and Lam, S.M., 2005. *Cosmetic surgery of Asian face*, 2nd ed. Thieme Medical Publishers, New York.

Nerad, J., 2010. *Techniques in ophthalmic plastic surgery.* Saunders: Elsevier, Chap. 11.

Neuhaus, R. and Baylis, H., 1982. Complications of lower eyelid blepharoplasty. In: A.N. Putterman, ed. *Cosmetic oculoplastic surgery.* New York: GrundStratton.

Rohrich, R.J., Ghavami, A. and Mojallal, A., 2011. The five-step lower blepharoplasty: blending the eyelid-cheek junction. *Plastic and Reconstructive Surgery*, 128, pp. 775-83.

Scoppettuolo, E., Chadha, V., Bounce, C., Olver, J.M., Wright, M., 2008. British oculoplastic surgery society (BOPSS) national ptosis survey. *Br J Ophthalmol.*, 92, pp. 1134-8.

Yoo, D.B., Peng, G.L. and Massry, G.G., 2013. Effacing the orbitoglabellar groove with transposed upper eyelid fat. *Ophthalmic Plastic and Reconstructive Surgery*, 29, pp. 220-4.

Drooping Eyelids (Ptosis) 27

Don Julian De Silva, Robert Schwarcz

Chapter Overview

Pearls and Pitfalls

Pearls

- The two muscles that elevate the upper eyelid are the levator aponeurosis (striated muscle) and Müller's muscle (smooth muscle).
- There are three important measurements for the assessment of ptosis: margin reflex distance (MRD), levator function, and skin crease.
- Ptosis can be graded in terms of severity, mild ptosis MRD1 is >1 mm, severe ptosis MRD is ≤0 mm.
- The two most common causes are involutional and congenital ptosis; other causes of ptosis must be excluded before these diagnoses are made.
- The treatment of involutional ptosis is surgery that can be of three types: anterior approach levator advancement, posterior approach (mullerectomy), or Fasanella-Servat procedure (tarsectomy).
- Levator aponeurosis advancement is the most common operation for correction of involutional ptosis.
- The Fasanella-Servat procedure is a straightforward and traditional surgery that involves the excision of the superior tarsus and Mllüller's muscle, although results can be less predictable with this technique.

Pitfalls

- There are many different causes of ptosis, which include life-threatening pathology; these must be excluded in all cases.
- Common complications from ptosis surgical correction include asymmetry, undercorrection, and overcorrection.

27.1 PRESENTATION: PTOSIS

Ptosis has been defined as drooping of the upper eyelid and may be classified by several different means including severity, etiology, onset, and levator function. The exact incidence of ptosis is not known; however, the condition is common and has equal frequency among different races and between the sexes.

27.2 ANATOMY—KEY POINTS

- The upper eyelid is a mobile structure that protects the eye from injury and enables the even distribution of the tears on blinking. The eyelid consists of three principal layers: anterior lamellar (skin, subcutaneous tissue, orbicularis oculi muscle), middle lamellar (orbital septum), and the posterior lamellar (tarsal plates, striated and smooth muscle, and conjunctiva).

- *Anterior lamellar*: The eyelid skin is the thinnest in the body; beneath the skin is the loose subcutaneous tissue of the eyelids with increased elastic fibers and minimal fat. The orbicularis oculi muscle is an elliptical muscle that surrounds the globe. It is divided into two principal parts: the innermost palpebral part that is present in the eyelids and an outer orbital part. The function of the orbicularis oculi is to close the eyelids like a purse string. The muscle is innervated by the temporal and zygomatic branches of the facial nerve from its deep surface and is not injured by transcutaneous eyelid surgery. The orbicularis muscle is the antagonist to the levator aponeurosis (striated muscle) and Horner's muscle (smooth muscle), both of which open the upper eyelids.
- *Middle lamellar*: The orbital septum forms a fibrous divide between the skin and the orbital cavity and is a continuation of the periosteum at the orbital rim. The septum lies posterior to the medial palpebral ligament and anterior to the lateral palpebral ligament and blends with the levator aponeurosis above the superior tarsal border. The orbital septum provides an important functional barrier in the eyelid that protects the spread of infection from superficial skin tissues to the orbital cavity.
- *Posterior lamellar*: The tarsal plates are a dense fibrous tissue that gives the eyelids a defined shape and structure. The tarsus in the upper lid measures approximately 10 mm in height and 20 mm in length. It is attached medially via the medial palpebral ligament to the lacrimal crest and laterally to Whitnall's ligament. Attached at the superior edge of the upper tarsus are the smooth muscle fibers of the levator superior tarsal muscle (Müller's muscle) and the aponeurosis of the levator palpebral superioris.

- *Muscle*: There are three retractors that open the upper eyelid:
  - The levator muscle is the primary retractor of the upper eyelid (Figs. 27.1A and B); it opens the eyelid during voluntary elevation. The muscle is innervated by the third cranial nerve.
  - Müller's muscle is responsible for sympathetic elevation of the eyelid during the "fight-or-flight response" and opens the eyelid during involuntary elevation.
  - The frontalis muscle lifts the eyebrows and indirectly lifts the upper eyelid. The frontalis is a weak elevator of the upper eyelid; however, it has an important role in elevating the eyelid in patients with very poor levator muscle function (e.g. severe congenital ptosis).
- *The levator complex*:
  - The upper eyelid is elevated by two muscles: the levator palpebral superioris (striated muscle) and the superior tarsal muscle (smooth muscle). The levator palpebral superioris originates from the lesser wing of the sphenoid bone and is approximately 55 mm in length. It becomes the levator aponeurosis just above the optic foramen. The muscle transitions to an aponeurosis tendon approximately 15 mm from the superior tarsus, attaching to the superior transverse ligament of Whitnall, which acts as a check ligament of the levator. Whitnall's ligament extends from the trochlea medially to the lacrimal gland capsule and frontal periosteum laterally. It changes the direction of aponeurotic pull. The aponeurosis inserts into the anterior aspect of the superior tarsus and sends some fibers to the skin to form the upper eyelid crease. The aponeurosis extends in both medial and lateral expansions termed horns, which may have a pathological role in upper eyelid retraction in conditions such as thyroid eye disease. The lateral horn indents the lacrimal gland partially dividing the gland into a smaller palpebral and thicker orbital portion. The lateral horn is attached to the marginal tubercle of the zygomatic bone and the medial horn fuses with the medial palpebral ligament. The levator palpebral superioris is innervated by the superior branch of the oculomotor nerve and elevates the eyelid by 12–15 mm from full closure of palpebral fissure to wide-eyed staring.
  - The superior tarsal muscle (Müller's muscle) is a vascularized smooth muscle that is innervated by the sympathetic nervous system. The muscle originates from the inferior surface of the levator aponeurosis and inserts into the superior tarsal plate. The muscle is approximately 20 by 20 mm with a 1 mm tendon and elevates the upper eyelid by approximately 2 mm. Müller's muscle is responsible for setting the upper lid level in conjunction with the levator palpebral superioris. Increased stimulation of the sympathetic nervous system

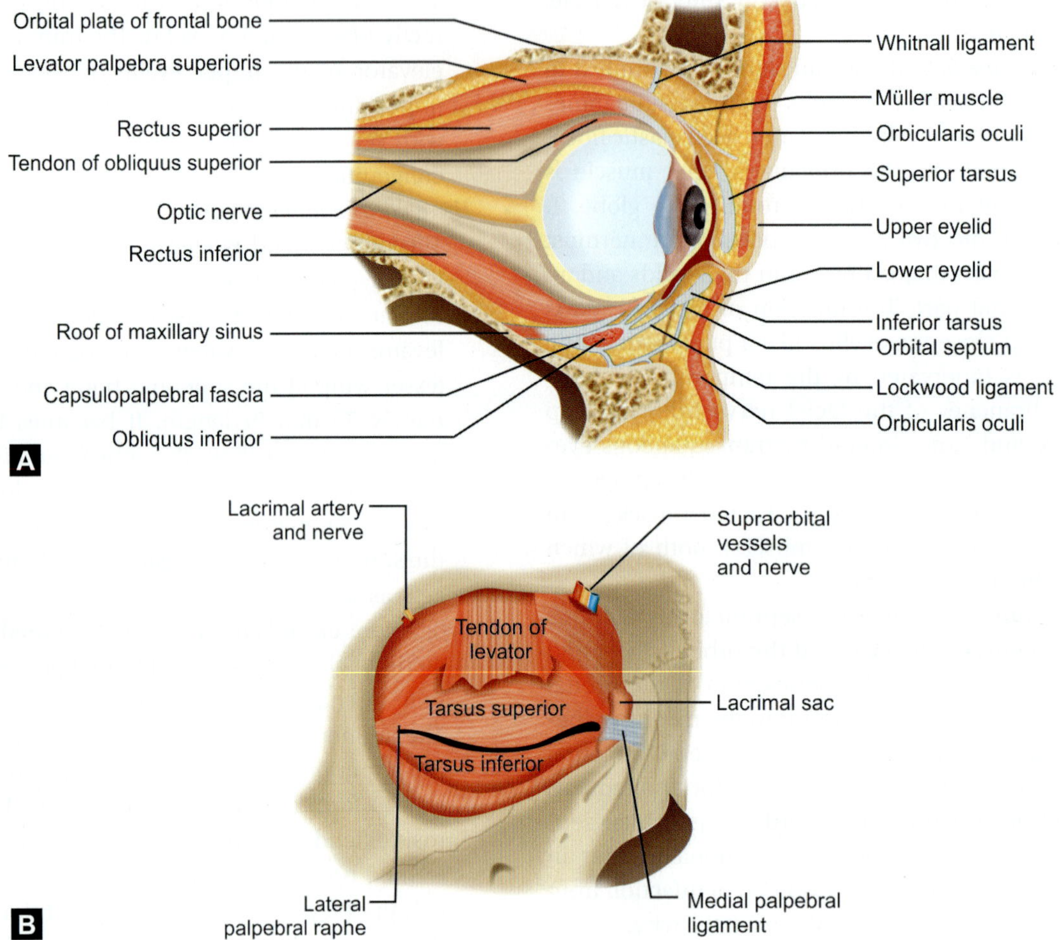

Figs. 27.1A and B: Eyelid anatomy. (A) Elevators of the upper eyelid: sagittal section. (B) Elevators of the upper eyelid: coronal section. *Source*: Gray (1918).

such as stress or adrenaline elevates the eyelid, whereas damage to the sympathetic innervation results in 1–2 mm ptosis.

- *Eyelid measurements*:
  - The normal upper eyelid rests just below the upper limbus.
  - The normal distance between the upper and lower eyelids (palpebral distance) is 9 mm (however, this is not necessarily an accurate measurement of eyelid position as the measurement is reliant on the position of the lower eyelid).
  - There are three important measurements for the assessment of ptosis: MRD, levator function, and skin crease.
  - The position of the upper eyelid is most accurately defined quantitatively by the MRD1 measurement from the central corneal light reflex to the upper lid margin. This distance is normally 4–5 mm.
  - Ptosis can be graded in terms of severity, mild ptosis MRD1 is >1 mm, severe ptosis MRD is ≤0 mm (Scoppettuolo, et al., 2008).
  - Levator function is evaluated by measuring the change in position of the eyelid from maximum downgaze to upgaze, normally it is >12 mm. A measurement of >10 mm is considered very good, 8–10 mm considered good, 5–7 mm considered fair, and ≤4 mm is considered poor (Edmonson and Wulc, 2005).
  - Skin crease is the distance from the upper eyelid margin to the supratarsal crease. Normally, it is 6–8 mm in men and 8–10 mm in women but can vary ethnically.
- *Blood supply and lymphatic drainage of the upper eyelids*:
  - The eyelids have a profuse blood supply from the lateral and medial palpebral arteries that form a

marginal and peripheral arterial arch in the upper and lower eyelids. The lateral palpebral arteries are derived from the lacrimal artery and the medical palpebral arteries from the ophthalmic artery. The venous drainage is to the superior orbital vein and the facial vein.

- The lymphatic drainage of the medial one-third of the upper eyelid is to the submandibular lymph nodes and from the lateral two-thirds to the superficial parotid lymph nodes (Nerad, 2010).

27.3 PTOSIS CAUSES

- *Involutional ptosis*: Gradual onset ptosis.
- *Third cranial nerve palsy*: Ptosis, eye downward, and outward, with reduced ocular movements.
- *Sympathetic nerve palsy*: Acute onset ptosis with small pupil.
- *Myasthenia gravis and ptosis*: Variable bilateral ptosis with signs of reduced ocular motility.
- *Mechanical ptosis*: Mass effect weighing down on the eyelid.
- *Congenital ptosis*: Patient born with congenital ptosis.
- Other unusual types of ptosis.

27.4 DIAGNOSTIC SUMMARY

1. Ptosis is defined as droopy upper eyelid that may result in aesthetic deformity or loss of vision.
2. Visual loss affects the superior visual field first, with severe ptosis there maybe a loss of central vision.
3. The two most common causes are involutional and congenital ptosis; other causes of ptosis must be excluded before these diagnoses are made.

- *Involutional ptosis* (Fig. 27.2A):
  - Gradual onset ptosis from middle age.
  - The most common cause of ptosis is involutional ptosis, which occurs as part of aging of the eyelid, with disinsertion of the levator aponeurosis from its attachment to the tarsal plate with stretching and thinning of the aponeurosis.
  - It may be unilateral or bilateral.
  - It worsens with tiredness and is associated with compensatory brow overaction.
  - Clinical diagnosis is made by exclusion of other types of ptosis.
- *Third cranial nerve palsy and ptosis* (Fig. 27.2C):
  - Partial or complete ptosis.
  - The eye is turned downward and outward (by the action of unaffected muscles supplied by IV and VI cranial nerves).
  - Ptosis is associated with reduced ocular movements.
  - The III cranial nerve palsy may be complete or partial (or if long standing may result in aberrant nerve regeneration).
  - Cause must be investigated urgently with imaging [computed tomography (CT) or magnetic resonance imaging (MRI)] and blood tests dependent on the clinical signs.
  - Investigations include imaging of neck [ultrasound, magnetic resonance arteriography (MRA), computed tomography arteriography (CTA)] to exclude carotid artery dissection, and chest radiograph in smokers to exclude Pancoast tumor.
- *Sympathetic nerve palsy and ptosis*:
  - Acute onset ptosis may be caused by traumatic injury to the sympathetic innervation of the Müller's muscle.
  - Injury to the sympathetic nerves in the neck due to trauma or iatrogenic injury resulting from neck surgery including central venous cannulation.
  - Signs include partial ptosis, with small constricted pupil.
  - Pupil will be smaller than the normal side. In the dark normal pupil dilates, but a Horner's pupil remains constricted.
  - It is important to exclude Horner's pupil in all young people presenting with ptosis.
  - Life-threatening causes of ptosis include carotid dissection, which may present only with Horner's pupil.
- *Myasthenia gravis and ptosis*:
  - Variable bilateral ptosis with other signs of reduced ocular motility.
  - Bilateral ptosis of gradual onset, which is variable in severity and gets worse during repeated exercise (termed fatigue).
  - May have systemic symptoms including difficulty swallowing, general tiredness, other autoimmune disease, or a positive family history.
  - Antibody test for acetylcholine receptors is sensitive in over 80% in patients with ocular myasthenia.
- *Mechanical ptosis* (Fig. 27.2D):
  - Caused by a lesion of anterior eyelid skin or posterior conjunctival tissue as a consequence of gravity.
  - Diagnosis is made on clinical features and biopsy of the lesion.
- *Congenital ptosis* (Fig. 27.2B):
  - A common cause of ptosis that is present at birth and characterized by dystrophy of the levator muscle.

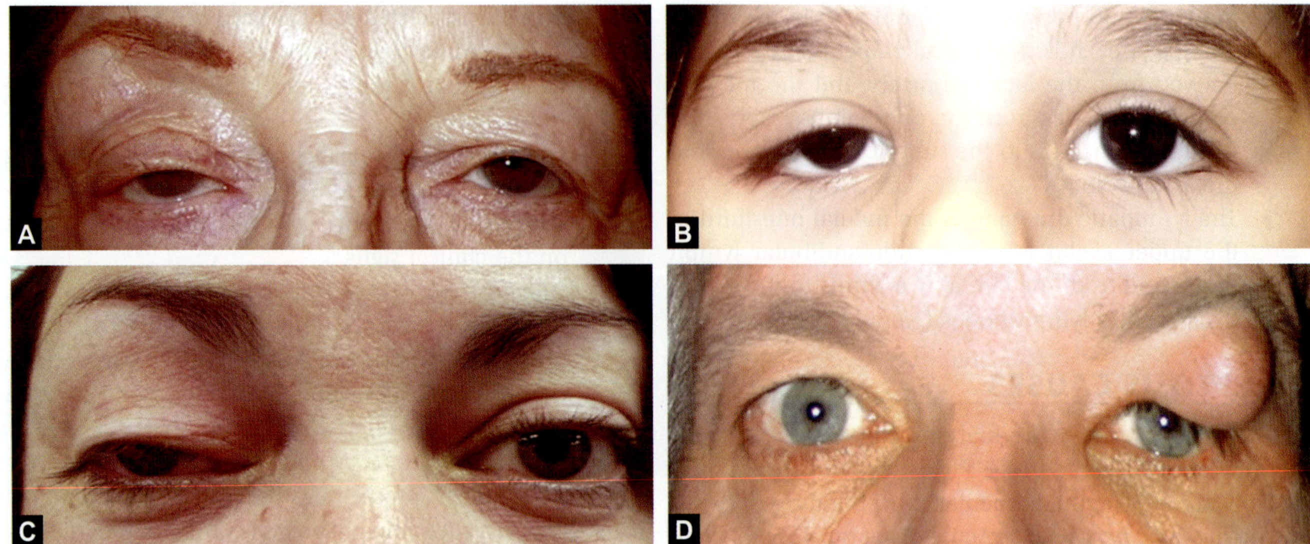

Figs. 27.2A to D: Diagnosis of ptosis. (A) Involutional ptosis: bilateral asymmetrical ptosis obscuring visual axis, brow compensatory elevation, and high skin crease. (B) Congenital ptosis: mild unilateral ptosis, clear visual axis, and high supratarsal skin crease. (C) Partial third nerve ptosis: unilateral partial ptosis, and eye turned downward (depression) and outward (abduction). (D) Mechanical ptosis: large left upper eyelid lump of unknown etiology causing mechanical ptosis.

- Variable severity from mild ptosis (normal visual acuity) to severe ptosis (reduced visual acuity).
- Reduced levator function (assessed by evaluating lid excursion from down gaze to upgaze).
- Clinical diagnosis that is made upon the exclusion of other causes of ptosis.

27.5 INVOLUTIONAL PTOSIS

Epidemiology and Pathogenesis

There is disinsertion of the levator aponeurosis from its attachment to the tarsal plate with stretching and thinning of the aponeurosis.

Clinical Features

- *Features in clinical history*:
  - Patients with involutional ptosis often complain of a droopy upper eyelid and a sleepy appearance.
  - Patients may tilt their head backward and adopt a chin-up position to improve their sight or use a finger to physically lift the eyelids.
  - Gradual onset ptosis.
  - May have a history of wearing contact lens.
- *Typical findings in examination*:
  - Unilateral or commonly bilateral (with different severity in the two eyes).
  - Moderate ptosis (3–4 mm) that may worsen in downgaze.
  - Levator function is normal (>12 mm).
  - High eyelid crease (10–15 mm).
  - Patient may have brow over action to elevate eyelid.

Investigations

Clinical assessment of the degree of ptosis and exclusion of other causes of ptosis is sufficient, and no other investigations are usually required.

Preferred Treatment

The treatment of involutional ptosis is surgery that can be of three types: anterior approach levator advancement, posterior approach (mullerectomy), or Fasanella-Servat procedure (tarsectomy).

- Levator aponeurosis advancement is the most common operation for correction of involutional ptosis (Fig. 27.3A). The procedure involves a skin crease incision, identification of the levator aponeurosis, and advancement on the tarsus to elevate the upper eyelid higher. The procedure is often completed under local anesthesia with or without sedation, which enables the height of the ptotic eyelid to be adjusted and matched to the other normal side. Despite careful intraoperative adjustment of the lid height asymmetry between the two eyes may occur.
- The Fasanella-Servat procedure (tarsectomy) is a straightforward and traditional surgery that involves

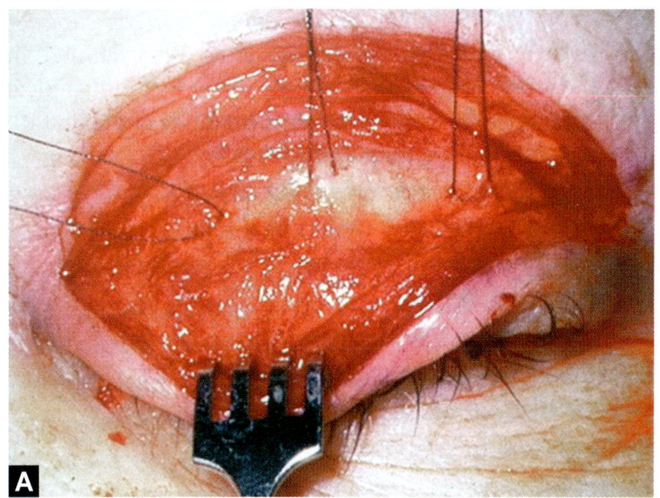

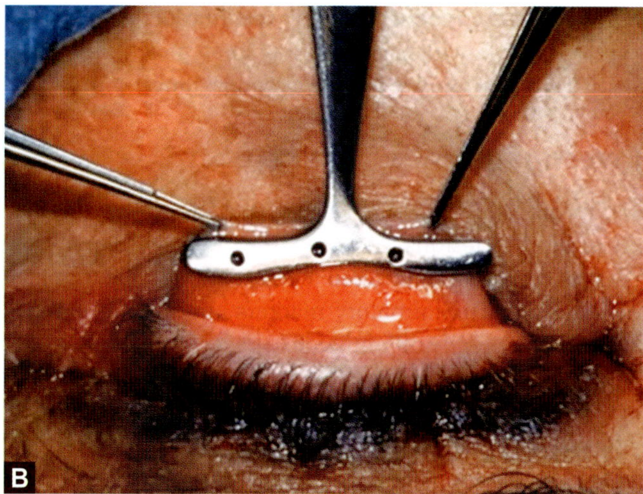

Figs. 27.3A and B: Intraoperative photographs. (A) Anterior approach levator advancement. Levator is advanced on the upper eyelid tarsal plate with three sutures, each is individually adjusted to control the shape and contour of the upper eyelid. (B) Posterior approach levator advancement. A Putterman clamp is used to shorten the posterior lamella and conjunctiva. Müller's muscle and approximately 3 mm of the tarsal edge is excised.

the excision of the superior tarsus and Müller's muscle, the procedure is an option for patients with mild ptosis with good levator function, although results can be less predictable with this technique. The eyelid is everted and a clamp used to grasp the conjunctiva, Müller's muscle, and approximately 3 mm of the tarsal edge (Fig. 27.3B). The clamped tissue is then excised and a single suture passed along the length of the eyelid to reattach the upper eyelid posterior lamella.

- Posterior approach or mullerectomy is an alternative surgical procedure that is effective in correcting mild-to-moderate ptosis with normal levator function. The procedure is completed without a skin incision, and the degree of resection of the conjunctiva and Müller's muscle is guided by a preoperative phenylephrine testing, unlike the Fasanella-Servat procedure the tarsus is preserved. A clamp is used to excise a measured amount of the conjunctiva and Müller's muscle, and the remaining posterior lamella is reattached with a single suture.

Complications of Treatment

Common complications include asymmetry, undercorrection, and overcorrection.

Complications of Disease

Reduced superior field of vision and encroachment on the central vision occurs without treatment (Anderson and Dixon, 1979).

27.6 THIRD CRANIAL NERVE PALSY

Epidemiology and Pathogenesis

The levator muscle is innervated by the third cranial nerve. Central lesions result in bilateral ptosis and are rare. Peripheral lesions can be caused by trauma, neoplasm, aneurysms, inflammation, or ischemia and usually lead to unilateral ptosis.

Any orbital space-occupying lesion (e.g. metastatic tumor, thyroid eye disease) can result in compression of the third cranial nerve and a combination of ptosis, reduced ocular movements, and orbital signs.

Clinical Features

- *Features in clinical history*:
  - The patient presents with rapid onset ptosis with double vision (diplopia).
- *Typical findings in examination*:
  - Unilateral ptosis.
  - Eye is turned downward (depression) and outward (abduction).
  - Reduced or absent ocular movements (except depression and abduction).
  - Diplopia as a consequence of reduced ocular movements.
  - Orbital signs include reduced visual acuity, pain, proptosis, diplopia, and exposure keratopathy (dry eye).

- Aberrant regeneration of the third cranial nerve develops with time resulting in atypical upper eyelid elevation with atypical ocular movements.

Investigations

- Imaging (CT or MRI) is performed to exclude space occupying lesions.
- Blood tests are ordered dependent on the clinical signs, e.g. inflammatory markers and autoantibodies are checked if inflammatory space occupying lesion is suspected.

Preferred Treatment

- Treatment is guided by the etiology of the third cranial nerve palsy.
- Spontaneous resolution may occur.
- Before surgical ptosis correction, complex strabismus surgery may be required to avoid intractable diplopia.
- The ptosis may be surgically corrected utilizing a sling to the frontalis muscle (innervated by the seventh cranial nerve).

Complications of Treatment

Correction of the ptosis is limited by the degree of loss of innervation to the levator muscle and relatively immobile upper eyelid. With severe third nerve palsy overcorrection carries increased risk of exposure keratopathy. With or without prior strabismus surgery, patient may have intractable diplopia as a result of reduced ocular movements, although there are alternative management options including the use of an opaque contact lens.

Complications of Disease

- It is essential to identify the etiology of the third cranial nerve as there are potential vision-threatening and life-threatening consequences without treatment (Kline and Bajandas, 2001).

27.7 SYMPATHETIC NERVE PALSY (HORNER'S SYNDROME)

Epidemiology and Pathogenesis

Injury to the sympathetic innervation to the eye results in a rare and characteristic array of signs. The injury to the sympathetic nerve may occur at three places:

- *Central nervous system*: Other coexistent brainstem signs may be present.
- *Preganglionic injury to the spinal cord or superior cervical ganglion*: Neoplasm must be excluded in this group. Compression in the chest including apical lung cancer or congenital abnormalities of the first rib needs to be excluded.
- *Postganglionic injury after the superior cervical ganglion*: Neoplasm is rare in this group.

Clinical Features

- *Features in clinical history*:
    - There maybe a history of neck trauma resulting in carotid artery dissection.
    - Smoking is a risk factor for developing lung neoplasm (Pancoast tumor) that compresses the sympathetic nerve.
- *Typical findings in examination*:
    - Typically there is acute onset mild ptosis with anisocoria (difference between the pupil sizes).
    - Abnormal pupil is small in size and fails to dilate in dark light.
    - Subtle signs include lower lid elevation and ipsilateral anhydrosis.

Investigations

- Imaging of neck (ultrasound, MRA, CTA) to exclude carotid artery dissection.
- Chest radiograph/CT chest in smokers to exclude Pancoast tumor.
- Pharmacological testing may help determine if a sympathetic lesion is pre- or postganglionic. Topical cocaine (4–10%) prevents reuptake of noradrenaline, resulting in pupil dilation if there is an intact postganglionic nerve.

Preferred Treatment

The potentially life-threatening consequences of carotid artery dissection require urgent treatment by vascular surgeons including angioplasty and anticoagulative therapy.

Complications of Treatment

Once the life-threatening etiology has been treated, ptosis can be corrected surgically with levator advancement or mullerectomy procedure.

Complications of Disease

Depending on the etiology of the Horner's syndrome, life-threatening consequences can occur in patients without treatment (Kline and Bajandas, 2001).

27.8 MYASTHENIA GRAVIS AND PTOSIS

Epidemiology and Pathogenesis

Myasthenia gravis is an autoimmune disease with reduced number of acetylcholine receptors at the neuromuscular junction.

Clinical Features

- *Features in clinical history*:
  - Highly variable ptosis.
  - Generalized symptoms of fatigue, weakness, dysarthria, and dysphasia may occur.
- *Typical findings in examination*:
  - Variable bilateral ptosis that may change during the assessment.
  - Associated abnormal ocular motility including fatigue with repetitive movements.
  - Diplopia may be present.
  - Eye signs are the presenting features in 85% of patients.

Investigations

- *Ice test*: Apply ice pack to ptosis for several minutes and reassess degree of ptosis. Improvement with ice suggests a diagnosis of myasthenia (Kline and Bajandas, 2001).
- Tensilon test is the standard diagnostic test, in which intravenous edrophonium is given, as an anticholinesterase inhibitor it improves the ptosis and fatigue (Kline and Bajandas, 2001).
- Antibody test for acetylcholine receptors is sensitive in over 80% of patients with ocular myasthenia (Kline and Bajandas, 2001).
- Chest radiograph/CT scan to exclude thyoma.

Preferred Treatment

- Medical treatments include oral acetylcholinesterase inhibitors (pyridostigmine) and immunosuppressant's (steroids, cyclosporine, azathioprine).
- Surgical correction of ptosis can be used as an adjunct and includes levator advancement and frontalis sling suspension.
- Thymectomy is indicated for patients with thyoma.

Complications of Treatment

Recurrence or progression of autoimmune disease and variable ptosis may occur.

Complications of Disease

- Patients may develop a myasthenia crisis, a potentially life-threatening emergency in which the respiratory muscles become very weak.
- Majority of patients have a normal life expectancy (Kline and Bajandas, 2001).

27.9 MECHANICAL PTOSIS

Epidemiology and Pathogenesis

Any substantial lesion on the upper eyelid may cause ptosis.

Clinical Features

- *Features in clinical history*:
  - Characterized by the presence of a mechanical lesion on the eyelid, resulting in a gravitational effect on the eyelid and ptosis.
  - Most commonly on the anterior lamella including excess skin, fat, and skin tumors.
  - Rarely of the posterior lamella, important to evert the upper eyelid to exclude neoplastic lesions.
- *Typical findings in examination*:
  - Lesion may be readily apparent on the eyelid skin.
  - Lesion may be on the conjunctival surface of the eyelid, only apparent on lid eversion.

Investigations

Excisional or incisional biopsy.

Preferred Treatment

Specific to the etiology of the lump, e.g. excision of benign and malignant neoplasms.

Complications of Treatment

Dependent on the etiology of the lesion.

Complications of Disease

Dependent on the etiology of the lesion, e.g. sebaceous or squamous cell carcinoma can progress with systemic metastases (Nerad, 2010).

27.10 CONGENITAL PTOSIS

Epidemiology and Pathogenesis

The majority of children with *congenital ptosis* have a developmental dystrophy of the levator muscle.

Clinical Features

- *Features in clinical history*:
  - Ptosis presents at birth, although the patient may present for assessment at a later age.
  - Ptosis is unilateral in the majority of cases (70%).
- *Typical findin gs in examination*:
  - Variable severity from mild ptosis (normal visual acuity) to severe ptosis (reduced visual acuity).
  - Reduced levator function.
  - Faint or absent supratarsal skin crease.
  - One-third of patients have ocular motility abnormalities such as strabismus (squint) and lid lag on downgaze.
  - Other rarer causes of congenital ptosis include blepharophimosis syndrome that includes characteristic-shortened palpebral fissures (blepharophimosis), widened intercanthal distance (telecanthus), and eyelid abnormalities.

Investigations

Clinical assessment and exclusion of other causes of ptosis.

Preferred Treatment

- Ptosis with good vision does not require surgery.
- Severity of ptosis and levator dysfunction are the principles for timing of surgical intervention and surgical technique.
- Severe ptosis, which results in the upper eyelid covering the visual axis, requires urgent surgical intervention to prevent long-term reduction in visual acuity (amblyopia). The eye and neural connections important for sight require visual stimulation and can be damaged if the visual axis is obstructed before 8 years of age.
- Children often undergo ptosis correction at the age of entering school (4 years) for social and mental wellbeing.
- Mild-to-moderate ptosis can be treated with surgical advancement of the levator muscle.
- Severe ptosis with poor levator function is treated with frontalis sling surgery in which the frontalis muscle is used to elevate the upper eyelid. There are a variety of nonautologous (e.g. silicone) and autologous (e.g. fascia lata) materials that can be used as a sling.
- Children often have comorbidity with refractive errors and strabismus, and these also require treatment and regular assessments.

Complications of Treatment

- Surgical correction of ptosis in children under general anesthesia can result in overcorrection or undercorrection. Overcorrection with a high upper eyelid (high MRD > 4 mm) results in corneal exposure (keratopathy) that can become complicated with a corneal ulcer, permanent corneal scar, and reduced visual acuity. Undercorrection may result in the eyelid obscuring the visual axis that requires further surgery.
- Asymmetry of the eyelids and irregular lid margin (Congenital ptosis with severe ptosis and poor levator function requires frontalis sling surgery that can result in an irregular lid shape or upper eyelid margin), need for surgical revision.
- If used, nonautologous materials may become infected or exposed through the skin, requiring surgical revision.

Complications of Disease

Without the treatment of severe ptosis in a child, the long-term visual potential of that eye is impaired. The most important period of development is when the child is first developing vision and up until the age of 8 years. If the ptosis is corrected after this critical period, the eye will only have basic visual acuity (amblyopia) (Whitehouse, Grigg and Martin, 1995).

27.11 MYOGENIC PTOSIS

Myogenic ptosis includes oculopharyngeal dystrophy, myotonic dystrophy, and chronic progressive external ophthalmoplegia. Symptoms include progressive bilateral ptosis in association with generalized musculoskeletal signs. Most are diagnosed clinically, and treatment is generally nonsurgical with the use of ptosis props to elevate the eyelids (Kline and Bajandas, 2001).

REFERENCES

Anderson, R.L. and Dixon, R.S., 1979. Aponeurotic ptosis surgery. *Archives of Ophthalmology*, 97(6), pp. 1123-8.

Anderson, R.L. and Jordan, D.R., 1995. The aponeurotic approach to congenital ptosis. *Ophthalmic Surgery*, 21(4), pp. 237-44.

Edmonson, B.C. and Wulc, A.E., 2005. Ptosis evaluation and management. *Otoloaryngologic Clinics of North America*, 38, pp. 921-46.

Kline, L.B. and Bajandas, F.J., 2001. *Neuro-ophthalmology*. 5th ed. NJ: Slack Incorporated. Ch. 11. p. 173.

McCord, C. ed., 1995. Evaluation of the ptosis patient. In: *Eyelid surgery principles and techniques*, Philadelphia: Lippincott-Raven, Ch. 7, pp. 99-112.

Nerad, J., 2010. *Techniques in ophthalmic plastic surgery*. Philadelphia, PA: Saunders/Elsevier, Ch. 11, p. 299.

Scoppettuolo, E., Chadha, V., Bunce, C., Olver, J.M. and Wright, M., 2008. British Oculoplastic Surgery Society (BOPSS) National Ptosis Survey. *British Journal of Ophthalmology*, 92(8), pp. 1134-8. doi: 10.1136/bjo.2007.132746. Epub Jun 20, 2008.

Whitehouse, G.M., Grigg, J.G. and Martin, F.J., 1995. Congenital ptosis. *Clinical and Experimental Ophthalmology*, 23(4), pp. 309-14.

Correction of Ears (Otoplasty) 28

M Kicken, N van Heerbeek, Koen JAO Ingels

Chapter Overview

Pearls and Pitfalls

Pearls

- Prefer cartilage sparing and avoid cartilage cutting.
- Pay attention to the earlobe and consider setback to avoid a "telephone ear" deformity.
- Work predominantly on the posterior side of the auricle and avoid cartilage cuts or sutures on the anterior side.

Pitfalls

- Try not to make the antihelix too sharp, which gives an unnatural aspect to the auricle.
- Avoid tension on the postauricular skin. Do not remove too much postauricular skin, because the underlying deformity is not caused by excess skin.
- Do not suture the concha too far anteriorly during conchal setback, as this may lead to stenosis of the entrance of the outer ear canal.

28.1 INTRODUCTION

Prominent ears are one of the most common congenital malformations in the head and neck region. The incidence is approximately 5% in the Caucasian race (Lohuis and Vuyk, 2006). This anatomical deformity can often be ascribed to an underdeveloped *antihelix* and/or hypertrophy of the conchal cartilage. In patients with an underdeveloped antihelix, the concha and the scapha are not delineated by a well-defined fold, leading to a protrusion of the upper part of the *helix*. Lateral protrusion of the ear lobule secondary to a prominent helical tail may be present in a proportion of the patients.

In most cases, prominent ears are familial (Rogers, 1968), and several relatives show a similar morphology. Children with this deformity are often ridiculed and are consequently very conscious of their appearance. This can have a negative impact on the self-confidence of the child, particularly between 5 and 7 years of age, when the child becomes aware of his/her appearance (Bradbury, Hewison and Timmons, 1992). Otoplasty offers a safe and effective method for addressing this aesthetic deformity. About 85% of the adult length of auricle is reached between 3 and 5 years of age (Adamson, Horton and Crawford, 1965). Hence, it is considered safe to perform surgery by the age of 6 years without having a significant impact on the dimensions of the ears (Adamson, Horton and Crawford, 1965).

28.2 ANATOMY

The *auricle*, also known as the pinna, contains mostly cartilage and skin. Different topographical parts are mentioned in Figure 28.1, which shows a schematic of the surface anatomy. Although the characteristic landmarks can be recognized in every anatomically normal auricle, every auricle has its own unique appearance, with the morphology being mirrored closely by the contralateral ear.

About one-third of the medial surface of the auricle is actually attached to the skull. Both anterior and posterior ligaments help the auricle to maintain its position.

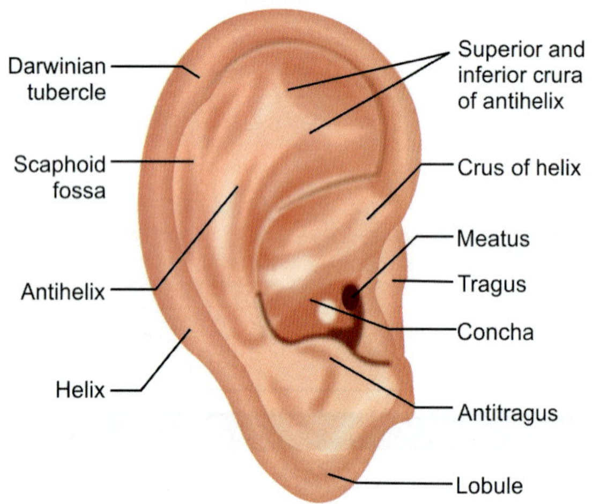

Fig. 28.1: Anatomy of the pinna.
Source: With permission from Vuyk, H.D. and Lohuis, P.J.F.M., 2006. *Facial plastic and reconstructive surgery*. London: Hodder Arnold. pp. 341-53.

Although some people can wiggle their ears, the auricular muscles (musculus auricularis superior, posterior, and anterior) are largely rudimentary in humans. They contribute to the soft-tissue mass, especially in the postauricular sulcus. They are associated with an increase in local blood supply, which is important to recognize during surgery.

28.3 MEASUREMENTS AND DIAGNOSIS

The average ear is 65 mm long and 35 mm wide. Some variation may occur, which means that the width of the ear is 50–60% of the height. In natural head position, the top of the auricular helix should be at the level of the lateral eyebrow, the inferior aspect lies at the level of the base of the nasal alae. The ear is situated roughly 6 cm from the lateral orbital rim and slopes 15–20°, with the cephalic margin more posteriorly.

The *auriculocephalic angle* is about 20–30° and determines the protrusion of the ear from the skull. It is the angle between the temporal surface of the scalp and a line connecting the posterior concha and scapha (Figs. 28.2A and B). If this angle becomes larger than 30°, the auricle catches the eye and prominent ears become manifest. In fact, the auriculocephalic angle determines how far the helix will diverge from the skull and thus creates the distance between the helix and the mastoid

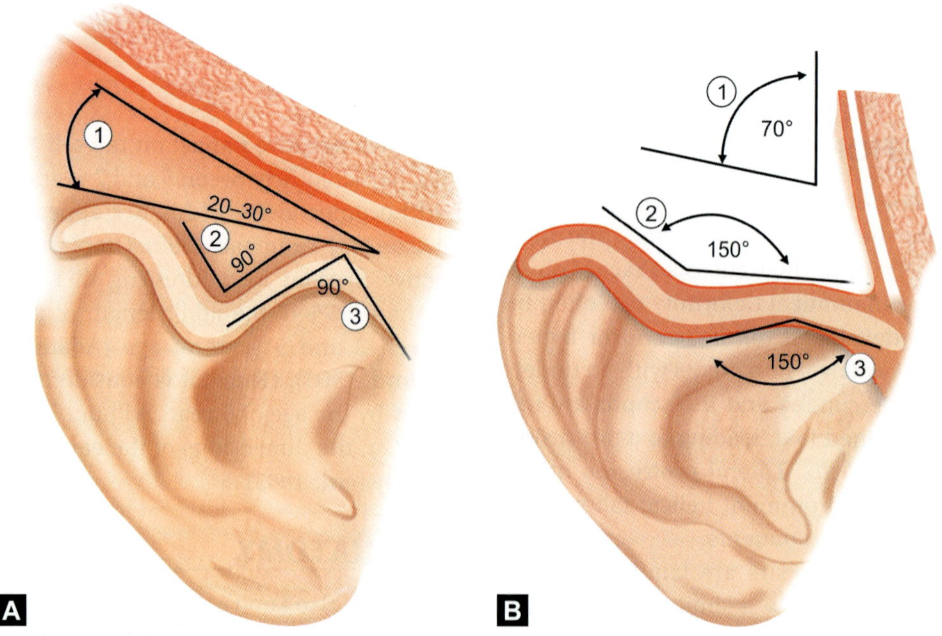

Figs. 28.2A and B: Angles in a normal (A) and a protruding ear (B).

process. Two important factors influence the auriculocephalic angle: the morphology and amount of conchal cartilage and the absence/presence of the antihelix. Both factors determine the *conchocephalic* and *conchoscaphalic angle* (Fig. 28.2A); they being 90° in the normal situation.

The distance between the scalp and the ear generally varies between 1.5 cm in the superior and 2.2 cm in the inferior part, respectively. This is because of the curvilinear nature of the helix on one hand and the skull being narrower in the region of the *lobule* on the other hand. A distance of <1.0 cm between the scalp and the ear looks unnatural.

The antihelical fold lies between the concha and scapha-helical units. The more defined the antihelical fold, the sharper the conchoscaphalic angle. When the conchocephalic and/or conchoscaphalic angle and thus the auriculocephalic angle become obtuse, the distance from helical rim to the scalp increases, which then leads to more prominent ears (Mallen, 1974). In the protruding ear in Figure 28.2B, the conchocephalic and conchoscaphalic angles are both 150°, and consequently, the auriculocephalic angle is 70°.

All these angles and distances are relative parameters and vary slightly from patient to patient. As a general rule, one can say that when seen from a frontal viewpoint, if a spectator can look into the concha or the helical rim appears too prominent behind the antihelix, then surgical correction may be considered.

28.4 PREVENTION

At present, it is not possible to prevent prominent ears in the antenatal period. The ear cartilage is still immature in the early neonatal period because of the influence of circulating maternal hormones, and it can be molded by splinting. A device called "Ear Buddies" (van Wijk, Breugem and Kon, 2012) has been shown to be effective in achieving this. In some cases, this might prevent surgery. The success rates can be up to 66% if intervention is started before the age of 6 weeks, especially in an ear with a large conchoscaphalic angle.

28.5 TREATMENT

It is important for the surgeon to analyze the structure and resilience of the ear cartilage by inspection and palpation, and by moving the different anatomical subunits toward the desired position, to determine the appropriate surgical technique for correction of protruding ears in a given patient.

Protruding ears are usually a result of one or more of the following anatomical deformities: (1) hypoplasia of the antihelix, (2) hyperplasia of the cavum or high conchal wall, (3) protruding ear lobule. Mostly, a combination of hypoplasia of the antihelix and hyperplasia of the cavum causes the deformity.

A variety of surgical techniques ranging from incision less otoplasty, cartilage scoring, suture techniques, conchal bowl retropositioning, or excision of conchal cartilage have been described to correct prominent ears (Siegert, 2004a). This suggests that no single technique can address all of the anatomical variants leading to this deformity. The surgeon often uses a combination of different techniques to treat an individual patient. The choice of surgical techniques is dictated by the surgeon's experience, preference, and the anatomical deformities leading to prominent ears (Table 28.1).

Incision

Incisions in the sulcus give unfavorable scars, and therefore, the skin is incised on the posterior surface of the auricle, about 1 cm lateral to the postaural groove. Some surgeons start by removing an ellipse of skin, but the authors prefer to remove skin at the end of the procedure when a better estimation of the amount of skin to be excised can be made. The surgeon should not rely

Table 28.1: Synopsis of otoplastic procedures for protruding ears (according to Siegert).

Malformation	*Characteristics*	*Technique*
Antihelix hypoplasia	Very soft cartilage	Sutures (Mustardé)
	Average cartilage	Sutures and posterior scoring (Converse)
	Strong cartilage	Sutures and anterior scoring (Crikelair modification)
Cavum hyperplasia	High antihelix	Cavum rotation
Protruding lobule	Prominent helix	Scoring
	Soft-tissue tension	Mattress suture and slight skin resection

solely on skin tension to correct protruding ears, even in patients with very weak auricular cartilage. This is because the skin tends to stretch under tension leading to a relapse of the original deformity. Moreover, too much tension on the skin may predispose the patient to hypertrophic scars or keloids.

Cutting

Conchal Setback

Sometimes it is sufficient to remove a layer of cartilage on the posterior surface of the concha in the area of the conchal eminence (*conchal shave*), thus allowing the concha to move closer to the skull (Yazar, et al., 2012). In other patients, some of the soft tissue in the postaural groove may need to be excised to allow the concha to lie closer to the scalp. The cartilage is then sutured to the periosteum of the mastoid process.

Cartilage Excision

The early otoplasty techniques were based on excision of part of auricular cartilage; these cartilage cuts risk creating noticeable sharp and unattractive edges. Therefore, cartilage excision techniques are best reserved for conchal wall hypertrophy. They are less suitable for creation of the antihelix, where sharp edges are more likely to draw the attention of the spectator.

Cartilage Scoring

Multiple parallel partial thickness cartilage incisions break the spring of the cartilage. This helps to create a permanent convexity on the incised surface. The scoring technique is based on the principle that cartilage bends away from the incised surface (as a result of the opposite, still intact contractile forces on the nonincised surface). Stenström (1963) was the first to utilize this principle to describe the cartilage-scoring technique for otoplasty. In the *Stenström technique*, the anterior surface of the antihelix is exposed through an incision on the posterior surface of the pinna. The skin and soft tissue are then raised over the posterior surface of the pinna, and the cartilage is incised a few millimeters lateral to the proposed antihelical fold. Next, the perichondrium is raised over the anterior surface of the pinna, and multiple, parallel, partial thickness, vertically oriented incisions are made into the cartilage with a knife (Fig. 28.3). Scoring can also be performed by making a 2–3 mm incision in the anterior skin just under the superior helical rim. A tunnel is then created under the skin and soft tissue over the proposed antihelix. With a "Dingman" rasp or a sharp 19 or 21 gauge hypodermic needle microincisions or scorings can then be made in the cartilage.

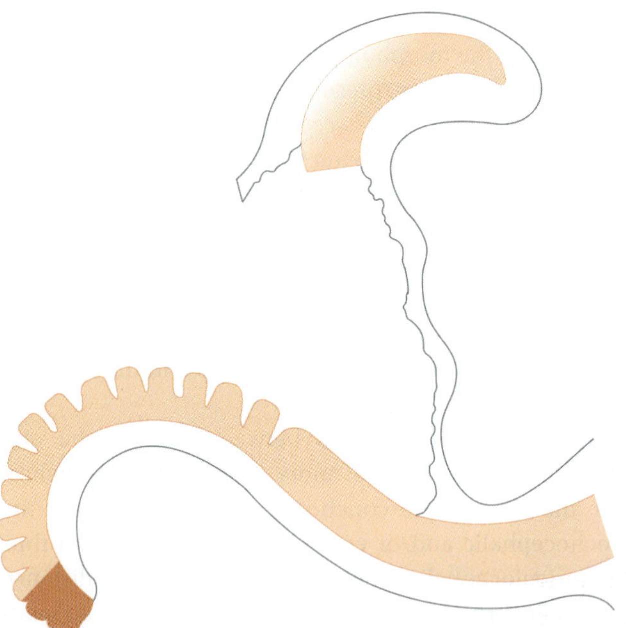

Fig. 28.3: The scoring technique.
Source: With permission from Vuyk, H.D. and Lohuis, P.J.F.M., 2006. *Facial plastic and reconstructive surgery*. London: Hodder Arnold. pp. 341-53.

Cartilage Sparing

Of the cartilage sparing and reshaping techniques, Mustardé and Furnas are most commonly used. With the Mustardé (1963) technique, it is possible to create a new antihelix by using several transcartilaginous mattress sutures (Fig. 28.4). Tattooing the skin and cartilage using a hypodermic needle whose tip has been dipped in Bonish blue or methylene blue dye marks the boundaries of the proposed antihelix. The needle is passed through the entire thickness of the pinna, thus marking the cartilage and guiding the transcartilaginous sutures. The skin incision is made on the posterior surface of the pinna as described previously. The skin and soft tissues are raised over the posterior surface of the auricular cartilage. The perichondrium over the posterior surface of the auricular cartilage is not raised, which helps to prevent the sutures from cutting through the cartilage. These sutures are placed making sure that they are not exposed through the

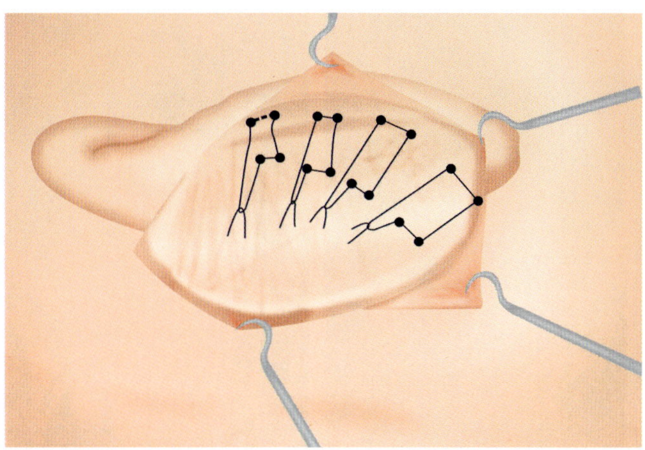

Fig. 28.4: Mattress sutures according to Mustardé.

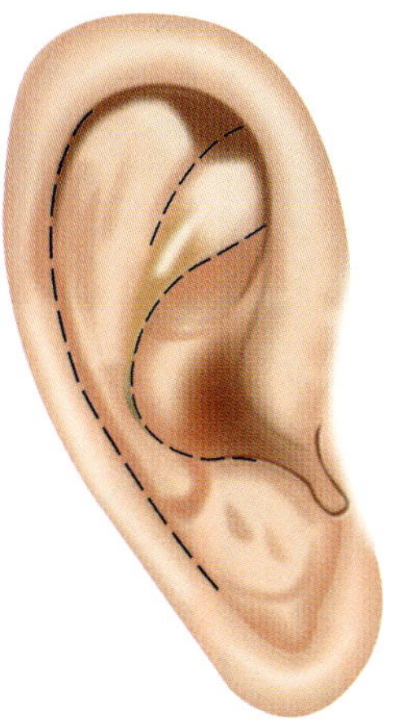

Fig. 28.5: Positioning of the three cartilage incisions as described in the Converse technique.

thin anterior skin. Tying the sutures progressively (3 to 5 sutures are used on average) helps to fold the cartilage and create an antihelix. It is common to use permanent sutures of braided polyethylene terephthalate (Mersilene) or Goretex to prevent relapse.

Incisionless Otoplasty

Incisionless otoplasty is a technique where the auricular skin is entered via puncture holes through which tunnels are made over the cartilage that needs to be bent (Fritsch, 2004). The cartilage is then scored along the proposed antihelix with a sharp needle (Gauge 21) or rasp. Eventually, buried mattress sutures are applied to the auricular cartilage to keep the cartilage securely in the new position.

Combination of Techniques

All kinds of the above-mentioned techniques or variations might be combined to achieve the desired surgical result. One of the best-known combinations is described by Converse, et al. (1955). In the *Converse technique*, a single postauricular skin incision is made to expose the cartilage. Postauricular cartilage incisions are made along the antihelix as shown in Figure 28.5. By making these incisions, a vertical oriented strip of cartilage is created in the region of the antihelix. Postauricular permanent sutures are then used to create a more pronounced antihelix. Patients in Figures 28.6A to D were treated using this technique.

Protruding Lobule

A *prominent lobule* is often considered to be a problem of excess skin. This can be treated by excision of a rhomboid-shaped piece of skin on the posterior part of the lobule. Others prefer a suturing technique by placing nonabsorbing sutures between the cavum conchae on one side and the soft-tissue lobule on the other side (Siegert, 2004b). The knot is buried in a stab incision on the posterior surface of the ear (Fig. 28.7).

Abnormal cartilage framework, especially prominence of the cauda helicis, can play a role in lobular prominence. After isolation of this most distal part of the helix, it can be turned around and sutured on itself to decrease prominence of the lobule. This technique is demonstrated in a video clip, which can be accessed at http://www.aroundthenose.com/dissection-manual-login/. Some authors prefer to excise a wedge along the posterior edge of the auricular cartilage just superior to the cauda helicis. This helps to break the spring of the cartilage, which can then be repositioned, sometimes without the aid of sutures. Protruding lobules are often considered difficult to correct. They may sometimes result due to overcorrection of the concha giving a "telephone shape" to the auricle.

28.6 COMPLICATIONS

Hematoma and Infection

Like all surgical procedures, there is a risk of postoperative hematoma formation and infection after otoplasty. Gentle tissue handling and adequate coagulation can minimize the risk of hematoma. The risk of postoperative hematoma is low, although it is reported to be up to 6.5% (Limandjaja, et al., 2009). Postoperative pain should warn the surgeon regarding a developing hematoma and infection. Most authors describing postoperative complications

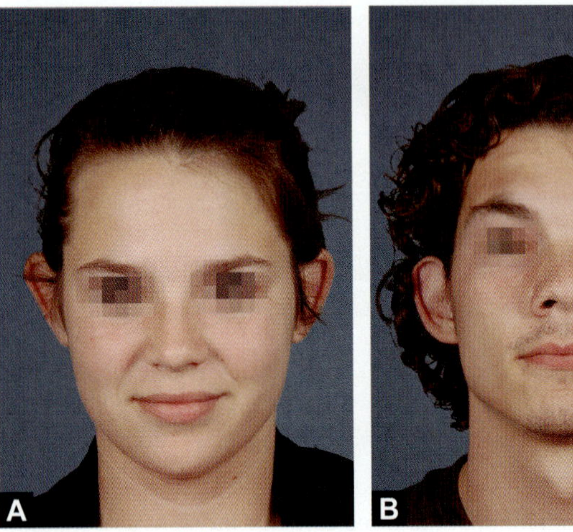

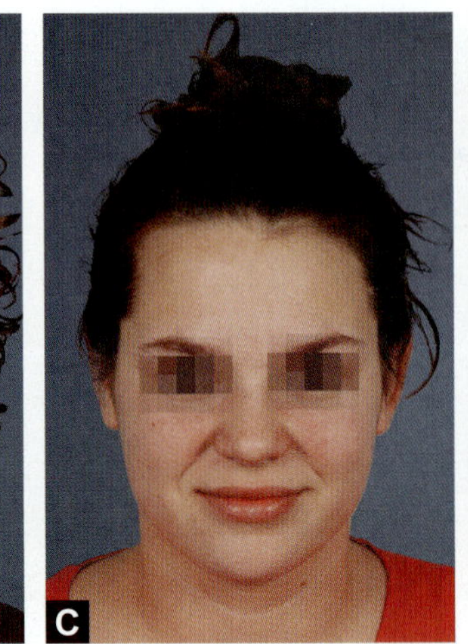

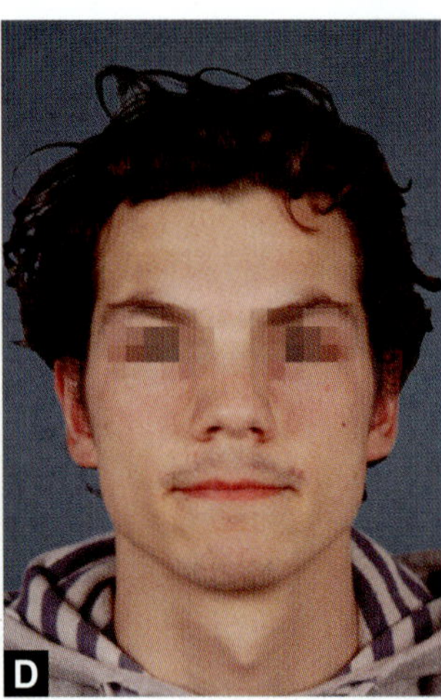

Figs. 28.6A to D: Siblings with antihelix hypoplasia. (A) and (B) before surgery; (C) and (D) after surgery.

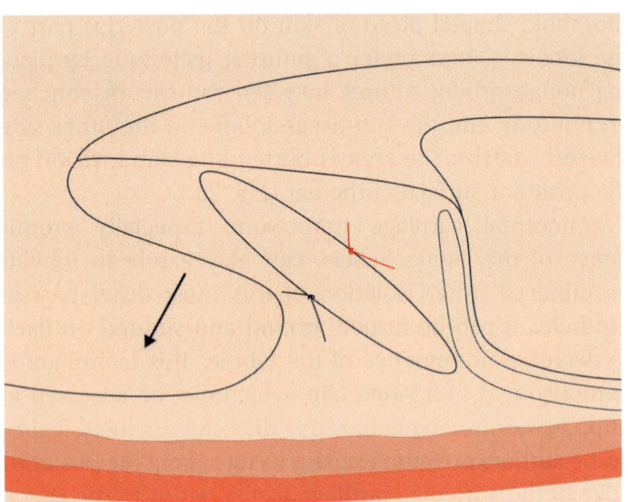

Fig. 28.7: Approximation of the lobule by the suturing technique.

have not seen postoperative infections (Limandjaja, et al., 2009). Some surgeons prefer antibiotic prophylaxis to prevent postoperative infection. Signs of infection usually present 3–4 days after surgery and include pain (sometimes absent), swelling, and development of an abscess. If there is any suggestion of infection, it must be treated aggressively to prevent perichondritis/chondritis, cartilage necrosis, and cauliflower ear deformity. A hematoma must be drained as soon as possible and quilting sutures applied to the pinna over a silastic sheet placed on the anterior and posterior surfaces of the pinna.

Unsatisfactory Cosmetic Outcome

Preoperative photographic documentation is routinely performed in all cases and is used to point out any pre-existing asymmetries to the patient. As a part of the informed consent, patients are counseled that slight postoperative asymmetries are inevitable as the final result is partly dependent on the way the tissues heal.

Telephone ear deformity results from overcorrection of the middle third of the ear and/or undercorrection of the cranial helix and lobule. As a result, the upper and lower third of the ear bend anteriorly and are more distant from the skull as compared to the central part.

When seen from the frontal view, the helical rim should be visible beyond the antihelix (at least from upper to midhelix and preferably all the way to the lower helix). Overcorrection results in an unnatural looking "glued ear" appearance in which the ear seems to stick to the skull. Other familiar failures are undercorrection and recurrences. The overall incidence of unsatisfactory outcome lies between 3% and 21% (Limandjaja, et al., 2009).

Suture extrusion sometimes occurs after Mustardé technique, occasionally many years after surgery. Incidence varies between 0% and 22.2% (Limandjaja, et al., 2009). Extruded sutures must be removed because they predispose to infection. The skin wound can then be treated with topical antibiotic ointment. In most cases, scar formation will keep the auricle in the intended position. If relapse of the original deformity occurs, it may require revision surgery in up to 12% of patients (Limandjaja, et al., 2009).

Skin Necrosis

Most surgeons apply a contour dressing in the first few postoperative days to prevent hematoma formation. Acroflavin-soaked cotton wool or paraffin gauze is commonly used to fill the contours on both surfaces of the ear

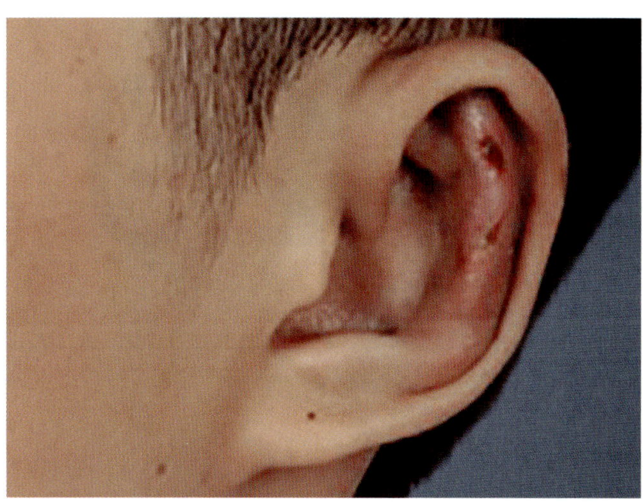

Fig. 28.8: Pressure necrosis of the skin on the anterior surface of the pinna secondary to tight bandage following pinnaplasty. *Photograph courtesy*: Dr Sandeep Uppal, Singapore.

followed by a light pressure bandage to help achieve this goal. Necrosis of the skin over the newly created antihelical fold or superior and inferior crura may develop in a small proportion of patients due to a tight head bandage or a bandage that has been applied for too long a period (Fig. 28.8). Although uncommon, one paper has reported a 17.2% incidence of skin necrosis (Limandjaja, et al., 2009).

Keloid Formation

Keloids form more often in the earlobe region than in any other place in the head and neck. The risk of keloid formation is higher in Africans and Asians. The risk of keloid formation increases with an increase in the wound closure tension. It is therefore important that the surgeon should not excise excessive amount of skin from the postauricular region. The mainstay of treatment for management of keloids is surgical excision followed by serial injection of triamcinolone. In therapy-resistant cases, radiotherapy may be used (Naylor and Brissett, 2012).

REFERENCES

Adamson, J.E., Horton, C.E. and Crawford, H.H., 1965. The growth pattern of the external ear. *Plastic and Reconstructive Surgery*, 36, pp. 466-70.

Bradbury, E.T., Hewison, J. and Timmons, M.J., 1992. Psychological and social outcome of prominent ear correction in children. *British Journal of Plastic Surgery*, 45, pp. 97-100.

Converse, J.M., Nigro, A., Wilson, F. and Johnson, N., 1955. A technique for surgical correction of lop ears. *Plastic and Reconstructive Surgery*, 15, pp. 411-8.

Fritsch, M.H., 2004. Incisionless otoplasty. *Facial Plastic Surgery*, 20(4), pp. 267-70.

Limandjaja, G.C., Breugem, C.C., Mink van der Molen, A.B. and Kon, M., 2009. Complications of otoplasty: a literature review. *Journal of Plastic, Reconstructive & Aesthetic Surgery*, 62(1), pp. 19-27.

Lohuis, P.J.F.M. and Vuyk, H.D., 2006. Otoplasty. In: P.J. Lohuis, H.D. Vuyk, eds. *Facial plastic and reconstructive surgery*. London: Hodder Arnold. pp. 341-53.

Mallen, R.W., 1974. Otoplasty. *Canadian Journal of Otolaryngology*, 3(1), pp. 74-8.

Mustardé, J.C., 1963. Correction of prominent ears using simple mattress sutures. *British Journal of Plastic Surgery*, 16, pp. 170-8.

Naylor, M.C. and Brissett, A.E., 2012. Current concepts in the etiology and treatment of keloids. *Facial Plastic Surgery*, 28(5), pp. 504-12.

Rogers, B.O., 1968. Microtic, lop, cup and protruding ears: four directly inheritable deformities? *Plastic and Reconstructive Surgery*, 41, pp. 208-31.

Siegert, R., 2004a. Synopsis of otoplasty. *Facial Plastic Surgery*, 20(4), pp. 299-300.

Siegert, R., 2004b. Correction of the lobule. *Facial Plastic Surgery*, 20(4), pp. 293-8.

Stenström, S.J., 1963. A 'natural' technique for correction of congenitally prominent ears. *Plastic and Reconstructive Surgery*, 32, pp. 509-18.

van Wijk, M.P., Breugem, C.C. and Kon, M., 2012. A prospective study on non-surgical correction of protruding ears: the importance of early treatment. *Journal of Plastic, Reconstructive & Aesthetic Surgery*, 65(1), pp. 54-60.

Yazar, M., Basat, S.O., Biçer, A., Yazar, S.K., Güven, E., Kuvat, S.V. and Emekli, U., 2012. Creating a neoconchal complex using the adjustable conchal sliding technique in prominent ear correction. *Journal of Craniofacial Surgery*, 23(5), pp. 1414-7.

Correction of Small Ears (Microtia) 29

Yogesh Bajaj, Rishi Talwar

Chapter Overview

Pearls and Pitfalls

Pearls

- Children with microtia should have an urgent hearing assessment.
- Bilateral microtia patients should be prescribed hearing aids as early as possible.
- Microtia is commonly associated with other abnormalities, and a general pediatrician and a geneticist should assess affected children.
- Radiological assessment is necessary to assess the middle ear, course of the facial nerve, and exclude congenital cholesteatoma.
- Bone-anchored hearing aid is a good option for hearing amplification.

Pitfalls

- Microtia surgery performed by the occasional microtia surgeon is likely to result in poor outcomes for the patient.

29.1 INTRODUCTION

Microtia in simple terms means a small/deformed ear. The incidence of microtia is one in 6000 births. Microtia (Fig. 29.1) may occur as an isolated congenital anomaly or associated with other anomalies. Microtia usually coexists with atresia of the ear canal and anomalies of the middle ear. Generally, these are not associated with inner ear malformations. Management of microtia and associated canal atresia and middle ear malformations is surgically very challenging.

29.2 EMBRYOLOGY OF EXTERNAL EAR

By 6th week of embryonic life, six hillocks have developed in the mesodermal tissue of the first and second arch. These hillocks begin to fuse by the 7th week to produce the primitive pinna. The first (mandibular) arch contributes to 1, 2, and 3 hillocks, and the second (hyoid) arch contributes to 4, 5, and 6 hillocks. It is widely accepted that hillock 1 forms the anterior portion of the ear lobe, hillock 2 forms the tragus, hillock 3 forms the ascending helix, hillock 4 forms the antihelix, hillock 5 produces the helix, and hillock 6 forms the posterior lobule (Park, 1999). The concha develops from the first branchial groove. At birth the pinna is nearly 70% of the size of pinna in an adult. By 6 years of age, the shape and size are 90% of adult size. In the initial stages of the development, the ear is formed in the neck and gradually migrates on to the head by 10th week of fetal life.

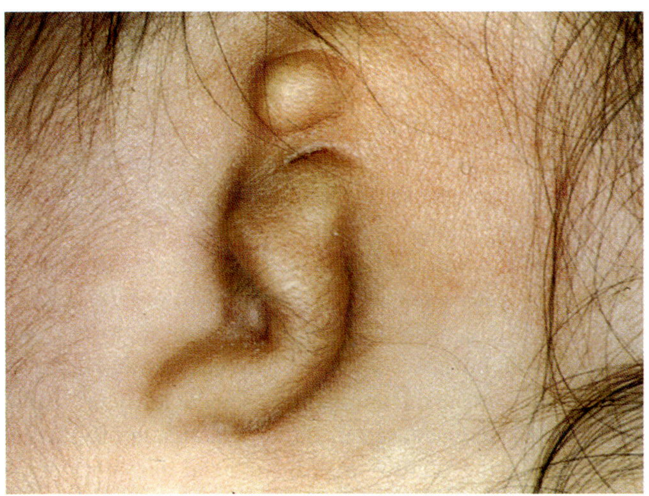

Fig. 29.1: Microtia.

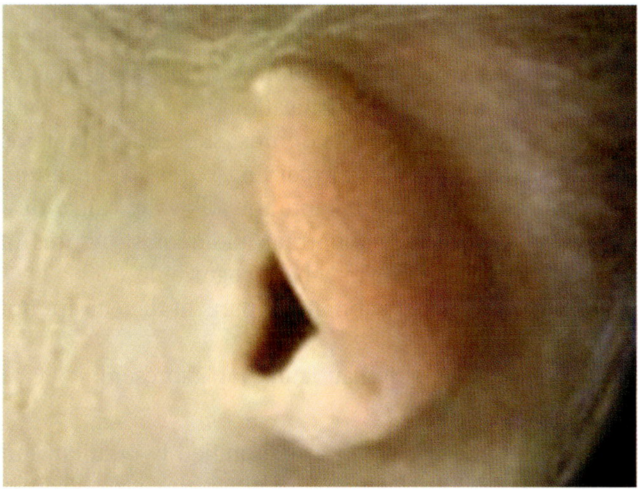

Fig. 29.2: Cup ear.

Abnormal development at various stages can lead to different anomalies. If the hillocks do not fuse completely, it can lead to clefts. Hypergenesis can lead to formation of tubercles, tags, and polyotia. Any abnormality of development at 7–8 weeks of age can lead to microtia or anotia. Developmental anomalies at a later stage can lead to deformities like prominent ears or cup ears.

Malformations of the inner ear are associated with middle or external ear anomalies in only 8% children, since the inner ear is formed at a different period of intrauterine development.

29.3 EPIDEMIOLOGY AND ETIOLOGY

Microtia is unilateral in 90% cases and bilateral in 10% of cases. It is more common on the right side than the left and more common in males than in females. It is more common in Asians and Hispanics rather than blacks and whites. Microtia can be sporadic or be a part of a syndrome. In majority of the cases, the cause for microtia is unknown. In about 15% cases, a genetic or environmental causes, i.e. maternal diabetes, thalidomide exposure, and fetal alcohol syndrome, can be identified. Very small numbers of isolated cases have been reported as familial (autosomal dominant/recessive/x-linked inheritance). There have been reports of identical twins, where only one twin has microtia. This clearly indicates that an intrauterine event rather than a genetic process leads to the deformity of the ear. The current thinking is that hemorrhage from stapedial artery during intrauterine development can lead to deformed pinna (Poswillo, 1973).

Common syndromes associated with microtia are Treacher Collins, Crouzon, Branchio-oto-renal, Noonan syndrome, fetal alcohol syndrome, Sticklers, and CHARGE.

29.4 NORMAL PINNA

The average length of pinna in an adult male and adult female is 63 and 59 mm, respectively. For a male child, the length of the ear at 6 months is 48 mm, which increases to 55 mm at 5 years and further to 59 mm at 10 years of age. In female children, the length is slightly less as compared to male children. On an average, the adult ear protrudes 19 mm from the mastoid bone. The longitudinal axis of the ear slopes backward in line with the slope of the bridge of the nose. The normal pinna lies between the level of the eyebrow and nasal columella.

29.5 TYPES OF MICROTIA

There is a wide variation in the shape of the underdeveloped external ear. Anotia is a total absence of the pinna and an associated low hairline. Majority of microtia patients have a small dependent ear lobe underneath a deformed cartilaginous remnant (Fig. 29.1). Some patients have two separate ear remnants, indicating failure of fusion of cartilage hillocks arising from first and second branchial arches. These patients can have an associated facial nerve weakness and a higher risk of facial nerve injury during reconstruction because of the superficial course of nerve. Conchal type microtia or cup ear (Fig. 29.2) is another variation in microtia. In this deformity, the tragus, external auditory canal, and a considerable amount of other ear tissue are present, but the ear is folded upon itself at the upper pole.

29.6 CLASSIFICATION OF MICROTIA

There are multiple classification systems available for grading microtia. The classification proposed by Marx in 1926 still forms the basis of most subsequent systems (Gault and Rothera, 2008). According to this classification, external ear deformities fall into the following categories:

- *Grade I*: Auricle is abnormal, different structures of each part of the ear may be recognizable.
- *Grade II*: Auricle is abnormal; parts of the ear are not recognizable.
- *Grade III*: Very small auricular tag is present.
- *Grade IV*: Anotia.

The Marx classification was modified by Aguilar and Jahrsdoerfer (1988), which simplifies the classification further:

- *Grade I*: Any normal ear that is simply smaller in size in any given dimension.
- *Grade II*: Any ear with structural deficiencies, i.e. absent lobule, absent scapha, broadened helix, missing helix, missing concha, or missing antihelix.
- *Grade III*: Any ear showing classic peanut deformity with no recognizable structures present or anotia.

In essence, as per this classification, in Grade I, the ear is smaller but otherwise normal and needs no correction. Grades II and III deformities can be treated surgically.

29.7 CLASSIFICATION OF EXTERNAL AUDITORY CANAL ATRESIA

The original classification was proposed by Altmann in 1955 and divided external auditory canal atresia into mild, moderate, and severe deformities.

- *Mild or Type I atresia*: The tympanic membrane is present but smaller in area than normal; the bony ear canal is either normal or slightly reduced in size. This might be associated with ossicular abnormalities.
- *Moderate or Type II atresia*: There is either a partial or total failure of the bony canal to develop, i.e. a solid piece of bone lateral to the middle ear. The middle ear cavity is normal, but the course of facial nerve might be abnormal.
- *Severe or Type III atresia*: There is complete absence of external auditory canal and very small middle ear cavity.

29.8 ASSESSMENT OF THE PATIENT

Microtia can be an isolated anomaly or associated with other malformations. A detailed history and physical examination is essential to rule out any associated abnormalities. The history should include antenatal history specifically for any exposure to drugs/toxins. The child's general development especially the genitourinary system and spine need to be assessed for abnormalities. The ear canal is graded as per severity, i.e. normal, stenotic, blind ending, or absent. There is no correlation between a deformed *pinna* and middle ear abnormality. Developmentally, the external ear develops before the middle ear. Microtia is usually associated with a middle ear abnormality, but an isolated middle ear anomaly can be associated with a normal pinna. The facial nerve function should be evaluated in detail, because a proportion of patients with microtia may have facial nerve paralysis.

Patients with microtia can have moderate-to-severe hearing loss, which needs to be assessed as a priority soon after birth. This is usually done by brain stem-evoked response audiometry as soon as practically possible. Delaying the testing or adopting a wait and see strategy is not in child's best interest. In the majority of cases, sensorineural function is normal, and the canal atresia causes a conductive hearing loss of 45–60 dB. In children with bilateral abnormalities, hearing aids (air or bone conduction) need to be prescribed within 6 months after birth to avoid any delays in speech or language development. In children with unilateral atresia, the status of hearing in the nonatresia ear needs to be clearly established. Unilateral microtia children should ideally be kept under regular audiology follow-up for early identification of hearing loss due to otitis media with effusion (OME).

All patients with atresia need a high-resolution computerized tomography (CT) scan of the temporal bones for the detailed evaluation of middle ear and course of the facial nerve. It is important to know the relationship of the facial nerve to the oval window. If the vertical segment of facial nerve is anteriorly displaced, the access to middle ear is restricted for ossiculoplasty, and the risk of facial nerve injury is also increased. The scans also give information on ossicular and inner ear anatomy. Any abnormality of the semicircular canals or abnormal communication between the perilymph and cerebrospinal fluid can be identified. The CT scan can be performed either in the neonatal period or at the time of potential surgical correction. In patients with canal atresia, repeat scans are not required as the chances of cholesteatoma formation are rare in this situation. *Congenital stenosis* carries a much greater risk of *cholesteatoma* as compared to *congenital aural atresia* (Cole and Jahrsdoerder, 1990). In children with meatal stenosis, CT scan should be done between

5 and 10 years of age to exclude cholesteatoma. The CT scan can also predict bone thickness at the site of implantation for the titanium fixtures.

29.9 TREATMENT OPTIONS

Children with microtia are usually diagnosed soon after birth and referred to an otolaryngologist for further management. At this stage, it is important to provide psychological support to the parents to alleviate their guilt and fear. The next important step is to evaluate the child's hearing threshold. If the hearing needs to be amplified, it should to be done on an urgent basis to aid normal speech and language development.

Parents should be offered genetic counseling to explore the etiology of microtia and rule out any syndromic associations or systemic involvement. These children need to be under regular follow-up to identify the development of OME in the normal ear. If OME is detected in the nonmicrotic ear, this needs to be treated medically or surgically as required. If the ear with atresia shows symptoms and signs suggestive of acute otitis media, prompt antibiotic treatment should be started to reduce the risks of intratemporal or intracranial complications.

Audiological Treatment

Unilateral microtia does not need any urgent medical or surgical intervention in the neonatal period. Hearing assessment is mandatory to make sure that the hearing is normal in the contralateral ear and the child develops normal speech and language. The options for the child with hearing loss due to unilateral microtia include sitting in the front of the class with the better ear facing the teacher. Another option is using a hearing aid. The choice of type of hearing aid depends on the presence of an ear canal. In the presence of an external auditory canal, the preferred hearing aid is the air conduction aid as it provides less distortion and broader frequency response. Bone conduction hearing aid is an option for patients where the external auditory canal is stenosed (Fig. 29.3). The abutment for bone conduction hearing aid should be implanted at least 65 mm from the microtic ear (Fig. 29.4) to aid in future reconstruction (Bajaj, et al., 2005). Also, a contralateral routing of signal aid can be offered.

Bilateral microtia is managed differently. In neonates with bilateral disease, early hearing aids are mandatory and should be in place ideally by 3 months of age. The evaluation of hearing should be done within first few months, and initially a soft headband bone conduction hearing aid should be provided to the child. The soft band is an elastic band with a sound processor, which transmits the sound transcutaneously to the middle and inner ear.

Surgical Treatment

Cosmetic correction of microtia is not essential, and some patients/parents might choose not to undergo any surgical treatment. The two main cosmetic surgical approaches are autogenous reconstruction of the residual structures and the use of a prosthetic implant. Ideally the discussion about cosmetic reconstruction should happen in a multidisciplinary setting in a microtia clinic. The team members should include ENT surgeons, plastic surgeons,

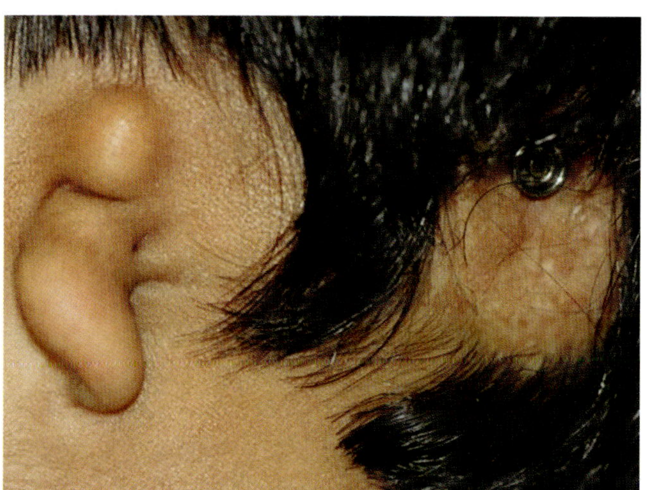

Fig. 29.3: Microtia and bone-anchored hearing aid abutment.

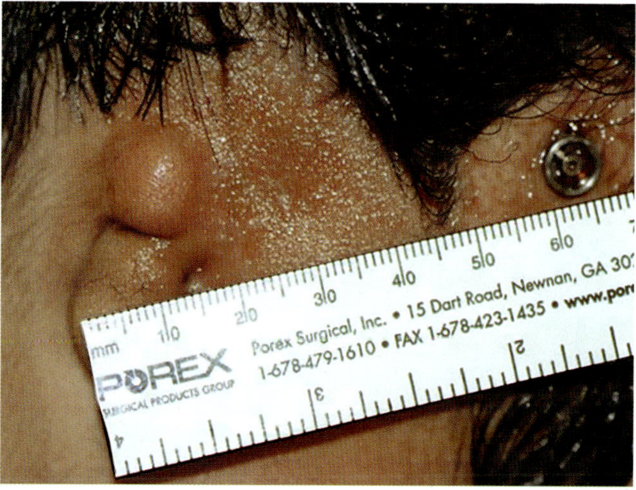

Fig. 29.4: Correct positioning of bone-anchored hearing aid in relation to microtia.

audiologist, and geneticists. It is essential that the parents understand the pros and cons of both treatment options before making a final decision for an irreversible course of action.

Having an otherwise healthy child with a congenital deformity of the ear is psychologically traumatic for the parents, and there is usually a sense of urgency on their part for surgical correction. For psychological reasons, parents might be keen to intervene early especially in severe cases; however, delaying the procedure allows the child himself to make a more mature and informed decision. It is essential that the families meet other children who have undergone both the treatment options. None of the cosmetic treatment options for auricular reconstruction is ideal, and doing nothing is always an option.

Autogenous reconstruction of the auricle using a rib cartilage is the gold standard treatment for cosmesis. This was pioneered by Tanzer in 1959 and modified by Brent in 1974 and Nagata in 1993. The timing of surgical reconstruction depends on the age of maturity of the pinna, availability of adequate rib cartilage, and the psychological impact of the disease. Since the pinna is 95% of adult size by 6 years of age and the minimum age for harvesting adequate rib cartilage is 6 years, the preferred age of operation is from 7 to 10 years of age. Ideal age is 10 years, as by this time adequate amount of costal cartilage is available and the chest deformity postharvest is less. The autogenous reconstruction is best carried out on a virgin field, as previous operation can interfere with the blood supply. Auricular reconstruction can be done as single-stage or multiple-stage procedures. At present, the most popular technique used is the two-stage technique.

The three main components of this procedure are as follows:

- Creating the costal cartilage framework and placing it at the site of pinna
- Rotating the lobule and creating the tragus
- Elevating the helical rim.

The most common techniques used for reconstruction are Brent technique and the Nagata technique, which will be discussed here.

Brent Technique

This technique introduced in 1974 (Brent, 1974) and modified in 1992 (Brent, 1992) involves four surgical stages.

- *First stage*: In this stage, the framework of the pinna is formed using contralateral rib cartilage graft. For unilateral cases, a template is made by placing an X-ray film or a cardboard piece against the normal ear to measure all the anatomical landmarks (Fig. 29.5). The position of the proposed pinna is marked (Fig. 29.6). Usually, the contralateral sixth, seventh, and eighth ribs cartilage graft are harvested and carved according to the template. This is then placed in a subcutaneous pocket at the proposed site of the pinna, and suction drains are used to help drape the skin on it.
- *Second stage*: This step aims to reposition the ear lobe. The existing soft tissue of the microtic ear is mobilized and shaped as the ear lobe.
- *Third stage*: The next step is to elevate the framework of the pinna. A small incision is made few millimeters behind the framework margin, and it is dissected off

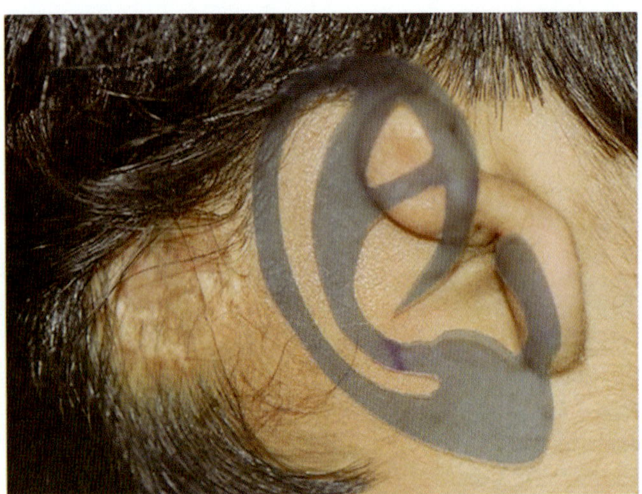

Fig. 29.5: X-ray film used to construct a template for carving rib cartilage.

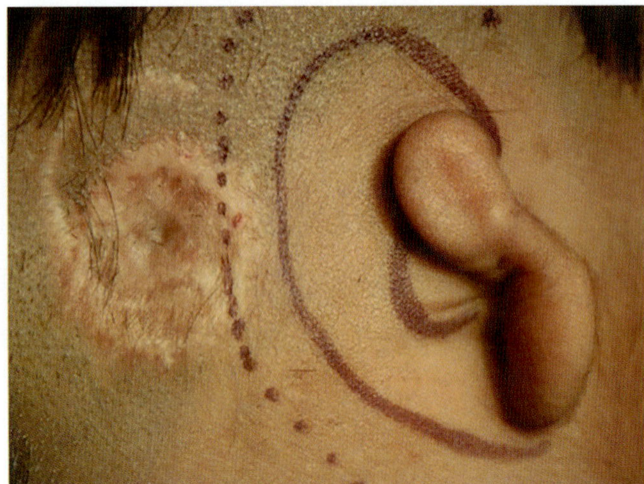

Fig. 29.6: Marking the position of proposed pinna.

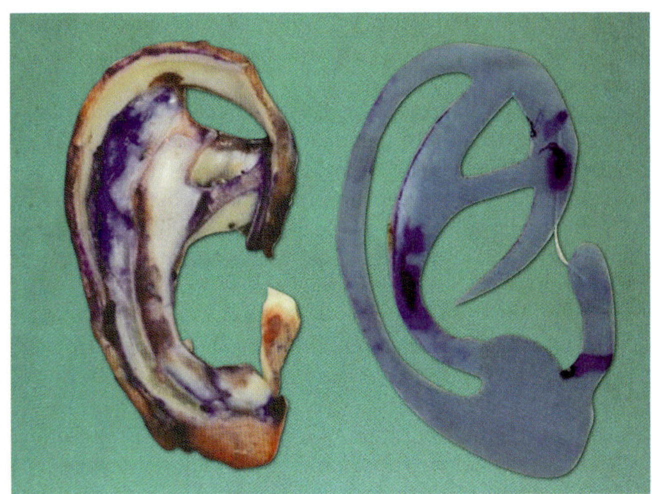

Fig. 29.7: Pinna framework constructed using rib cartilage.

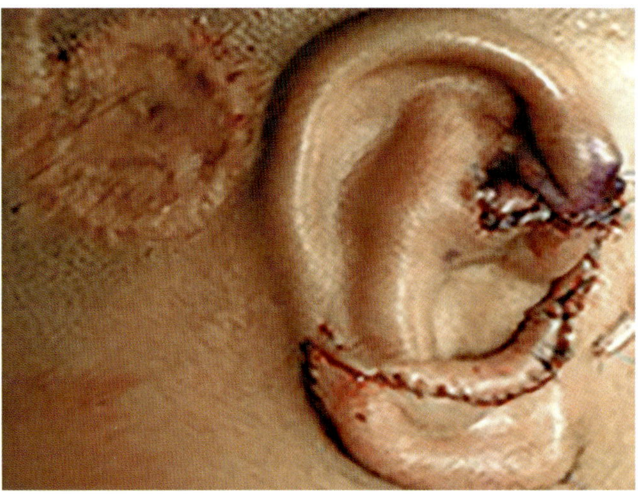

Fig. 29.8: Cartilage framework has been placed into a subcutaneous pocket, and the ear lobe has been transposed into the correct position.

and lifted. A small piece of cartilage is placed between this framework and the mastoid bone to achieve projection of the pinna. Split skin graft is placed in the postaural groove.

- *Fourth stage*: During this step, the surgeon reconstructs the tragus. Composite skin/cartilage graft is harvested from the normal ear concha and shaped as the tragus. It is then sutured in the correct anatomical position.

Nagata Technique

This technique (Nagata, 1993) has two stages.

- *First stage*: In this stage, the framework of the pinna and tragus is reconstructed and the ear lobe is transposed. Ipsilateral costal cartilages of sixth, seventh, eighth, and ninth ribs are harvested to form the framework (Fig. 29.7). The framework is slipped into the subcutaneous pocket, and the lobe is transposed inferior to it (Fig. 29.8).
- *Second stage*: During this stage, the surgeon elevates the cartilaginous framework by using a small piece of cartilage in the postaural groove. The postaural groove is covered with temporoparietal fascia and skin graft.

The success of the surgical procedure is based on comparison with the appearance of the normal ear. Brent reported patient satisfaction of 83–100%, whereas Nagata reported an overall satisfaction of 64%. Research on tissue engineered cartilage framework for the pinna is in progress (Shasti, et al., 2014).

Prosthetic Pinna

This is another choice that should be offered to the patient/parents while discussing cosmetic options for the pinna. The prosthesis is made up of silicone using the normal ear as a template (Fig. 29.9). For children with bilateral atresia, parent's ear can be used as a template. For this option, the prosthetic ear can be either a stick on prosthesis or clipped on to osseointegrated anchors. For the latter, titanium fixtures are implanted at the site of proposed pinna along with an anchoring device to provide a structural connection between the skull and the prosthetic ear (Tjellstrom, 1990). The usual indications are patient choice, failed surgical reconstruction, hypoplasia of bone and soft tissue, and low hairline. The main benefits of prosthetic option are reduced cost and good cosmetic appearance. The downside of prosthesis is that it needs replacement every 2–5 years. It also discolors and becomes brittle over time. Moreover, the abutments in the bone need to be looked after. For a prosthetic ear, all the remnants of the microtic ear have to be excised; hence, reconstruction with rib cartilage in the future is not an option. Various studies have reported that there is no adverse reaction at the site of the implants in 89.6% of cases. As per feedback from patients, bone-anchored technique was preferable to adhesion technique (Somers, et al., 1998).

Autogenous and prosthetic reconstructions have been compared in some studies. One study reported that the results with autogenous reconstruction were not as good

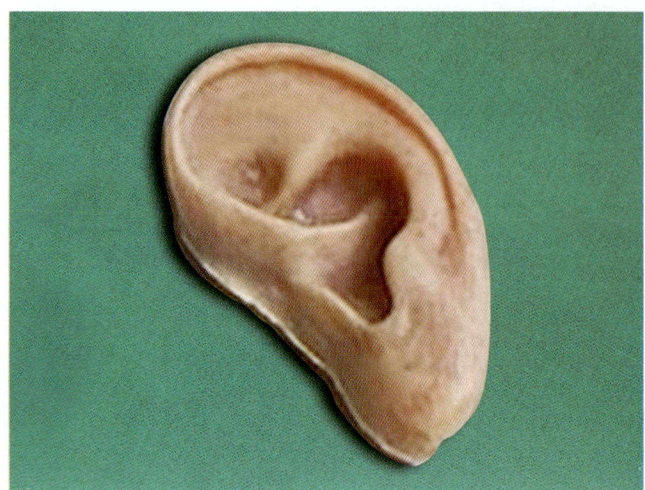

Fig. 29.9: Prosthetic pinna.

as those from prosthesis (Granstrom, et al., 2001). Other studies have reported that results of autogenous reconstruction are improving. The technique is surgically demanding and is only available at very few centers around the world (Somers, et al., 1998). The major advantage of autogenous reconstruction is that the reconstructed ear becomes an integral part of the body and does not need any maintenance or replacement.

REFERENCES

Aguilar, E.A. and Jahrsdoerfer, R.A., 1988. The surgical repair of congenital microtia and atresia. *Otolaryngology—Head and Neck Surgery*, 98, pp. 600-6.

Bajaj, Y., Wyatt, M.E., Gault, D., Bailey, C.M. and Albert, D.M., 2005. How we do it: BAHA positioning in patients with microtia requiring auricular reconstruction. *Clinical Otolaryngology*, 30, pp. 468-71.

Brent, B., 1974. Ear reconstruction with an expansile framework of autogenous rib cartilage. *Plastic and Reconstructive Surgery*, 53, pp. 619-28.

Brent, B., 1992. Auricular repair with autogenous rib cartilage grafts: two decades of experience with 600 cases. *Plastic and Reconstructive Surgery*, 90, pp. 355-74.

Cole, R.R. and Jahrsdoerder, R.A., 1990. The risk of cholesteatoma in congenital aural stenosis. *Laryngoscope*, 100, pp. 576-8.

Gault, D. and Rothera, M., 2008. Management of congenital deformities of the external and middle ear. In: M. Gleeson, G.G. Browning, M.J. Burton, R. Clarke, J. Hibbert, A.S. Jones, V.J. Lund, L.M. Luxon and J.C. Watkinson, eds. *Scott-Brown's otorhinolaryngology, head and neck surgery*. London: Edward Arnold. pp. 965-89.

Granstrom, G.P.B., Bergstrom, K., Odersjo, M. and Tjellstrom, A., 2001. Osseointegrated implants in children: experience from our first 100 patients. *Otolaryngology—Head and Neck Surgery*, 125, p. 85.

Nagata, S., 1993. A new method of total reconstruction of the auricle for microtia. *Plastic and Reconstructive Surgery*, 92, pp. 187-201.

Park, C., 1999. Lower auricular malformation: their representation, correction and embryologic correlation. *Plastic and Reconstructive Surgery*, 104, pp. 29-40.

Poswillo, D., 1973. The pathogenesis of the first and second branchial arch syndrome. *Journal of Oral Surgery*, 35, pp. 302-27.

Shasti, M., Jacquet, R., McClellan, P., Yang, J., Matsushima, S., Isogai, N., Murthy, A. and Landis, W.J., 2014. Effects of FGF-2 and OP-1 in vitro on donor source cartilage for auricular reconstruction tissue engineering. *International Journal of Pediatric Otorhinolaryngology*, Mar;78(3), pp. 416-22.

Somers, T., De Cubber, J., Govarets, P., and Offeciers, F.E., 1998. Total auricular repair: bone anchored prosthesis or plastic reconstruction? *Acta Oto-Rhino-Laryngologica Belgica*, 52, pp. 317-27.

Tjellstrom, A., 1990. Osseointegrated implants for replacement of absent or defective ears. *Clinics in Plastic Surgery*, 17, pp. 355-66.

Facial Weakness 30

Jennifer Kim

Chapter Overview

Pearls and Pitfalls

Pearls

- Weakness of the forehead muscles indicates a peripheral facial nerve problem, whereas sparing of the forehead muscles is diagnostic of a central lesion.
- The most common cause of peripheral facial weakness is Bell's palsy (BP), but a careful history and examination must be performed to exclude other rare causes.
- Identification of the anatomic landmarks (posterior belly of the digastric muscle, mastoid process, tympanic bone, and external auditory canal cartilage) is paramount for safe identification of the main trunk of the facial nerve.
- In reoperations or when the identification is obscured (by the tumor), try the retrograde approach.
- Facial rehabilitation therapy plays an integral role in optimizing the quality of nonsurgical and surgical interventions in patients affected by facial nerve injuries.

Pitfalls

- Failure to rule out neoplasm as cause of gradually progressive facial paralysis.
- Failure to individualize facial reanimation options depending on patient's preference, patient factors, and surgeon expertise.
- Failure of systematic data collection including standardized photographs, video documentation, and clinician and patient reported outcome scales would make it difficult to assess outcomes.

30.1 INTRODUCTION

Acute facial paralysis is a common diagnostic problem encountered by the otolaryngologist but relatively uncommon in the general population with an incidence of 15–30/100,000 reported in the literature (Morris, et al., 2002). Starting in the facial nucleus, the facial nerve is a complex motor and sensory nerve with a convoluted course through the temporal bone before it exits the stylomastoid foramen to innervate the muscles of the face. From pontine artery infarcts affecting the facial nucleus to lacunar infarct affecting fibers in the internal capsule to cerebellopontine angle tumors compressing the nerve to traumatic insults to the nerve along its course; there is an extensive list of causes of facial nerve paralysis with the most common being BP.

Historically, BP has been considered idiopathic and a diagnosis of exclusion, although some have demonstrated

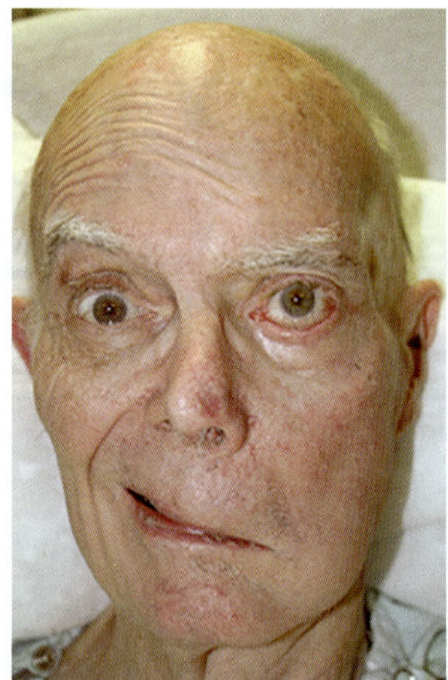

Fig. 30.1: Patient with left-sided facial nerve paralysis.

a link to herpes simplex virus (Adour, et al., 1978; Murakami, et al., 1996). The condition results in partial or complete inability to voluntarily move facial muscles on the affected side of the face. The functional, psychological, and social dysfunctions related to facial paralysis are devastating to those afflicted (Fig. 30.1).

Paralysis of the forehead results in brow ptosis, which can be of benefit in weighing down the paralyzed upper lid or cause problems with hooding and visual obstruction and entropion of the upper lashes further irritating the eye. The loss of the normal eye blink and incomplete closure leads to dry eye and exposure keratitis and potentially devastating ophthalmologic complications if the cornea is not protected. Paralysis of the orbicularis oculi also leads to ectropion of the lower eyelid, which is critical part of the eye blink and tear film distribution. Midface descent further impacts the lower lid ectropion leading to eversion of the lower lid punctum resulting in epiphora due to secondary loss of contact between the punctum and medial canthal tear lake with the globe. Nasal obstruction results from valve collapse with loss of dilator nasal muscle tone and weight of midface descent. Paralysis of the orbicularis oris and buccinator causes oral incompetence affecting mastication and speech. Patients have difficulty keeping a lip seal that results in spillage and enunciating bilabial consonants. Losing the ability to smile has profound impact on one's nonverbal communication and self-image. The overall effect of facial paralysis on static and dynamic facial appearance and function has major psychosocial impact. It is imperative that the physician recognizes and addresses psychosocial manifestations and offers professional referral for counseling.

30.2 EPIDEMIOLOGY AND CLASSIFICATION OF FACIAL PARALYSIS

Rowlands, et al. (2002) report the largest population-based study of BP and cite their epidemiologic findings, which confer with most findings published previously. Specifically, they include incidence rates of 20–25 cases per 100,000 population annually, increasing incidence with advancing age, and no seasonal variance. They also reported no difference in incidence rates based on gender, but other studies have reported increased prevalence in pregnant women (43 cases per 100,000) and people with diabetes mellitus (Adour, Bell and Wingerd, 1974). Facial nerve palsy is uncommon in children under age 2 years and similar to adults in regard to causes and recovery rates (Cha, et al., 2010). Paralysis occurs with equal frequency on the right and left side of the face, and bilateral facial palsy is extremely rare with a prevalence of 0.3–2% of the facial palsies. In the United States, the annual incidence of newly diagnosed cases is 40,000–50,000 (Morris, et al., 2002).

A list of causes of facial paralysis is outlined in Table 30.1.

Bell's Palsy/Idiopathic Facial Paralysis

Bell's palsy is the most common cause of facial paralysis (Holland and Weiner, 2004). There are some distinguishing characteristics in the history. These include an abrupt onset with complete and unilateral facial paralysis within 24–72 hours, as well as ipsilateral periauricular numbness or pain, decreased taste sensation, decreased production of tears, and/or hyperacusis. The usual course results in symptoms resolving spontaneously without treatment in 6 months' time.

Ramsay-Hunt Syndrome

Facial paralysis with otic involvement related to reactivation of a latent varicella zoster viral infection in the geniculate ganglion (Ramsay-Hunt syndrome) is uncommon with an incidence of 5/100,000 per year but the second most frequent etiology in nontraumatic peripheral facial paralysis (Adour, 1994). Ramsay-Hunt syndrome is a clinical diagnosis made on history and examination

Table 30.1: Causes of facial nerve palsy.

Causes	*Examples*
Idiopathic	Bell's, Melkersson-Rosenthal syndrome
Trauma	Temporal bone fracture, facial trauma, birth trauma, iatrogenic injury
Infection	Otitis media, mastoiditis, herpes zoster oticus (Ramsay-Hunt syndrome), encephalitis, mumps, syphilis, Lyme disease, acquired immunodeficiency syndrome, tuberculosis, cat scratch, Hansen's disease (leprosy), varicella zoster, influenza, parotitis, malignant external otitis
Metabolic	Diabetes mellitus, hypertension, pregnancy
Neoplastic	Parotid neoplasms, facial nerve tumor, carcinoma (invading or metastatic), schwannoma, glomus jugulare tumor, neurofibromatosis type 2, meningioma, leukemia, histiocytosis
Iatrogenic	Local anesthesia, cerebellopontine angle tumor surgery, parotid surgery, mastoid surgery, dental surgery, embolization, facelift surgery, forceps delivery
Congenital	Agenesis or hypoplastic facial nerve, Goldenhar's syndrome, Moebius syndrome
Neurologic	Stroke, multiple sclerosis, Guillain-Barre syndrome, opercular syndrome
Inflammatory	Temporal arteritis, periarteritis nodosa, amyloidosis, sarcoidosis, systemic lupus erythematosis

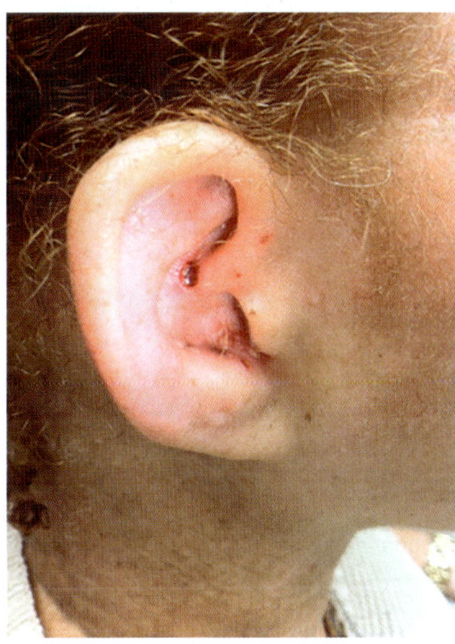

Fig. 30.2: Patient with vesicular, erythematous rash of the pinna secondary to Ramsay-Hunt syndrome.

finding of facial palsy with associated painful, vesicular, erythematous rash of the pinna or mouth (Fig. 30.2). There may also be associated hearing loss and vertigo. Early recognition is imperative, as a number of studies have shown improved recovery rate and extent of recovery with timely treatment with combination of acyclovir and high-dose corticosteroids (Murakami, et al., 1997).

Complication of Otitis Media

Facial nerve paralysis is an uncommon but significant complication of chronic otitis media (COM). Although the incidence of facial nerve paralysis has decreased with the use of antibiotics, prevention thereof remains a challenging problem. It has been reported that the frequency of facial nerve paralysis in COM ranges from 0.16% to 5.1% (Yetsier, Tosun and Kazkayasi, 2002).

The pathogenesis of otitic facial paralysis remains unclear. Osteitis, bone erosion, external compression, edema, and inflammation of the nerve are possible causes. Treatment recommendations have focused on both antibiotic treatment and surgery, including myringotomy, mastoidectomy, and nerve decompression, to re-establish the physiological state of the facial nerve.

Trauma

A common cause of facial paralysis is trauma, which includes blunt, penetrating, and iatrogenic forms. Most commonly, traumatic injuries to the facial nerve are caused by temporal bone fractures. Less than 5% of all temporal bone fractures involve the otic capsule; of these, half are associated with facial nerve injury (Nash, et al., 2010). Blunt trauma usually leads to nerve edema and contusion and only rarely causes nerve transection.

Facial nerve injury during middle ear or mastoid surgery occurs with <1% frequency, and most commonly occurs in the tympanic segment near the oval window because it is the most common site for fallopian canal dehiscence (Vrabec and Coker, 2006).

Neoplasms

Neoplastic causes of facial paralysis may include a history of multiple cranial nerve involvement, progressive onset of symptoms, and associated hearing loss. The most common tumor affecting facial nerve function is the acoustic neuroma, or vestibular schwannoma. The most common tumor of the facial nerve itself is the facial schwannoma (Snyderman, et al., 1988). Meningiomas and hemangiomas are benign neoplasms that can cause paralysis.

Malignant parotid neoplasms are another fairly common cause of facial paralysis. Onset of paralysis is typically insidious and progressive unlike most other causes. This may occur from direct nerve invasion or compression.

30.3 ANATOMY AND PATHOPHYSIOLOGY OF FACIAL NERVE PARALYSIS

Mavrikakis (2008) reviewed anatomy of the facial nerve, which is a complex motor and sensory nerve consisting of special visceral afferent, general visceral efferent, and special visceral efferent fibers. The nerve originates with the motor nucleus of the facial nerve that is located in the ventrolateral pons (Fig. 30.3). The facial nerve then passes through the internal auditory meatus with the auditory nerve. Then, it courses through a narrow bony canal through the petrous portion of the temporal bone and out the stylomastoid foramen. On emerging from the stylomastoid foramen it runs forward in the substance of the parotid gland, crosses the external carotid artery, and divides behind the ramus of the lower jaw into upper and lower divisions. The temporofacial trunk further divides into temporal, zygomatic, and buccal branches to innervate the upper two-thirds of the face, and the lower cervicofacial trunk divides into marginal mandibular and cervical branches to the lower face and neck.

The facial nerves innervate facial muscles, which control a number of functions, such as eye blink and tear distribution, lacrimation, salivation, eating, drinking, speech, smiling, and expressing emotions. They also innervate the stapedial muscle to the stapes and carry taste sensations from the anterior two-thirds of the tongue.

Bell's palsy is the most common etiology of facial paralysis and attributed to acute inflammation and edema of the facial nerve in the bony canal, which leads to

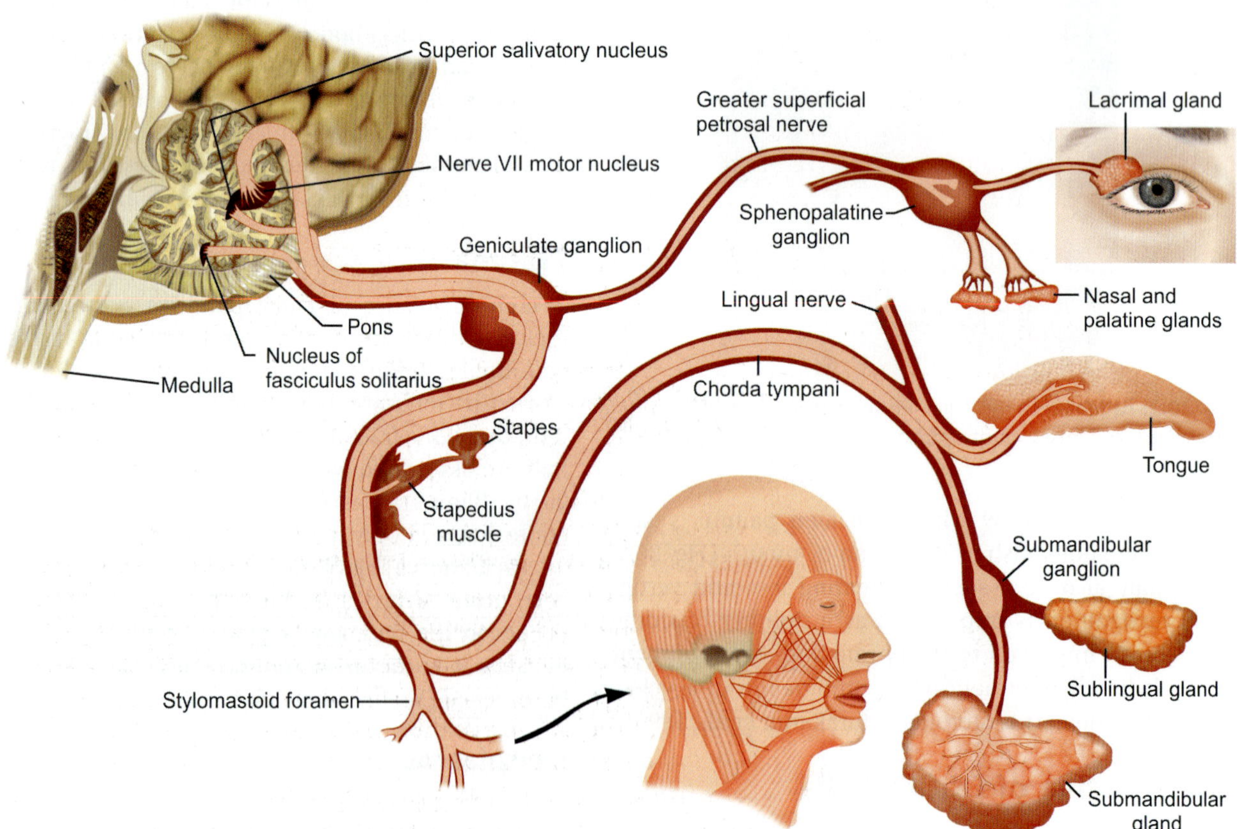

Fig. 30.3: Anatomy of facial nerve.

compression ischemia. An observation that supports the hypothesis of an inflammatory etiology is that the facial nerve shows enhancement on magnetic resonance imaging (MRI) in patients with acute BP (Gupta, et al., 2013).

There is an extensive list of other causes with differing pathophysiology. If not inflammation, the most common causes of paresis are direct neural injury whether due to stretch, transection, or tumor invasion.

There are two classification schema used to describe nerve injuries. The first was published by Seddon in 1942 and separated injuries into three categories—neuropraxia, axonotmesis, and neurotmesis—largely based on the scale of injury from microscopic to macroscopic. Neuropraxia is a compression injury where the nerve is viable and recovers when the axoplasmic blockade is removed. Axonotmesis involves Wallerian degeneration distal to the lesion with preservation of endoneural sheaths of the motor axons. In neurotmesis there is loss of the endoneural tubules. In 1978, Sunderland expanded upon this idea, subdividing neurotmesis into three additional grades. The Seddon classification is useful to understand the anatomic basis for injury, whereas the Sunderland classification adds information useful for prognosis and treatment strategies.

- *Grade 1*: Neuropraxia
  - Conduction disruption with intact axon and preserved supportive structures and no distal Wallerian degeneration.
  - *Prognosis*: Normally full recovery in days to weeks without surgical intervention.
- *Grade 2*: Axonotmesis
  - Disrupted axon with intact endoneurium; Wallerian degeneration takes place after 1–2 weeks.
  - *Prognosis*: Variable recovery, worse prognosis for proximal injuries, and injuries that do not successfully reimplant in the muscle within 18 months.
- *Grade 3*: Neurotmesis with preservation of perineurium
  - Endoneurium is disrupted.
  - *Prognosis*: 60–80% recovery.
- *Grade 4*: Neurotmesis with preservation of epineurium
  - *Prognosis*: Nerve grafting is required.
- *Grade 5*: Neurotmesis with complete transection of nerve trunk
  - *Prognosis*: Bypass/jump grafting is required.

30.4 ASSESSMENT OF THE FACIAL PARALYSIS PATIENT

As with any new patient encounter, a detailed history and physical examination is obtained. Subsequently, focused questions and examination are performed to identify the cause and topographic location of the injury to guide further management (Fig. 30.4). It is important to ascertain the rate and duration of onset of facial paralysis, whether it is partial or complete, involving one or all nerve branches, associated symptoms of pain, numbness, taste disturbance, or hyperacusis. Intense ear pain and a vesicular eruption are hallmarks of herpes zoster infection.

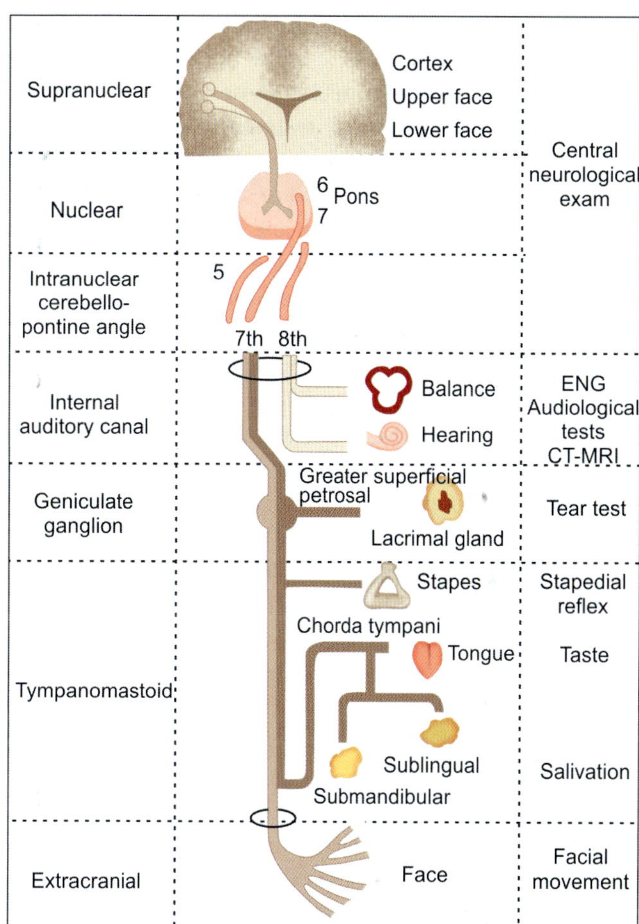

Fig. 30.4: Topographic location of the injury and appropriate clinical test/investigation for diagnosis.

History of autoimmune disease or any unexplained symptoms of rashes, orofacial edema, and arthritis is important to elicit. Autoimmune disease should be considered for any history of recurring, bilateral, or alternating facial paralysis.

Slowly progressive facial paralysis most likely represents neoplasia. Tumors may be malignant or benign and include primary or metastatic squamous cell carcinoma of parotid gland and/or facial nerve, sarcomas, schwannomas, and hemangiomas.

The physical examination includes a complete head and neck evaluation with careful attention to the ear examination and cranial nerves. Assessment for trauma, local infection, tumor, or central nervous system disease is imperative.

A focused physical examination should note how many branches, and which branches, are involved. Involvement of only one or two branches suggests trauma or a parotid gland tumor. A thorough ear examination is indicated. Middle ear infection, cholesteatoma, and malignant external otitis all have been associated with facial paralysis. Examine the parotid gland and neck for fullness or masses. It is important to perform full cranial nerve examination especially when considering nerve substitution procedures. Assess hypoglossal nerve function as well as trigeminal nerve by having patients clench their teeth and palpate the temporalis and masseter muscles.

The most commonly used facial nerve grading scale is the House-Brackmann (HB) scale (House and Brackmann, 1985). The HB scale is used to approximate the quantity of volitional motion the patient has based on their clinical facial presentation. Although the HB scale is based on clinical observation, and variation among observers exists, the HB scale allows us to grossly describe the characteristics and degree of facial nerve motion using a subjective analysis scale, which is easily and reliably applied. The HB scale has six grades. Each grade is reported as a fraction (i.e. 1/6 = grade I). A grade I presentation is perfectly normal. Grade II is a slight or mild weakness. Grade III is a moderate weakness with good (normal) eye closure. Grade IV is a moderate weakness with no volitional eye closure. Grade V is a severe weakness. Grade VI is a total facial paralysis (Table 30.2). It is fair to say that grade III is best obtainable level once the facial nerve has been severed and repaired.

Most patients with acute onset of facial paralysis characteristic of Bell's do not require any laboratory testing or imaging studies. However, patients who have persistent weakness without significant improvement, involvement of other cranial nerves, or a second episode of palsy require further investigations.

Laboratory testing is necessary if the patient has signs of systemic involvement, such as fever, weight loss, rash, or progressive facial weakness without significant improvement over > 4 weeks. A number of tests may be helpful:

- Complete blood count with differential helps rule out lymphoreticular malignancy, the first manifestation of which may be peripheral facial palsy.

Table 30.2: House-Brackmann facial paralysis scale.

Grade	*Impairment*
I	Normal
II	Mild dysfunction (slight weakness, normal symmetry at rest)
III	Moderate dysfunction (obvious but not disfiguring weakness with synkinesis, normal symmetry at rest). Complete eye closure with maximal effort, good forehead movement
IV	Moderately severe dysfunction (obvious and disfiguring asymmetry, significant synkinesis). Incomplete eye closure, moderate forehead movement
V	Severe dysfunction (barely perceptible motion)
VI	Total paralysis (no movement)

Note: House-Brackmann facial paralysis scale is used to evaluate facial paralysis at the nerve trunk, and it is not a descriptive scale to describe injury to specific distal facial nerve branches.

- Serum antibodies against herpes zoster and *Borrelia burgdorferi* (the agent of Lyme disease) can be checked if the patient has signs such as vesicular lesions on the external ear or lives in an area where Lyme disease is endemic.
- Serum calcium and angiotensin-converting enzyme levels should be tested if sarcoidosis is suspected; these levels are high in sarcoidosis.

Computed tomography (CT) or MRI is indicated in the following cases:

- No improvement in facial paresis after 1 month
- Hearing loss
- Multiple cranial nerve deficits
- Signs of limb paresis or sensory loss.

Magnetic resonance imaging with gadolinium is the test of choice to rule out cerebellopontine angle tumor, stroke, multiple sclerosis, or other structural lesions (Gupta, et al., 2013). High-resolution temporal bone CT is recommended if a temporal bone fracture is suspected. If hearing loss is suspected, then audiologic testing can be performed to measure hearing loss and work-up for acoustic neuroma.

30.5 ELECTRODIAGNOSTIC STUDIES

Electrophysiologic tests are complementary, and when used appropriately in cases of complete paralysis, they can describe the extent of degeneration with serial testing. One of the primary objectives of measuring facial nerve function is to differentiate those patients who will spontaneously recover to an acceptable degree from those who could benefit from surgical intervention. Electroneuronography (ENoG) and electromyography (EMG) are most useful in determining the prognosis of a facial nerve injury and guiding treatment (Mannarelli, et al., 2012). They both are electrophysiologic measures that indirectly quantify facial nerve function.

The ENoG is the electrical stimulation of the facial nerve at or near the stylomastoid foramen with measurements taken from the nasolabial fold. The ENoG is the only "relatively objective" measure of facial nerve integrity. It compares the normal side to quantify and prognosticate. Since Wallerian degeneration takes 3 days, the first ENoG test session is delayed until 72 hours postonset of paralysis. However, at the other end of the timing window is maximum of 21 days. In essence, the ENoG should be performed for the first time at about 72 hours postonset and again at 3–5-day intervals until a trend and confirmation can be obtained. If the trend and confirmation are determined prior to 21 days postonset, surgical intervention may be an option. If the ENoG is not obtained prior to 21 days postonset, it is of little clinical use. Specifically, an ENoG obtained 4 weeks after onset of facial paralysis is difficult, if not impossible, to interpret.

Electromyography is the recording of motor unit action potentials. The EMG is useful in the very early phase of degeneration (<1 week), as the presence of motor units indicates an intact nerve with incomplete injury. Thereafter, it is limited in being able to differentiate neuropraxia from complete degeneration during the acute phase. In long-standing paralysis, needle EMG may be employed to confirm any subclinical signs of reinnervation, thus acting as a prognostic indicator for the possibility of recovery. The presence of myogenic fibrillation potentials and the absence of voluntary motor units indicate complete nerve degeneration; the presence of both fibrillation potentials and motor units indicates an incomplete lesion; the appearance of polyphasic motor units signifies a regenerating nerve (Valls-Sole, 2007).

30.6 MANAGEMENT

The management of this complex group of patients requires determination of the etiology and duration of the paralysis, as well as an estimation of the prognosis for spontaneous recovery. Reversible and irreversible injuries require very different management as do acute versus chronic paralysis. An understanding of the timing of injury is important because there is a critical window of 12–18 months during which reinnervation of motor endplates is ideal. In general, the management of patients after 2 years of facial paralysis is based on static suspension procedures, regional myofascial procedures, and free tissue transfer, often in combination or tandem. Ophthalmologic consultation is important for any facial paralysis patient with eye symptoms.

The most common clinical scenarios that present are facial paralysis due to BP, iatrogenic injury, and related to neoplasm.

Bell's Palsy

Treatment of BP is still controversial. Therapy is difficult to evaluate, because as many as two-thirds of patients with BP spontaneously recover and achieve near-normal function within several months (Peitersen, 2002). In his study following the natural course of 2,500 BP patients, follow-up showed that in 85% of patients function returned within 3 weeks and in the remaining 15% after 3–5 months. In 71% of patients, normal mimetic function was obtained. Many patients begin to improve as early as 10 days after the onset, even without treatment. Older patients are less likely to recover completely. His survey of the literature showed that no kind of therapy, including steroids, improved prognosis.

However, the treatment regimens for BP therapy are still deliberated, with several randomized controlled trials showing mixed results. A recent Cochrane review of eight randomized controlled trials with over 1,500 patients (Salinas, et al., 2010) validated the benefit of treating BP patients with corticosteroids for recovery of facial nerve function as well as a significant reduction in motor synkinesis.

Antiviral agents against herpes simplex virus have also been extensively used to treat BP, and their effectiveness has been increasingly disputed based on recent studies. A 2009 Cochrane systematic review of seven high-quality trials with 1987 participants concluded that antiherpetic antivirals provide no significant benefit compared with placebo in generating complete recovery from BP, whereas a study in Korea found a statistically significant improvement in patients with severe facial palsy when given famciclovir plus steroids within 1 week of presentation versus steroids alone (Lee, et al., 2013).

Gantz, et al. (1999) outline the role of surgical decompression in BP. Those patients with complete clinical facial paralysis, >90% degeneration on ENoG, and no evidence of voluntary action muscle potentials on EMG testing were candidates for surgical decompression. Those patients undergoing decompression within the first 2 weeks of the onset of paralysis showed a 91% chance of a good outcome versus a 42% chance of obtaining a HB scale grade I or II if treated with steroids.

The literature shows no consensus for the benefit of, or indication for, surgery in the treatment of BP (Bodenez, et al., 2010). Risks associated with surgical decompression include seizures, unilateral hearing loss, cerebrospinal fluid leak, and facial nerve injury. Surgical decompression of the facial nerve therefore remains highly controversial and should only be considered in refractory cases, given the low-quality and inconclusive nature of the reports on its use.

Most recently, the American Academy of Otolaryngology–Head and Neck Surgery Foundation set forth clinical practice guidelines to improve the accuracy of diagnosis for BP, to improve the quality of care and outcomes for patients with BP, and to decrease harmful variations in the evaluation and management of BP Baugh, et al., (2013). Their recommendations included prescribing oral steroids within 72 hours of symptom onset for adult BP patients and offering oral antiviral therapy in addition but not alone also within 72 hours of onset of symptoms. They made no recommendation regarding the surgical decompression for patients with BP.

Trauma

Injury to the facial nerve can occur along many locations and in various scenarios such as blunt injury, laceration, temporal bone fracture, and iatrogenic insult. Oftentimes, the status of facial nerve continuity is not known. Immediate evaluation of the motor function of the facial nerve following the injury provides key information. If paresis (weakness) is present, then the injury is incomplete and spontaneous return of facial function should be anticipated.

Temporal bone fractures are the most common traumatic etiology of facial paralysis. They are classified as longitudinal versus transverse based on its relationship to the long axis of the petrous pyramid. High-resolution CT of the temporal bone is obtained to evaluate the course of the facial nerve throughout the temporal bone in attempt to localize site of injury and help determine operative approach based on findings. If a patient has complete paralysis upon presentation, serial ENoGs may be obtained and surgical decompression considered if there is >90% degeneration of axons. Management of traumatic nerve injuries is to restore continuity of fresh nerve endings under no tension. If there is any gap, an interposition cable graft is used to bridge the nerve endings. Nerve endings may be coapted microsurgically with 9-0 Neurolon or fibrin glue.

Neoplasms

Benign and malignant tumors can involve the facial nerve anywhere along its course from the cerebellopontine angle, intratemporally, or extracranially with the most common nerve tumor being the facial schwannoma. The dilemma in benign cases is the timing of management. As the tumor grows, more motor axons will degenerate and compromise the opportunity for neural reinnervation. It is important to educate the patient that facial function will never be restored to one's preoperative state, and the best outcome would be HB grade III. An educated decision needs to be made with the patient as to when to sacrifice one's current state of facial function at the expense of salvaging and restoring some facial function before the tumor takes it out completely. Furthermore, the larger the tumor grows it brings along greater challenges in operative resection and risks.

Skull base tumors bring about situations where facial nerve status is not certain after surgery where there is extensive manipulation in and around the facial nerve at the cerebellopontine angle. With facial nerve monitoring, the proximal facial nerve stimulation threshold at the end of surgical removal is predictive of long-term facial nerve function (Lalwani, et al., 1994). At 1 year, 98% (87 of 89) of the patients with electrical thresholds of 0.2 V or less had grade I or II facial nerve function compared with only 50% (8 of 16) of those with thresholds between 0.21 and 0.6 V (Lalwani, et al., 1994). If it is known that the facial nerve is transected, attempts can be made to place an interposition graft or be prepared to perform a nerve substitution. End-to-end coaptation of the hypoglossal and facial nerve results in significant donor site morbidity and problems with mass movement and synkinesis. Lingual morbidity and excellent functional outcomes have been reported by effects of the jump interposition graft for the hypoglossal–facial anastomosis (Hammerschlag, 1999) and split hypoglossal–facial neurorrhaphy (Shipchandler, Seth and Alam, 2011).

Malignant Tumors

In settings of malignancy, the facial nerve is either compromised by invasion or resection for oncologic reasons.

The nerve is grafted whenever possible. When multiple branches are involved, the medial antebrachial cutaneous nerve of the arm is suitable given its branching pattern and caliber match. Priority should be given to restore reinnervation to the zygomatic and buccal branches to the lower lid, midface, and smile as the upper lid can be reanimated well with lid weights and the marginal mandibular and cervical branches are not as critical to function.

Many patients will receive adjuvant therapy. The effect of high-dose radiation therapy on facial nerve grafts is controversial. Some authors believe radiotherapy is so detrimental to the outcome of facial nerve graft function that dynamic or static slings should be performed instead of facial nerve grafts in all patients who are to receive postoperative radiation therapy. Unfortunately, the facial function achieved with dynamic and static slings is almost always inferior to that after facial nerve grafts. Brown, et al. (2000) compared facial nerve function in irradiated and unirradiated nerve grafts. They found that radiotherapy was not a negative prognostic factor and revealed no difference in facial nerve function achieved between irradiated and unirradiated nerve grafts.

Eye Protection

One of the greatest concerns with facial palsy is the involvement of the eye due to exposure. Eye care focuses on the protection of the cornea from drying, or abrasions due to insufficient lid closure or tearing. Extra precaution is imperative in those who also have anesthesia of the cornea. Frequent rewetting drops and ointment are necessary. Taping and moisture chambers are also effective.

Physical Therapy

The facial rehabilitation team plays an integral role in maximizing the quality of facial reanimation. Neuromuscular re-education, a process of facilitating the return of intended facial movement patterns and eliminating unwanted patterns of facial movement and expression, provide patients with disorders of facial paralysis or facial movement control opportunity for the recovery of facial movement and function (Vanswearingen, 2008). Facial rehabilitation comes in the form of neuromuscular re-education, surface electromyographic biofeedback, mime therapy, and video self-modeling.

One of the primary goals of facial rehabilitation is synkinesis management. Synkinesis results in varying degrees after any nerve injury or reanimation procedure. Specific neuromuscular reeducation exercises teach the patient how to symmetrically move the facial muscles while simultaneously controlling associated synkinesis (Robinson, et al., 2012).

Botulinum Toxin

Many patients with facial paralysis recover with synkinesis. Many caregivers do not realize that synkinesis can be an equally debilitating condition as facial paralysis and that the patient could be helped. The aberrant regeneration of the facial nerve introduces a new set of problems with mass movement, tight and painful muscle spasms, and continued lack of smile. Contralateral hyperkinesis refers to the exaggerated contraction of the intact side of the face, which is thought to be both a behavioral and reflex adaptation to compensate for the paralyzed side. This overcompensation is a key component of the overall facial disharmony that results from facial paralysis. There are familiar patterns of facial nerve recovery in synkinesis: palpebral narrowing, poor zygomatic excursion, prominent nasolabial fold, or midfacial tightness (Figs. 30.5A and B).

Botox therapy has dramatically improved the management of patients with facial-movement disorders. It is now a first-line agent for the treatment of facial synkinesis. The effect of botulinum toxin injection on both sides of the face for synkinesis and contralateral hypertrophy at the same time showed significant suppression of the facial synkinesis and improvement of facial symmetry with resulting elevated quality of life, social interaction, personal appearance, and food intake (Figs. 30.5A and B).

Botox therapy is an effective adjunctive treatment in the reanimation of any facial paralysis patient. Many patients fail to recover forehead and depressor function after nerve reanimation procedures. Treatment of the contralateral intact side is a relatively noninvasive option to restore overall symmetry and improve function.

30.7 SURGICAL REANIMATION PROCEDURES

Facial reanimation is a process involving numerous procedures that are tailored to the individual based on patient factors, such as etiology of facial paralysis, patient desires and expectations as well as the skills and abilities of the treating surgeon. It is important to properly risk-stratify patients to get optimal results for each individual;

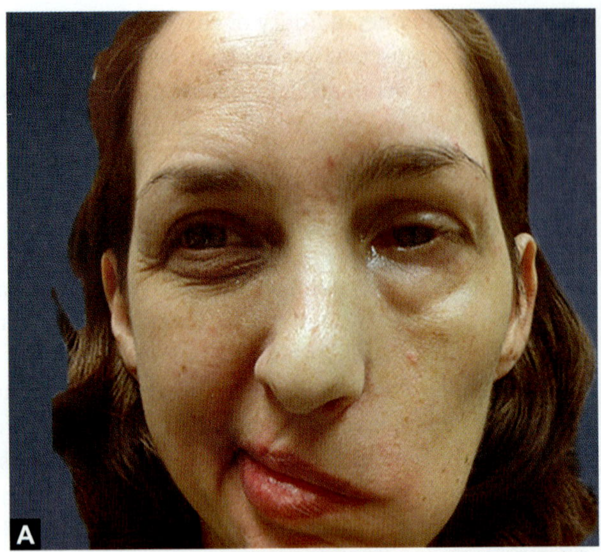

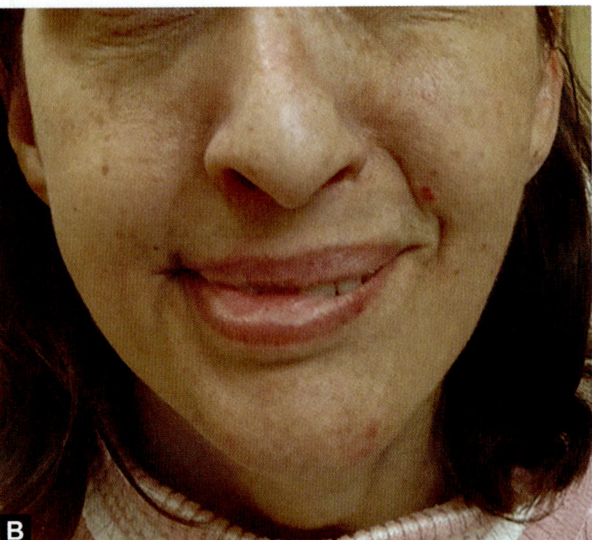

Figs. 30.5A and B: (A) Patient with familiar patterns of facial nerve recovery in synkinesis: palpebral narrowing, poor zygomatic excursion, prominent nasolabial fold, or midfacial tightness. (B) Same patient after botulinum toxin therapy.

appropriate strata may at least include age, overall health, residual hearing, which segment of the nerve is injured, and the patient's desires. There are functional as well as esthetic goals, which are equally important in facial reanimation.

The major goals of facial reanimation are to restore eyelid function to protect the globe and restore resting and dynamic symmetry of the lower face for smile and perioral competence. It is helpful to divide the face zonally in considering facial reanimation procedures.

Eye Reanimation

Early intervention to reanimate the eye is reasonable given the potential long-term corneal complications and reversibility of the procedures. Eyelid weight placement with platinum is typically the first step to address paralytic lagophthalmos. It is also reasonable to consider Botox injection for temporary levator chemodenervation as well as blepharotomy to create an intentional blepharoptosis.

Lower eyelid retraction is also important to address especially in older patients who often start with diminished lower lid tone at baseline. Lower lid treatments may range from simple canthopexy to lateral tarsal strip procedures to adding structural lower lid support with cartilage grafting in addition to midface lifting. Taping of the lower lid upward is a simple way to provide temporary support if timely recovery is anticipated.

Neural Procedures

The primary surgical methods for restoring the function of the facial nerve include neurotization, direct nerve repair, nerve grafting, cross-facial nerve grafting, nerve crossover, regional muscle transfer, and microneurovascular free muscle transfer. The most successful outcomes of reanimation result from procedures that restore neural input to a functionally intact muscle. Thus, duration of paralysis and timing of intervention are critical factors in reanimation surgery.

Primary Repair

The best prognosis for facial nerve regeneration comes from early repair of the transected nerve by primary epineural coaptation. The nerve endings are freshened under an operating microscope, and 10-0 Neurolon sutures are used to approximate the epineurium without tension. If there is loss of nerve and tension-free coaptation is not possible, interposition nerve grafts are incorporated. Donor nerves include greater auricular, sural, and other sensory as well as motor nerves.

Nerve Substitution

Where no proximal stump of the facial nerve exists for coaptation, then nerve substitutions with an alternative cranial nerve should be considered. The traditional hypoglossal to facial nerve end-to-end substitution procedure resulted in significant morbidity related to speech

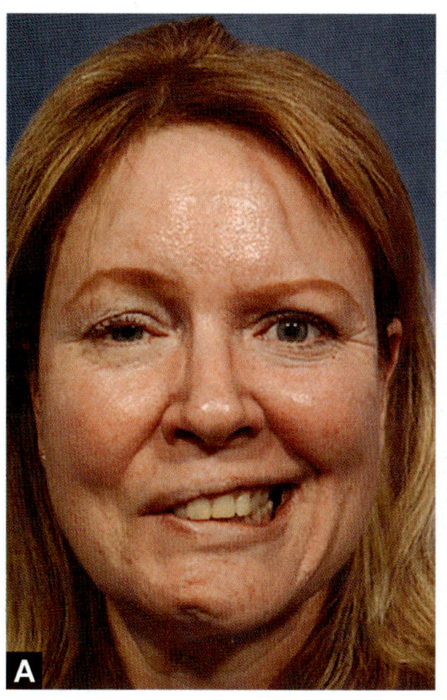

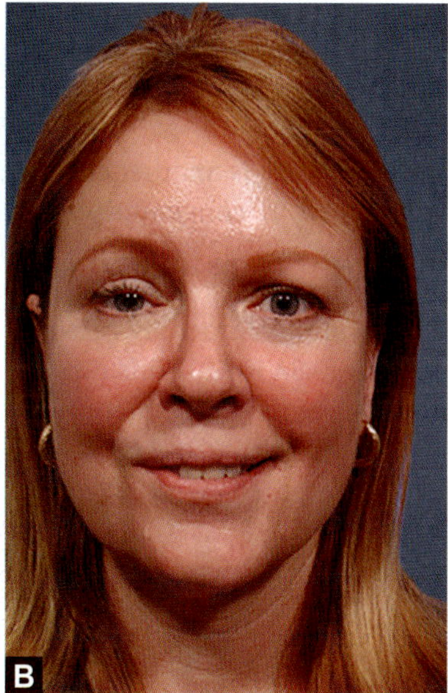

Figs. 30.6A and B: (A) Preoperative photograph of a patient with left-sided facial nerve paralysis with asymmetrical smile excursion. (B) Postoperative photograph of the patient showing smile excursion achieved at 1 year after masseteric to facial nerve substitution.

and swallow and mass facial movement. Advances in technique including partial hypoglossal transection and the use of jump grafts have minimized secondary deficits (Hammerschlag, 1999). In some cases, direct inset of the main trunk of the facial nerve without a jump graft is possible after drill out and mobilization of the facial nerve from the mastoid bone.

Recent literature has popularized use of the masseteric nerve (Klebuc, 2011). Klebuc reports improved excursion owing it to the masseteric nerve as a pure motor nerve with high myelinated fiber count. Furthermore, its proximity allows for direct coaptation and shorter reinnervation time. Sacrifice of the nerve to the masseter is well tolerated without functional deficit. Figures 30.6A and B show a patient with smile excursion achieved at 1 year after masseteric to facial nerve substitution.

The contralateral facial nerve is also a source of input using one of the zygomatic or buccal branches and is the only option, which offers mimetic reinnervation. However, the long distance to travel and the slow rate of nerve regeneration at 1 mm per day introduces the factor of time in duration of paralysis.

The clinical challenge arises in patients where the continuity of the nerve or the potential for recovery is unknown. The important early decision is whether or not to apply reinnervation techniques prior to 12–18 months of paralysis, since muscle that is denervated for >12–18 months will show decreased acetylcholinesterase receptor activity and muscle fiber volume as well as development of intramuscular fibrosis. These sequelae minimize the possibility of functionally reinnervating these muscles. Here the concept of babysitting was introduced by Terzis and Tzafetta (2009), wherein an ipsilateral hypoglossal jump graft provides innervation to preserve the facial neuromuscular junctions while awaiting cross-facial nerve graft to reach across the face. A second stage 9–12 months later helped to coapt the distal cross-facial nerve grafts with selected branches of the affected facial nerve.

Muscle Transfer

There are instances where the native facial musculature is not present, as in cases of extensive tumor resection or nonviable muscle, as in cases with long-standing paralysis. In these circumstances, regional muscle transfers or free tissue transfers are considered.

The masticators are powerful muscles located close to the mouth and innervated by the mandibular division of the trigeminal nerve. Both the masseter and temporalis muscles have been used for dynamic smile restoration. In recent years, the orthodromic temporalis tendon transfer has become the favored regional muscle procedure providing both resting symmetry and volitional commissure excursion with activation by clenching (Byrne, et al., 2007). It is a single-stage procedure with immediate benefits. This procedure transfers the temporalis tendon to the extra-anatomical site at the perioral muscles either with a lengthening myoplasty or intervening fascia grafts to obtain the ideal resting tension length that will achieve maximal excursion (Labbe, Bussu and Iodice, 2012; Boehane, 2013) (Fig. 30.7).

Microneurovascular muscle transfer is another option in long-standing facial paralysis or in congenital cases such as Moebius syndrome (Evans, et al., 2005). The gracilis muscle is the most commonly transferred muscle due to low donor site morbidity and contractility providing commissure excursion (Figs. 30.8A to C). This procedure can be single stage or two staged. If mimetic input is desired, then a two-staged procedure is performed using the cross-facial sural nerve graft followed by the gracilis transfer 9–12 months later. The masseteric nerve can be used to transfer the muscle as a single-stage procedure, but this option theoretically does not restore spontaneous smile. However, there are reports of cortical plasticity or adaptation where patients achieve spontaneous smile with trigeminal nerve input (Scott, et al., 2005).

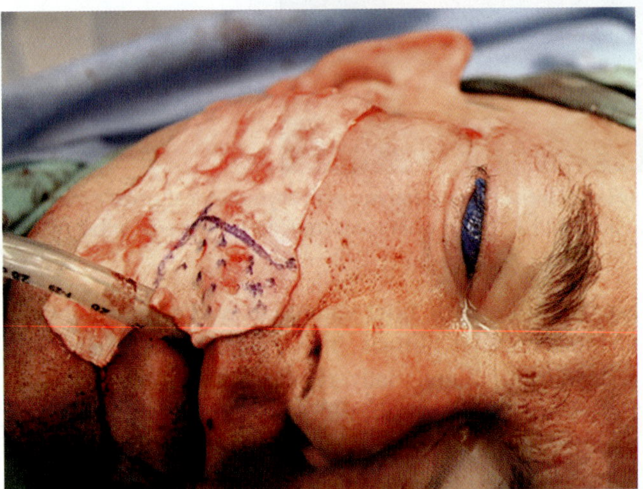

Fig. 30.7: Transfers of temporalis tendon to the perioral region may be achieved with intervening fascia grafts to achieve smile excursion symmetry.

Static Procedures

Static techniques are employed to suspend the soft-tissue structures of the face, but they do not provide facial reanimation. They are often adjunctive maneuvers performed in conjunction with dynamic techniques to enhance facial symmetry, particularly in treating brow ptosis, nasal valve collapse, lagophthalmos and lower lid laxity.

However, static procedures may also be performed alone for patients who are not candidates for dynamic reanimation procedures (because of physical debilitation, advanced age, poor prognosis, or patient's preference) but who would still benefit from the restoration of facial symmetry (Figs. 30.9A and B).

Adjunctive Procedures

As the ultimate goal of facial rehabilitation lies in maximally restoring functional and esthetic symmetry, adjunctive procedures may include asymmetric rhytidectomy, contralateral depressor muscle transection, and suture

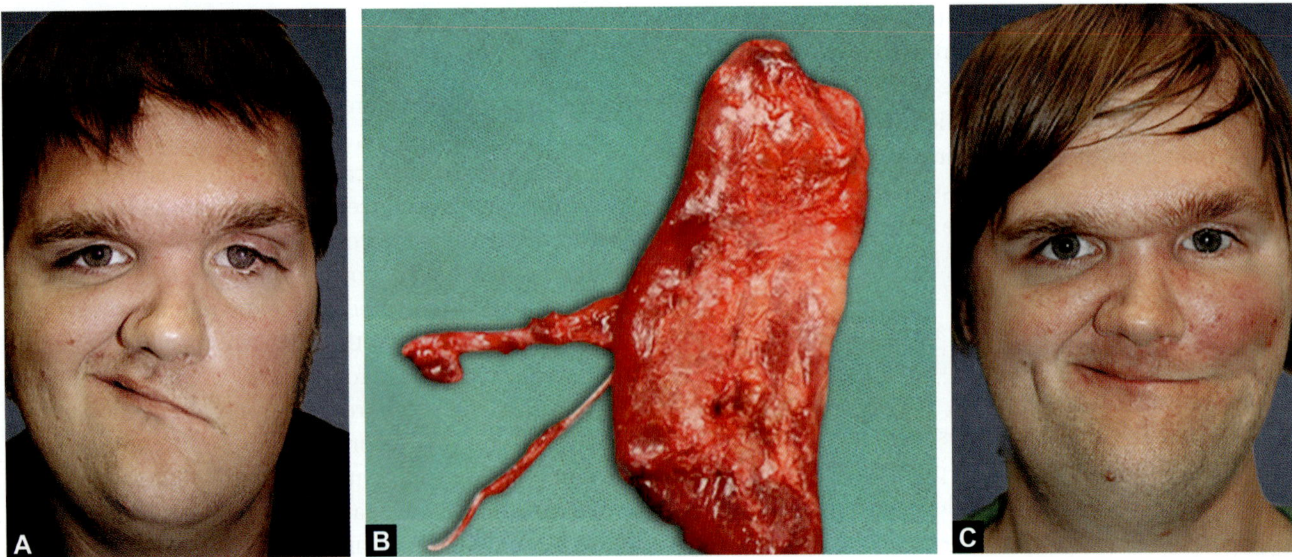

Figs. 30.8A to C: (A) Preoperative photograph of a patient with left facial palsy. (B) Gracilis free muscle flap. (C) Patient after gracilis muscle transfer with much improved smile symmetry and commissure excursion.

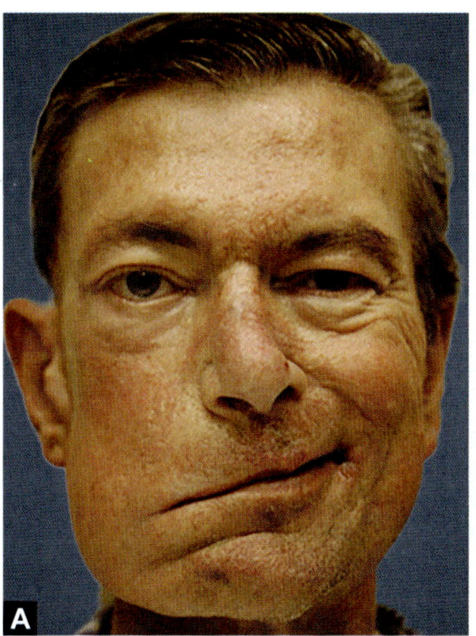

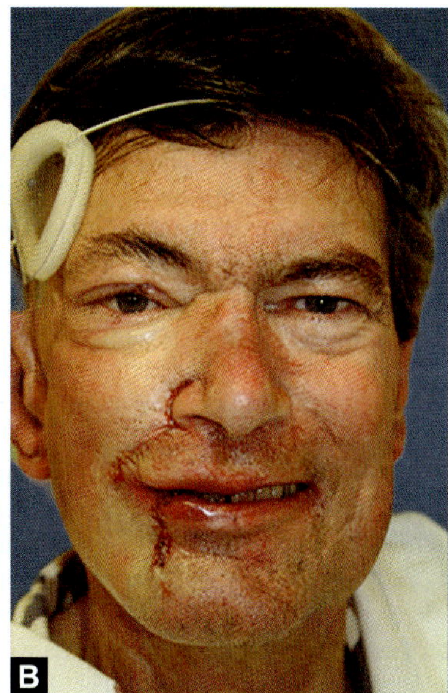

Figs. 30.9A and B: (A) Preoperative photograph of a patient with right-sided facial nerve palsy. (B) Postoperative photograph of the patient after static procedures to restore facial symmetry.

suspension of the nasal valve. Facial paralysis and/or synkinesis also results in three-dimensional contour asymmetries, which may be improved with autologous fat transfer or fillers to improve volume asymmetry.

SUMMARY

Facial paralysis has proved a difficult disease process to diagnose and manage. This difficulty is due in part to the wide range of causes that lead to the condition and the challenge in designing valid, prospective clinical trials for treatment. Clinicians must be aware of the numerous etiologies and realize that the cause can usually be identified with a thorough history and physical examination, thereby guiding management. Management options are also varied and depend on each individual patient factors, desires, and abilities of the treating surgeon to restore meaningful facial movement and improve quality of life.

REFERENCES

Adour, K.K., 1994. Otological complications of herpes zoster. *Annals of Neurology*, 35(Suppl), pp. S62-4.

Adour, K.K., Bell, D.N. and Wingerd, J., 1974. Bell's palsy Dilemma of diabetes mellitus. *Archives of Otolaryngology*, 99(2), pp. 114-7.

Adour, K.K., Byl, F.M., Hilsinger, R.L., JR, et al., 1978. The true nature of Bell's palsy: analysis of 1,000 consecutive patients. *Laryngoscope*, 88, pp. 787-801.

Baugh, R.F., Basura, G.J., Ishii, L.E., Schwartz, S.R., Drumheller, C.M., Burkholder, R., Deckard, N.A., Dawson, C., Driscoll, C., Gillespie, M.B., Gurgel, R.K., Halperin, J., Khalid, A.N., Kumar, K.A., Micco, A., Munsell, D., Rosenbaum, S. and Vaughan, W., 2013. Clinical practice guideline: Bell's palsy. *Otolaryngology–Head and Neck Surgery*, 149(3 Suppl), pp. S1-27.

Boahene, K.D., 2013. Principles and biomechanics of muscle tendon unit transfer: application in temporalis muscle tendon transposition for smile improvement in facial paralysis. *Laryngoscope*, 123, pp. 350-5.

Bodenez, C., Bernat, I., Willer, J.C., et al., 2010. Facial nerve decompression for idiopathic Bell's palsy: report of 13 cases and literature review. *Journal of Laryngology and Otology*, 124(3), pp. 272-8.

Brown, P.D., Eshleman, J.S., Foote, R.L. and Strome, S.E., 2000. An analysis of facial nerve function in irradiated and unirradiated facial nerve grafts. *International Journal of Radiation Oncology Biology Physics*, 48(3), pp. 737-43.

Byrne, P.J., Kim, M., Boahene, K., et al., 2007. Temporalis tendon transfer as part of a comprehensive approach to facial reanimation. *Archives of Facial Plastic Surgery*, 9, pp. 234-41.

Cha, H.E., Baek, M.K., et al., 2010. Clinical features and management of facial nerve paralysis in children: analysis of 24 cases. *The Journal of Laryngology and Otology*, 124(4), pp. 402-6.

Evans, A.K., Licameli, G., Brietzke, S., Whittemore, K. and Kenna M., 2005. Pediatric facial nerve paralysis: patients, management and outcomes. *International Journal of Pediatric Otorhinolaryngology*, 69(11), pp. 1521-8.

Gantz, B.J., Rubinstein, J.T., Gidley, P. and Woodworth, G.G., 1999. Surgical management of Bell's palsy. *Laryngoscope*, 109, pp. 1177-88.

Gupta, S., Mends, F., Hagiwara, M., Fatterpekar, G. and Roehm, P.C., 2013. Imaging the facial nerve: a contemporary review. *Radiology Research and Practice*.

Hammerschlag, P.E., 1999. Facial reanimation with jump interpositional graft hypoglossal facial anastomosis and hypoglossal facial anastomosis: evolution in management of facial paralysis. *Laryngoscope*, 109, pp. 1-23.

Holland, N. and Weiner, G.M., 2004. Recent developments in Bell's palsy. *British Medical Journal*, 329, p. 553.

House, J.W. and Brackmann, D.E., 1985. Facial nerve grading system. *Otolaryngology—Head and Neck Surgery*, 93, pp. 146-7.

Klebuc, M.J., 2011. Facial reanimation using the masseter-to-facial nerve transfer. *Plastic and Reconstructive Surgery*, 127(5), pp. 1909-15.

Labbe, D., Bussu, F. and Iodice, A., 2012. A comprehensive approach to long-standing facial paralysis based on lengthening temporalis myoplasty. *Acta Otorhinolaryngologica Italica*, 32, pp. 145-53.

Lalwani, A.K., Butt, F.Y., Jackler, R.K., Pitts, L.H. and Yingling, C.D., 1994. Facial nerve outcome after acoustic neuroma surgery: a study from the era of cranial nerve monitoring. *Otolaryngology—Head and Neck Surgery*, 111(5), pp. 561-70.

Lee, H.Y., Bryun, J.Y., Park, M.S. and Yeo, S.G., 2013. Steroid-antiviral treatment improves the recovery rate in patients with severe Bell's palsy. *American Journal of Medicine*, 126(4), pp. 336-41.

Mannarelli, G., Griffin, G., Kileny, P. and Edwards, B., 2012. Electrophysiological measures in facial paresis and paralysis. *Operative Techniques in Otolaryngology-Head and Neck Surgery*, 23(4), pp. 236-47.

Mavrikakis, I., 2008. Facial nerve palsy: anatomy, etiology, evaluation, and management. *Orbit*, 27(6), pp. 466-74.

Morris, A.M., Deeks, S.L., Hill, M.D., Midroni, G., Goldstein, W.C., Mazzulli, T, et al., 2002. Annualized incidence and spectrum of illness from an outbreak investigation of Bell's palsy. *Neuroepidemiology*, 21, pp. 255-61.

Murakami, S., Hato, N., Horiuchi, J., et al., 1997. Treatment of Ramsay Hunt syndrome with acyclovir-prednisone: significance of early diagnosis and treatment. *Annals of Neurology*, 41(3), pp. 353-7.

Murakami, S., Mizobuchi, M., Nakashiro, Y., et al., 1996. Bell palsy and herpes simplex virus: identification of viral DNA in endoneurial fluid and muscle. *Annals of Internal Medicine*, 124, pp. 27-30.

Nash, J.J., Friedland, D.R., Boorsma, K.J. and Rhee, J.S., 2010. Management and outcomes of facial paralysis from intratemporal blunt trauma: a systematic review. Laryngoscope, 120 (7), pp. 1397-404.

Peitersen, E., 2002. Bell's palsy: the spontaneous course of 2,500 peripheral facial nerve palsies of different etiologies. *Acta Otolaryngologica Supplementum*, 549, pp. 4-30.

Robinson, M., Baiungo, J., Hohman, M. and Hadlock, T., 2012. Facial rehabilitation. *Operative Techniques in Otolaryngology*, 23, pp. 288-96.

Rowlands, S., Hooper, R., et al., 2002. The epidemiology and treatment of Bell's palsy in the UK. *European Journal of Neurology*, 9(1), pp. 63-7.

Salinas, R.A., Alvarez, G., Daly, F. and Ferreira, J., 2010. Corticosteroids for Bell's palsy (idiopathic facial paralysis). *Cochrane Database of Systematic Reviews*, 3, CD001942.

Scott, D., Lifchez, M.D., Hani, S., Matloub, M.D., Arun, K. and Gosain, M.D., 2005. Cortical adaptation to restoration of smiling after free muscle transfer innervated by the nerve to the masseter. *Plastic and Reconstructive Surgery*, 115(6), pp. 1472-9.

Seddon, H.J., 1942. A classification of nerve injuries. *British Medical Journal*, 2(4260), pp. 237-9.

Shipchandler, T.Z., Seth, R. and Alam, D.S., 2011. Split hypoglossal-facial nerve neurorrhaphy for treatment of the paralyzed face. *American Journal of Otolaryngology*, 32, pp. 511-6.

Snyderman, C., May, M., Berman, M.A. and Curtin, H.D., 1988. Facial paralysis: traumatic neuromas vs. facial nerve neoplasms. *Otolaryngology—Head and Neck Surgery*, 98, pp. 53-9.

Sunderland, S., 1978. *Nerve and nerve injury*. 2nd ed. New York, Churchill Livingstone.

Terzis, J.K. and Tzafetta, K., 2009. The babysitter' procedure: minihypoglossal to facial nerve transfer and cross-facial nerve grafting. *Plastic and Reconstructive Surgery*, 123, pp. 865-76.

Valls-Sole, J., 2007. Electrodiagnostic studies of the facial nerve in a peripheral facial palsy and hemifacial spasm. *Muscle & Nerve*, 36(1), pp. 14-20.

Vanswearingen, J., 2008. Facial rehabilitation: a neuromuscular reeducation, patient-centered approach. *Facial Plastic Surgery*, 24(2), pp. 250-9.

Vrabec, J.T. and Coker, N.J., 2006. Acute paralysis of the facial nerve. In: B. Bailey, J. Johnson, eds. *Head and neck surgery-otolaryngology*. Philadelphia, PA: Lippincott. pp. 2139-54.

Yetsier, S., Tosun, F. and Kazkayasi, M., 2002. Facial nerve paralysis due to chronic otitis media. *Otology & Neurotology*, 23(4), pp. 580-8.

Pigmented and Nonpigmented Lesions of the Face 31

M Veenstra, GAM Krekels

Chapter Overview

Pearls and Pitfalls

Pearls

- Biopsy any skin lesion that enlarges or persists longer than 2 months.
- Always trust your gut-feeling when you examine pigmented lesions.

Pitfalls

- Patient is likely to be mismanaged if a dermatologist is not consulted for a doubtful diagnosis of skin lesion.
- To underestimate the destructing effect of a basal cell carcinoma.

31.1 BASAL CELL CARCINOMA

Epidemiology and Pathogenesis

- Basal cell carcinoma (BCC) is the most common skin cancer in humans and occurs worldwide. Basal cell carcinoma is more common in men than women (1.5–2:1) and occurs most frequently on the head and neck (Bolognia, Jorizzo and Rapini, 2008). Its incidence increases with age.
- Basal cell carcinomas are rapidly becoming an important public health issue worldwide because of the rapidly increasing number of patients with a history of BCC, the total number of BCC patients, and the costs of their treatment and follow-up. In the Netherlands, between 1973 and 2008, age-adjusted incidence rates (European Standard Population) increased approximately threefold from 40 to 148 per 100,000 in males and from 34 to 141 in females (Flohil, 2011). Basal cell carcinomas are also a health problem in the United States, being the most common cancer with an estimated annual incidence of 0.1–0.5% (Tang, 2012). Van de Geer et al. describe nonmelanoma skin cancer (BCC and squamous cell carcinoma) as a chronic disease, a disease that has a long duration and generally progresses slowly, as defined by the World Health Organization. Progression should, in this case, be regarded as development of new tumors. Therefore, a new skin cancer management strategy is indispensable (Van der Geer, et al., 2010).
- The increasing incidence of BCCs might be related to fashion changes, including clothing and hairstyle but also increasing sun exposure due to use of tanning lamps and travel behavior (Bolognia, Jorizzo and Rapini, 2008). However, aging, increased detection and skin cancer awareness might also partly explain the increased incidence of BCC. Skin phenotype remains the most important factor for the development of BCC, but the amount of ultraviolet (UV) radiation exposure is also an important factor (Bolognia, Jorizzo and Rapini, 2008).

- Next to environmental factors, the patched (*PTCH*) gene plays an important role in the pathogenesis of BCC. Under normal conditions, it controls proliferation and differentiation of cells, and disruption of its normal function is required for the development of BCC. Up to 70% of sporadic BCC is caused by mutation in *PTCH and 10–20%* by mutation in Smoothened.
- The *nevoid basal cell carcinoma syndrome (NBCCS),* also known as *Gorlin syndrome,* is a separate entity, caused by mutations in the *PTCH* gene. This rare disease has an autosomal dominant inheritance pattern and is characterized by numerous BCCs of the skin; cutaneous epidermoid cysts; odontogenic keratocysts of the jaws; palmar and plantar pits; and calcified dural folds. It has a high level of penetrance and variable expressiveness, and has an incidence of approximately 1 in 19,000 (Jones, 2011; Pandeshwar, Jayanthi and Mahesh, 2012).
- Basal cell carcinomas are stroma-dependent and locally invasive without producing metastasis (with rare exceptions) (Bolognia, Jorizzo and Rapini, 2008). Besides the *PTCH* gene, *p53* tumor suppressor gene mutations are frequently encountered in BCCs. Both *PTCH* and *p53* genes are the major targets of UV radiation for BCC induction and frequently display characteristic UV-induced mutations. Inhibiting mutations of *p53* and in the Sonic Hedgehog pathway, inhibiting mutations in *PTCH,* and activating mutations in Smoothened result in BCC. Constituent expression of the Sonic Hedgehog pathway, which can occur through either inhibiting the *PTCH* gene or activating the Smoothened gene, has been shown in mouse models to result in tumors that demonstrate features of BCCs (Kwasniak and Garcia-Zuazaga, 2011). It has also been shown that there is an association between *MC1R* (melanocortin-1 receptor) variants with risk of developing BCC. A combination of fair complexion and *MC1R* variants greatly increases this risk.

Clinical Features

- No universally accepted classification exists for BCC and at least 26 different subtypes have been described. Variants of BCC include nodular, superficial, morpheaform, cystic, basosquamous, micronodular, and fibroepithelioma of Pinkus (Bolognia, Jorizzo and Rapini, 2008).
- Nodular BCC is the most common type of BCC accounting for approximately 60% of all primary BCCs (Fig. 31.1). Nodular BCC presents as a raised, translucent papule or nodule with telangiectasias, and has a propensity for the face. As the lesion enlarges, ulceration may occur. Pigmented BCC is a variant of nodular BCC, usually with a few flecks of brown pigment. However, the tumor may be completely black or blue-black and therefore difficult to differentiate form nodular melanoma. Nodular BCCs may become large and extend deeply, destroying an eyelid, nose, or ear. In large lesions, tissue destruction and ulceration may dominate the picture, so that the inexperienced clinician may not recognize the true nature of the ulcer (Bolognia, Jorizzo and Rapini, 2008).
- Superficial BCC commonly presents as an erythematous macule or thin plaque (Fig. 31.2), and it may be difficult to differentiate clinically from actinic keratosis (AK), squamous cell carcinoma in situ [squamous cell carcinomas (SCC) in situ], or a benign inflammatory lesion. Although this common variant of BCC is more often found on the trunk and extremities, the head and neck may also be affected. The mean age at diagnosis of 57 years is younger than in other BCCs. Areas of spontaneous regression characterized by atrophy and hypopigmentation may be present. The diameter of the lesion varies from a few millimeters to several centimeters. Multiple lesions may be present. Variable amounts of pigment can be present, which may lead to confusion with a melanocytic lesion.

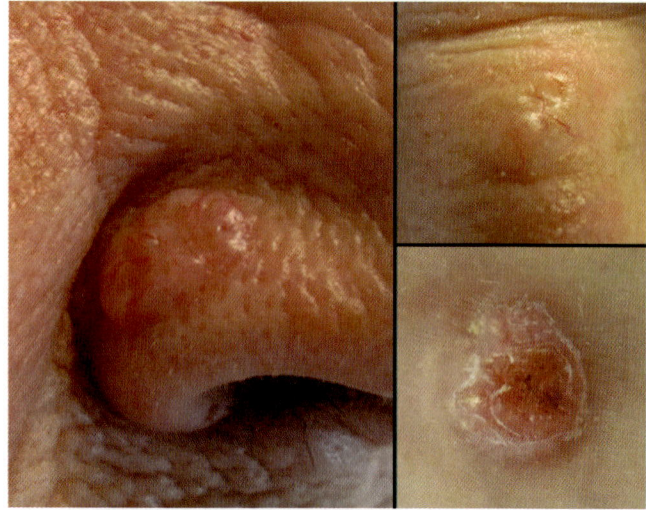

Fig. 31.1: Primary nodular basal cell carcinomas.

The growth pattern is primarily horizontal, but these tumors can become deeply invasive, with induration, ulceration, and nodule formation. Extensive subclinical lateral spread accounts for the significant recurrence rate of these tumors after routine surgical treatment (Bolognia, Jorizzo and Rapini, 2008).

- Morpheaform, also known as sclerosing BCC is a more aggressive type of BCC and commonly presents as a flat, skin-colored, slightly atrophic lesion, or as a plaque without well-defined borders (Fig. 31.3). Its name is derived from an appearance similar to a morphea-plaque. Lesions are often found on the midface and are difficult to differentiate from a scar. The actual size of the carcinoma is often much greater than the clinical extent of the tumor (Richman and Penneys, 1988; Bolognia, Jorizzo and Rapini, 2008).

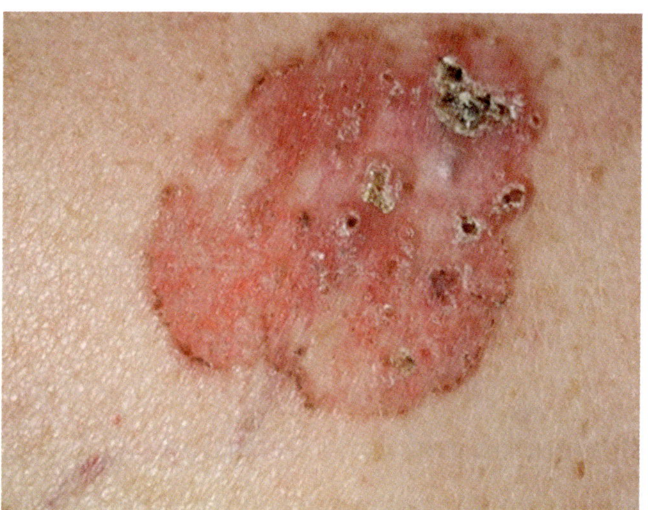

Fig. 31.2: Primary superficial basal cell carcinoma.

Pathological Diagnosis

Basal cell carcinomas are characterized by proliferation of basaloid keratinocytes in various configurations with a variable fibromyxoid stroma. Epidermal origin is usually evident and an inflammatory infiltrate is sometimes present. The cells are characterized by large, relatively uniform nuclei and scant cytoplasm. Cellular borders are indistinct and desmosomes are inapparent. Apoptotic cells are common. The fibromyxoid stroma is intimately associated with the tumor islands, often showing increased cellularity. A characteristic feature of BCC is retraction of the stroma around the tumor islands, creating microscopically visible clefts. Although this feature may not be seen in all instances, it is useful when present and aids in differentiating histologic simulators (Bolognia, Jorizzo and Rapini, 2008).

Preferred Treatment

Surgical

- *Surgical excision*: Standard surgical excision is effective for most primary BCCs. It has been demonstrated that 4 mm margins are adequate for removal of BCC in 98% of cases of nonmorpheaform BCC < 2 cm in diameter. For facial lesions, simple excision with narrow margins is often not adequate for effective removal (Kimyai-Asadi, 2005).
- *Mohs' Micrographic Surgery* (MMS): It provides the lowest recurrence rates and is the gold standard treatment for primary facial BCCs with an aggressive histopathological subtype and for recurrent BCC in the face (Kwasniak and Garcia-Zuazaga, 2011).

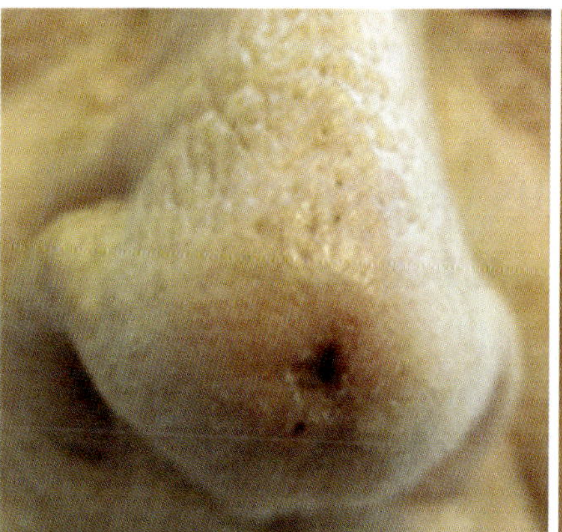
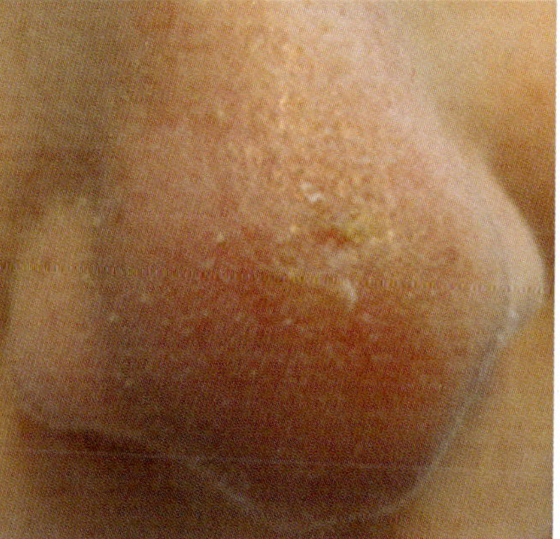
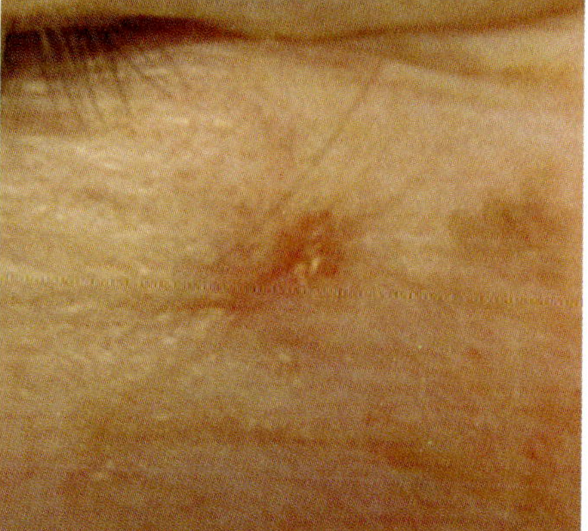

Fig. 31.3: Primary morpheaform basal cell carcinomas.

Nonsurgical

- *Photodynamic therapy* (PDT): It is most often used for the treatment of superficial BCCs. Nodular BCCs can also be treated but higher recurrence rates are found (Bath-Hextall, 2007).
- *Topical imiquimod*: Topical imiquimod cream can be used for low-risk superficial BCC, with the main advantage being a superior cosmetic result. Cure rates for nodular BCC range from 53% to 75%, with higher cure rates for superficial BCC (Peris, 2005). Imiquimod is a toll-like receptor 7 (TLR7) agonist, and it induces interferon-α (IFN-α) and other cytokines and promotes Th1-type immunity. In general, adverse side effects are limited to local skin reactions.
- *Topical fluorouracil*: Topical 5-fluorouracil has been used for the treatment of superficial BCCs. Side effects are usually limited to local skin reactions.
- *Radiotherapy*: This is the preferred treatment for BCCs in patients who are unwilling or unfit for surgery. Disadvantages of radiotherapy include lack of margin control, poor cosmesis in some patients, prolonged course of therapy, and increased risk for future skin cancers. Radiation therapy is associated with higher recurrence rates than surgery for BCC (Bath-Hextall, 2007). Scars from radiation therapy tend to worsen with time, in contrast to surgical scars, which improve over time.
- *Oral vismodegib*: Recently, vismodegib has been introduced for the treatment of BCC. Vismodegib is an oral inhibitor of the Hedgehog pathway. The Hedgehog pathway is a newly identified area in which mutations or dysregulation can occur, leading to the development and progression of tumors. As reviewed by Cirrone et al., this medicine is an effective therapy with good response rates for patients with unresectable BCC or where resection would be cosmetically disadvantageous (Cirrone and Harris, 2012).

Treatment Outcomes

- Danial et al. estimate that the distant metastatic rate of BCCs range from 0.0028% to 0.55% (Danial, 2013). Apart of this rare complication of the disease, BCC has a good prognosis.
- The subtype of the BCC is a predictor for the risk of residual disease or recurrence after conventional excision. Morpheaform BCC is most likely to have involved margins after excision, this happens in about 30% of cases (Abbas and Borman, 2012).
- Besides subtype, choice of management is of major importance for the risk of recurrence and irradicality. In Australia, Leibovitch et al. researched recurrence rates after MMS and found that recurrence at 5 years was diagnosed in 1.4% of primary and in 4% of recurrent tumors. On the other hand, standard excision has a 5-year recurrence rate of 3.2–10% for primary tumors, and >17% for recurrent BCC. Main predictors for tumor recurrence after Mohs' surgery are previous tumor recurrence, longer tumor duration before MMS, infiltrating histology, and more Mohs' rounds positive for tumor (Leibovitch, et al., 2005).

Complications of Disease

- Mortality from BCC is quite rare and might occur in immunocompromised patients. The age-adjusted mortality rate has been estimated at 0.12 per 100,000 and mortality risk is related to increasing age, Caucasian race, and male gender.
- Agressive giant BCCs can be mutilating and may ultimately lead to loss of function of vital organs (Fig. 31.4).
- Cases of metastatic BCC are more likely to occur when tumors have aggressive histologic patterns (morpheaform, infiltrating, metatypical, basosquamous). Perineural space invasion may be an indicator of aggressive disease. Metastases often involve regional lymph nodes, lungs, bone, and skin (Bolognia, Jorizzo and Rapini, 2008).

Prevention and Early Detection

- Lowering UV exposure appears to be having a positive effect in lowering skin cancer incidence.
- Regular use of sunscreens helps to lower the risk.
- Medical students need to receive more training in recognizing skin cancer and examining patients with this condition.

31.2 SQUAMOUS CELL CARCINOMA

Epidemiology and Pathogenesis

- Incidence rates of cutaneous squamous cell carcinoma (CSCC) have increased 3–10% per year worldwide over the last decades, in all age groups. In the United States alone, there are over 250,000 cases of invasive CSCC diagnosed annually (Bolognia, Jorizzo and Rapini, 2008). Cutaneous squamous cell carcinoma

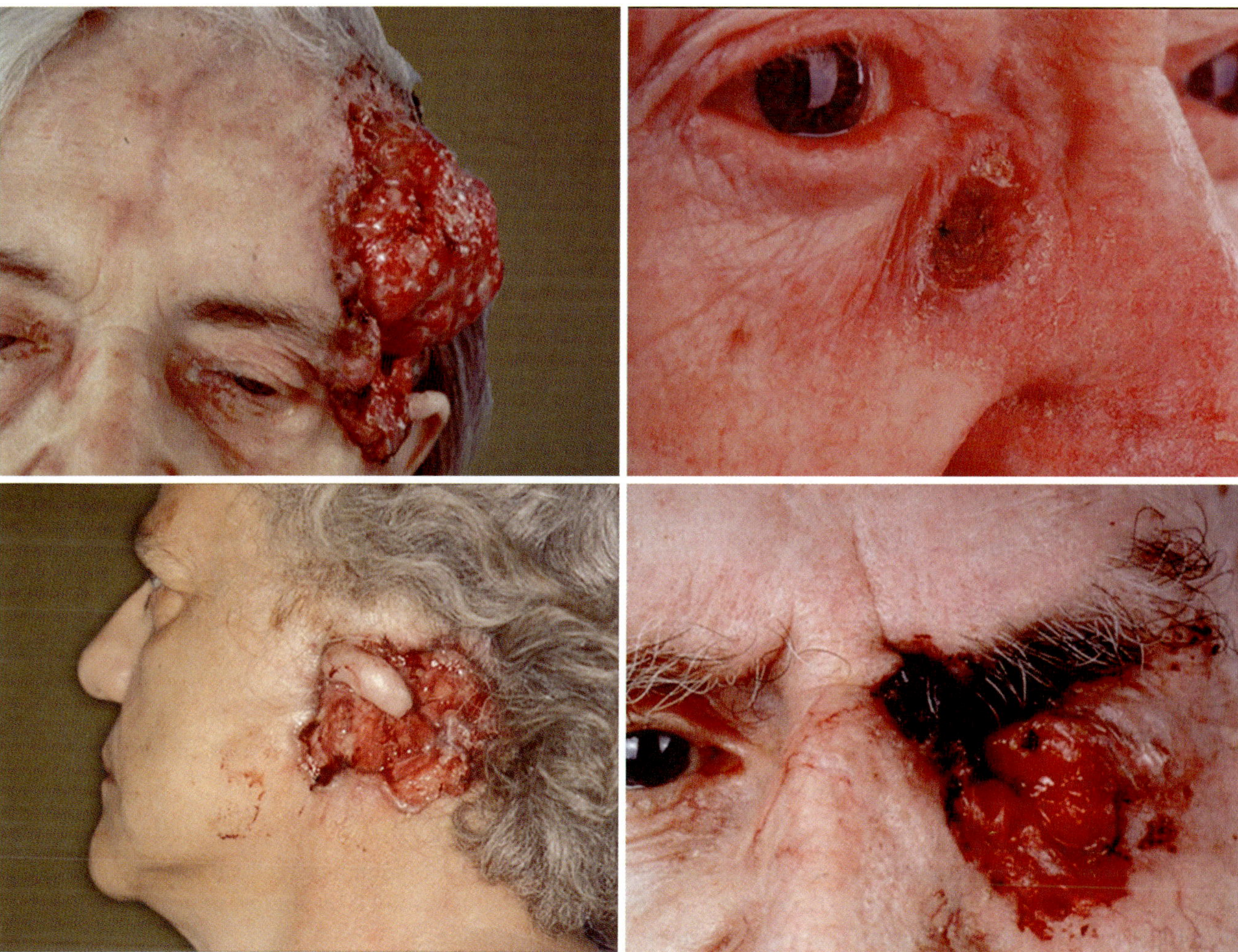

Fig. 31.4: Multiple large basal cell carcinomas.

is found more frequently in men (3:1 male: female) and its incidence increases dramatically with age.

- Cutaneous squamous cell carcinomas normally arise in chronically sun-exposed skin and originate from epidermal keratinocytes. Sites of chronic trauma, scars, inflammation, radiation, or chemical exposure are prone to develop CSCCs (Fig. 31.5).
- Cutaneous squamous cell carcinomas develop through a series of progressive stages including AK, carcinoma in situ (Bowen's disease), invasive cancer, and eventually metastasis. Premalignant lesions associated with cutaneous SCC include AK and Bowen's disease (CSCC in situ).
- The risk for an individual AK to progress into an invasive cancer is low, probably <1 in 1,000 per year. The risk of CSCC in situ progressing to invasive cancer is considered to be higher. Cutaneous squamous cell carcinomas in areas of chronically sun-exposed skin exhibit a relatively indolent behavior and the development of metastases is infrequent (less than 5%). Squamous cell carcinomas occurring on the lip, ear, and genitalia are more prone to metastasize (up to 30%) and therefore have a higher mortality rate. Most metastases are found in regional lymph nodes, but distant hematogenous spread can also be observed.
- The incidence of metastasis also increases with increasing size and in immunosuppressed patients. Lesions arising in scars and sites of inflammation are perhaps the most prone to metastasize.
- Cumulative sun exposure is the most important etiological factor in the development of CSCCs. Ultraviolet radiation can damage DNA, making squamous cells more vulnerable to uncontrolled cell growth and division. For example, UV radiation can induce mutations

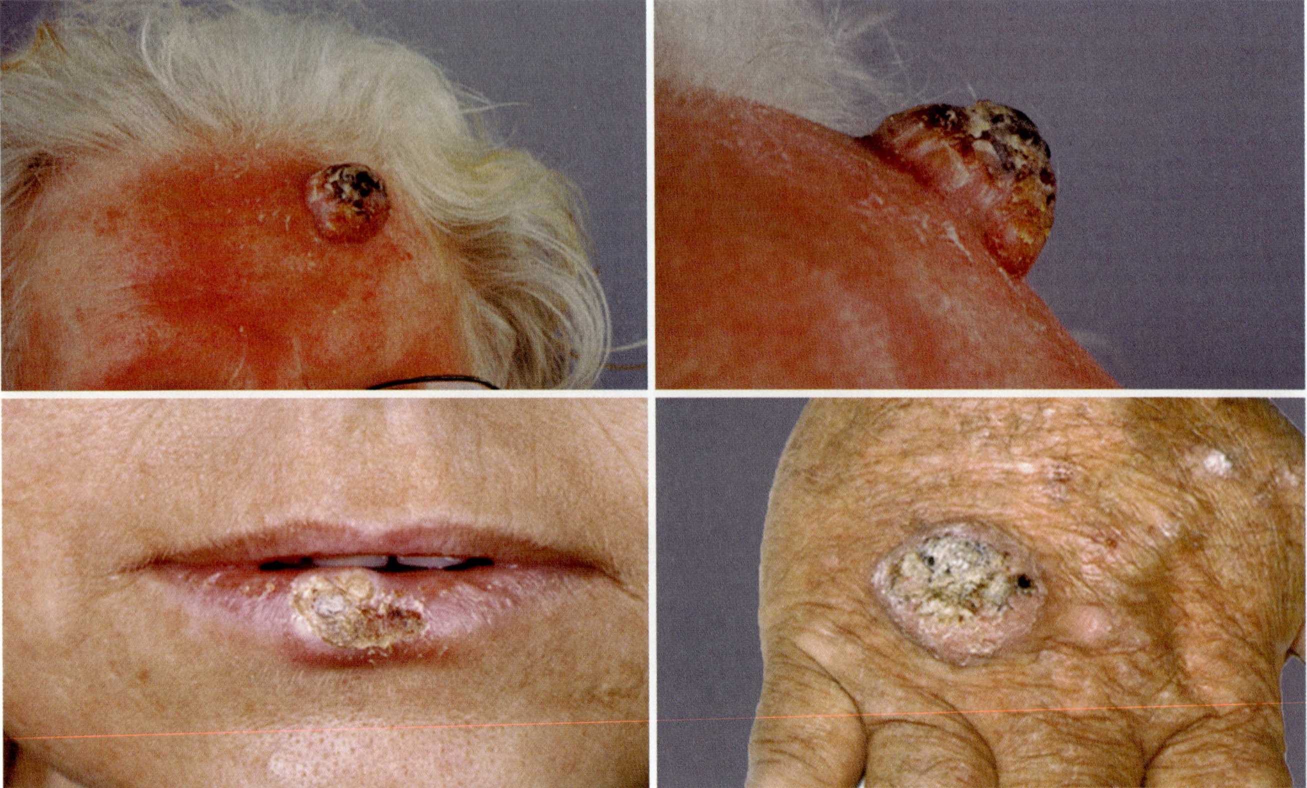

Fig. 31.5: Primary cutaneous squamous cell carcinomas.

in the *p53* gene, a gene that is involved in DNA repair and cell cycle arrest (Brash, 1991). Other risk factors for CSCCs are ionizing radiation and viral infections (human papillomavirus) (Alam and Ratner, 2001).

- Invasive SCCs can have different degrees of differentiation. Highly differentiated tumors show features of keratinization and often invade the dermis with a broad-rounded tumor margin. Papillomatous extensions and cords of slightly atypical squamous epithelia grow down into the dermis. Verrucous SCC, which very rarely metastasizes, is considered a special variant of highly differentiated SCC. Poorly differentiated SCCs show more anaplastic cytologic features and the squamous cell phenotype can sometimes only be verified via immunohistochemistry with antikeratin antibodies.

TNM Classification

In Tables 31.1 to 31.4, the newest TNM classification is elaborated.

TNM staging is incorporated within. Further modifications for 8th edition American Joint Committee on Cancer cutaneous squamous cell carcinoma staging system will be determined by studies that rely on evidence based medicine.

31.3 INTERMEZZO AK AND BOWEN'S DISEASE

- Atypical keratinocytes within AKs are confined to the epidermis. There is no risk of metastasis until these lesions evolve into invasive carcinoma.
- Actinic keratoses are some of the most frequently encountered lesions in clinical practice (Fig. 31.6). Individuals at high risk for the development of AKs are older people, those with lighter skin types and those with a history of chronic sun exposure.
- The primary lesion is a rough erythematous papule with white to yellow scales. Patients may report tenderness. Actinic keratoses may vary in size from a few millimeters to large confluent patches several centimeters in diameter, especially in heavily sun-exposed individuals. A clue to their presence is background solar damage, i.e. dyspigmentation, telangiectasias, and erythema.

Table 31.1: Definition of cutaneous squamous cell carcinoma tumor (T) staging system in 7th edition of American Joint Committee on Cancer manual.

TX	Primary tumor cannot be assessed
T0	No evidence of primary tumor
Tis	Carcinoma in situ
T1	Tumor ≤2 cm in greatest dimension with <2 high-risk features*
T2	Tumor >2 cm in greatest dimension with or without one additional high-risk feature,* or any size with ≥2 high-risk features*
T3	Tumor with invasions of maxilla, mandible, orbit, or temporal bone
T4	Tumor with invasion of skeleton (axial or appendicular) or perineural invasions of skull base

Source: Farasat, S., et al., 2011. A new American Joint Committee on Cancer staging system for cutaneous squamous cell carcinoma: creation and rationale for inclusion of tumor (T) characteristics. *Journal of the American Academy of Dermatology*, 64(6), pp. 1051-9.

*High-risk features include depth (>2 mm thickness; Clark level ≥ IV); perineural invasion; location (primary site ear or non-glabrous lip); and differentiation (poorly differentiated or undifferentiated).

Table 31.2: Definition of cutaneous squamous cell carcinoma nodal (N) staging in 7th edition of American Joint Committee on Cancer manual.

NX	Regional lymph nodes cannot be assessed
N0	No regional lymph node metastasis
N1	Metastasis in single ipsilateral lymph node, ≤3 cm in greatest dimension
N2	Metastasis in single ipsilateral lymph node, >3 cm but not >6 cm in greatest dimension; or in multiple ipsilateral lymph nodes, none >6 cm in greatest dimension; or in bilateral or contralateral lymph nodes, none >6 cm in greatest dimension
N2a	Metastasis in single ipsilateral lymph node, >3 cm but not >6 cm in greatest dimension
N2b	Metastasis in multiple ipsilateral lymph nodes, none >6 cm in greatest dimension
N2c	Metastasis in bilateral or contralateral lymph nodes, none >6 cm in greatest dimension
N3	Metastasis in lymph node, >6 cm in greatest dimension

Source: Farasat, S., et al., 2011. A new American Joint Committee on Cancer staging system for cutaneous squamous cell carcinoma: creation and rationale for inclusion of tumor (T) characteristics. *Journal of the American Academy of Dermatology*, 64(6), pp. 1051-9.

Table 31.3: Seventh edition American Joint Committee on Cancer definition of cutaneous squamous cell carcinoma distant metastasis (M) staging.

MX	Distant metastasis cannot be assessed
M0	No distant metastasis
M1	Present distant metastasis

Source: Farasat, S., et al., 2011. A new American Joint Committee on Cancer staging system for cutaneous squamous cell carcinoma: creation and rationale for inclusion of tumor (T) characteristics. *Journal of the American Academy of Dermatology*, 64(6), pp. 1051-9.

- Lesions are typically clustered in areas of highest sun exposure, such as the tops of the ears, upper forehead, nasal bridge, malar eminences, dorsal hands, extensor forearms, and scalp in bald individuals (Bolognia, Jorizzo and Rapini, 2008).
- Treatment options are cryosurgery in solitary lesions and PDT in extensive lesions. Superficial lesions can be treated by topical therapy by using 5-fluorouracil or imiquimod 5% cream. In case of hypertrophic AKs curettage is advised. Laser resurfacing is also a useful therapeutic option for widespread actinic keratoses (Ostertag, 2006). Chemical peels may also be utilized.

Table 31.4: Final 7th edition American Joint Committee on Cancer stage grouping for cutaneous squamous cell carcinoma.

Stage	*T*	*N*	*M*
0	In situ	N0	M0
I	T1	N0	M0
II	T2	N0	M0
III	T3	N0 or N1	M0
	T1 or T2	N1	M0
IV	T1, 2, or 3	N2	M0
	Any T	N3	M0
	T4	Any N	M0
	Any T	Any N	M1

Source: Farasat, S., et al., 2011. A new American Joint Committee on Cancer staging system for cutaneous squamous cell carcinoma: creation and rationale for inclusion of tumor (T) characteristics. *Journal of the American Academy of Dermatology*, 64(6), pp. 1051-9.

Bowen's Disease

- Cutaneous squamous cell carcinoma in situ is commonly called Bowen's disease (Fig. 31.7). The most common presentation of CSCC in situ is an erythematous scaling patch or slightly elevated plaque that

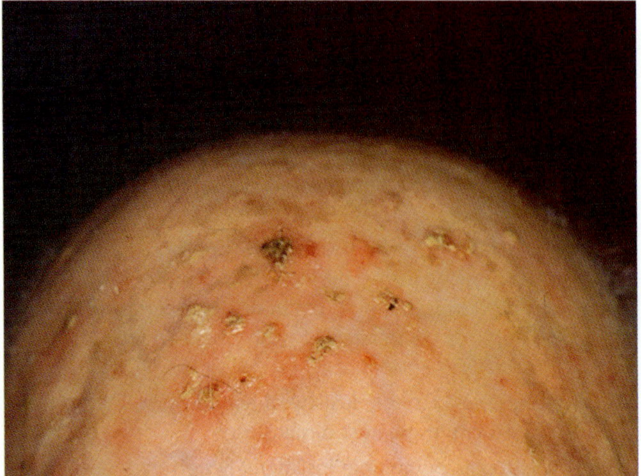

Fig. 31.6: Actinic keratosis on the scalp.

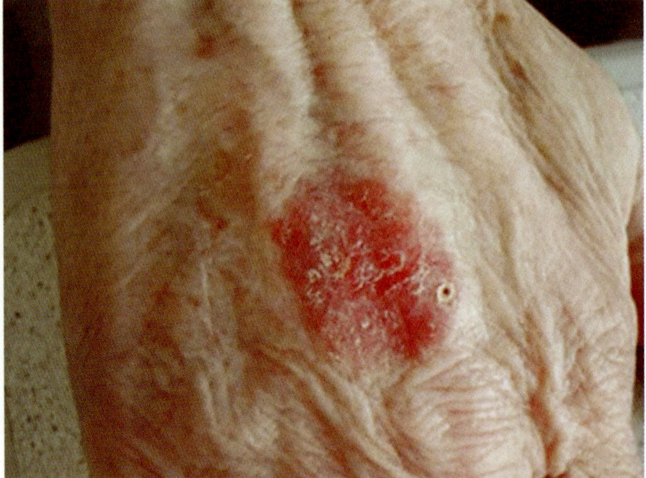

Fig. 31.7: Morbus Bowen on dorsal surface of hand.

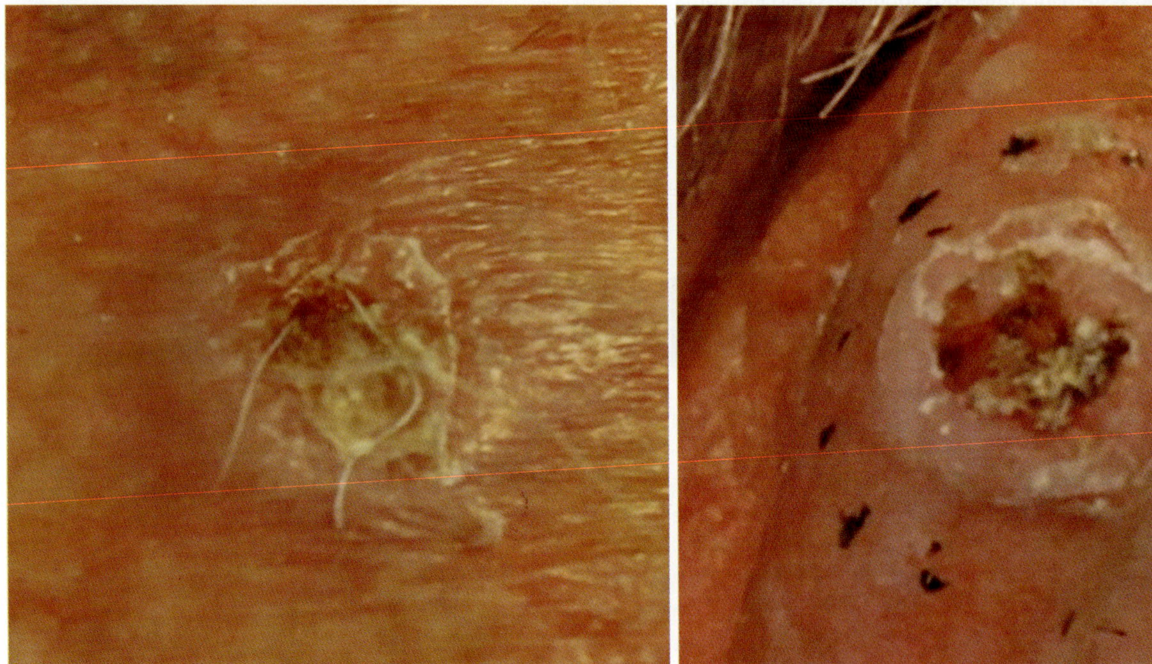

Fig. 31.8: Primary cutaneous squamous cell carcinomas situated on the neck (left) and helix (right).

arises on sun exposed skin of an elderly individual. Lesions may be crusted. It may also arise as a keratotic papule or nodule that arises within a background of sun-damaged skin.

- Bowen's disease may arise de novo or from a preexisting AK.
- Cutaneous squamous cell carcinoma occurs mostly on head, neck, and upper extremities (Fig. 31.8).
- There is often a history of tenderness as the lesion slowly or rapidly enlarges to become more nodular.
- Lesions may ulcerate.
- Cutaneous squamous cell carcinoma may resemble BCC, atypical fibroxanthoma, neuroendocrine carcinoma, amelanotic melanoma, adnexal tumors, prurigo nodularis, verruca, and irritated seborrheic keratosis.

Investigations

Histopathological Diagnosis

- Well-differentiated CSCCs generally arise in the setting of epidermal changes consistent with AK. There is a downward proliferation of lobules and detached islands of glassy, brightly eosinophilic keratinocytes containing nuclei with some degree of pleomorphism and mitosis. Tumor nests are irregular and more or less differentiated depending on the grade of the tumor. In the better-differentiated types, horny pearls are easily found. Single-cell keratinization as well as dyskeratoses is also seen. Cell pleomorphism is evident. The tumor sometimes grows surrounding the nerves, either partly or completely. This perineural infiltration is considered as a sign of bad prognosis. Biopsies should also be checked for tumor invasion of vessels since CSCCs can infiltrate both blood and lymphatic vessels.

Preferred Treatment

Surgical

- *Surgical excision; standard excision*: As per National Comprehensive Cancer Network (NCCN) treatment guidelines, standard surgical excision with a 4–5 mm margin (in which a sampling but not the entire marginal surface is evaluated pathologically) is considered adequate for non-high-risk CSCC. The only scenario in which standard excision is recommended for high-risk CSCC is for tumors >2 cm on the trunk and extremities with no other high-risk factors that can be excised with a 1.0 cm clinical margin with a primary closure (LeBoeuf and Schmults, 2011). For all other high-risk CSCC, Mohs' surgery or excision with "complete circumferential peripheral and deep margin assessment" (CCPDMA) is advised. Complete circumferential peripheral and deep margin assessment refers to procedures in which a surgeon excises the tissue and a pathologist assesses the entire circumferential and deep margin. In Mohs' surgery, the surgeon performs his complete margin assessment (LeBoeuf and Schmults, 2011). In this case, a standard of 5 mm margin is accepted for all types of SCC.
- *Slow-MMS*: (Slow-) Mohs' surgery or resection with CCPDMA is the recommended therapy for all high-risk CSCC (with the single exception above), as well as tumors located in cosmetically or anatomically sensitive areas. LeBoeuf states that standard excision reportedly cures 92% of primary tumors, while Mohs' cures 97%; standard excision has a 77% cure rate for recurrent disease, while Mohs' cures 90–94%. With the presence of high-risk features, cure rates across all modalities decrease, but are still superior with Mohs' (LeBoeuf and Schmults, 2011).
- *Mohs' surgery*: This is discussed in detail in Chapter 32.

Nonsurgical

- *Radiotherapy*: Radiation therapy is the preferred treatment option for CSCCs in case surgery is contraindicated. Advantage of radiotherapy is the avoidance of an invasive procedure in a patient who may not be able to tolerate or is unwilling to undergo surgery. Disadvantages include lack of margin control, poor cosmesis in some patients, prolonged course of therapy, and increased risk for future skin cancers. Scars from radiation therapy tend to worsen with time, in contrast to surgical scars, which improve over time. Radiation is often used as an adjuvant modality following treatment of aggressive or high-risk SCC with surgery, especially when perineural involvement is identified, although no controlled studies have proven its usefulness.

Treatment Outcome(s)

Complete circumferential peripheral and deep margin assessment is critical for achieving cure of high-risk CSCCs. The rate of local recurrence with clear margins is 5%. Nodal metastasis occurs in 5% of cases, as distant metastasis only occur in 1% of cases. Disease specific death is 1% (LeBoeuf and Schmults, 2011). Especially the size and location of the tumor are risk factors. Large lesions of >2 cm in diameter recur at a rate of 15%. Major tumors metastasize at a rate of 30%. Cutaneous squamous cell carcinomas of the lip and ear are also at higher risk, with rates of recurrence and metastasis ranging from 10% to 25%. Lesions occurring in chronically diseased or injured skin are associated with a risk of metastasis of approximately 40% (Alam and Ratner, 2001).

Complications of Disease

Cutaneous squamous cell carcinomas of the head and neck most commonly metastasize to parotid and cervical lymph nodes. Metastasis of CSCCs is associated with lower survival rates. Aggressive local surgery, lymph node dissection, and postoperative radiation therapy are often needed. Discussion of chemotherapy for metastatic disease, usually undertaken by oncologists, is beyond the scope of this book.

Prevention and Early Detection

- Lowering UV exposure appears to be having a positive effect in lowering skin cancer incidence.
- Regular use of sunscreens helps to lower the risk.
- Medical students need to receive more training in skin cancer examination.

31.4 MELANOMA SKIN CANCER

Epidemiology and Pathogenesis

- Over the last decades, the incidence of cutaneous malignant melanoma has increased tremendously worldwide, with the highest incidence in Australia and New Zealand. Because of improved early detection, mortality rates have increased at a significantly lower rate than the incidence rates (annual increase of 3–7% in fair-skinned populations) (Bolognia, Jorizzo and Rapini, 2008). In the United States, the lifetime risk of melanoma increased from 1 in 1,500 persons in 1935, to 1 in 75 persons in 2000 (Volkovova, 2012). Melanoma is the most common type of cancer in young adults. Taking this together, melanoma is a significant public health problem.
- According to their configuration, anatomic site of origin and prognosis, several subtypes of melanoma can be defined (Table 31.5).
- The sequence of events in which normal melanocytes transform into melanoma cells is incompletely understood. It probably involves a multistep process of progressive genetic mutations that alter cell proliferation, differentiation, and death and impact susceptibility to the carcinogenic effects of UV radiation.
- Germline genetic mutations and polymorphisms can predispose individuals to melanoma. The major high-penetrance melanoma susceptibility gene locus associated with familial melanoma is CDKN2A (in 25% percent of familial melanoma kindred), which encodes p16 and p14ARF, proteins that exert regulatory effects on cell cycle progression through the retinoblastoma protein (Rb) and *p53* pathways, respectively.
- In those with phenotypic susceptibility, UV light exposure is the most important risk factor for melanoma. Excessive childhood exposure and blistering sunburns are more important factors than cumulative regular sun exposure, which too plays a role in development of melanoma.
- Phenotypic factors associated with melanoma risk are melanocytic nevi, skin color, and skin type. Large numbers of common nevi and the presence of atypical nevi are strong risk factors for melanoma. Although primary cutaneous melanoma may develop in precursor melanocytic nevi, >70% of cases are believed to arise de novo.
- Other risk factors are a personal or family history of melanoma, extensive tanning bed use, genetic syndromes with skin cancer predisposition (e.g. xeroderma pigmentosum) and iatrogenic (immunosuppressive drugs used in transplant medicine or extended PUVA therapy) or acquired (e.g. HIV) immunosuppression.

Table 31.5: Overview of the distribution of the different types of melanoma (Volkovova, 2012).

Type of malignant melanoma	*Proportion of all melanomas (%)*
Superficial spreading malignant melanoma	70
Nodular melanoma	15–30
Lentigo maligna melanoma	4–10
Acral lentiginous melanoma	2–8

Clinical Features

- *Superficial spreading malignant melanoma* is usually seen in adults and develops most frequently on the upper back of both men and women and on the legs of women, although it may develop anywhere on the body (Volkovova, 2012) (Fig. 31.9).
- *Nodular melanoma* is a dome-shaped, pedunculated, or nodular lesion that may occur anywhere on the body (Fig. 31.10). It is commonly dark brown or reddish brown but may occasionally be amelanotic. Nodular melanomas tend to rapidly invade the dermis from the onset with no apparent horizontal growth phase. These tumors are frequently misdiagnosed, because they may resemble blood blisters, hemangioma, dermal nevi, or polyps (Volkovova, 2012).
- *Lentigo maligna melanoma* originates from lentigo maligna (Fig. 31.11). Untreated lentigo maligna tends to exhibit horizontal or radial growth with epidermal involvement for many years (often decades) before it enters the vertical growth phase and invades the dermis to become lentigo maligna melanoma. This change is often indicated clinically by the development of focal papular or nodular areas (Volkovova, 2012).
- *Acral lentiginous melanoma* occurs on the palmar and plantar surfaces, the digits and subungual areas (Volkovova, 2012).

Diagnosis

- Early detection is a key factor in improving survival from melanoma. The clinical diagnosis of cutaneous melanoma continues to be based on simple visual inspection. The American Cancer Society uses the ABCDE mnemonic. With this mnemonic the following

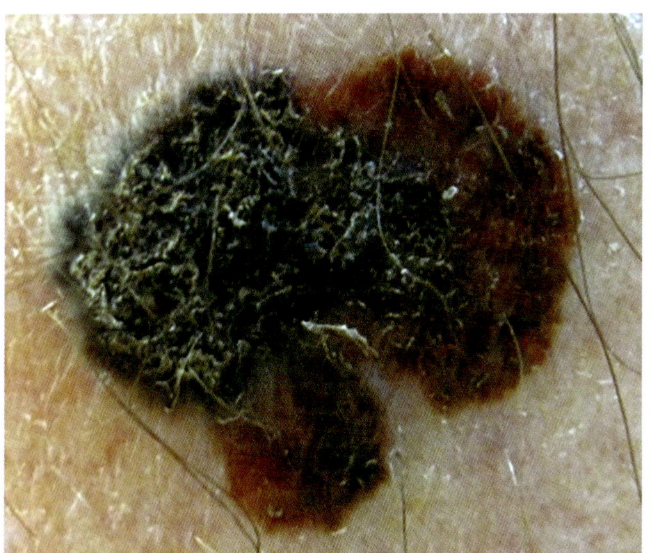

Fig. 31.9: Superficial spreading malignant melanoma.

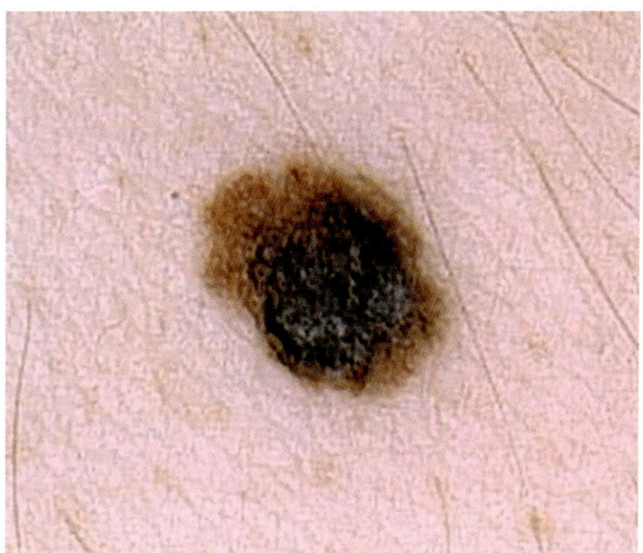

Fig. 31.10: Nodular melanoma.

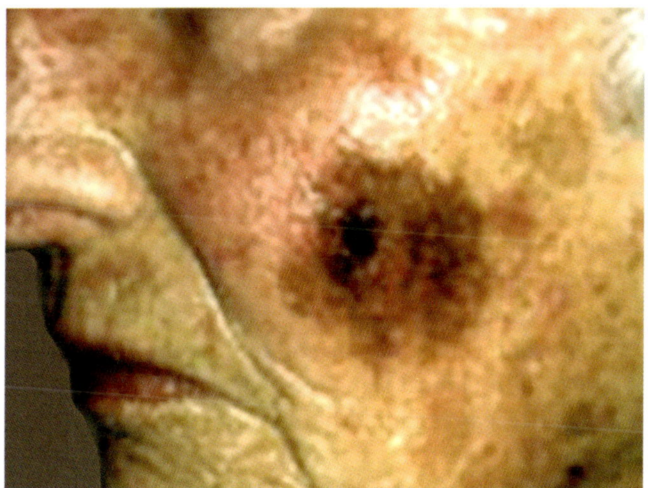

Fig. 31.11: Lentigo maligna melanoma.

criteria are evaluated: ***A***symmetry, ***B***order irregularity, ***C***olor variegation, ***D***iameter >5 mm, and ***E***volving to connote the importance of change. A history of change in the color, shape, or size of a pigmented skin lesion over the course of months is the most sensitive clinical sign for melanoma (Fig. 31.12) (Bolognia, Jorizzo and Rapini, 2008).

- Complete skin examination has to be done, as melanoma can arise on any cutaneous surface. High-risk individuals with a personal or family history of melanoma, many nevi, and/or dysplastic nevi should undergo longitudinal dermatologic evaluation. Dermoscopy, also known as skin surface microscopy or epiluminescence microscopy (ELM), is a helpful noninvasive tool in this setting. In this way, morphologic structures within the epidermis, the dermal–epidermal junction, and the superficial dermis can be better visualized. Most importantly, early stages of melanoma can be differentiated from benign lesions. Dermoscopy increases diagnostic sensitivity when used by dermatologists formally trained in the use of this technique (Bolognia, Jorizzo and Rapini, 2008).

Differential Diagnosis

- A variety of conditions may simulate melanoma, either clinically of histopathologically, or both. Awareness of these simulators is of great practical importance to avoid overdiagnosis of melanoma.
- Melanocytic lesions that simulate melanomas clinically and/or histopathologically are acral nevi, black (hypermelanotic) nevi, blue nevi, atypical nevi, halo nevi, hyperplasia of melanocytes in sun-damaged skin, melanosis of mucosal regions, and so on. Nonmelanocytic simulators of melanoma may be Paget's disease, Bowen's disease, pigmented BCC, seborrheic keratosis, subungual hematoma, thrombosed hemangioma, angiokeratoma, pyogenic granuloma, and tinea nigra (Bolognia, Jorizzo and Rapini, 2008).

Histopathological Diagnosis

- This remains the gold standard for melanoma diagnosis. Criteria for the histopathological diagnosis of melanoma include asymmetry, poor circumscription

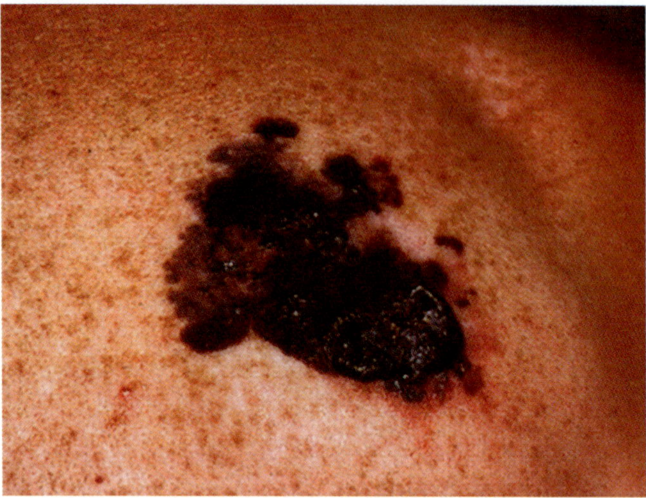

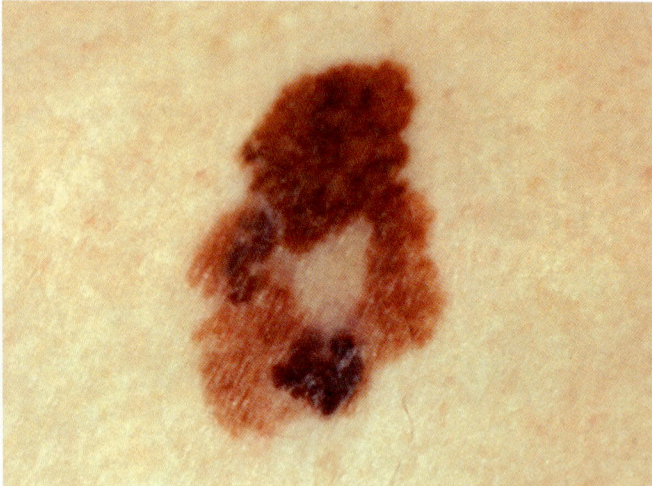

Fig. 31.12: Malignant melanoma.

of intraepidermal melanocytic component, no maturation of melanocytes with progressive descent into the dermis, nests of melanocytes variable in size and shape, some nests of melanocytes become confluent, atypical melanocytes with pleomorphic nuclei, mitotic figures, necrotic melanocytes, signs of regression, and "dusty" melanin within tumor cells (Bolognia, Jorizzo and Rapini, 2008).

- Staging is done by the TNM classification. At the moment, the seventh edition of the American Joint Committee on Cancer (AJCC) Cancer Staging Manual is available. Important criteria included are Breslow depth and Clark level, both pathological descriptions of how deeply tumor cells have invaded. The Breslow depth is a continuous variable, while Clark levels differentiate between different groups of invasion depth. In Tables 31.6 and 31.7, the newest TNM classification for melanoma is elaborated.

Preferred Treatment

- Excisional biopsy with narrow margins (2 mm) is the preferred method of biopsy, as it prevents sampling error (e.g. missing a focus of melanoma arising in a precursor benign lesion) and enables the pathologist to assess the overall architecture of the lesion and accurately microstage the tumor (Bolognia, Jorizzo and Rapini, 2008).
- Following histologic diagnosis, the primary melanoma site should be re-excised with an appropriate margin determined by the Breslow depth. Melanoma cells can migrate away from the tumor origin and may extend wider or deeper than is visibly apparent. The major goal is to prevent local recurrence or persistent disease. Current recommendations are excision margins of 0.5 cm for in situ melanoma, 1 cm for melanoma <1 mm, 2 cm for melanoma 1–4 mm, and 2–3 cm for melanoma >4 mm in depth (Bolognia, Jorizzo and Rapini, 2008).
- In case of a Breslow depth of >1 mm, sentinel lymph node biopsy is advised. This provides valuable prognostic information, and identifies patients with metastatic lymph nodes for early therapeutic lymph node dissection (Bolognia, Jorizzo and Rapini, 2008).
- In case of clinical signs for metastatic disease, additional research should be performed (e.g. scans and laboratory tests). After surgery, the management options for patients with stage III melanoma involving regional lymph nodes include observation, high-dose interferon-a-2b, enrolment in a clinical trial, and adjuvant radiation in select cases to reduce risk of regional recurrence (Fox, 2013a). Several treatment options for stage IV melanoma (with the presence of distant metastasis) are high-dose interleukin-2, conventional chemotherapy, biochemotherapy, and novel therapies, such as ipilimumab and vemurafenib. Additional therapies are currently under investigation in the form of clinical trials (Fox, 2013b).
- A dermatologist should be consulted for clinical assessment and biopsy of suspicious skin lesions, for surveillance, early detection and surgical or topical treatment, and for skin surveillance to detect possible new primary melanoma.

Table 31.6: Definitions of TNM for the revised 7th edition AJCC melanoma staging classification.

T classification		
Primary tumor (T)	*Thickness (mm)*	*Ulceration status/mitoses*
T0	No evidence of primary tumor	
Tis	Melanoma in situ	
T1	≤1.0	Without ulceration and mitosis <1/mm² With ulceration or mitoses ≥1/mm²
T2	1.01–2.0	Without ulceration With ulceration
T3	2.01–4.0	Without ulceration With ulceration
T4	>4	Without ulceration With ulceration
TX	Primary tumor cannot be assessed (e.g. curettage or severely regressed melanoma)	
N classification		
Regional lymph nodes (N)	*Number of metastatic nodes*	*Nodal metastatic mass*
NX	Patients in whom the regional nodes cannot be assessed (e.g. previously removed for another reason)	
N0	No regional metastases detected	
N1	1 node	Micrometastasis* Macrometastasis†
N2	2–3 nodes	Micrometastasis* Macrometastasis† In transit met(s)/satellite(s) without metastatic nodes
N3	4 or more metastatic nodes, or matted nodes, or in transit met(s)/satellite(s) with metastatic node(s)	
M classification		
Distant metastasis (M)	*Site*	*Serum LDH*
M0	No detectable evidence of distant metastases	
M1a	Distant skin, subcutaneous, or nodal metastases	Normal
M1b	Lung metastases	Normal
M1c	All other visceral metastases	Normal
	Any distant metastases	Elevated

Source: Nading, M.A., Balch, C.M. and Sober, A.J., 2010. Implications of the 2009 American Joint Committee on Cancer melanoma staging and classification on dermatologists and their patients. *Seminars in Cutaneous Medicine and Surgery*, 29(3), pp. 142-7.
(AJCC: American Joint Committee on Cancer Staging; LDH: Lactate dehydrogenase; TNM: Tumor nodes metastases).
*Micrometastases are diagnosed after sentinel lymph node biopsy and completion lymphadenectomy (if performed).
†Macrometastases are defined as clinically detectable nodal metastases confirmed by therapeutic lymphadenectomy or when nodal metastasis exhibits gross extracapsular extension.

Treatment Outcome(s) and Complications of Disease

The prognosis of a patient with melanoma is dependent on stage at diagnosis. Prognosis for patients with localized melanoma and no nodal or distant metastases is generally good. Major independent prognostic factors for survival are tumor thickness, ulceration, age, sex, anatomic site, number of involved lymph nodes, regional lymph node tumor burden, and site of distant metastases (Bolognia,

Table 31.7: Anatomic stage/prognostic groups for the revised 7th edition AJCC melanoma staging classification.

Anatomic stage/prognostic groups							
*Clinical staging**				*Pathologic staging†*			
Stage 0	Tis	N0	M0	0	Tis	N0	M0
Stage IA	T1a	N0	M0	IA	T1a	N0	M0
Stage IB	T1b	N0	M0	IB	T1b	N0	M0
	T2a	N0	M0		T2a	N0	M0
Stage IIA	T2b	N0	M0	IIA	T2b	N0	M0
	T3a	N0	M0		T3a	N0	M0
Stage IIB	T3b	N0	M0	IIB	T3b	N0	M0
	T4a	N0	M0		T4a	N0	M0
Stage IIC	T4b	N0	M0	IIC	T4b	N0	M0
Stage III	Any T	≥N1	M0	IIIA	T1-4a	N1a	M0
					T1-4a	N2a	M0
				IIIB	T1-4b	N1a	M0
					T1-4b	N2a	M0
					T1-4a	N1b	M0
					T1-4a	N2b	M0
					T1-4a	N2c	M0
				IIIC	T1-4b	N1b	M0
					T1-4b	N2b	M0
					T1-4b	N2c	M0
					Any T	N3	M0
Stage IV	Any T	Any N	M1	IV	Any T	Any N	M1

Source: Nading, M.A., Balch, C.M. and Sober, A.J. 2010. Implications of the 2009 American Joint Committee on Cancer melanoma staging and classification on dermatologists and their patients. *Seminars in Cutaneous Medicine and Surgery*, 29(3), pp. 142-7.
(AJCC: American Joint Committee on Cancer).
*Clinical staging includes microstaging of the primary melanoma and clinical/radiographic evaluation for metastases. By convention, it should be used after complete excision of the primary melanoma with clinical assessment for regional and distant metastases.
†Pathologic staging includes microstaging of the primary melanoma and pathologic information about the regional lymph nodes after partial or complete lymphadenectomy. Pathologic stage 0 or stage IA patients are the exception; they do not require pathologic evaluation of their lymph nodes.

Jorizzo and Rapini, 2008). For example, women with stage I/II disease tend to have a better survival rate than men. Location of the primary melanoma on the trunk, head or neck portends a poorer prognosis than a location on the extremities. Lesions, which are ulcerated and/or associated with regional or distant metastasis, tend to fare worse. Advancing age is inversely related to survival from melanoma (Bolognia, Jorizzo and Rapini, 2008).

Survival rates conducted by Nading, Balch and Sober are seen in Tables 31.8 and 31.9.

Melanoma is considered to be a chronic life-threatening disease that may affect patients' lives considerably (Holterhues, 2011). Although the prognosis of thin melanoma is relatively good, prognosis decreases with increased thickness of the lesions. The diminished prognosis is mainly due to the well-established tendency of melanoma to metastasize, which accounts for 75% of all deaths associated with skin cancer. In addition, melanomas are highly resistant to most forms of chemotherapy and radiation; therefore, cure of the disseminated disease is uncommon.

Melanoma is a devastating disease. Once in an advanced stage, few therapeutic options are left. Despite a tremendous amount of research performed on melanoma, it remains an unpredictable disease (Palmer, 2011).

Table 31.8: Survival rates for 4,861 T1 melanoma patients (1.00 mm or less) subgrouped by thickness and mitotic rate of the primary melanoma.

Thickness (mm)	*Mitosis (mm²)*	*N*	*Survival rate ± SE*	
			5 Years	10 Years
0.01–0.50	<1.0	1194	0.991 ± 0.004	0.974 ± 0.086
0.01–0.50	≥1.0	327	0.970 ± 0.012	0.952 ± 0.017
0.51–1.00	<1.0	1472	0.977 ± 0.005	0.930 ± 0.010
0.51–1.00	≥1.0	1868	0.935 ± 0.006	0.871 ± 0.012

Source: Nading, M.A., Balch, C.M. and Sober, A.J., 2010. Implications of the 2009 American Joint Committee on Cancer melanoma staging and classification on dermatologists and their patients. *Seminars in Cutaneous Medicine and Surgery*, 29(3), pp. 142-7.

Table 31.9: 2008 AJCC melanoma staging database: 5- and 10-year survival rates for stage III melanoma substages.

Stage	*N*	*Survival Rate ± SE*	
		5 Years	10 Years
IIIA	1196	0.78 ± 0.02	0.68 ± 0.02
IIIB* (including N2c)	1391	0.59 ± 0.02	0.43 ± 0.02
IIIB (excluding N2c)	992	0.54 ± 0.02	0.38 ± 0.03
IIIC	720	0.40 ± 0.02	0.24 ± 0.03

Source: Nading, M.A., Balch, C.M. and Sober, A.J. 2010. Implications of the 2009 American Joint Committee on Cancer melanoma staging and classification on dermatologists and their patients. *Seminars in Cutaneous Medicine and Surgery*, 29(3), pp. 142-7.
(AJCC: American Joint Committee on Cancer).
*399 N2c patients (intralymphatic metastases) had 5- and 10-year survival rates of 69% and 52%.

Prevention and Early Detection

- Continued efforts in primary prevention (i.e. sun protection) and secondary prevention (i.e. early detection) are warranted.
- Further scientific advances in our ability to distinguish between biologically aggressive and indolent melanomas are required to direct our strategies for melanoma prevention and assess the impact of our efforts (Bolognia, Jorizzo and Rapini, 2008).

REFERENCES

Abbas, O.L. and Borman, H., 2012. Basal cell carcinoma: a single-center experience. *ISRN Dermatology*, 2012, p. 246542.

Alam, M. and Ratner, D., 2001. Cutaneous squamous-cell carcinoma. *The New England Journal of Medicine*, 344(13), pp. 975-83.

Bath-Hextall, F.J., et al., 2007. Interventions for basal cell carcinoma of the skin. *Cochrane Database of Systematic Reviews*, 1, p. CD003412.

Bolognia, J., Jorizzo, J.L. and Rapini, R.P., 2008. *Dermatology*. 2nd ed. In: J.L. Bolognia, J.L. Jorizzo, R.P. Rapini, eds.; associate and artwork editor, J.V. Schaffer. St. Louis, MO/London: Mosby Elsevier.

Brash, D.E., et al., 1991. A role for sunlight in skin cancer: UV-induced p53 mutations in squamous cell carcinoma. *Proceedings of the National Academy of Sciences of the United States of America*, 88(22), pp. 10124-8.

Cirrone, F. and Harris, C.S., 2012. Vismodegib and the hedgehog pathway: a new treatment for basal cell carcinoma. *Clinical Therapeutics*, 34(10), pp. 2039-50.

Danial, C., et al., 2013. Markedly improved overall survival in 10 consecutive metastatic basal cell carcinoma patients. *The British Journal of Dermatology*, 169(3), pp. 673-6.

Farasat, S., et al., 2011. A new American Joint Committee on Cancer staging system for cutaneous squamous cell carcinoma: creation and rationale for inclusion of tumor (T) characteristics. *Journal of the American Academy of Dermatology*, 64(6), pp. 1051-9.

Flohil, S.C., et al., 2011. Incidence, prevalence and future trends of primary basal cell carcinoma in the Netherlands. *Acta Dermato-Venereol*, 91(1), pp. 24-30.

Fox, M.C., et al., 2013a. Management options for metastatic melanoma in the era of novel therapies: a primer for the practicing dermatologist: part I: Management of stage III disease. *Journal of the American Academy of Dermatology*, 68(1), pp. 1e1-9; quiz 10-12.

Fox, M.C., et al., 2013b. Management options for metastatic melanoma in the era of novel therapies: a primer for the practicing dermatologist: part II: Management of stage IV disease. *Journal of the American Academy of Dermatology*, 68(1), pp. 13e1-13; quiz 26-8.

Holterhues, C., et al., 2011. Impact of melanoma on patients' lives among 562 survivors: a Dutch population-based study. *Archives of Dermatology*, 147(2), pp. 177-85.

Jones, E.A., et al., 2011. Basal cell carcinomas in Gorlin syndrome: a review of 202 patients. *Journal of Skin Cancer*, 2011, p. 217378.

Kimyai-Asadi, A., et al., 2005. Efficacy of narrow-margin excision of well-demarcated primary facial basal cell carcinomas. *Journal of the American Academy of Dermatology*, 53(3), pp. 464-8.

Kwasniak, L.A. and Garcia-Zuazaga, J., 2011. Basal cell carcinoma: evidence-based medicine and review of treatment modalities. *International Journal of Dermatology*, 50(6), pp. 645-58.

LeBoeuf, N.R. and Schmults, C.D., 2011. Update on the management of high-risk squamous cell carcinoma. *Seminars in Cutaneous Medicine and Surgery*, 30(1), pp. 26-34.

Leibovitch, I., et al., 2005. Basal cell carcinoma treated with Mohs surgery in Australia II. Outcome at 5-year follow-up. *Journal of the American Academy of Dermatology*, 53(3), pp. 452-7.

Nading, M.A., Balch, C.M. and Sober, A.J., 2010. Implications of the 2009 American Joint Committee on Cancer Melanoma Staging and Classification on dermatologists and their patients. *Seminars in Cutaneous Medicine and Surgery*, 29(3), pp. 142-7.

Ostertag, J.U., et al., 2006. A clinical comparison and long-term follow-up of topical 5-fluorouracil versus laser resurfacing in the treatment of widespread actinic keratoses. *Lasers in Surgery and Medicine*, 38(8), pp. 731-9.

Palmer, S.R., et al., 2011. Circulating serologic and molecular biomarkers in malignant melanoma. *Mayo Clinic Proceedings*, 86(10), pp. 981-90.

Pandeshwar, P., Jayanthi K. and Mahesh D., 2012. Gorlin-Goltz syndrome. *Case Reports in Dentistry*, 2012, p. 247239.

Peris, K., et al., 2005. Imiquimod treatment of superficial and nodular basal cell carcinoma: 12-week open-label trial. *Dermatologic Surgery*, 31(3), pp. 318-23.

Richman, T. and Penneys, N.S., 1998. Analysis of morpheaform basal cell carcinoma. *Journal of Cutaneous Pathology*, 15(6), pp. 359-62.

Tang, J.Y., et al., 2012. Inhibiting the hedgehog pathway in patients with the basal-cell nevus syndrome. *The New England Journal of Medicine*, 366(23), pp. 2180-8.

Van der Geer, S., et al., 2010. Need for a new skin cancer management strategy. *Archives of Dermatology*, 146(3), pp. 332-6.

Volkovova, K., et al., 2012. Associations between environmental factors and incidence of cutaneous melanoma. Review. *Environmental Health*, 11(Suppl 1), p. S12.

Mohs' Micrographic Surgery 32

M Veenstra, GAM Krekels

Chapter Overview

Pearls and Pitfalls

Pearls

- Correct indications for Mohs' surgery lead to less recurrences.

Pitfalls

- Applying Mohs' surgery to previously incompletely excised tumors can be challenging as the extensiveness of the tumor is easily overestimated.

32.1 INTRODUCTION

Mohs' surgery is a specialized technique that is used for the removal of cutaneous neoplasms. The technique was developed in the 1930s by Dr Frederic E Mohs and first published in 1941 (Mohs, 1941). The goal of Mohs' surgery is to completely remove a cutaneous neoplasm while sparing the healthy surrounding tissue. During Mohs' surgery, a tumor is initially excised with a small margin and tissue margins are directly and completely examined microscopically using horizontal frozen section technology. In case all margins are tumor free, the skin defect is closed. When tissue margins still contain tumor, an oriented re-excision is performed of the specific positive region followed by histological re-examination of the new tissue margins. This procedure is repeated until all margins are 100% free of tumor cells. Because tissue margins are completely examined microscopically, the technique is officially called Mohs' micrographic surgery (MMS).

32.2 MOHS' SURGERY VERSUS CONVENTIONAL EXCISION

- The major difference between MMS and conventional excision, both of which are treatment options for basal cell carcinoma and squamous cell carcinoma, is the histologic processing of the specimen. When performing a conventional excision, histological sections are manipulated into paraffin embedded sections using the "bread loaf" technique. This means vertical sections are made and merely a small part of the total margins is examined. In Mohs' surgery, all margins are examined by horizontal histologic sections. Mohs' surgery uses frozen section technology to obtain a faster outcome. With Mohs' surgery, 100% of the margins are controlled in order to achieve optimal cure rates (Bolognia, Jorizzo and Rapini, 2008).
- Mohs' surgery is the gold standard in the treatment of high-risk cutaneous neoplasms. By precise micrographic tissue mapping, a high cure rate is reached (Baxter, Patel and Varma, 2012). This is especially useful on the face because of its high tissue-sparing ability. Although this technique offers the highest cure rates for all nonmelanoma skin cancers, it is time and cost prohibitive to use this highly technical modality for the management of all skin cancers, particularly those that are at low risk of recurrence. Therefore, Mohs' surgery is commonly reserved for cancers that are at high risk of recurrence when treated with less rigorous management options.

Indications

Indications for Mohs' surgery are the following (http://emedicine.medscape.com/article/876110-overview#a3; Finley, 2003):

- Primary basal cell carcinoma with clinically indistinct borders.
- Recurrent or incompletely excised basal cell carcinoma.
- Other cosmetically and functionally important areas where tissue preservation is of the utmost concern (digits, genitals).
- Lesions located in high-risk anatomical locations, these are areas involving mainly embryonic fusion planes (e.g. eyelids, nose, ear, nasolabial folds, upper lip, vermillion border, columella, periorbital, temples, preauricular and postauricular areas, and scalp) called the H-zone.
- Tumors with an aggressive histologic subtype [e.g. sclerosing (morpheaform), basosquamous, perineural and perivascular invasion, and infiltrating, adenoidal, or multicentric tumors].
- Tumors with aggressive clinical behavior (e.g. rapidly growing, perineural invasion, and >2 cm in diameter).
- Tumors arising in sites of previous irradiated skin.
- Tumors arising in immunocompromised patients.
- Tumors arising in chronic scars (Marjolin's ulcer).
- In patients with an underlying genetic syndrome, e.g. basal cell nevus (Gorlin) syndrome, xeroderma pigmentosum, and Bazex-Dupré-Christol syndrome.
- Unusual cutaneous tumors that are contiguous in highly cosmetically sensitive areas (e.g. dermatofibrosarcoma protuberans, microcystic adnexal carcinomas, porocarcinoma, and pilomatrix carcinomas).

Technique

During Mohs' surgery, the clinically evident tumor is marked with a small margin of normal-appearing skin (the margin may range from 1 mm to 10 mm and depends on histological subtype, likelihood of subclinical tumor extensions, and areas where tissue sparing is essential (Bolognia, Jorizzo and Rapini, 2008). In case of a recurrent tumor, all tissue involved by previous treatments, including the primary site and reconstruction scar, are resected. References to diagrams are made to ensure correct site identification. After local anesthesia, marking stitches are placed in surrounding tissue adjacent to the tumor. Tumor debulking is done by curettage or, in case of deeper tumors, by excision. This informs the surgeon of the subclinical extent of the tumor and aids in better tissue processing because the specimen becomes flatter. Subsequently, the first Mohs' stage is done. The tissue is excised using an incision that is beveled inwards at an angle of 45°, followed by horizontal excision of the base of the specimen. The specimen is cut into four pieces and marked with red and blue inks along the vertical and horizontal cuts, respectively. In the Mohs' laboratory, the specimen is flattened and processed into horizontal frozen sections. In this way, all margins of the specimen are captured in the histopathological sections. The Mohs' surgeon assesses these sections and performs further resection when tumor residue is present. Further tissue is only excised at the place where residual tumor was found during histopathological examination. Eventually, tumor-free margins are achieved and the defect can then be closed.

Figures 32.1A to G shows the different stages of the Mohs' procedure.

Reconstruction

When dealing with a tissue defect resulting from excision of facial cutaneous malignancy, the surgeon chooses from the reconstruction ladder to repair the defect. Most used closure techniques are direct closure or a single-stage local flap, as they lead to a more desirable color and texture match with the surrounding skin. Other options include healing by second intention, a split-thickness skin graft, or a full-thickness skin graft, but are more likely to lead to color and texture mismatch with the surrounding tissues and a less than ideal aesthetic result. Rarely wedge repairs, two-stage flaps, composite grafts, free flaps, and combination closures may be utilized.

Slow-Mohs' Surgery

An alternative for MMS is formalin-fixed paraffin-embedded tissue micrographic surgery, also known as Slow-Mohs' surgery. It is mostly used for treating cutaneous squamous cell carcinoma but basal cell carcinoma, and other cutaneous tumors can also be treated with slow-Mohs' surgery. In this procedure, marking stitches are placed in surrounding tissue adjacent to A, B, C, and D. The tumor is excised in toto and marked with a marking stitch at A. The wound is then dressed with a Mepitel and Spongostan pad, and a pressure bandage is applied before the patient is sent home. Side A to B is marked with red dye, B to C is marked with blue dye, C to D is marked with green dye, and D to A is marked with

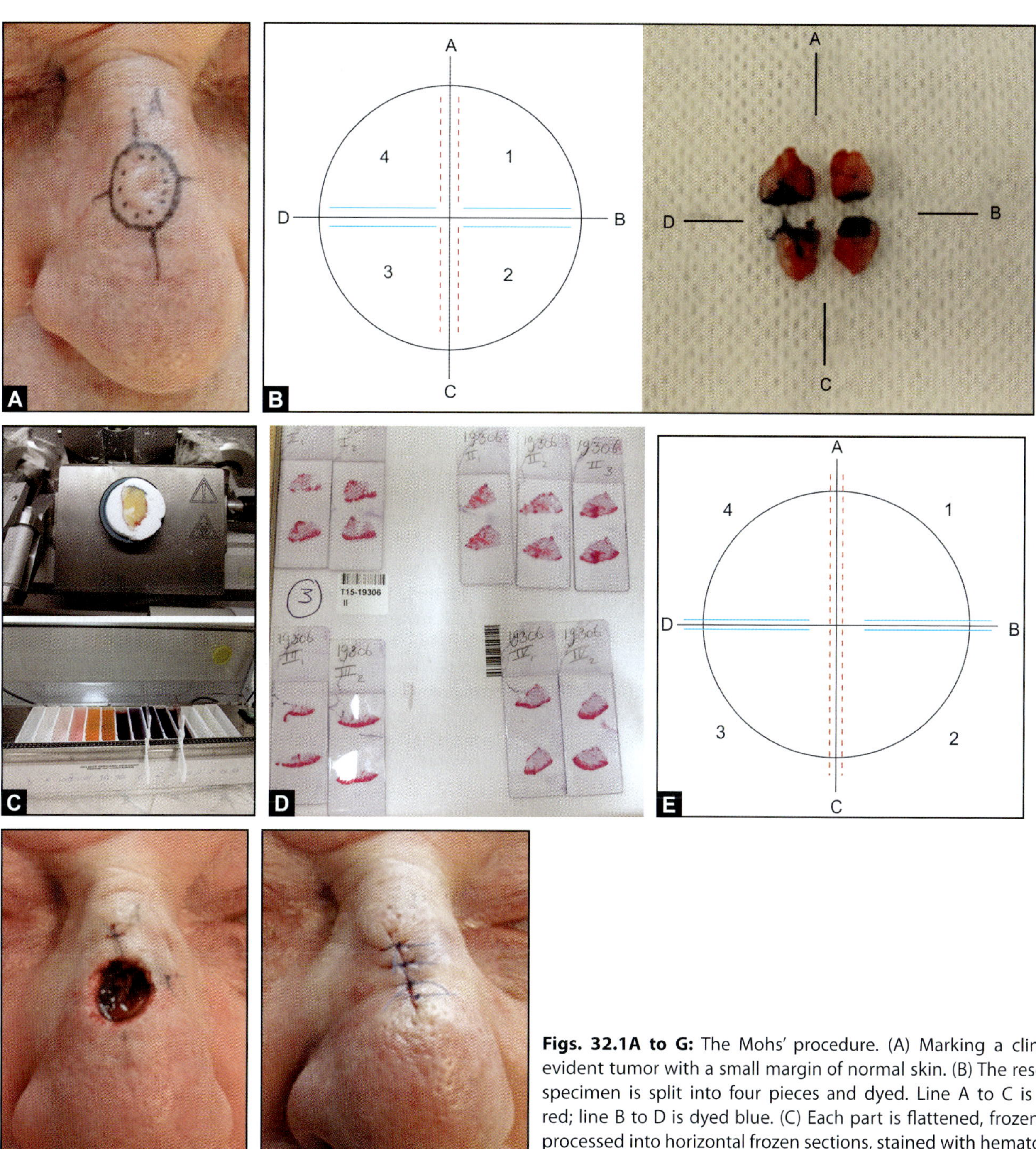

Figs. 32.1A to G: The Mohs' procedure. (A) Marking a clinically evident tumor with a small margin of normal skin. (B) The resected specimen is split into four pieces and dyed. Line A to C is dyed red; line B to D is dyed blue. (C) Each part is flattened, frozen, and processed into horizontal frozen sections, stained with hematoxylin and eosin. (D) The four parts are each processed into four frozen sections on separate glasses. (E) The way of coloring is drawn on the Mohs' form. (F) The defect after Mohs. (G) After reconstruction.

yellow dye. Also the bottom of the section is colored with black ink. In the pathology laboratory, the specimen is distributed in several pieces: sides AB, BC, CD, and DA are sliced as well as the bottom of the specimen. In this way, all margins of the specimen are captured in formalin-fixed paraffin-embedded sections. Processing of the tissue takes a few days, and analysis is performed by the pathologist. The patient usually returns 1 week after surgery and further tissue is excised if needed. In case the surgical wound is tumor free, the defect is closed. The use of horizontal paraffin-embedded sections lengthens the duration of the procedure but facilitates accurate assessment of histological sections in selected tumors.

Complications

Postoperative bleeding is the most common complication in dermatologic surgery. The use of anticoagulants is a contributing factor. Management of acetylsalicylic acid during dermatologic surgery varies among countries. For example, in the Netherlands acetylsalicylic acid is continued during surgery. Patients using acenocoumarol need to adapt their schedule to ensure the international normalized ratio (INR) is ≤2.5 during surgery. To prevent bleeding, adequate hemostasis during surgery is important. Significant bleeding that compromises wound integrity requires exploration of the wound to visualize the bleeding vessel. Once identified, the vessels can be ligated or cauterized to achieve hemostasis.

Wound infection is a rare complication (<5% of cases) (Elliott, Thom and Litterick, 2012). Predisposing factors for infection are lengthy procedures (2 hours or more), hematoma, seroma, necrosis, and wound dehiscence (Bath-Hextall, 2007). Prophylactic or postoperative antibiotics are used in cases considered to be at high risk of wound infection like complex procedures on the nose or ear (Elliott, Thom and Litterick, 2012). Bacterial wound infections require antibiotic treatment.

Nerve damage can be caused by surgical treatment and may be transient and reversible or permanent. Thorough knowledge of the anatomy, with special attention to known danger zones, is required to anticipate vital structures as they are approached. Transection of supratrochlear or supraorbital nerves or the mental nerve is less common and causes functional disability, which is usually permanent. Transection of the temporal branch of the facial nerve causes eyebrow droop, loss of normal forehead furrows, and the inability to raise the eyebrow. The consequences of motor nerve injury may be treated with reconstructive procedures to restore functionality, such as a brow lift or a blepharoplasty. In other cases, nerve anastomosis or transplantation may be indicated. Sensation is often at least partially restored within 6 months (Bath-Hextall, 2007).

REFERENCES

Bath-Hextall, F.J., et al., 2007. Interventions for basal cell carcinoma of the skin. *Cochrane Database of Systematic Reviews*, 1, p. CD003412.

Baxter, J.M., Patel, A.N. and Varma, S., 2012. Facial basal cell carcinoma. *BMJ*, 345, p. E5342.

Bolognia, J., Jorizzo, J.L. and Rapini, R.P., 2008. *Dermatology*. 2nd ed. In: J.L. Bolognia, J.L. Jorizzo, R.P. Rapini, eds.; associate and artwork editor, J.V. Schaffer. St. Louis, MO; London: Mosby Elsevier.

Elliott, T.G., Thom, G.A. and Litterick K.A., 2012. Office based dermatological surgery and Mohs surgery: a prospective audit of surgical procedures and complications in a procedural dermatology practice. *The Australasian Journal of Dermatology*, 53(4), pp. 264-71.

Finley, E.M., 2003. The principles of Mohs micrographic surgery for cutaneous neoplasia. *The Ochsner Journal*, 5(2), pp. 22-33.

Mohs, F.E., 1941. Chemosurgery: a microscopically controlled method of cancer excision. *Archives of Surgery*, 42(2), pp. 279-95.

Local Flaps for Facial Reconstruction

33

Sarah J Novis, Shan R Baker

Chapter Overview

Pearls and Pitfalls

Pearls

- In flap design, both the defect and tissue movement must be considered.
- Skin excisions and repairs are performed parallel to the relaxed skin tension lines (RSTLs) whenever possible to minimize the wound closure tension and optimize the appearance of scars.
- Aesthetic regions should be considered in flap design, and the preferred reconstruction often uses a flap within the same aesthetic region with incisions positioned along aesthetic borders.

Pitfalls

- Local flaps must have ample blood supply to survive. Inadequate blood supply can lead to flap loss.
- If the defect was caused by excision of a malignancy, it must be ensured that all tumors have been excised prior to reconstruction.
- Defects should be analyzed in terms of missing tissue layers. Each layer of absent tissue should ideally be replaced with like tissue to provide adequate support of the local flap. Failure to replace all layers may compromise the functional and/or aesthetic results.

A *local cutaneous flap* is as an area of skin and subcutaneous tissue with a direct vascular supply that is transferred from its in situ position to a site located immediately adjacent to or near the flap. Local flaps are an important part of *facial reconstruction*, and an understanding of flap physiology and biomechanics is necessary to achieve optimal wound repair. This chapter introduces principles of flap physiology and design, with a discussion of some select flaps and their uses in facial reconstruction.

33.1 PRINCIPLES OF FLAP DESIGN

Flap design is dependent on the intrinsic mechanical properties of skin. There are directional variations in skin extensibility, such that skin is more extensible when the vector of strain is in a certain direction (Larrabee, 1990). These vectors are referred to as the *lines of maximum extensibility* (LME). It is desirable to recruit skin along the LME for repair of skin defects. Perpendiculars to the LME are the RSTLs. The RSTL are the areas of the aging face, which manifest as skin creases or wrinkles and are caused by the orientation of collagen fibers in the skin. Skin excisions and repairs are performed parallel to the RSTL whenever possible to minimize the wound closure tension and optimize the appearance of scars.

In flap design, both the defect and tissue movement must be considered. The primary defect refers to the wound that is to be closed with a local cutaneous flap. Creation of a flap will result in a secondary defect at the donor site when the flap is transferred to repair the primary defect. The goal of flap design is to place the secondary defect in a favorable location, which is often accomplished by harvesting the flap from areas with greater skin laxity. The transfer of the flap to the defect is the primary tissue movement. This creates secondary movement, which displaces surrounding skin toward the center of the primary defect. Care must be taken to avoid distortion of adjacent mobile facial structures by secondary tissue movement. Facial structures such as the eyelids, lips, and nostrils, which have visible margins, are especially susceptible to distortion. Undermining the skin can reduce wound closure tension and distribute skin deformation more widely.

Blood supply is also an important consideration in flap design. It is essential for a local flap to have ample blood supply to survive. Local flaps are transferred with a pedicle, which provides the vascular supply to the flap. The pedicle can consist of skin, subcutaneous fat, muscle, or a combination of these. *Random pattern flaps* are supplied by the vascular plexus of the skin and do not have a named blood vessel supplying the flap. *Axial pattern flaps*, such as the paramedian forehead flap, depend on a named artery for the majority of their blood supply. The majority of local flaps described in this chapter are based on a random pattern blood supply.

The concept of aesthetic regions is important to flap design, as the aesthetic regions provide individual uniqueness to the face and are key to planning a reconstruction. *Aesthetic regions* are facial areas with similar skin characteristics, such as color, thickness, amount of subcutaneous fat, texture, and hair growth. The principle aesthetic regions of the face are the forehead, eyelids, cheeks, nose, lips, mentum, and auricles (Fig. 33.1). Aesthetic regions are separated by aesthetic borders, which consist of ridges or valleys created by the facial skeleton or musculature. Facial landmarks such as the anterior hairline, eyebrows, melolabial creases, vermilion border, and mental crease identify the aesthetic borders. Some of these regions with complex topography are further divided into *aesthetic units*. For example, the nose is divided into nine aesthetic units (Fig. 33.2) (Burget and Menick, 1985). When using local flaps, the preferred method of reconstruction is frequently to use a flap that can be designed within the same aesthetic region as the primary defect. Incisions are positioned along aesthetic borders whenever possible to minimize the appearance of scars. This means that some defects may be extended to an aesthetic border or in some cases enlarged to occupy an entire aesthetic unit. When a defect involves two or more aesthetic regions, it is often best to compartmentalize the repair and use skin flaps from each region to construct the separate components of the defect.

33.2 DEFECT ANALYSIS

Decisions regarding reconstruction must take multiple factors into consideration (Baker, 1994; Clevens and

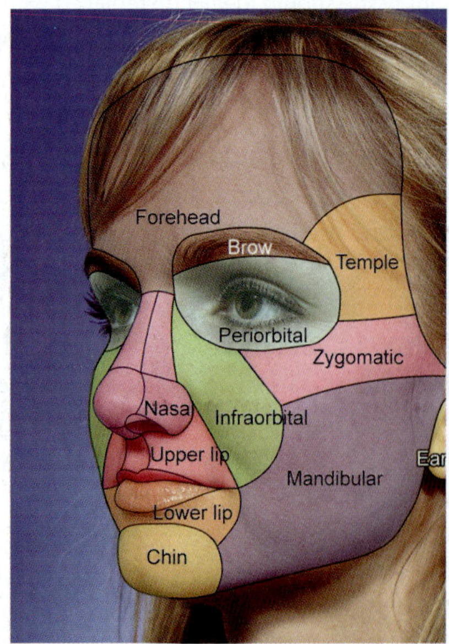

Fig. 33.1: Facial aesthetic regions.

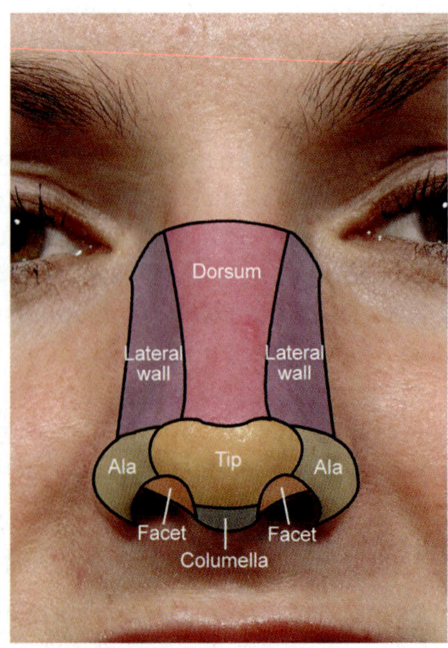

Fig. 33.2: Nasal aesthetic units.

Baker, 1997). If the defect was caused by excision of a malignancy, it must be ensured that all tumors have been excised. Similarly, risk of recurrence must be considered, which may alter the recommended reconstruction. In consideration of the repair, the defect must first be carefully evaluated in terms of its missing tissue layers, topography, and aesthetic region or unit involvement. Ideally, each layer of absent tissue should be replaced with like tissue.

33.3 TYPES OF LOCAL FLAPS

Multiple methods for classifying local flaps exist, including those based on blood supply, location, configuration, and method of transfer or movement. In this chapter, flaps will be discussed in relation to their method of movement.

Advancement Flaps

Advancement flaps involve linear movement of the flap toward the defect. There is some stretching of the skin in advancement flaps, making them best suited to areas of greater skin elasticity. While the simple linear closure is an example of an advancement flap, with side-to-side movement to close the defect, this requires no additional incisions or excision of standing cutaneous deformities. Advancement flaps most often involve incisions to allow for sliding movement of tissue in a single vector. This results in the distal border of the flap having the greatest wound closure tension. Advancement flaps for facial reconstruction may be categorized as unipedicle, bipedicle, V-Y/Y-V, and island flaps. Bipedicle advancement flaps are used infrequently in facial reconstruction and will not be discussed further in this chapter.

Unipedicle Advancement Flaps

Unipedicle advancement flaps are created by parallel incisions, which allow a sliding movement of tissue in a single vector toward a defect. The flap is created adjacent to the defect with one border of the defect becoming the leading border of the flap. It is important to undermine the soft tissue around the pedicle to facilitate movement. Unipedicled advancement flaps create two standing cutaneous deformities, unlike pivotal flaps, which only create one. These deformities are due to unequal lengths of the borders of the wound. This length mismatch can be corrected by creating triangular skin excisions along the periphery of the wound (Burow's triangle) or alternatively by distributing the redundant tissue evenly over the length of the repair in cases of minimal mismatch. The standing cutaneous deformity (SCD) can be excised anywhere along the length of advancement flaps, allowing for placement of excisions in RSTL or in borders between aesthetic regions. Bilateral unipedicle advancement flaps are often designed on opposite sides of a defect to advance toward each other, creating an H- or T-shaped wound closure (H-plasty or T-plasty). The two flaps can be of different lengths, with the flap length determined by the elasticity and redundancy of tissue at the donor site. Bilateral advancement flaps are commonly used in reconstruction of forehead defects as they produce good aesthetic results when incisions for the flaps are placed in the horizontal forehead creases or along the border of the eyebrow (Figs. 33.3A to C). Bilateral advancement flaps can also be used for reconstruction of central lip defects with incisions for the flaps placed along the vermilion-cutaneous border and either the nasal sill or mental crease.

V-Y and Y-V Advancement Flaps

The *V-Y advancement flap* is unique from other facial flaps in that the V-shaped flap achieves its advancement by recoiling rather than by being pulled forward into the defect. This makes V-Y advancement flaps especially useful for lengthening or release from a contracted state. The affected or distorted area of skin is incorporated into the V-shaped flap, and the skin borders adjacent to both sides of the secondary defect are then advanced toward each other and sutured, forming a Y-configuration of the suture line (Figs. 33.4A to D). The V-Y flap may also be designed as an island flap, which is discussed later in this chapter.

The *Y-V advancement flap* involves creation of a V-shaped flap, which is stretched or pulled toward a linear incision made at the apex of the triangular flap. The flap is advanced into this linear incision and closed in a V-configuration, leaving the maximum wound closure tension at the apex of the flap.

Pivotal Flaps

Pivotal flaps are moved toward the defect by moving the flap around a fixed point at the base of the pedicle. Pivotal flaps can be classified as four types: rotation, transposition, interpolated, and island. Except for island flaps skeletonized to their nutrient vessels, the flap becomes shorter as the angle of the pivot increases. A 90° pivot reduces the effective length by 15% and a 180° pivot reduces the effective length by 40% (Gorney, 1977). This

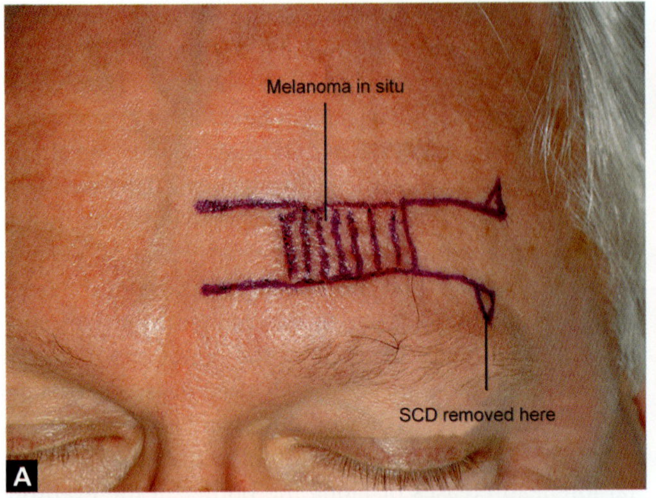

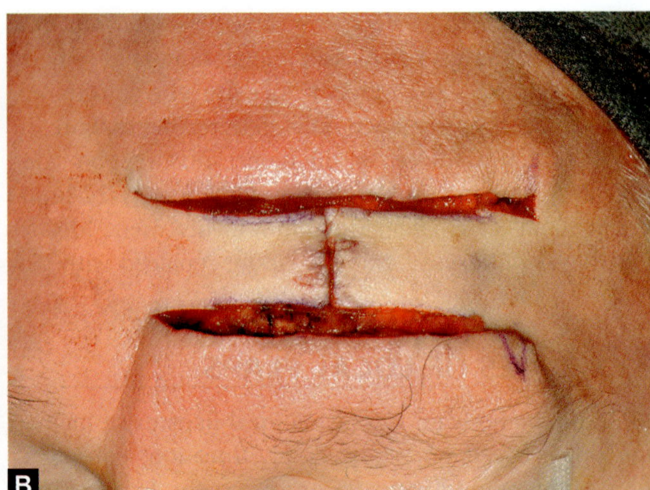

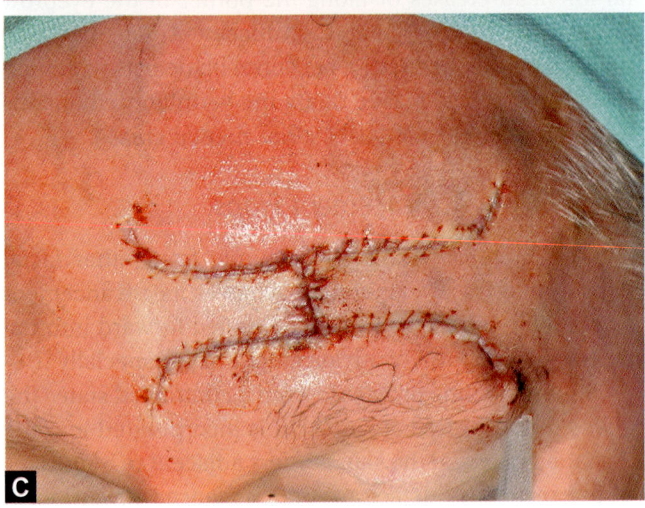

Figs. 33.3A to C: (A) Melanoma in situ. Bilateral advancement flaps designed for repair (H-plasty). (B and C) Melanoma excised and wound repaired.

decrease in length must be accounted for when designing the flap. In addition, pivoting of the flap around a fixed point results in an SCD, which increases in size with a greater degree of pivoting. For this reason, it is recommended to limit the arc of pivot to 90° whenever possible.

Rotation Flaps

Rotation flaps are pivotal flaps with a curvilinear configuration (Figs. 33.5A and B). These flaps are best suited to closure of triangular defects, as a portion of the SCD is used to cover the defect. The wound closure tension of rotational flaps depends on the amount of advancement incorporated in the flap. The component of advancement will create a vector of greatest wound closure tension from the base of the flap to a distal point of the curvilinear border. When no advancement is utilized, the greatest wound closure tension is perpendicular to the periphery of the flap rather than across its length (Larrabee, 1990). These tension vectors can be changed by creating a back cut at the base of the flap, which shifts the position of the pivotal point and thus changes both the wound closure tension as well as the location of the SCD. Care must be taken to position the distal tip of the flap so that it is not subjected to excessive wound closure tension and vascular compromise.

Rotation flaps have inherent discrepancy between the length of the flap's border compared to the length of the primary and secondary defect. It is often necessary to equalize this discrepancy by excising a Burow's triangle along the periphery of the curvilinear incision. Another solution to the length discrepancy is to change the movement of the flap from one that is purely pivotal to one that is both pivotal and advancement. Stretching the flap will lengthen the flap border so that it approaches the sum length of the primary and secondary defect. When

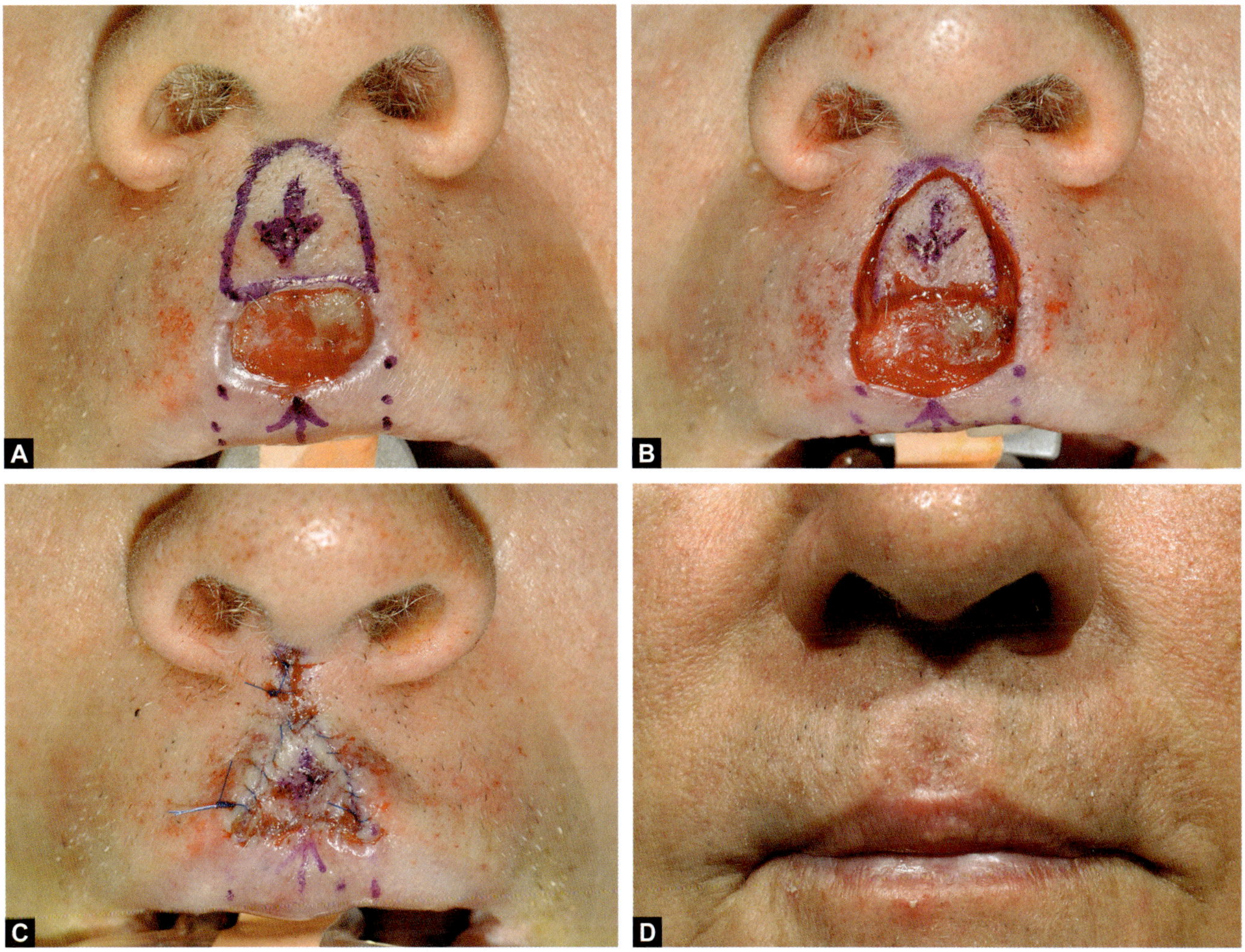

Figs. 33.4A to D: (A) 1.0 x 0.75 cm cutaneous defect of the upper lip. V-Y island advancement flap designed for repair. (B and C) Flap incised and advanced into recipient site. (D) Three months postoperative.

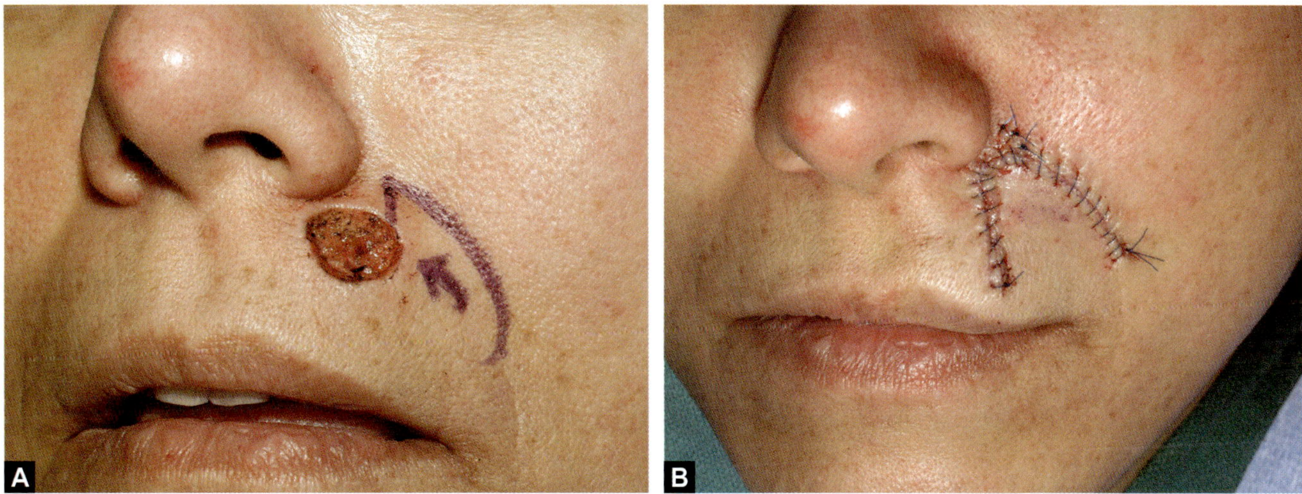

Figs. 33.5A and B: (A) 1.5 x 1.0 cm cutaneous defect of the upper lip. Rotation flap designed for repair. (B) Flap in place.

designing rotation flaps for facial reconstruction, the length of the curvilinear border of the flap should be four times the width of the defect. The defect's shape should ideally have a triangular configuration with a height to width ratio of 2:1. In addition, the height of the triangular defect should be 0.5–1 times the radius of the curve of the flap to make the arc of the flap's incision a completely symmetrical curve. Rotation flaps are commonly used for reconstruction of scalp defects as well as lateral lip defects and large defects of the lateral cheek.

Transposition Flaps

Transposition flaps are the most commonly used flaps in facial reconstruction. Transposition flaps are pivotal flaps, which have a linear configuration in contrast to the curvilinear configuration of rotation flaps. Transposition flaps may be designed like rotation flaps so that one border of the flap is also a border of the defect. It may also be designed with borders that are removed from the defect so that only the base of the flap is continuous with the defect (Figs. 33.6A to D). The area of greatest wound closure tension is at the closure site of the secondary defect adjacent to the base of the flap, but it can vary depending on the amount of stretching. The versatility of transposition flaps arises from the ability to construct a flap at some distance from the defect with its axis independent from the linear axis of the defect. This allows recruitment of skin at variable distances from the defect, and selection of donor sites with the greatest skin elasticity or redundancy. This also allows selection of a variable harvest site to provide the best possible scar camouflage or to hide

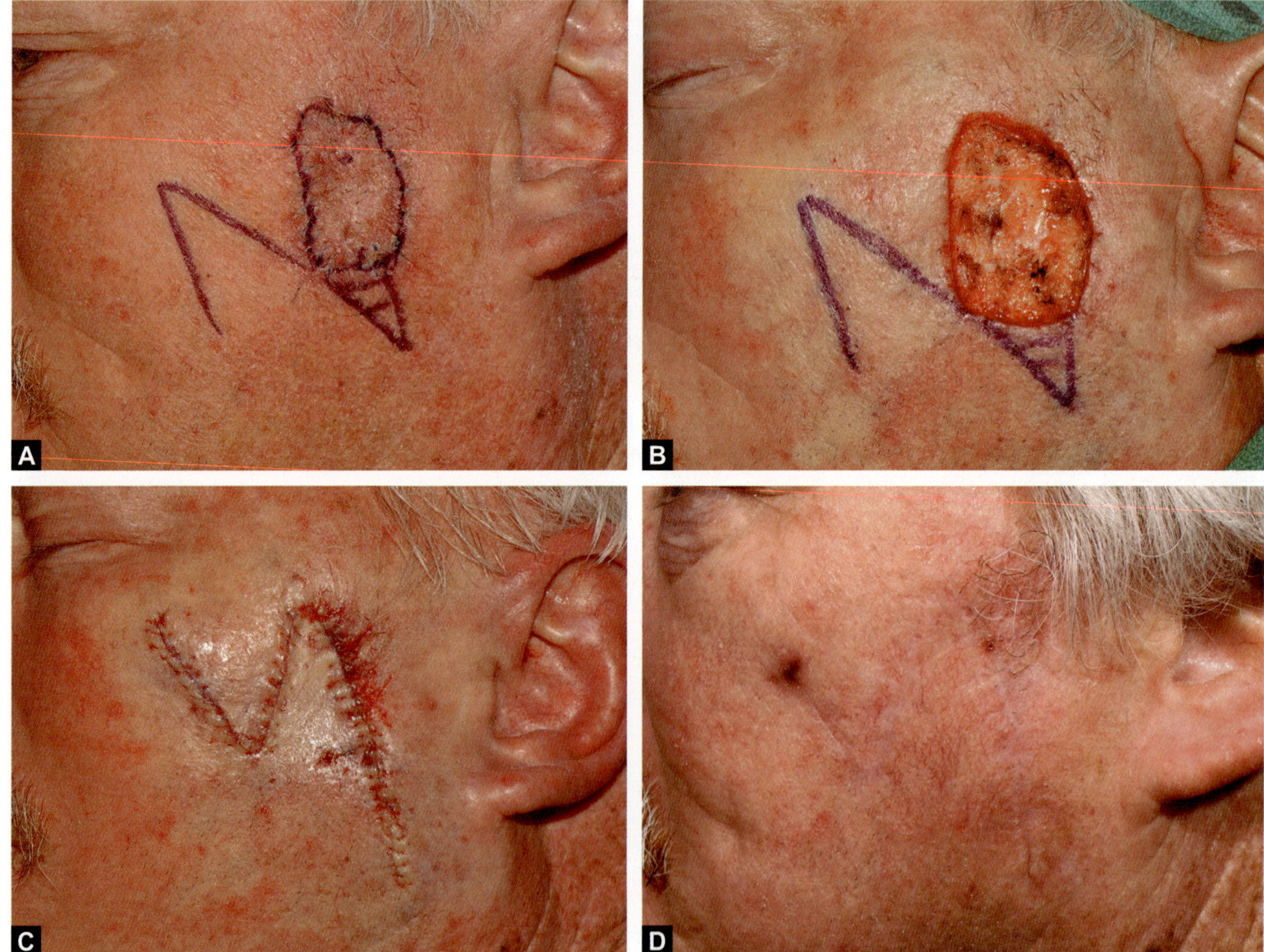

Figs. 33.6A to D: (A) 3 x 2 cm melanoma in situ outlined for excision. Transposition flap designed for wound repair following excision. Anticipated standing cutaneous deformity marked for excision (horizontal lines). (B and C) Melanoma excision and flap transferred to recipient site. (D) Two months postoperative.

the scar in aesthetic borders. The bilobed and rhombic flaps are common types of transposition flaps, which will be discussed in further detail.

Rhombic flaps are based on a defect that is an equilateral parallelogram. The defect must be modified to form a rhombus with angles of 60° and 120°. The flap is designed by first extending a line that bisects the 120° angle and is equal in length to one of the sides of the defect. A second line is drawn parallel to one of the adjacent borders of the defect and is again equal to all other sides. This configuration gives four potential flaps that can be designed for any rhombic defect. The preferred flap must be selected based on wound closure tension and placement of the resulting scar (Park and Little, 2007). The major disadvantage of rhombic flaps is that approximately half of the resulting scar line is not parallel to the RSTL. Rhombic flaps are used mostly in cheek reconstruction, as this area has thin skin and less prominent creases, allowing for better aesthetic results (Figs. 33.7A to C).

Bilobed flaps are double transposition flaps that share a single base. Bilobed flaps function as modified Z-plasties that result in greater distribution of wound closure tension than single lobe transposition flaps. Each lobe of the flap has a separate pivot point, giving each an SCD. In classic bilobed flaps, the axis of each lobe is separated by an angle of 90°, but the modified bilobed flap most commonly used in nasal reconstruction consists of two lobes separated by 45° (Zitelli, 1989). Bilobed flaps are often used for both nasal and cheek reconstruction, with excellent results (Figs. 33.8A to D).

Interpolated Flaps

Interpolated flaps also are transferred by pivotal movement and have a linear confirmation but differ from transposition flaps in that their base is not contiguous with the defect. This requires that the pedicle of an interpolated flap crosses over or under the intervening tissue. Pedicles

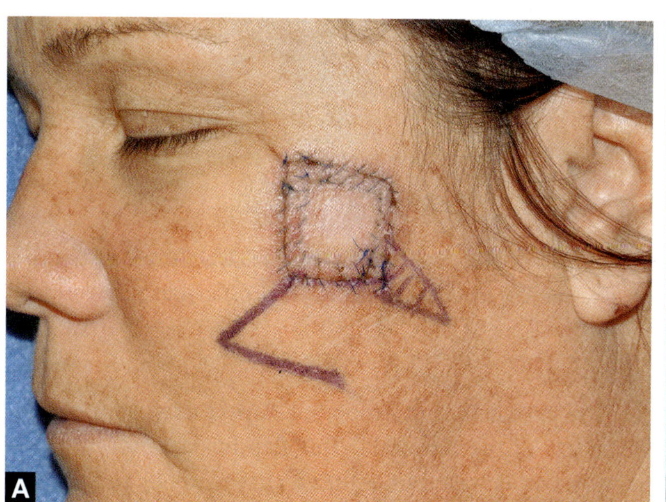

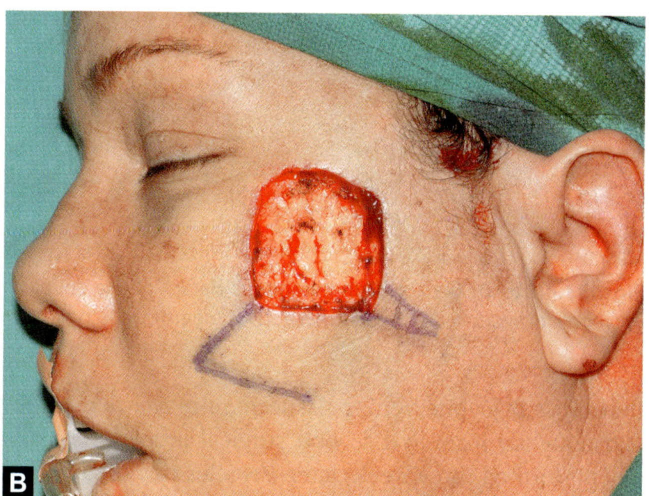

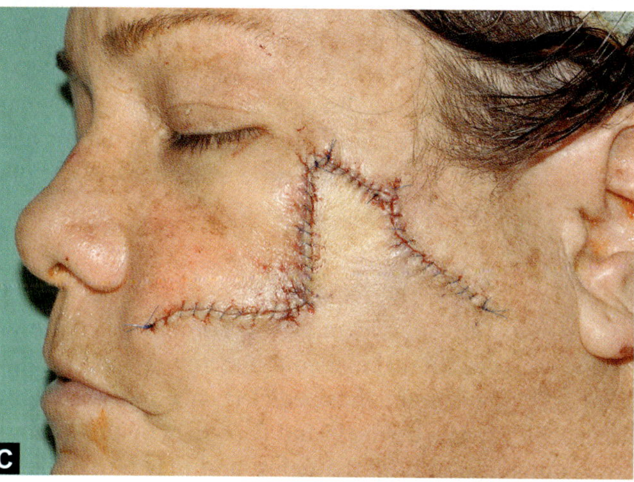

Figs. 33.7A to C: (A) 3 x 3 cm melanoma in situ outlined by sutures. Rhombic flap designed for repair of wound following excision of melanoma. (B and C) Melanoma excised. Flap transferred to recipient site.

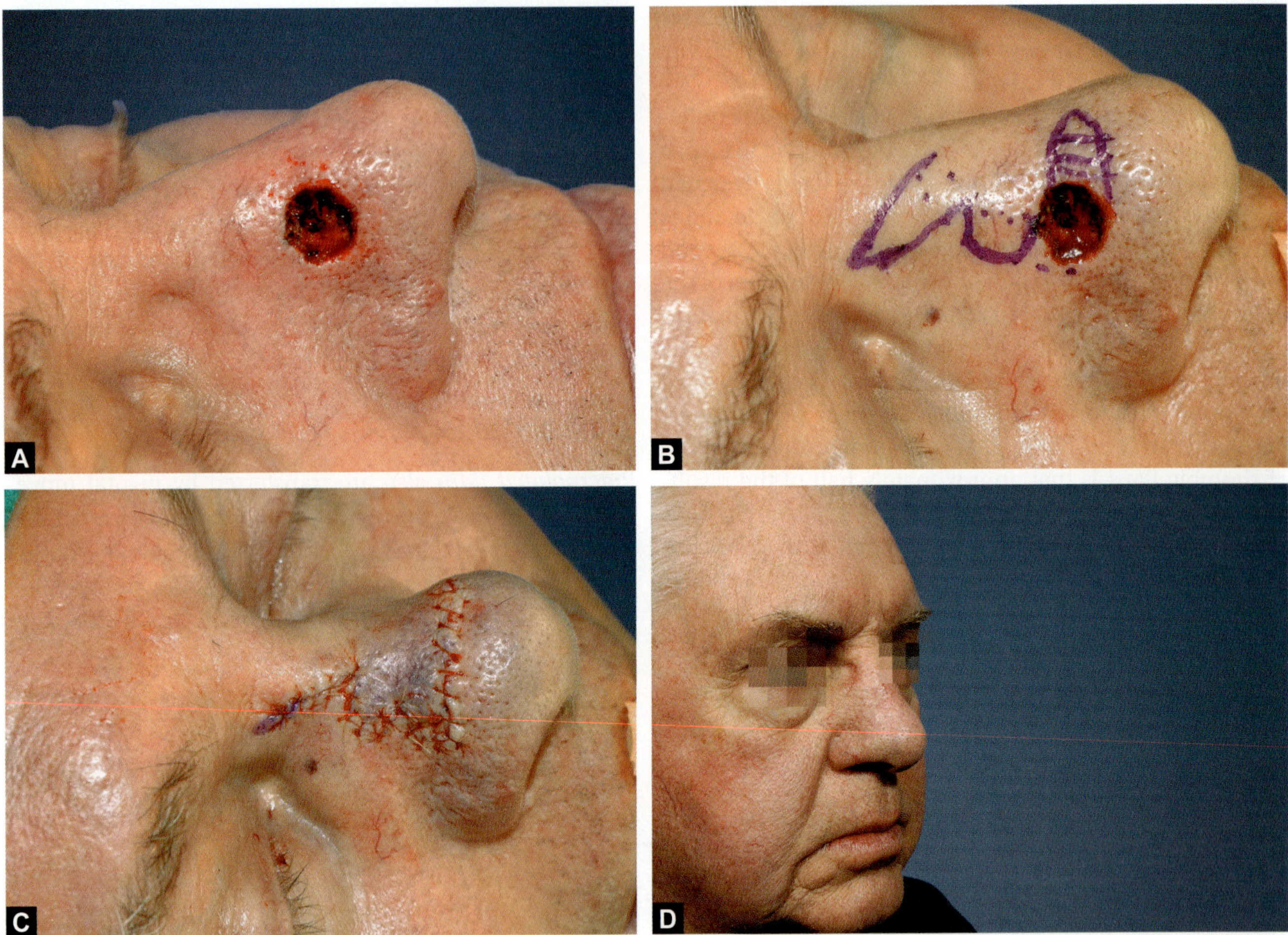

Figs. 33.8A to D: (A) 1 x 1 cm cutaneous defect of the caudal nasal sidewall. (B) Medially based bilobed cutaneous flap designed for repair of wound. (C) Flap in place. (D) Three months postoperative.

that cross over intervening tissue require the flap to be subsequently inset in a second surgical procedure, usually performed three weeks later. Pedicles can sometimes be de-epithelialized and brought under the intervening skin as an island flap to allow for single-staged reconstruction, but this may compromise the vascular pedicle or create a contour deformity. The two most commonly used interpolated flaps are the *paramedian forehead flap* and the *melolabial flap*.

The paramedian forehead flap is used for reconstruction of large nasal defects and is based on an axial blood supply from the supratrochlear artery and vein (Figs. 33.9A to G). These vessels are located in the subcutaneous tissue plane and extend along the axis of the flap. They provide ample blood supply to the skin and allow for flap thinning cephalic to the level of the eyebrow, enabling better nasal contouring (Menick, 1990; Baker and Ashford, 1993).

The melolabial interpolated flap is useful for reconstruction of the nasal ala. This flap has a random blood supply and is based on either a cutaneous or subcutaneous pedicle. Given the random blood supply, the cheek flap cannot be safely thinned of as much of its subcutaneous tissue as the forehead flap. The cheek flap is ideal for nasal ala reconstruction as it crosses over, rather than through, the intervening alar facial sulcus so that the aesthetic boundary between the nose and cheek is not distorted (Figs. 33.10A to I).

Island Flaps

Island flaps are incised along all borders to create an island of skin with no cutaneous attachments to the adjacent skin. The island flap is pedicled only on the underlying subcutaneous tissue. Island flaps may be designed in any configuration to fit the defect and may have a linear

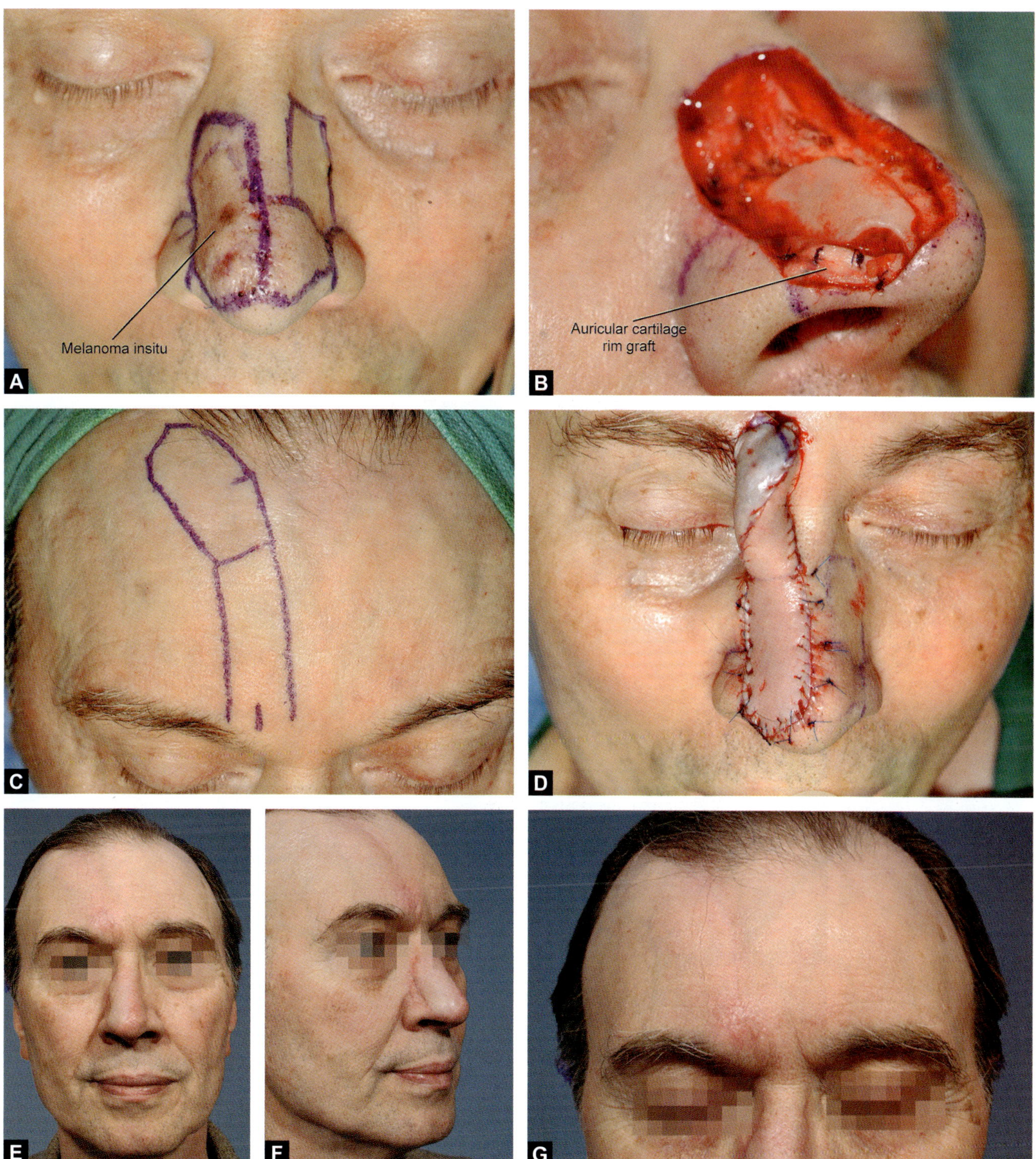

Figs. 33.9A to G: (A) Melanoma in situ marked for excision. (B) Melanoma excised. Auricular cartilage rim graft placed caudal to alar cartilage for structural support. (C) Interpolated paramedian forehead flap designed for repair of nose. (D) Flap in place. (E and F) Six months postoperative following flap inset. (G) Forehead donor site after 6 months.

or nonlinear axis depending on their shape. Island flaps may be transferred by advancement or pivoting and can be classified as either type of flap depending on the movement. Island advancement flaps are commonly

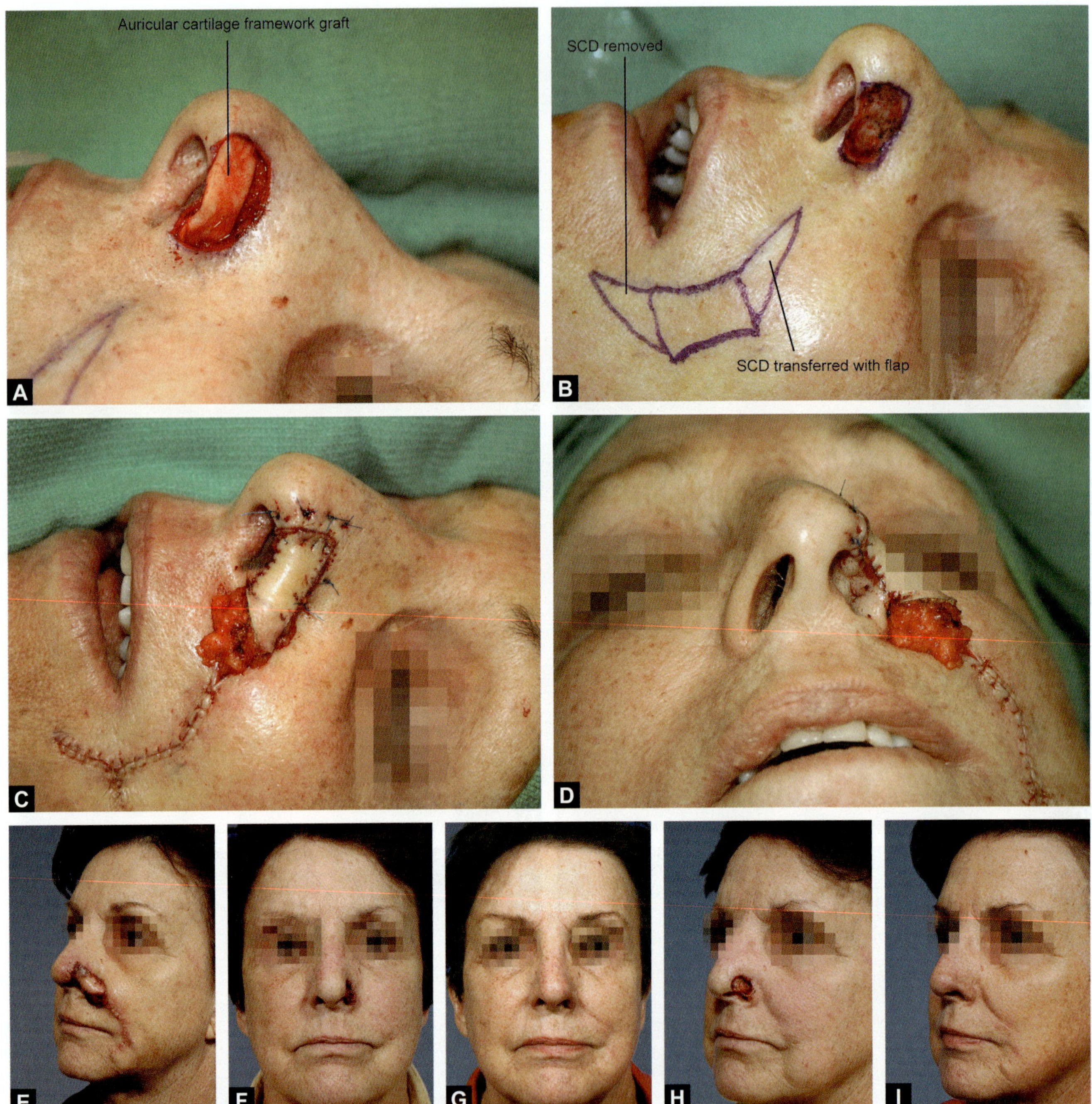

Figs. 33.10A to I: (A) Cutaneous defect of left ala. Auricular cartilage framework graft in place. (B) Interpolated subcutaneous tissue pedicled melolabial flap designed for wound repair. Anticipated standing cutaneous deformities (SCD) following donor site closure marked. Inferior SCD excised, superior SCD travels with flap pedicle. (C and D) Flap in place. (E) One week postoperative following first surgical stage. (F to I) Preoperative and 6 months postoperative.

used in facial reconstruction and are useful for both lateral upper lip defects and medial cheek defects adjacent to the nasal ala (Figs. 33.11A to D). The most commonly used pivotal island flaps are for nasal defects and consist of either cheek or forehead skin.

Hinge Flaps

Cutaneous *hinge flaps* are often used for reconstruction of facial defects that require both external and internal lining surfaces. Hinge flaps are designed in a linear or

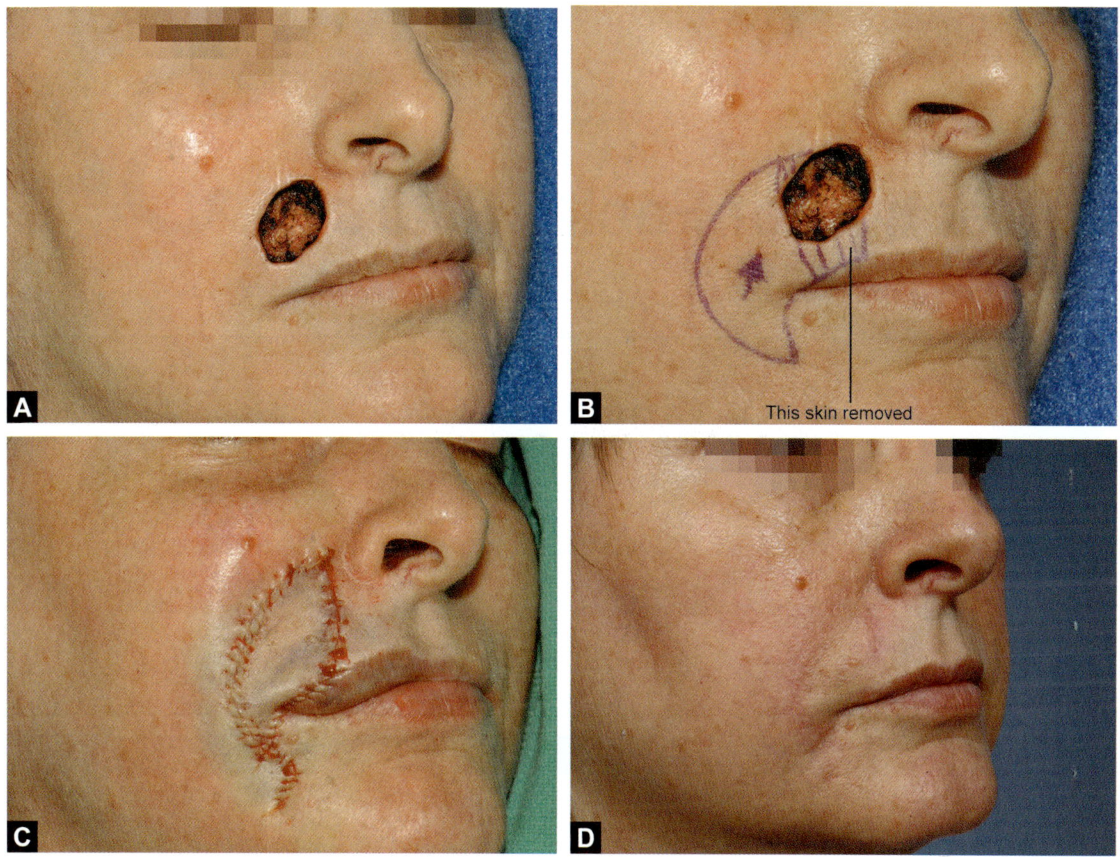

Figs. 33.11A to D: (A) 2 x 2 cm cutaneous defect of the lateral lip. (B) V-Y subcutaneous tissue pedicled advancement flap designed for repair. (C) Flap in place. (D) Three months postoperative.

curvilinear shape with the pedicle based on one border of the primary defect. The flap is dissected in the subcutaneous plane and turned over into the defect like a page in a book. A second flap or graft is necessary to provide coverage of the secondary defect, as well as the exposed surface of the hinge flap. Hinge flaps are commonly used for repair of full-thickness nasal defects in which the nasal skin adjacent to the defect is sufficient to develop a flap for internal nasal lining (Burget and Menick, 1989; Johnson, et al., 1994; Baker, 2011).

REFERENCES

Baker, S.R., 1994. Local cutaneous flaps. *Otolaryngologic Clinics of North America*, 27(1), pp. 139-59.

Baker, S.R., 2011. *Principles of nasal reconstruction*. 2nd ed. New York: Springer.

Baker, S.R. and Ashford, E.L., 1993. Mid-forehead flaps. *Operative Techniques in Otolaryngology—Head and Neck Surgery*, 4, pp. 24-30.

Burget, G.C. and Menick, F.J., 1985. The subunit principle in nasal reconstruction. *Plastic and Reconstructive Surgery*, 76(2), pp. 239-47.

Burget, G.C. and Menick, F.J., 1989. Nasal support and lining: the marriage of beauty and blood supply. *Plastic and Reconstructive Surgery*, 84(2), pp. 189-202.

Clevens, R.A. and Baker, S.R., 1997. Conceptual considerations in head & neck reconstruction. Defect analysis and options for reconstruction. *Otolaryngologic Clinics of North America*, 30(4), pp. 495-517.

Gorney, M., 1977. Tissue dynamics and surgical geometry. In: L.M. Vistnes, D.A. Kernakan, eds. *Biological aspects of reconstructive surgery*. Boston: Little and Brown.

Johnson, T.M., Baker, S., Brown, M.D. and Nelson, B.R., 1994. Utility of the subcutaneous hinge flap in nasal reconstruction. *Journal of American Academy of Dermatology*, 30(3), pp. 459-66.

Larrabee, W.F., Jr., 1990. Design of local skin flaps. *Otolaryngologic Clinics of North America*, 23(5), pp. 899-923.

Menick, F.J., 1990. Aesthetic refinements in use of forehead for nasal reconstruction: the paramedian forehead flap. *Clinics in Plastic Surgery*, 17(4), pp. 607-22.

Park, S.S. and Little, S., 2007. Rhombic flaps. In: S.R. Baker, ed. *Local flaps in facial reconstruction*. 2nd ed. St Louis: Mosby. pp. 151-63.

Zitelli, J.A., 1989. The bilobed flap for nasal reconstruction. *Archives of Dermatology*, 125(7), pp. 957-9.

34 Correction of Facial Scars

Michael G Brandt, Corey C Moore

Chapter Overview

Pearls and Pitfalls

Pearls

- Respectful tissue handling, revision of desiccated wound edges, meticulous reapproximation of tissue layers, maintaining overall wound cleanliness, and avoiding mechanical reinjury are core principles in achieving optimal scars.
- Avoid wound tension and maintain wound moisture.
- Hypertrophic scars can be improved through the use of silicone gel or silicone sheeting, compression therapy, and intralesional injection of triamcinolone.
- Keloid scars require excision with regular postoperative intralesional triamcinolone injections.
- Mild-to-moderate scar depression, wound edge misalignment, and texture irregularity can be improved with resurfacing techniques.
- Moderate-to-severe intrinsically and extrinsically unsatisfactory scars require scar revision (fusiform excision, irregularization, and/or reorientation).

Pitfalls

- En vogue scar therapies with limited empiric evidence.
- Resorting to expensive (i.e. laser) or potentially dangerous (i.e. external beam radiotherapy) treatments without trialing conservative and well-established techniques first.

34.1 INTRODUCTION

With substantial implications on self-esteem and social functioning, the morbidity of a facial scar extends far deeper than the skin. Predictably, both patients and surgeons seek to optimize facial scaring. This chapter provides an overview of wound healing and contemporary means of optimizing scar outcomes.

34.2 SKIN ANATOMY—KEY POINTS (BICHAKJIAN AND JOHNSON, 2007)

- *Skin* is composed of three layers: epidermis, dermis, and subcutaneous tissue (superficial to deep).
- Epidermis is composed of five layers: stratum corneum, stratum lucidum, stratum granulosum, stratum spinosum, stratum basale (superficial to deep).

    - Stratum spinosum contains squamous cells and is the site of origin of cutaneous squamous cell carcinoma.
    - Stratum basale contains basal keratinocyte cells, melanocytes, Langerhans cells, and Merkel cells—it is the site of origin of basal cell carcinoma and malignant melanoma.
- Dermis has two layers: Papillary dermis and Reticular dermis.
    - *Papillary dermis* contains mostly collagen.
    - *Reticular dermis* contains thicker collagen, elastin, hair follicles and their associated sweat and apocrine glands, eccrine glands, blood vessels, and nerves.
    - Skin injuries that extend below the superficial part of the reticular dermis result in fibrotic permanent scarring (Dunkin, et al., 2007).
- Subcutaneous layer is composed mainly of fat, connective tissue, blood vessels, and nerves.

34.3 NORMAL WOUND-HEALING PATHOPHYSIOLOGY

Wound-healing pathophysiology is important to the understanding of facial skin scarring. A comprehensive discussion of wound healing is however beyond the scope of this chapter and is well described elsewhere (Hebda, 2009; Leong and Philips, 2012). This chapter will focus on a brief overview of this topic as it pertains to facial skin scarring.

Wound healing occurs via three phases: inflammation, proliferation, and maturation. Wounds closed by primary intention (i.e. sutured together) will heal promptly through these three phases, whereas wounds that heal by secondary intention (i.e. allowed to granulate) will have a protracted proliferative phase.

The inflammatory phase of wound healing involves the initial attainment of hemostasis and a reactive period lasting for approximately 5 days. During this time the wound experiences increased vascular permeability, migration of cells by chemotaxis, secretion of cytokines and growth factors, and activation of the migrating cells (Leong and Philips, 2012).

The proliferative phase of wound healing typically begins on the 4th day following injury—overlapping partly with the inflammatory phase (Leong and Philips, 2012). This phase persists for approximately 2 weeks (Leong and Philips, 2012). As the inflammatory phase comes to an end, wound repair begins to occur through angiogenesis, fibroplasia, and epithelialization (Leong and Philips, 2012). Granulation tissue is the hallmark of this phase and is composed of a capillary bed, fibroblasts, macrophages, and loose arrangement of collagen, fibronectin, and hyaluronic acid (Leong and Philips, 2012). Although not entirely isolated to this issue, excessive fibroplasia/collagen formation during this phase can result in hypertrophic or keloid scarring.

The maturation phase of wound healing begins to occur 1 week postinjury and persists for many months thereafter (Leong and Philips, 2012). Scars mature for up to 12 months. During this time synthesized collagen is reorganized, the wound contracts, and rapidly gains in overall strength. A skin wound achieves 10% of its preinjury strength at 2 weeks, 20% strength at 3 weeks, 40% at 4 weeks, 70% at 6 weeks, and plateaus at approximately 80% strength at 12 months (Levenson, et al., 1965).

34.4 EVIDENCE-BASED TECHNIQUES TO IMPROVE SCAR OUTCOMES

While the scar evaluation and outcome literature are fraught with inconsistent evaluation tools (Brandt, et al., 2009), a scar is generally considered "acceptable" if it is well camouflaged relative to its surrounding skin. It is typically narrow, in the same vertical plane as the surrounding skin, parallel to relaxed skin tension lines (RSTLs), masked within natural anatomic wrinkles and creases, or located at natural junctions between facial aesthetic units. Numerous techniques have been employed to improve scar outcomes with various degrees of efficacy demonstrated. Only those measures with reasonable empiric support and/or minimal morbidity will be reviewed here.

Primary closure of a wound is the first step in achieving optimized scar outcomes. Respectful tissue handling, revision of lacerated or fragmented wound edges, meticulous reapproximation of tissue layers, maintaining overall wound cleanliness, and avoiding mechanical reinjury (friction, scratching) of the wound are core principles in achieving optimal scars (Marcus, 2007; Ogawa, 2010). Reducing skin stretch tension (i.e. tension across a wound) is an important first step in minimizing the risk of wide, hypertrophic, or keloid scarring (Ogawa, et al., 2012). Intraoperative methods of decreasing wound tension include undermining and layered wound closure.

Table 34.1: Initial wound-healing strategies.
Optimize systemic factors
Primary meticulous wound closure
Postoperative wound taping, occlusion, and moisture maintenance for 7 days
Silicone gel/sheeting, ultraviolet protection, and scar massage

Postoperative wound taping and/or the use of topical silicone gel/sheeting may result in a lower incidence of hypertrophic or keloid scarring (Ogawa, 2010). Maintaining wound moisture and occlusion until epithelialization is complete are additional techniques with demonstrated efficacy in speeding overall wound healing and may be especially valuable for skin grafts or in wounds that heal via secondary intention (Chaby, et al., 2007). The same principle holds true for healing by primary intention. A moist environment is essential for normal proliferation and migration of epithelial cells across the wound edges. Crusting on the wound surface due to drying impairs wound edge reapproximation, epithelialization, and leads to unfavorable scars. Although frequently employed and anecdotally supported, scar massage is not yet evidence based (Shin and Bordeaux, 2012). Scar massage is however benign and may empower the patient in providing them with a therapy they can employ themselves and is thus a reasonable option in the management of postsurgical scarring.

It is prudent to recognize that wound healing does not occur in isolation, and the patient must be optimized to ensure proper skin repair. Accordingly, patients should be encouraged to maintain adequate nutrition, control chronic systemic illness (i.e. diabetes and renal failure), minimize medications that may inhibit healing (i.e. isotretinoin, corticosteroids, and aspirin), and minimize exposure to nicotine (Hom and Dresner, 2009). Judicious sun (ultraviolet) protection is an important routine practice, but also essential to the prevention of permanent wound pigment changes (Velangi and Rees, 2001) (Table 34.1).

34.5 UNSATISFACTORY AND PATHOLOGIC SCARRING

Poor scar outcomes are multifactorial and occur due to both intrinsic and extrinsic features to the scar itself (Table 34.2). Unsatisfactory intrinsic features to a scar influence its general appearance, i.e. how thin/thick a scar appears. Extrinsic features relate to the location and position of the scar, i.e. parallel to RSTLs, within an aesthetic facial unit, etc. Numerous techniques and strategies have been employed that influence intrinsic and extrinsic features of a scar with the overall goal of improving scar camouflage. These techniques will be discussed in turn.

The first step in evaluating an unacceptable scar is determining if the scar is intrinsically pathologic, i.e. hypertrophic, keloid, or an unrecognized malignancy. Distinguishing a hypertrophic from a keloid scar can be challenging, especially if the scar is the presenting illness and not simply the result of a previous surgical intervention in the ongoing care of a well-known patient. By definition, a hypertrophic scar is a fibroproliferative disorder of the skin that does *not* grow beyond the boundaries of the original wound, whereas a keloid does grow beyond the boundaries of the original wound or has an unrecognized origin (Ogawa, 2010). Clinically, if the scar in question is suspicious of pathology (hypertrophy, keloid, or possibly a cutaneous malignancy), an incisional or punch biopsy is prudent in directing its subsequent management. Histologically, a keloid can be distinguished from

Table 34.2: Factors impacting on scar acceptability.

Intrinsic factors

- Pathologic scars:
  - Hypertrophic scars
  - Keloid scars
  - Unrecognized skin pathology and/or malignancy
- Nonpathologic scars:
  - Iatrogenic:
    - Misaligned wound edges
    - Trap-door deformities
    - Evidence of surgery (i.e. suture marks)
  - Consequence of normal wound healing:
    - Wide scar
    - Discoloration relative to surrounding skin
    - Raised/depressed scar
    - Texture/surface irregularities

Extrinsic factors

- Scar location—anatomic structure, position relative to aesthetic units/subunits
- Scar position—angle relative to relaxed skin tension lines
- Distortion of surrounding anatomic structures (dynamically or at rest)

a hypertrophic scar due to the presence of thick eosinophilic (hyalinizing) collagen bundles (Ogawa, 2010). Once the scar pathology has been determined, actions can be taken to improve its overall outcome.

Hypertrophic and Keloid Scars

Ogawa (2010) presented an evidence-based algorithm for the management of hypertrophic and keloid scarring. Prevention is of primary paramount importance and can occur through the methods previously described—minimizing wound tension, avoiding mechanical reinjury, etc. Failing preventative techniques, a hypertrophic scar will improve naturally over the course of a year. Evidence-based noninvasive methods to accelerate hypertrophic scar maturation include the application of silicone gel/silicone sheet and the use of compression therapy (Ogawa, 2010). Invasive techniques including intralesional injection of triamcinolone, or the use of pulsed dye laser (PDL) therapy, may assist in the regression of hypertrophic scarring (Ogawa, 2010).

Triamcinolone injections are a mainstay therapy in the management of hypertrophic scarring and are thought to work through the inhibition of proliferating fibroblasts, the enhancement of collagenase production, and the reduction in collagenase inhibitors (Cupp and Gaball, 2012). The injection is placed at the level of the dermis within the thick portion of the scar. Resistance to injection is the rule, and pressure is typically needed during the first series of injections. A starting conservative concentration of 10 mg/mL is reasonable and is repeated every 4–6 weeks for 3–6 months. Judicious use of triamcinolone is important, with most facial scars unable to accommodate volumes > 1 mL. Blanching of the scar is common during the injections and is not a worrisome feature. Injections are painful and can be reduced with the application of an icepack to the region prior to injection. Anecdotally, patients report decreased discomfort with repeated injections (likely due to improved scar compliance and patient's experience). It is important to recognize that triamcinolone injections are not without risk, and the development of telangiectasias, skin thinning, and lipoatrophy (if injected into the subcutaneous tissue) may occur.

Pulsed dye laser 585-nm therapy has demonstrated inconsistent efficacy in improving hypertrophic scarring (Ogawa, 2011). Some evidence exists that PDL therapy reduces scar erythema, scar volume, and overall texture (Elsaie and Choudhary, 2010). Typical treatment protocols involve one to two treatments at an energy of 4.5–5.5 J/cm^2 at a spot size of 10 mm, 6–7 J/cm^2 at a spot size of 7 mm, or 6.5–7.5 J/cm^2 at a spot size of 5 mm (Elsaie and Choudhary, 2010). Adverse effects include temporary purpura and scar hyperpigmentation among dark-skinned patients (Elsaie and Choudhary, 2010). Given the limited adverse effects, PDL therapy can be considered in the management of hypertrophic scars with more quality empiric evaluations needed to support it as a foundational therapy.

Keloid therapy is quite divergent from the treatment of *hypertrophic scars* with noninvasive therapies demonstrating minimal efficacy (Ogawa, 2010). Facial keloids tend to be focal and isolated and are thus amendable to therapy (Ogawa, 2010). Treatment tends to involve surgical removal with adjuvant therapy or nonsurgical therapies. Nonsurgical therapies include the use of intralesional corticosteroids, cryotherapy, radiation, and injectable and topical antitumor/immunosuppressive agents (Ogawa, 2010). While the use of the above therapies individually as monotherapies have demonstrated efficacy, combined multimodal treatments are synergistically more efficacious. Of the treatments suggested, surgery with postoperative intralesional triamcinolone has been the most thoroughly investigated and widely practiced. The keloid is excised and the wound is closed as per the techniques previously discussed. At the time of wound closure, 40-mg/mL *triamcinolone* is injected along the wound edges to a maximum of 120 mg (3 cc). The region is then reinjected at 4- to 6-week intervals for a period of 3–6 months. Long-term studies have demonstrated a 50% recurrence at 5 years when using this protocol (Ogawa, 2010). Additional multimodal intralesional injections of 5-fluorouracil (5-FU), bleomycin, and mitomycin-C have demonstrated some efficacy beyond that of intralesional triamcinolone but with less empiric evidence to suggest routine use.

Of the antimetabolic agents, 5-FU has received the most attention. The 5-FU is an antimetabolic agent, which appears to impair fibroblast collagen synthesis while not affecting general protein synthesis (Cupp and Gaball, 2012). The most efficacious described treatment protocol involves injecting 50 mg of 5-FU diluted in 1 mL of 1% lidocaine starting 2 weeks after excision and then every 4 weeks for 10 months (Haurani, et al., 2009). One-year outcomes demonstrated a 19% keloid recurrence rate (Haurani, et al., 2009). It must be noted that this treatment is off-label, and long-term outcomes have not been evaluated.

External beam radiotherapy and brachytherapy have been used as both monotherapy and in combination with surgery for the treatment of keloid scars (Ogawa, 2010). Although these approaches have demonstrated efficacy, a legitimate risk of radiation induced tumorigenesis persists. Until long-term studies have stratified the true risk of radiation-induced tumorigenesis, it remains a controversial therapy for a benign and largely aesthetic condition.

Cryotherapy modifies collagen synthesis and differentiation of keloidal fibroblasts and has been used as a monotherapy and in combination with intralesional triamcinolone in the management of keloid scars (Ogawa, 2010). Treatment protocols involve topical cryotherapy spray and intralesional needle "cryosurgery", both as monotherapies or immediately prior to triamcinolone injection. Typical protocols involve the application of liquid nitrogen using a cotton swab or via a handheld spray unit. The keloid is completely frozen (requiring several seconds to minutes of exposure depending on the size of the keloid) and then allowed to thaw for 15–20 seconds. The lesion can then be injected with triamcinolone. The process is repeated every 4 weeks for up to 10 months. Although this technique has demonstrated some efficacy, the clinical utility is limited to small lesions as treatments are painful and can result in hypopigmentation (Ogawa, 2010).

Nonpathologic Intrinsically Unsatisfactory Scars

Intrinsically unsatisfactory scars that are nonpathologic can be iatrogenic (i.e. misaligned wound edges and trap door deformities) or simply features of normal wound healing (i.e. scar irregularity, wide/long, and elevated/depressed). These scar features do not typically respond to noninvasive therapies, and more substantial deformities will require scar revision—simple fusiform excision or scar irregularization techniques. Mild-to-moderate scar depression, wound edge misalignment, and irregularity can be improved through the prudent employment of resurfacing techniques.

Scar resurfacing is most frequently utilized 6–8 weeks following primary wound closure among those scars demonstrating the aforementioned features.

Resurfacing is a well-established technique that is thought to promote accumulation of hyaluronic acid and proliferation of epidermal cells in the wound and thus improve the overall scar appearance (Katz and Oca, 1991). Resurfacing is done via dermabrasion (using of a rotary diamond fraise, brush fraise, or dermabrasion/sand paper) (Surowitz and Shockley, 2011), or alternatively, via ablative laser resurfacing (Jared, et al., 2012). Although these therapies have each individually demonstrated strong efficacy, there have been no trials to date that demonstrate superiority of a particular modality.

Dermabrasion is performed following the infiltration of local anesthesia. Local anesthetics without epinephrine are preferred, as they do not impede capillary bleeding—an overtly visible characteristic of the papillary dermis. The abraded wound is taken down into the papillary dermis to the appropriate level to allow for improved wound edge flattening, taking care to avoid penetration into the reticular dermis, which is necessary for wound re-epithelialization. A similar technique is employed using ablative laser therapies (i.e. CO_2), taking care to preserve the reticular dermis. Irrespective of modality, patients are started on prophylactic antiviral therapy 1 week prior to treatment, and the wound is kept moist postoperatively with occlusive dressings employed whenever possible. Common adverse effects include pain, skin erythema that persists for up to 3 months post-treatment, and possible scar hypopigmentation or postinflammatory hyperpigmentation (Leake and Baker, 2007; Surowitz and Shockley, 2011). The use of a rotary diamond fraise should be avoided in patients with communicable blood-borne illnesses such as hepatitis or human immunodeficiency virus due to the risk of airborne transmission.

Adjunctive therapies such as temporary and permanent injectable soft-tissue fillers (i.e. hyaluronic acid and autologous fat) can also be used to raise depressed scars.

Scars that are not amendable to resurfacing techniques may benefit from scar revision. Scars that are not extrinsically unsatisfactory (i.e. located perpendicular to RSTLs and poorly designed) can be simply excised using a fusiform excision. Placement of the fusiform excision along RSTLs or within the junction of aesthetic facial units, maintaining opposing angles of ≤30°, employing adequate undermining and the aforementioned closure techniques ensures optimal scar outcomes. Scars that are both intrinsically and extrinsically unsatisfactory can be managed as extrinsically unsatisfactory scars as discussed below.

Extrinsically Unsatisfactory Scars

Extrinsic features of a scar that influence its overall acceptability generally refer to poor scar placement or scar design. These are frequently beyond the control of the treating physician (i.e. post-traumatic injury and mid-cheek skin cancer excision). Extrinsically unsatisfactory scars will generally not respond to conservative noninvasive therapies (i.e. silicone gel sheeting and compression) and require scar revision.

Scar revision techniques allow for reorientation or irregularization of an unsatisfactory scar. The most common surgical approaches include: z-plasty, w-plasty, or geometric broken-line closure (GBLC).

Z-plasty is a versatile technique that allows for scar reorientation, irregularization, lengthening of scar contracture, and repositioning of facial features (i.e. nasal ala and lip vermillion). The classic technique involves the placement of incisions at the superior and inferior aspects of the scar in what results in a "Z" appearance—incisions are of equal length to the original scar. Classic z-plasty angles correspond to predictably increased scar lengths and reorientation of the initial scar (Table 34.3). Once incised, the created wound is composed of two triangular flaps that are simply transposed (Figs. 34.1A to C). The wounds are closed in a tension-free fashion abiding by the aforementioned principles. Multiple z-plasties can be used along long or curvilinear scars to allow for improved irregularization or reorientation.

Table 34.3: Z-plasty angles and their corresponding increase in scar length and reorientation angle (relative to the original position of the scar).

Z-plasty angle	*Length increase*	*Reorientation angle*
30°	25%	45°
45°	50%	60°
60°	75%	90°

W-plasty is a technique employed where scar irregularization and mild reorientation is beneficial, but where lengthening does not occur. Optimal scar candidates for this technique are long, perpendicular to RSTLs, and those that traverse convex curvatures. The technique involves careful preplanning with the positioning of interdigitating triangular flaps (several small "Ws") on both sides of the original scar. Each triangular flap should be approximately 3–5 mm in length and oriented along RSTLs whenever possible. The ends of the scar excision should be <30° to prevent standing cutaneous cone deformities. The scar is excised along these W incisions with complete removal of the previous scar and adequate undermining to allow for a tension-free closure. In situations where there is scar depression (i.e. atrophic scars), the deep portion of the previous scar may be left behind after the epidermis has been removed to serve as a permanent dermal graft/filler. The wound is then carefully closed primarily with taping applied.

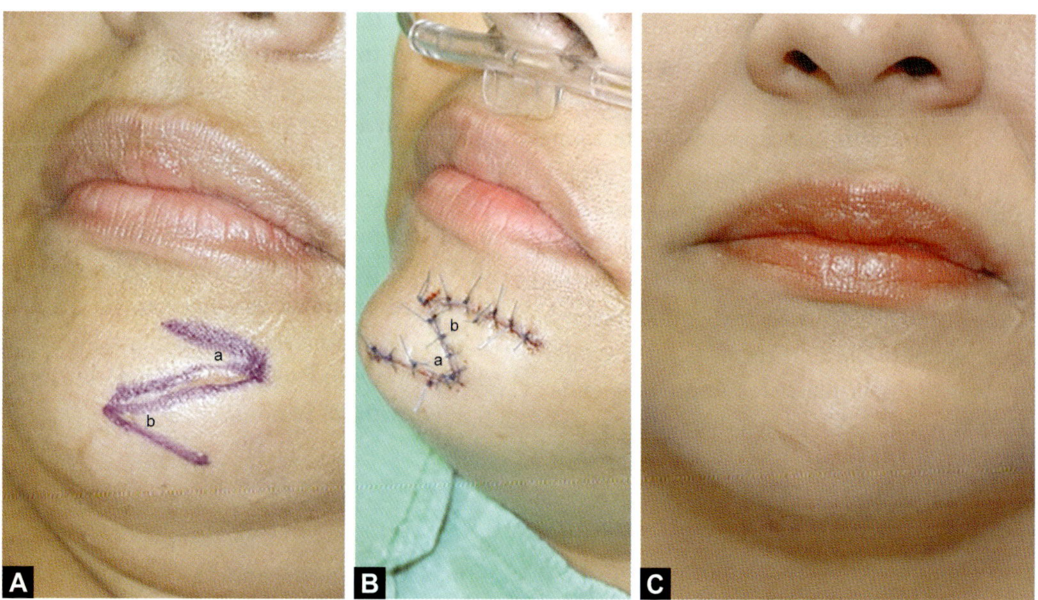

Figs. 34.1A to C: Z-plasty irregularization technique for a large chin scar. (A) Preoperative planning. (B) Intraoperative wound closure after the transposition of the Z-plasty flaps—note the new positions of flaps a and b. (C) Appearance of scar 1-year following z-plasty scar revision.

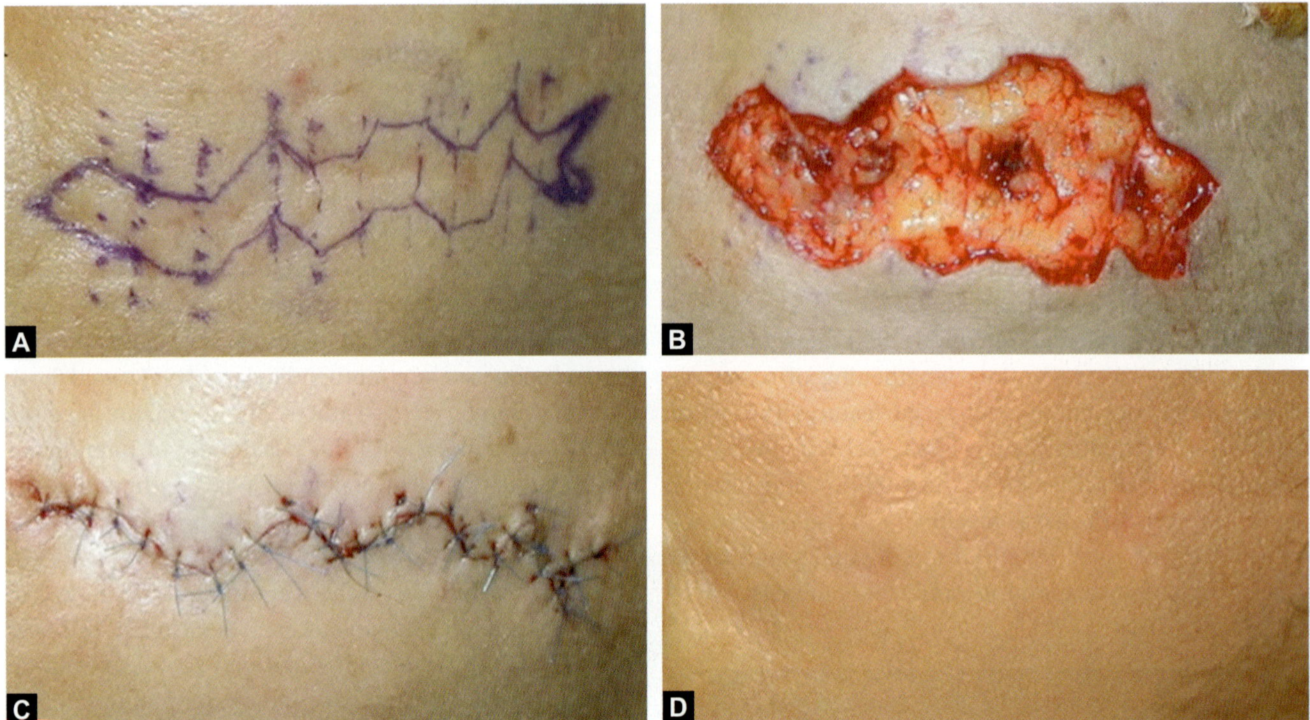

Figs. 34.2A to D: Geometric broken line closure (GBLC) of a traumatic cheek scar. (A) Preoperative planning. (B) Intraoperative appearance. (C) Wound closure. (D) Appearance of scar 1-year following GBLC scar revision.

The *GBLC* provides optimal scar camouflage without scar lengthening. It is not traditionally described as a means of reorienting a scar, but careful planning may allow it to be used in this way. Preplanning and design of the incisions using the GBLC technique are extensive (Figs. 34.2A to D). A variety of geometric shapes (i.e. triangles and squares) ranging in size from 3 mm to 7 mm and placed 3–5 mm from the scar margins are fashioned on one side of the scar. A mirror image of these geometric shapes is then fashioned on the contralateral side of the scar to allow for the interdigitating of these geometric shapes once the wound has been excised. Shapes with sharp edges (i.e. triangle) tend to heal more favorably than curvilinear shapes. The end result is an irregularly irregular scar. As with the W-plasty technique, the ends of the wound should remain <30° to avoid standing cutaneous cone deformities. The deep component of the scar is typically left behind as described for the W-plasty technique. Once the old scar has been removed, the wound edges are then carefully reapproximated and tape or an occlusive dressing is applied.

SUMMARY

Optimal facial scars are possible using the highlighted techniques. Meticulous attention to proper tissue handing and wound closure ensures the maximum opportunity for a wound to heal. Once healed, intrinsic wound pathologies can largely be modified with a combination of conservative and interventional techniques. Failing these techniques or in situations where wound reorientation or irregularization are required, scar revision procedures provide a means of achieving scar camouflage. In spite of thorough preplanning and fastidious surgical technique, there are limits as to what can be achieved with some scars—and some exacting patients. Thus, thorough frank discussions and appropriate goal setting must be conducted with all patients.

REFERENCES

Bichakjian, C.K. and Johnson, T.M., 2007. Anatomy of the skin. In: S.R. Baker, ed. *Local flaps in facial reconstruction*. 2nd ed. Philadelphia, PA: Elsevier/Saunders.

Brandt, M.G., et al., 2009. A prospective randomized evaluation of scar assessment measures. *The Laryngoscope*, 119(5), pp. 841-5.

Chaby, G., et al., 2007. Dressings for acute and chronic wounds: a systematic review. *Archives of Dermatology*, 143(10), pp. 1297-304.

Cupp, C. and Gaball, C.W., 2012. Utilizing topical therapies and mitomycin to reduce scars. *Facial Plastic Surgery*, 28(5), pp. 513-7.

Dunkin, C.S.J., et al., 2007. Scarring occurs at a critical depth of skin injury: precise measurement in a graduated dermal scratch in human volunteers. *Plastic and Reconstructive Surgery*, 119(6), pp. 1722-32; discussion 1733-4.

Elsaie, M.L. and Choudhary, S., 2010. Lasers for scars: a review and evidence-based appraisal. *Journal of Drugs in Dermatology: JDD*, 9(11), pp. 1355-62.

Haurani, M.J., et al., 2009. 5-Fluorouracil treatment of problematic scars. *Plastic and Reconstructive Surgery*, 123(1), pp. 139-48; discussion 149-51.

Hebda, P.A., 2009. Wound healing of the skin. In: D.B. Hom, et al., eds. *Essential tissue healing of the face and neck*. Shelton, CT: BC Decker.

Hom, D.B. and Dresner, H., 2009. General approach to a poorly healing problem wound: practical and clinical overview. In: D.B. Hom, et al., eds. *Essential tissue healing of the face and neck*. 1st ed. Shelto, CT: BC Decker.

Jared C.J., et al., 2012. A randomized controlled trial of fractional laser therapy and dermabrasion for scar resurfacing. *Dermatologic Surgery*, 38(4), pp. 595-602.

Katz, B.E. and Oca, A.G., 1991. A controlled study of the effectiveness of spot dermabrasion ("scarabrasion") on the appearance of surgical scars. *Journal of the American Academy of Dermatology*, 24(3), pp. 462-6.

Leake, D.S. and Baker, S.R., 2007. Scar revision and local flap refinement. In: S.R. Baker, ed. *Local flaps in facial reconstruction*. Philadelphia, PA: Elsevier Ltd.

Leong, M. and Philips, L.G., 2012. Wound healing. In: C.M. Townsend, ed. *Sabiston textbook of surgery: the biological basis of modern surgical practice*. 19th Ed. Philadelphia, PA: Elsevier Ltd.

Levenson, S.M., et al., 1965. The healing of rat skin wounds. *Annals of Surgery*, 161, pp. 293-08.

Marcus, B.C., 2007. Wound closure techniques. In: S.R. Baker, ed. *Local flaps in facial reconstruction*. Philadelphia, PA: Elsevier Ltd.

Ogawa, R., 2010. The most current algorithms for the treatment and prevention of hypertrophic scars and keloids. *Plastic and Reconstructive Surgery*, 125(2), pp. 557-68.

Ogawa, R., 2011. Mechanobiology of scarring. Wound Repair and Regeneration: Official Publication of the Wound Healing Society [and] the European Tissue Repair Society, 19(Suppl 1), pp. S2-9.

Ogawa, R., et al., 2012. The relationship between skin stretching/contraction and pathologic scarring: the important role of mechanical forces in keloid generation. *Wound Repair and Regeneration: Official Publication of the Wound Healing Society [and] the European Tissue Repair Society*, 20(2), pp. 149-57.

Shin, T.M. and Bordeaux, J.S., 2012. The role of massage in scar management: a literature review. *Dermatologic Surgery*, 38(3), pp. 414-23.

Surowitz, J.B. and Shockley, W.W., 2011. Enhancement of facial scars with dermabrasion. *Facial Plastic Surgery Clinics of North America*, 19(3), pp. 517-25.

Velangi, S.S. and Rees, J.L., 2001. Why are scars pale? An immunohistochemical study indicating preservation of melanocyte number and function in surgical scars. *Acta Dermato-Venereologica*, 81(5), pp. 326-8.

35 Frontal Sinus Fracture

Mahdi Shkoukani

Chapter Overview

Pearls and Pitfalls

Pearls

- A thorough review of the maxillofacial CT scan (axial, coronal and sagittal cuts) is needed for formulating a treatment plan. Extra attention should be given to the assessment of the posterior wall and the patency of frontal sinus outflow tract.
- CSF leak may take few days to develop in cases of minimally displaced posterior wall fractures.
- Endoscopic frontal sinusotomy helps to avoid a coronal incision in patients when the anterior wall is intact or minimally displaced but the frontal sinus outflow tract is obstructed.
- Contour deformity resulting from depressed fractures of frontal sinus anterior table (without frontal sinus outflow tract obstruction) may be filled with hydroxyapatite cement using the endoscopic forehead lift approach.
- In cases of cranialization, a large piece of temporal fascia is used to occlude the frontonasal recess to prevent ascending intracranial infection.

Pitfalls

- In cases of cranialization, failure to drill out any remnant mucosa in the frontal sinus will result in late frontal sinus mucocele.
- If part of superior orbital rim is covered with the mesh, failure to curve it over the rim and contour it properly will make it easily palpable postoperatively.

35.1 EPIDEMIOLOGY AND PATHOGENESIS

- Frontal sinuses are not present at birth. The frontal sinus is formed by pneumatization of anterior ethmoid air cells into the frontal bone. They appear at second year of life and begin their main phase of expansion from 5 years of age until they reach their final size in late childhood. One of the frontal sinuses is absent in about 4% of adult population (McLaughlin, Rehl and Lanza, 2001).
- The right and left frontal sinuses are usually asymmetric in shape and have a septum that divides the two sides. This septum is not necessarily in the midline. Each sinus drains into a nasofrontal recess through an opening that is located on the floor in a posteromedial position.
- Frontal sinus fractures represent about 2–15% of facial fractures (Xie, et al., 2000). There are numerous classifications (Gonty, Marciani and Adornato, 1999; Ioannides and Freihofer, 1999; Manolidis, 2004) of frontal sinus fractures but essentially these are based

on the frontal sinus wall involved in the fracture, and whether there is displacement of the fractured fragments: anterior wall fractures with or without displacement, posterior wall fractures with or without displacement, inferior wall fractures, fractures involving more than one wall, and "through and through" fractures (from the skin to the anterior cranial fossa). The fractures are further classified into those involving or sparing the frontal sinus outflow tract (Stanwix, et al., 2010).

- Isolated anterior wall fractures comprise about one-third of frontal sinus fractures, whereas the other two thirds comprise of a combination of multiple wall fractures (Swinson, Jerjes and Thompson, 2004). It is extremely rare to have an isolated posterior or inferior wall fracture.
- Frontal bone is considered one of the strongest bones in the craniofacial area. It has been shown that 800–1,000 lb. of force is required to fracture the frontal sinus (Nahum, 1975). This large amount of force often leads to multiple facial fractures, intracranial injuries, and orbital injuries. Patients with frontal sinus fractures often have naso-orbital ethmoid (NOE) fractures (34%), zygomaticomaxillary complex fractures (17%), and orbital wall fractures (27.5%). Close to 60% of patients with frontal sinus injury may present with associated orbital trauma (El Khatib, Danino and Malka, 2004; Gabrielli, et al., 2004; Gerbino, et al., 2000).
- The presence of a fracture of the posterior table indicates that the patient has sustained a severe injury. Posterior table fractures are associated with pneumocephalus in 25% of patients, CSF leak in 25%, and extradural hematoma in 10% (Gerbino, et al., 2000). These fractures are most commonly due to motor vehicle accidents followed by assaults and recreational accidents (Strong, Pahlavan and Saito, 2006).

35.2 CLINICAL FEATURES

Clinical History

- The presenting symptoms depend on the severity of the injury. Patients who sustain low-velocity injuries may have isolated anterior table fractures and may present with localized edema, bruising, or a depressed contour deformity of the forehead. However, patients with high-velocity injuries may have fractures involving all the three walls of the frontal sinus with associated NOE fractures, intracranial and orbital injuries. Other symptoms may include epistaxis, headache, vomiting, loss of consciousness, decreased visual acuity, or diplopia.
- Patients with breach of the dura mater may present with clear rhinorrhea. Numbness of the forehead may result from injury to the supraorbital and supratrochlear branches of the ophthalmic division of the trigeminal nerve.

Typical Findings on Examination

- A thorough head and neck examination should be completed with extra attention to the forehead, ophthalmic, and neurologic examination.
- Forehead edema, ecchymosis, abrasion, and/or open wounds are documented.
- Step deformity may be present on frontal bone examination. This may be seen as a forehead depression or bony fragments protrusion. Depression may not be apparent in the first 2 weeks post trauma due to associated edema.
- Presence of telecanthus and pig nose deformity suggests concomitant NOE fractures and needs to be confirmed by a CT scan of the facial bones. On examination, one can place the index finger of one hand on the medial canthal ligament and the contralateral hand is used to pull the upper and lower lids laterally. If the index finger feels any movement of the ligament, then that suggests an NOE fracture.
- Clear nasal discharge on bending down or with a Valsalva maneuver should alert the physician to CSF leak, in particular when posterior wall fracture or intracranial involvement is seen on imaging studies.

35.3 INVESTIGATIONS

- Computerized tomography—maxillofacial scan with three-dimensional (3D) reconstruction is the gold standard imaging technique currently for thorough evaluation of the craniofacial skeleton. Usually, it is ordered without intravenous (IV) contrast, so it may not have excellent soft tissue resolution. Anterior and posterior walls of frontal sinus are better appreciated on axial cuts (Figs. 35.1 and 35.2). The floor is better evaluated on coronal cuts (Fig. 35.3). The frontal sinus outflow tract is better appreciated on sagittal (Fig. 35.4) and coronal cuts. A 3D CT scan is not indicated in a straightforward case of frontal sinus fracture but the author may obtain it if concomitant NOE fracture is involved (Fig. 35.5).

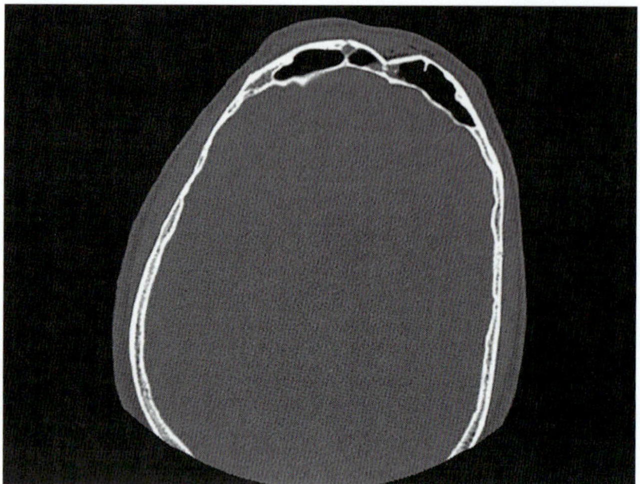

Fig. 35.1: Computerized tomography maxillofacial without intravenous-contrast axial cut showing frontal sinus anterior wall fracture.

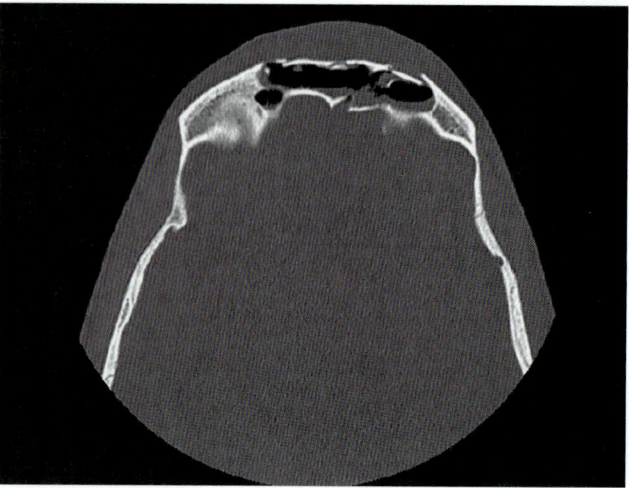

Fig. 35.2: Computerized tomography maxillofacial without intravenous-contrast axial cut showing frontal sinus anterior and posterior wall fractures.

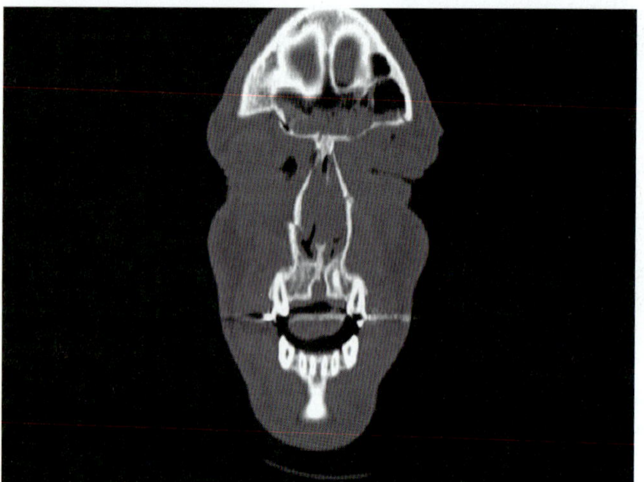

Fig. 35.3: Computerized tomography maxillofacial without intravenous-contrast coronal cut showing frontal sinus floor wall fracture.

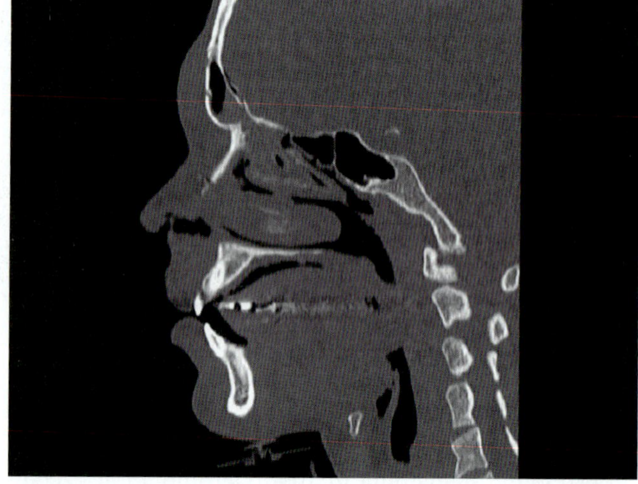

Fig. 35.4: Computerized tomography maxillofacial without intravenous-contrast sagittal cut showing frontonasal recess obstruction with soft tissue (edematous mucosa mixed with blood).

- Magnetic resonance imaging scan of the brain with IV gadolinium is ordered if intracranial involvement is suspected. A CT-head without contrast is ordered first if intracranial bleed is suspected.
- Nasal fluids should be checked for β-2-transferrin protein to confirm a CSF leak.

35.4 PREFERRED TREATMENT

- The significance of frontal sinus management comes from its proximity to brain and bilateral orbits. The elements considered in approaching frontal sinus fracture repair are the wall(s) involved with the fracture, their degree of displacement, the status of frontal sinus outflow tract, and status of CSF leak.
- The author prefers to observe all cases that involve fracture(s) of frontal sinus wall(s) with minimal or no displacement, absence of CSF leak, and absence of obstruction of frontal sinus outflow tract. Please refer to the Flowchart 35.1 for more details regarding the algorithm that the author uses to treat these fractures.
- In cases where there is minimal displacement of frontal sinus wall with suspicion of CSF leak, the fluid is

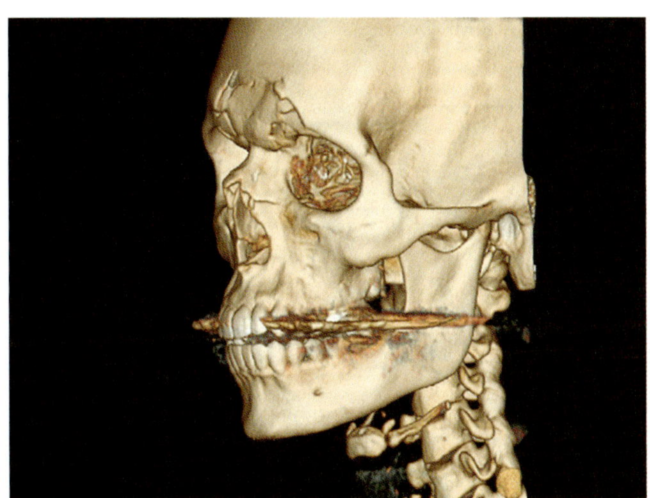

Fig. 35.5: A three-dimensional computerized tomography image with an oblique view of frontal sinus fracture with a concomitant naso-orbito-ethmoidal fracture.

checked for β-2-transferrin protein. While waiting for the results of the test, which may take up to 1 week, the patient is advised bed rest with head of bed elevated. The patient is told to avoid straining, bending forward, and nose blowing, and started on a stool softener. There had been some controversy in the literature regarding the use of antibiotics in patients with post-traumatic CSF leaks (Brodie, 1997; Villalobos, et al., 1998). Recently, a Cochrane review has shown that there is no evidence to support the use of antibiotics in post-traumatic CSF leak cases (Ratilal, et al., 2011).

If these measures fail in the first 3 days, a neurosurgery consultation is sought to place a lumber drain. Majority of cases resolve with conservative management within 1 week. However, a small proportion of cases need to be explored with a coronal incision and an osteoplastic flap approach as mentioned below. Most of these cases have a CSF leak coming out from a fracture through the posterior table. The best way to approach this is to cranialize the frontal sinus.

- Endoscopic approach is indicated if the inferior wall fracture causes an obstruction of frontal sinus outflow tract with no or minimal involvement of the anterior and posterior walls. Image guidance and development of dedicated frontal sinus drills and malleable instruments have made this more feasible. In these cases, an uncinectomy is performed followed by maxillary antrostomy and anterior ethmoidectomy. Next the frontal sinus is opened using Draf procedures I, II, or III.
- Occasionally, the endoscopic approach may address a CSF leak coming from posterior table in the inferior half of posterior wall. The mucosa is stripped around the bony defect and the dural defect is plugged with a medium thickness freeze-dried acellular human dermis or fascia lata obtained from the patient. Small dural tears may be repaired with bath plug technique using ear lobe fat graft tied to a Vicryl suture. Endoscopic techniques may avoid cranializing the sinus, as long as the nasofrontal recess remains open.
- Cranialization is indicated in cases of persistent CSF leak that fail conservative measures as mentioned above. The author recommends it in cases where there is CSF leak with a concomitant displacement of the posterior wall regardless of the status of the frontal sinus outflow tract.

Preoperatively, the author obtains a plain 6-foot Caldwell view X-ray with coin reference. The size of the frontal sinus on the X-ray film is near the actual size and this can be confirmed with size of the coin on the X-ray relative to the actual coin size. The plain film is cut around the outline of the frontal sinus before it gets sterilized on the day of surgery.

One-centimeter strip of hair centered at the marked incision is clipped (Fig. 35.6). The procedure entails infiltration of the skin with local anesthetic with epinephrine. A zigzag coronal incision extending between the roots of helix bilaterally is then made. The flap is elevated in the subgaleal plane. In the temple area, it is important to protect the frontal branch of the facial nerve by incising the superficial layer of the deep temporal fascia just superficial to the intermediate fat pad. The subgaleal plane is converted to a subperiosteal plane about 2 cm superior to the superior orbital rim. At this point, an anteriorly based pericranial flap is outlined starting from each zygomaticofrontal suture line and extending the periosteal incision superiorly with a number 15 blade, keeping it medial to the temporalis muscle (Fig. 35.7). The author extends the incision as posteriorly as possible and then connects both incisions with a transverse incision. The pericranial flap is elevated gently using a wide periosteal elevator. The periosteum will be stickier at the level of the arcus marginalis and extra attention is needed not to perforate the periosteum. Care is taken to preserve the supraorbital and supratrochlear neurovascular bundles. It should be noted that the supraorbital nerve might arise from a foramen rather than a notch up to 2 cm above the supraorbital rim in 10% of patients. Once the nasal root and superior

Flowchart 35.1: Management strategy for frontal sinus fractures (adapted from AOCMF website).

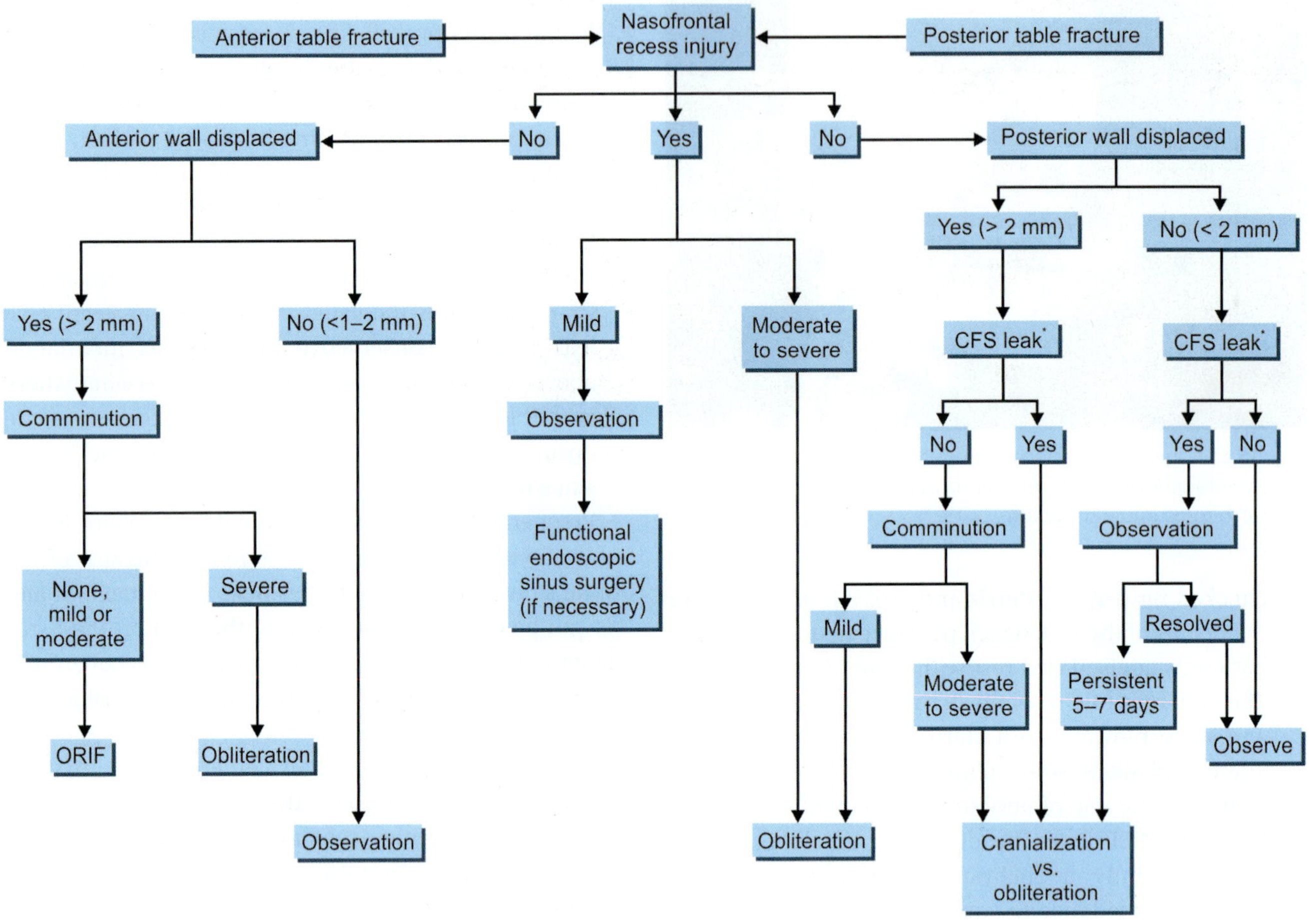

- Anterior table fracture → Nasofrontal recess injury ← Posterior table fracture
- Nasofrontal recess injury
  - No → Anterior wall displaced
    - Yes (> 2 mm) → Comminution
      - None, mild or moderate → ORIF
      - Severe → Obliteration
    - No (<1–2 mm) → Observation
  - Yes
    - Mild → Observation → Functional endoscopic sinus surgery (if necessary)
    - Moderate to severe → Obliteration
  - No → Posterior wall displaced
    - Yes (> 2 mm) → CFS leak*
      - No → Comminution
        - Mild → Obliteration
        - Moderate to severe → Cranialization vs. obliteration
      - Yes → Cranialization vs. obliteration
    - No (< 2 mm) → CFS leak*
      - Yes → Observation
        - Persistent 5–7 days → Cranialization vs. obliteration
        - Resolved → Observe
      - No → Observe

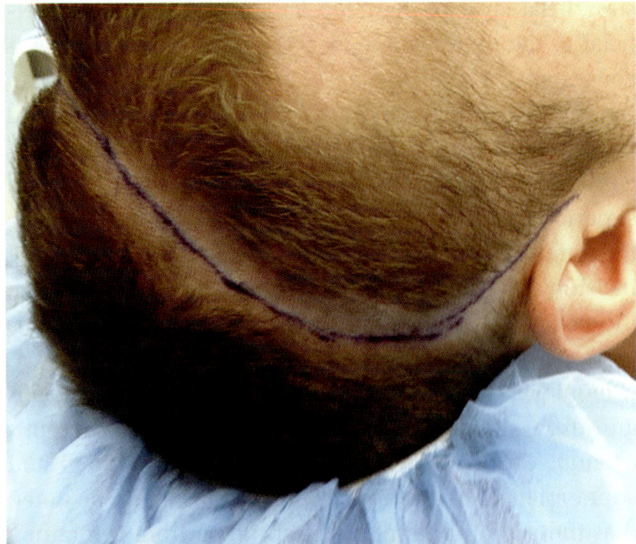

Fig. 35.6: A side view of bicoronal incision with 1 cm strip of hair had been clipped around the planned incision.

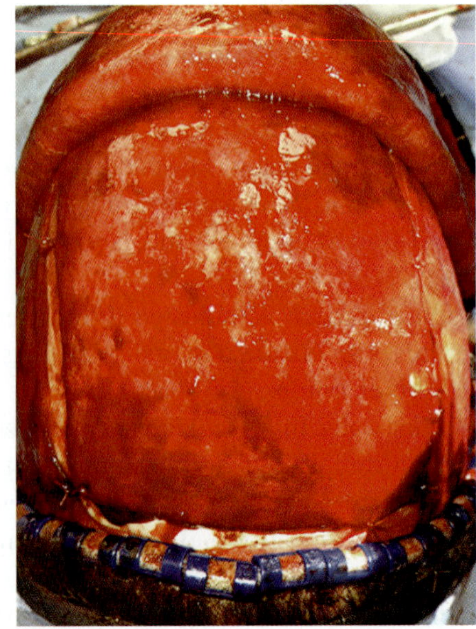

Fig. 35.7: An outlined anteriorly based pericranial flap.

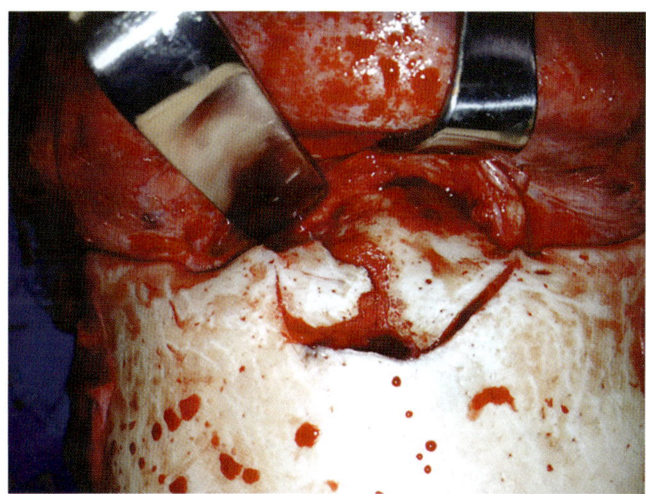

Fig. 35.8: An intraoperative view of a displaced anterior wall frontal sinus fracture.

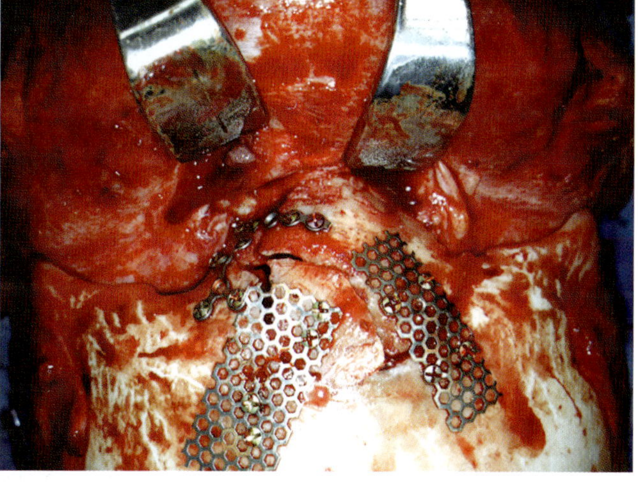

Fig. 35.9: An intraoperative view of a displaced anterior wall frontal sinus fracture status post-reduction with miniplates and small pieces of titanium mesh.

orbital rims are exposed adequately, the cut X-ray template is placed over the frontal bone using the orbital rims and nasal root as known landmarks. The periphery of the frontal sinus is marked on the frontal bone. Using a side-cutting burr, multiple perforations are made in the frontal sinus 2 mm inward from the outline of the sinus previously marked. The drill bit is angled about 45° off the frontal bone surface aiming toward the center of the sinus. All the perforations are then connected together using the side-cutting burr to completely separate the anterior wall from the rest of the frontal bone. At this point, the frontal sinus septum is what is holding the anterior wall, which can be taken down using an osteotome from a superior to inferior direction, and then drilled, down to the level of the posterior wall. Next, the mucosa covering the posterior surface of the anterior wall is curetted. The posterior table is inspected to characterize the fracture and identify the CSF leak. The posterior wall is denuded of all mucosa by drilling it with a burr. Caution is required not to push any bony segments intracranially. Also it is critical at this stage to identify the opening into the nasofrontal recess and strip the mucosa off it. The recess is then plugged with fascia obtained from the superficial layer of deep temporal fascia. Next, the neurosurgeon takes the posterior wall down to repair the dural defect. The anterior wall is placed back and secured using three miniplates (left, right, and superiorly). Next, two size 10 flat Jackson-Pratt drains are inserted, galea is closed with interrupted 2-0 Vicryl, and the skin is closed with staples up to the level of the superior portion of the helix. The inferior part of the incision is closed using a running 5-0 Prolene.

- Open reduction and internal fixation with miniplates are indicated when the fracture involves a posterior displacement of anterior wall of the frontal sinus. (Figs. 35.8 and 35.9) Failure to elevate and fix such fractures results in a cosmetic deformity of the forehead.
- The incision, plane of dissection, and approach to fractures of the anterior wall of frontal sinus are the same as that used for an osteoplastic flap. If the fracture line does not extend to the orbital rim, then there is no need to dissect the arcus marginalis or release the supraorbital nerve. If there is no suspicion of frontal sinus outflow tract obstruction, the fractured bone is reduced and fixated using multiple miniplates or titanium mesh (Fig. 35.9). Occasionally bone pieces have to be removed and secured ex vivo using titanium mesh before putting the mesh and reconstructed bony pieces on the frontal bone. In cases where there is suspicion that the nasofrontal recess is obstructed, the recess has to be inspected after removing few or all the fractured bony pieces. If the recess is blocked, then it must be repaired before repairing the fracture.
- If both anterior and posterior walls are displaced, a combination of cranialization and open reduction and internal fixation of anterior wall is carried out regardless of the status of the frontal sinus outflow tract.
- Nearly any scenario can be dealt with using one or more of the treatment options mentioned above. Obliteration of the frontal sinus with bone, muscle, fat, and hydroxyapatite has been mentioned in the

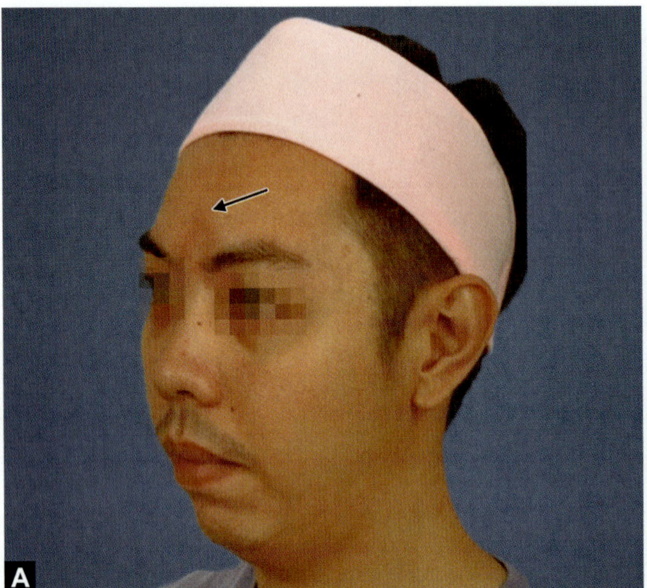
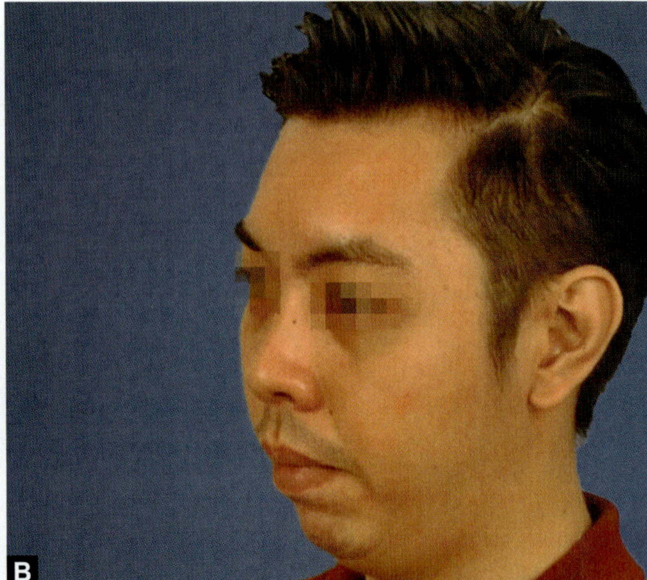

Figs. 35.10A and B: (A) Preoperative oblique view of the patient showing depressed fracture of the anterior table of frontal sinus. (B) Postoperative oblique view of the same patient after camouflage of the deformity with hydroxyapatite cement through the endoscopic forehead lift approach. (Figures courtesy: Dr Sandeep Uppal).

literature (D'Addario, Haug and Talwar, 2004). The author prefers not to obliterate the frontal sinuses and feels that there is no indication to do so. In the literature, obliteration is indicated when the frontal sinus outflow tract is damaged permanently (Weber, et al., 2000). The author believes that the nasofrontal recess can often be opened endoscopically, and if this proves difficult then an osteoplastic flap approach can be used.

- In the last 10–15 years, many authors have described endoscopic approach to the anterior wall fractures (Strong and Kellman, 2006). These fractures may be accessed via small incisions in the scalp similar to endoscopic brow-lift incisions. Using bone hooks, the fractured fragments may be lifted and fixated via percutaneously introduced self-drilling screws. Contour deformity resulting from depressed fractures of frontal sinus anterior table (without frontal sinus outflow tract obstruction) may be filled with hydroxyapatite cement using the endoscopic forehead lift approach (Figs. 35.10A and B).

35.5 COMPLICATIONS OF DISEASE

Early Complications

- *Forehead deformity*: It may develop in patients with a depressed fracture of the anterior wall of the frontal sinus if the patient does not undergo repair of the fracture.
- *Forehead/scalp numbness*: It may develop if the supraorbital and/or supratrochlear nerves are injured due to the trauma. In many cases, the sensation returns after edema has subsided, unless the nerve was transected due to the injury.

Late Complications

- *Intracranial complications*: These are not very common but carry a significant potential morbidity. Cerebrospinal fluid leak is the most common complication and is caused by displacement of the posterior table. These leaks are usually self-limiting with conservative treatment. Other potential complications include meningitis (~6% risk) and brain abscess.
- *Mucoceles or mucopyocele*: Mucoceles are epithelial-lined, mucous-containing cysts. Mucopyoceles are mucoceles that become infected. A recent retrospective review of cases in our institution has identified that mucoceles may develop on average of 15 years after trauma (Shkoukani, et al., 2013). These mucoceles may represent a complication of obstruction of the nasofrontal recess at the time of trauma or entrapped mucosa at the time of trauma or repair. The location is dependent on the location of entrapped mucosa. They may be limited to the frontal sinus or may spread intracranially or intraorbitally.

- *Scars*: They may form if there is laceration of the forehead skin at the time of injury. These can be revised 9–12 months post-trauma.

35.6 COMPLICATIONS OF TREATMENT

Early Complications

- *Hematoma/seroma*: It is uncommon for these to develop especially if drains are used. They can form subcutaneously if a coronal approach is used. It is important to leave the drains in-situ till the output drops down to 30 mL in 24 hours. A more serious complication is intraorbital hematoma in cases where the orbital wall is involved in the fracture or during repair. Anterior ethmoidal artery may get injured during endoscopic approach, which may lead to an intraorbital hematoma. This would be noted within minutes. Loss of red color vision is the first sign of impending blindness. If this is suspected, an immediate lateral canthotomy and inferior cantholysis should be performed followed by an ophthalmology consultation. If the pupil dilates then this is ominous sign that the optic nerve may have been injured permanently.
- *Infection*: Wound infection is uncommon in cases of coronal incision given the vascularity of the scalp. The author keeps his patients on antibiotic coverage as long as they have drains in place. In cases of cranialization and repair of CSF leak, the surgeon has to be vigilant to the development of meningitis and intracranial infections. Development of new symptoms such as fever, mental status change, or lethargy may point to development of intracranial complications.

Late Complications

- *Mucoceles/mucopyoceles*: A few steps can be taken to avoid the formation of a mucocele. First, the surgeon must drill out any sinus mucosa between bony fragments in cases of open reduction and internal fixation, even though the nasofrontal recess is still patent. In cases of obliteration, the entire frontal sinus mucosa should be drilled out with extra attention directed to the posterior wall mucosa where mucosa may follow the veins into the Breschet's canals, which connects the venous plexuses of the dura and the frontal sinus mucosa. Also, the nasofrontal recess should be plugged with fascia in cases of obliteration. In case of endoscopic approach, the surgeon should be experienced in performing Draf procedures to make sure that the frontal sinuses will drain intranasally.
- *Infection*: It may complicate a chronic mucocele. Obliterated sinuses without a tight closure of the frontonasal recess at the time of surgery may result in a mucopyocele secondary to exposure of the obliterated material to nasal flora.
- *Scar*: There will be a scar each time an incision is made. A favorable scar is the one that is narrow, flat, with no hypo- or hyperpigmentation. To avoid unfavorable scars, tissue needs to be handled gently and incisions closed without tension. Scar revision and dermabrasion may be performed if the scar is aesthetically unacceptable to the patient.
- *Alopecia*: It is relevant in cases of coronal incisions. There is no agreement in the literature whether to make incisions in the scalp parallel or perpendicular to the hair follicles. The author makes scalp incisions perpendicular to the hair follicles so that follicles next to the incision allow the hair shaft to grow through the scar (D'Addario, Haug and Talwar, 2004; Ende and Kabaker, 2010)

REFERENCES

Brodie, H.A., 1997. Prophylactic antibiotics for posttraumatic cerebrospinal fluid fistulae. A meta-analysis. *Archives of Otolaryngology—Head and Neck Surgery,* 123, pp. 749-52.

D'Addario, M., Haug, R.H. and Talwar, R.M., 2004. Biomaterials for use in frontal sinus obliteration. *Journal of Long-Term Effects of Medical Implants,* 14, pp. 455-65.

El Khatib, K., Danino, A. and Malka, G., 2004. The frontal sinus: a culprit or a victim? A review of 40 cases. *Journal of Craniomaxillofacial Surgery,* 32, pp. 314-7.

Ende, K.H. and Kabaker, S.S., 2010. *Hair restoration: medical and surgical techniques.* Philadelphia, PA: Mosby Elsevier.

Gabrielli, M.F., Gabrielli, M.A., Hochuli-vieira, E. and Pereira-Fillho, V.A., 2004. Immediate reconstruction of frontal sinus fractures: review of 26 cases. *Journal of Oral and Maxillofacial Surgery,* 62, pp. 582-6.

Gerbino, G., Roccia, F., Benech, A. and Caldarelli, C., 2000. Analysis of 158 frontal sinus fractures: current surgical management and complications. *Journal of Craniomaxillofacial Surgery,* 28, pp. 133-9.

Gonty, A.A., Marciani, R.D. and Adornato, D.C., 1999. Management of frontal sinus fractures: a review of 33 cases. *Journal of Oral and Maxillofacial Surgery,* 57, pp. 372-9; discussion 380-1.

Ioannides, C. and Freihofer, H.P., 1999. Fractures of the frontal sinus: classification and its implications for surgical treatment. *American Journal of Otolaryngology,* 20, pp. 273-80.

Manolidis, S., 2004. Frontal sinus injuries: associated injuries and surgical management of 93 patients. *Journal of Oral and Maxillofacial Surgery,* 62, pp. 882-91.

McLaughlin, R.B., JR., Rehl, R.M. and Lanza, D.C., 2001. Clinically relevant frontal sinus anatomy and physiology. *Otolaryngologic Clinics of North America,* 34, pp. 1-22.

Nahum, A.M., 1975. The biomechanics of maxillofacial trauma. *Clinical Plastic Surgery,* 2, pp. 59-64.

Ratilal, B.O., Costa, J., Sampaio, C. and Pappamikail, L., 2011. Antibiotic prophylaxis for preventing meningitis in patients with basilar skull fractures. *Cochrane Database of Systemic Reviews,* CD004884.

Shkoukani, M.A., Caughlin, B., PEREIRA, L., Carron, M., Folbe, A. and Mathog, R.H., 2013. Mucoceles of the paranasal sinuses: A 10 year single institution review. *Journal of Otology and Rhinology,* 2 (In Press).

Stanwix, M.G., Nam, A.J., Manson, P.N., Mirvis, S. and Rodriguez, E.D., 2010. Critical computed tomographic diagnostic criteria for frontal sinus fractures. *Journal of Oral and Maxillofacial Surgery,* 68, pp. 2714-22.

Strong, E.B. and Kellman, R.M., 2006. Endoscopic repair of anterior table—frontal sinus fractures. *Facial Plastic Surgery Clinics of North America,* 14, pp. 25-9.

Strong, E.B., Pahlavan, N. and Saito, D., 2006. Frontal sinus fractures: a 28-year retrospective review. *Otolaryngology—Head and Neck Surgery,* 135, pp. 774-9.

Swinson, B.D., Jerjes, W. and Thompson, G., 2004. Current practice in the management of frontal sinus fractures. *Journal of Laryngology and Otology,* 118, pp. 927-32.

Villalobos, T., Arango, C., Kubilis, P. and Rathore, M., 1998. Antibiotic prophylaxis after basilar skull fractures: a meta-analysis. *Clinical Infectious Diseases,* 27, pp. 364-9.

Weber, R., Draf, W., Keerl, R., Kahle, G., Schinzel, S., Thomann, S. and Lawson, W., 2000. Osteoplastic frontal sinus surgery with fat obliteration: technique and long-term results using magnetic resonance imaging in 82 operations. *Laryngoscope,* 110, pp. 1037-44.

Xie, C., Mehendale, N., Barrett, D., Bui, C.J. and Metzinger, S. E., 2000. 30-year retrospective review of frontal sinus fractures: the charity hospital experience. *Journal of Craniomaxillofacial Trauma,* 6, pp. 7-15; discussion 16-8.

Midface and NOE Fractures 36

Mahdi Shkoukani, Sandeep Uppal, Lucio Pereira

Chapter Overview

Pearls and Pitfalls

Pearls

- Midface and naso-orbito-ethmoidal (NOE) fractures require accurate diagnosis due to the complex anatomy of this area. This can be accomplished by performing systematic physical examination and review of high-resolution computerized tomography (CT) scans.
- Fracture classification systems are available and should be used not only to describe the fracture pattern, but also to allow for efficient physician communication.
- Correct the nasal dorsum height and reconstruct the facial pillars and beams while restoring the pretrauma occlusion.
- Public education regarding the role of airbags has significantly reduced the incidence of facial fractures and panfacial fractures after motor vehicle accidents (McGovern, et al., 2000).
- In depressed tripod fractures, the sphenozygomatic junction along the lateral wall of the orbit should be aligned before performing internal fixation as it serves as a useful guide to optimal three-dimensional (3D) reduction in fractured zygoma.
- Do not use the squamous portion of the temporal bone as fulcrum during reduction in depressed zygomatic arch fractures as it may lead to fracture of this bone.
- Overcorrection of the medial canthal position is recommended during open reduction and internal fixation of NOE fractures and medial canthal tendon injuries.

Pitfalls

- Failure to treat symmetry of the eyes and medial canthal tendon injuries during the first few weeks after trauma can lead to long-term facial deformity that is difficult to treat later.
- Failure to achieve optimal surgical exposure leads to suboptimal reduction and fixation of complex NOE fractures and medial canthal injuries.

36.1 CLINICAL FEATURES

Features in clinical history:

- Facial deformity and numbness
- Double vision and change in visual acuity
- Nasal obstruction and bleeding. May also have decreased sense of smell
- Clear rhinorrhea due to cerebrospinal fluid (CSF) leak
- Changes in dental occlusion

Typical findings on examination:

A thorough history is obtained and clinical examination performed in every patient to assess the extent of injuries and patient's fitness for any planned surgical procedure (Appendix 36.1). The following signs and symptoms may be present in any patient presenting with midface injuries.

- Inspection of the eyes may show displacement of the medial canthal tendon, periorbital edema, ecchymosis, chemosis, enophthalmos, restriction of eye movements due to muscle entrapment, epiphora, and globe injuries.
- It is very important to assess vision changes in these patients. Vision may be affected because of direct injury to the globe or due to optic nerve trauma. Optic nerve may be compressed by bony fragments or due to retro-orbital hematoma. Loss of red color vision is the first to occur in patients with compression of the optic nerve due to an expanding retro-orbital hematoma and indicates impending (<90 min) irreversible injury to the optic nerve. Both ipsilateral and consensual light reflex should be assessed. Loss of light reflex is a poor prognostic sign and indicates optic nerve injury.
- Nasal examination may show external nasal deviation due to nasal bone fracture and displacement. In NOE fractures, there is displacement of nasal bones posteriorly toward the fractured ethmoid complex. This leads to depression and widening of the root of the nose leading to telecanthus. Along with this, the nasal length gets shortened and the tip of the nose gets overrotated, exposing the nostrils (pig nose deformity). Fracture of the nasal septum leads to septal deviation and nasal obstruction. Loss of dorsal septal support may lead to saddle nose deformity. There may be bleeding and septal hematoma.
- Oral cavity inspection may show missing or damaged teeth, ecchymosis, open/cross bite, and impaction of the maxilla with decrease in anterior, posterior, and vertical height of the midface.
- Palpation may show step offs, laxity of the medial canthal tendon, and maxillary complex mobility.

36.2 INVESTIGATIONS

Imaging

High-resolution CT scan (axial, coronal, and sagittal views) (Figs. 36.1A to E) without contrast should be obtained on every patient with suspected facial fractures, except those with isolated nasal bone fractures. Coronal views are helpful for identifying orbital floor fractures and to evaluate the midface pillars. Axial views are good for identifying medial and lateral orbital walls, nasal, and NOE fractures, while sagittal cuts show posterior displacement of structures like the nasal dorsum, NOE complex, and maxilla. Sagittal cuts also help in the assessment of the posterior extent of orbital floor injuries. Three-dimensional reconstruction CT is available in many trauma centers and can help by giving a better and more intuitive picture of the extent of injury and the degree of displacement of fracture fragments and their relationship to each other. This can help guide the reconstruction in patients with severe midface and NOE fractures.

Beta-2 Transferrin

Anytime clear rhinorrhea is present; fluid should be sent to the laboratory for β-2 transferrin assay, which is very sensitive and specific for CSF.

36.3 CLASSIFICATION OF MIDFACE FRACTURES

Each area has its own classification, which is related to the pattern and degree of comminution. The most frequently used classifications are the Le Fort classification for maxillary fractures (Fig. 36.2) and the Markowitz classification of NOE fractures (Figs. 36.3A to C) (Markowitz, et al., 1991).

Le Fort Classification

The Le Fort classification is widely used and very important for documentation and communication between physicians. Pure Le Fort I, II, and III fractures are rare. Le Fort fractures are generally created secondary to low energy impact, which is different from most of the fractures we see in real life. Today the fracture pattern does not necessarily follow the classic Le Fort classification. As road traffic accidents lead to high-velocity facial skeletal injuries, it is increasingly common to encounter a combination of Le Fort I, II, and III fractures either unilaterally or bilaterally in the same patient. These are often associated with other facial fractures like unilateral or bilateral NOE and frontal bone fractures.

All types of Le Fort fractures have one thing in common. They all go through all three vertical buttresses of the face. Le Fort I fracture is a horizontal maxillary fracture

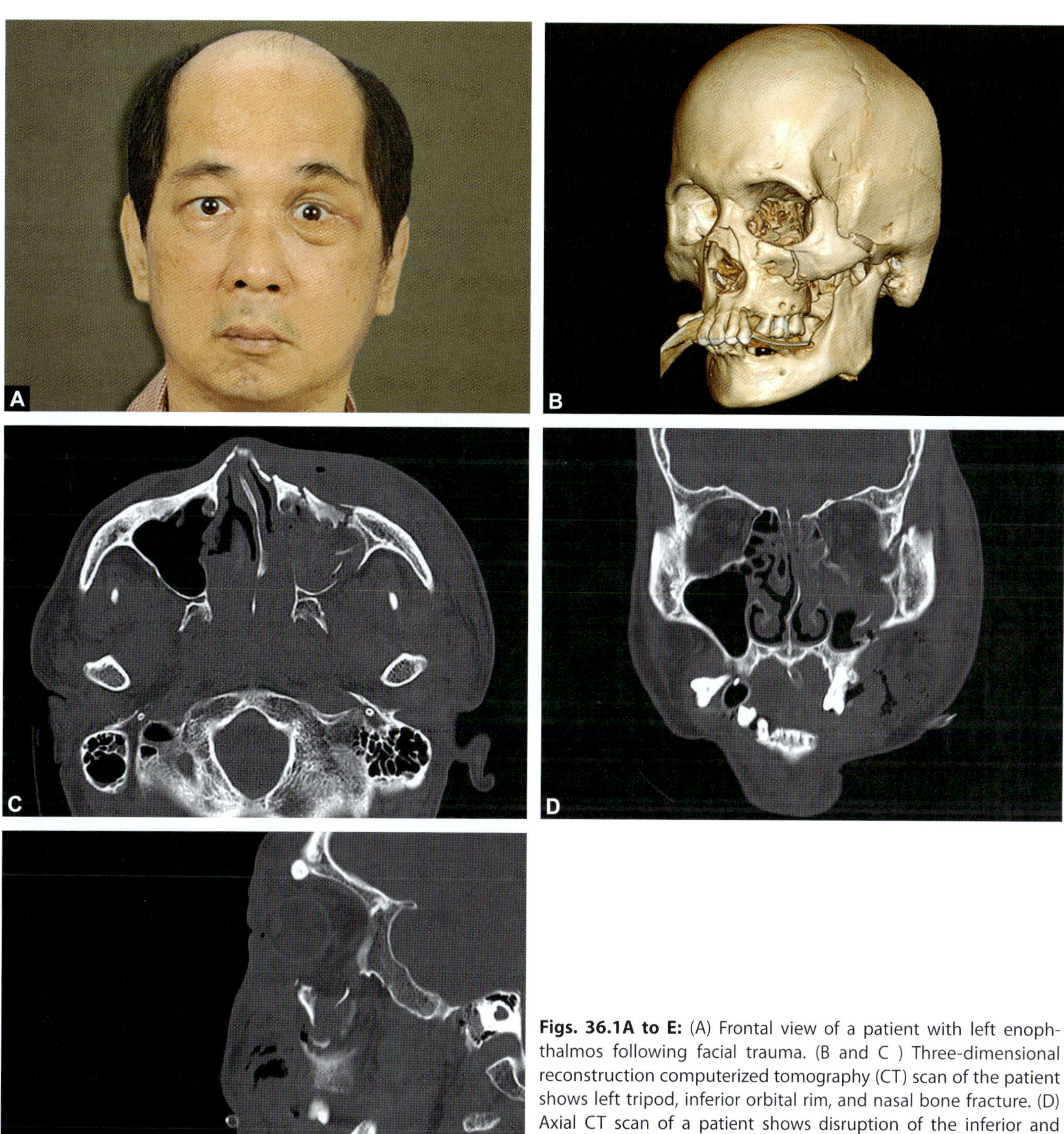

Figs. 36.1A to E: (A) Frontal view of a patient with left enophthalmos following facial trauma. (B and C) Three-dimensional reconstruction computerized tomography (CT) scan of the patient shows left tripod, inferior orbital rim, and nasal bone fracture. (D) Axial CT scan of a patient shows disruption of the inferior and lateral orbital walls. (D) Coronal CT scan shows left orbital floor fracture with herniation of orbital fat and inferior rectus muscle into the maxillary sinus. (E) Sagittal CT scan of the same patient shows orbital floor fracture.

with the fracture line starting at the pyriform aperture and then traversing the nasomaxillary (NM), zygomatico-maxillary (ZM), and pterygomaxillary (PM) pillars at their lower third.

Le Fort II, also described as pyramidal maxillary fracture, extends between the pterygoid plates on both sides. It crosses the lateral vertical (ZM) buttress, medial portion of infraorbital (IO) rim, behind the lacrimal bone, along

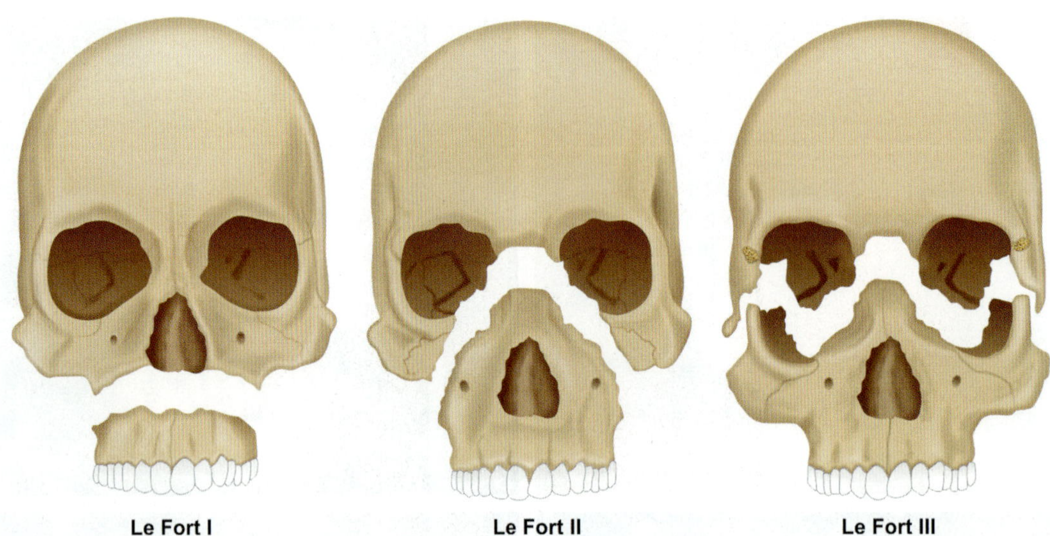

Fig. 36.2: Le Fort classification of midface fractures.

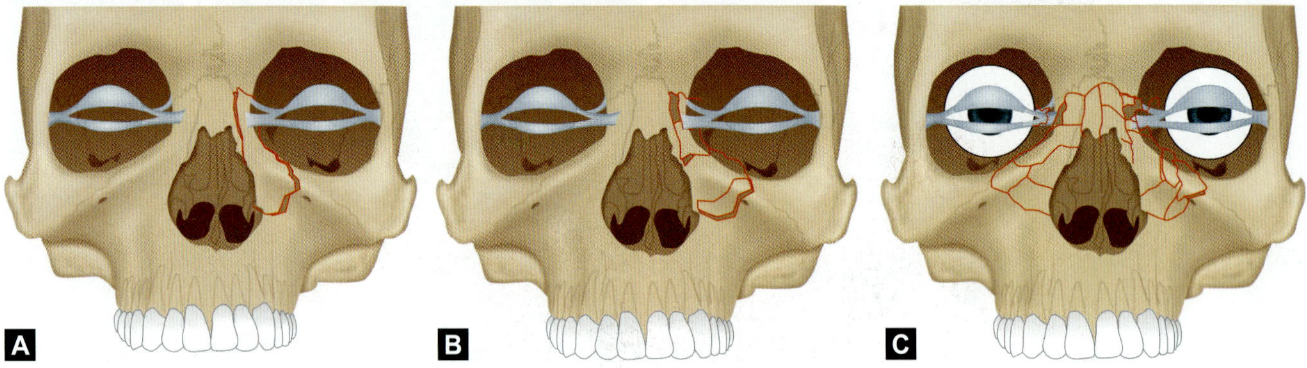

Figs. 36.3A to C: Markowitz classification of naso-orbito-ethmoidal (NOE) fractures. (A) Unilateral type I fracture. Medial canthal tendon is attached to a large fragment of bone, which may be used for reconstruction. (B) Unilateral type II fracture without nasal bone involvement. Medial canthal tendon is attached to a fragment of bone, which can be used for reconstruction. (C) Bilateral type III fracture, with severe comminution of bone in the NOE area and detachment of medial canthal tendon from bone. Bilateral type III fractures are often associated with comminution of nasal and ethmoid bones with loss of nasal pyramid height that requires bone grafting for reconstruction.

the medial orbital wall, and toward the nasal dorsum where it traverses and proceeds to the opposite side in a similar way.

Le Fort III is similar to II except that it crosses the upper third of the ZM pillar. Le Fort III fracture leads to craniofacial disjunction as the entire body of facial bones is separated from the cranial base. The fracture line extends from the frontozygomatic (FZ) suture, along the sphenozygomatic suture on the lateral orbital wall, to the inferior orbital fissure, across the floor and medial wall of the orbit toward the nasal dorsum. It then crosses across the nasal bones and follows a similar path on the opposite side.

The main findings in clinical examination are anterior open bite (Figs. 36.4A to D), vestibular and palatal ecchymosis, flat nasal bridge, and dish-shaped face. Palpation shows movement of the palate and the sutures involved.

Markowitz Classification of NOE Fractures

Naso-orbito-ethmoidal fractures involve the NM buttresses of the facial skeleton and are associated with disruption of the attachment of medial canthal tendon. They may be unilateral or bilateral. In Markowitz type I fractures, a single large NOE bone fragment bearing the medial canthal tendon can be identified. This can then be anchored to adjacent stable bone with plates and screws.

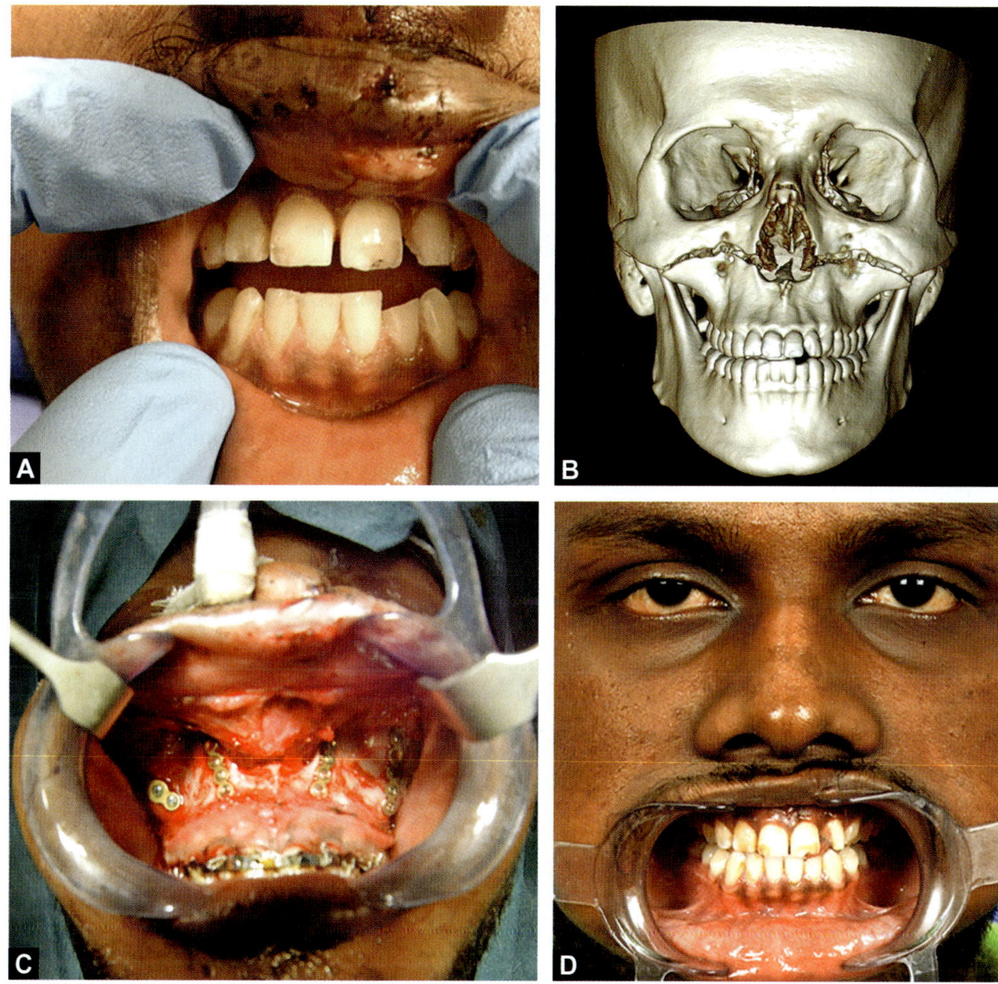

Figs. 36.4A to D: (A) Anterior open bite in a patient with Le Fort I fracture. (B) Three-dimensional reconstruction computerized tomography scan showing Le Fort I fracture. (C) Miniplate fixation of the nasomaxillary and zygomaticomaxillary buttresses through upper buccal sulcus incision. (D) Patient with normal occlusion in the postoperative period.

Types II and III fractures result from more substantial injury leading to comminution of the NOE area, which is often associated with nasal bone fracture and loss of dorsal nasal height. In type II fractures, the medial canthal tendon remains attached to a fragment of bone, which allows the surgeon to stabilize the medial canthus with wires or a miniplate on the fractured segment. In type III fractures, there is detachment of the medial canthal tendon from bone, which makes the reconstruction more complicated and technically challenging.

36.4 PREFERRED TREATMENT

The choice of soft tissue approach and method of fixation is dictated by the presence of facial lacerations, extent and pattern of the fractures, and the structures involved.

In a patient with multiple facial fractures, the main principle is to reduce the fractures from a stable to an unstable area to restore the vertical height, width, and anteroposterior (AP) dimensions of the face. In the top down approach, the reduction and fixation start superiorly (from an intact frontal bone) and then move to the more inferior aspects of the facial skeleton. In the bottom up approach, the reconstruction starts inferiorly (from an intact mandible) and then moves to more superior aspects. If the occlusal surface of either the mandible or maxilla is intact, this is used to reconstruct the other dental arch through maxillomandibular fixation. Reconstruction of the rest of the facial skeleton then follows. In certain situations, where the midface skeleton is severely comminuted, reconstruction starts from the intact/stable lateral skeleton and proceeds medially.

NOE Fractures

Early treatment of NOE fractures is extremely important since delayed post-traumatic deformities in this area are very difficult to correct.

Coronal approach provides the best access to these fractures, with good cosmetic results. In select cases, associated with nearby lacerations, the open sky approach can be used. The Gull wing approach is another option with similar limitations. When using the coronal approach, the surgeon has to be careful to preserve the frontal branch of the facial nerve, and the supraorbital and supratrochlear nerves. If skull base reconstruction is thought to be necessary, then a pericranial flap should be raised at the time of the coronal approach.

Minimally displaced fractures can be treated by careful reduction and rigid fixation using titanium micro- and miniplates. The medial canthal tendon is attached to the anterior lacrimal crest and reset to its normal position with proper reduction in the lacrimal bone fragment.

Comminuted fractures are always a challenge. If the bony fragments are not too small, and the medial canthus tendon remains attached to a reasonably sized bony piece, they can be reduced and plated. Otherwise replacing the medial canthus to its preinjury position will require bone graft reconstruction and repair of the medial canthal tendon with transnasal wire fixation. This can be accomplished by drilling two holes in the segment attached to the ligament and two additional holes on the contralateral side. Then the two ends of the wire are passed through the two holes, using a spinal needle or an owl needle if necessary. The wire is then tightened on the contralateral side. It is important to overcorrect the canthus, which requires drilling the holes more posterior and superior than the natural position.

In case of severe posterior displacement of the nasal dorsum, a bone graft should be used to restore nasal projection and correct a saddle nose deformity. The graft can be secured to the frontal bone with a miniplate.

Orbital Fractures

Orbital fractures can occur in combination with other facial fractures (Figs. 36.1A to E), or they can be an isolated finding (Figs. 36.5A to F). Isolated orbital wall fractures are called blowout fractures and can occur in the orbital floor, medial wall or, rarely in the orbital roof. When present in combination with ZM complex or NOE fractures, reduction in these other fractures results in reduction in the orbital fracture. If after reduction there is still an orbital wall defect, this can be repaired.

The main indications for repair of orbital blowout fractures are mechanical restriction of gaze associated with diplopia, and enophthalmos (Figs. 36.1A to E) or hypophthalmos (>2–3 mm). If these are present in the acute phase, despite the presence of swelling, there is a high chance of globe malposition after the swelling has resolved. Other findings associated with enophthalmos are displacement of >50% of the orbital floor or orbital volume change >1.5 mL. An area of 1.5–2 cm^2 displaced by 2–3 mm can cause a defect large enough to produce significant enophthalmos (Gassner, et al., 2003). The surgery can be done within 2 weeks after the swelling has subsided, but it should not be delayed for >3–4 weeks, when some permanent changes such as fat atrophy and consolidation of the displaced fragments may occur. Urgent surgery is necessary in the cases of traumatic optic neuropathy or oculocardiac reflex (secondary to muscle entrapment). Urgent surgery is also indicated in children with white-eye syndrome.

The approach to orbital floor and medial wall blowout fractures should permit visualization of the fracture, as well as the stable bone around it. The transconjunctival (Figs. 36.6A and B), subciliary, and IO approaches are most frequently used for the orbital floor, and the Lynch incision or transcaruncular approach for the medial wall. The authors prefer to avoid the IO approach unless there is a previous laceration in that area. This approach is associated with the disruption of lymphatics, which leads to pin cushioning of lower lid area.

After the fracture site is exposed, the orbital contents should be dissected out of the maxillary sinus and brought back into the orbit. Once this step is done, the orbital wall should be repaired. There are several options to repair the orbital walls including titanium mesh, porous polyethylene, bone grafts, silicone, Marlex mesh, and resorbable materials. Titanium and porous polyethylene are commonly used materials and, if properly placed, can provide good structural support, with low infection rate and no resorption. Any material can extrude if not stabilized properly. More extensive and comminuted fractures, especially if associated with ZM complex and NOE fractures, may require bone grafts.

After reduction and fixation, eye movement should always be checked to make sure that there is no residual entrapment by performing the forced duction test (Fig. 36.7). Conjunctiva over the sclera is grasped lateral

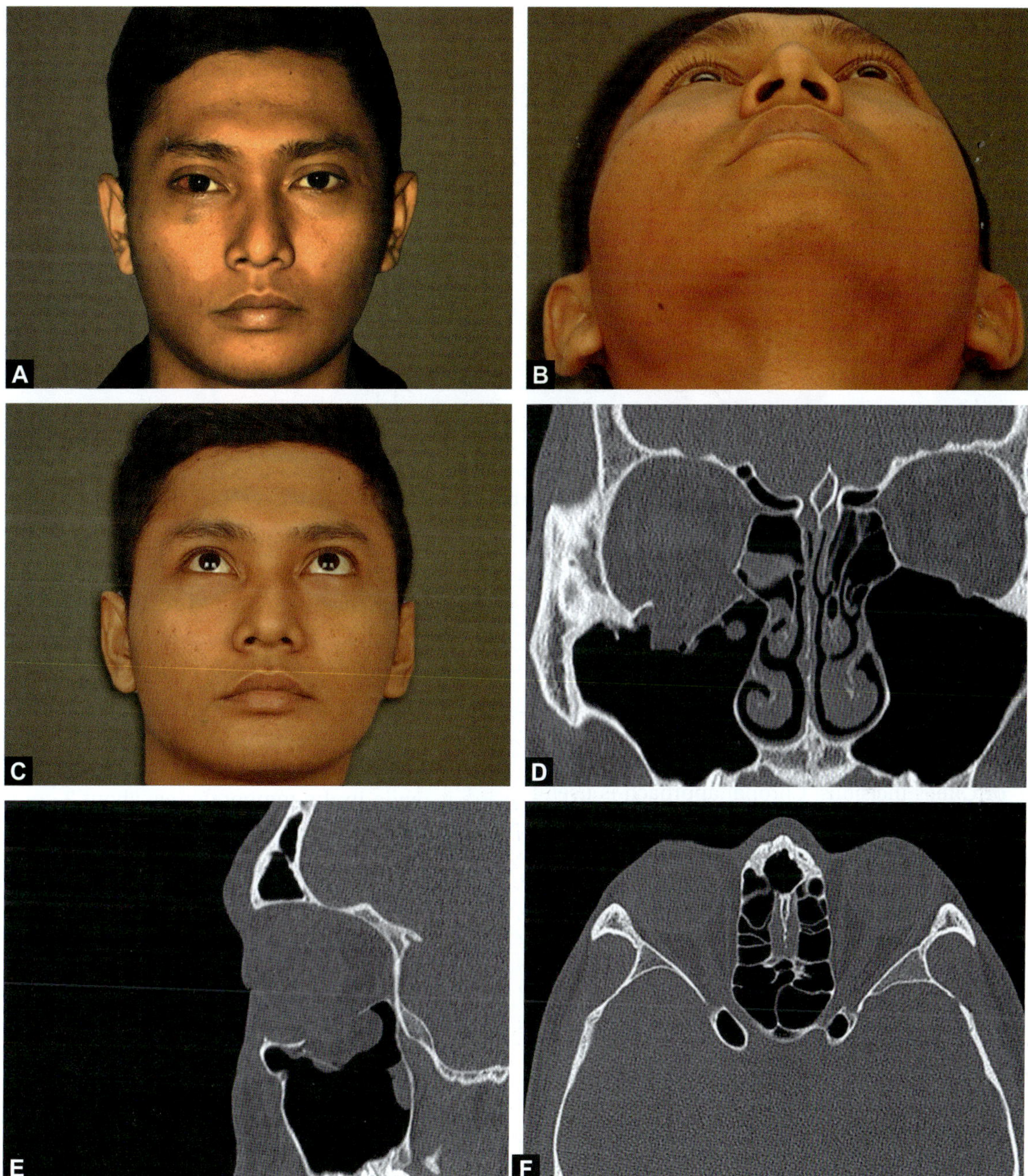

Figs. 36.5A to F: (A) Clinical photograph of a patient who was kicked in the right eye by a horse resulting in an isolated right orbital floor fracture. Right periorbital ecchymosis and subconjunctival hemorrhage are noted. (B) Note right-sided enophthalmos. (C) There is superior restriction of right globe movement because of entrapment of right inferior rectus muscle. (D) Coronal computerized tomography (CT) scan showing herniation of the right orbital fat into the maxillary sinus. (E) Sagittal CT scan showing the anteroposterior extent of the orbital floor fracture. (F) Axial CT scan showing intact medial and lateral orbital walls.

or inferior to the cornea using a smooth forceps. The globe is then moved medially, laterally, superiorly, and inferiorly. Any restriction to the smooth movement of globe is a sign of muscle entrapment, which should be addressed immediately.

Zygomatic Complex Fractures

Zygomatic complex fractures can be classified according to the degree of displacement and segmentation. Low-energy injuries (Figs. 36.8A to F) result in minimally

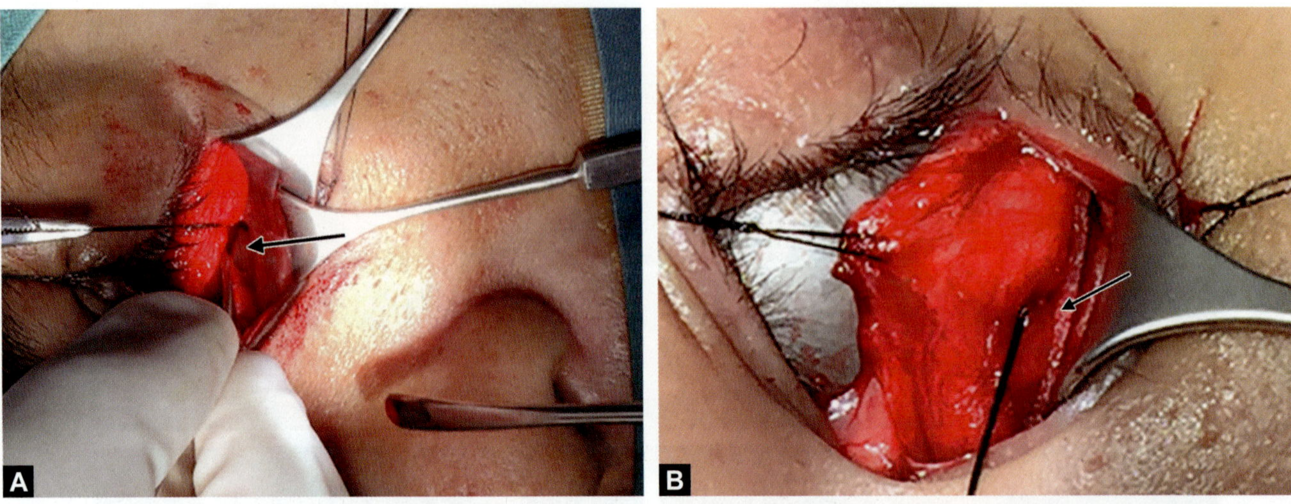

Figs. 36.6A and B: (A) Intraoperative photograph showing left orbital floor fracture (arrow) through a transconjunctival approach. (B) Porous polyethylene implant (arrow) was used to repair the orbital floor fracture in this patient.

displaced fracture, while high-energy fractures are associated with greater degree of comminution and displacement (Manson, et al., 1990). Nondisplaced or minimally displaced fractures usually do not need to be treated surgically.

Surgical approach is through lateral eyebrow, blepharoplasty or supratarsal, transconjunctival, infraciliary, intraoral, or Gillies incisions. Coronal approach is useful (Figs. 36.9A to D) when there is severe comminution, associated facial fractures, or when extensive bone grafts are required. It is preferred to treat fractures through a pre-existing laceration (Fig. 36.10) if it provides adequate exposure.

The complexity of the treatment will depend on the degree of displacement and comminution. Low-energy fractures with minimal displacement can be treated with one-point fixation at the FZ suture (Kim, et al., 2011). This technique is less invasive but does not allow direct inspection of the other sites of fracture. After reduction is accomplished through the lateral eyebrow or upper lid blepharoplasty approach, the surgeon has to make sure that the ZM and IO areas are reduced before plating the FZ fracture site. If there is any question regarding reduction in all fracture sites or if the fracture is unstable, the ZM and/or IO sites should be approached surgically and plated. The sequence of plating is also important. One should start plating the fragment to a stable portion of the skeleton and should start from superior to inferior, and also from lateral to medial. Before plating, it is essential to verify that a good reduction has been achieved. The three main sutures have to be aligned as well as the sphenozygomatic suture on the lateral orbital wall and ZM suture on the orbital floor. The ZM can be approached sublabially and IO via a transconjunctival or subciliary incision. Isolated zygomatic arch fractures are usually treated by open reduction through the Gillies approach or Keen approach without internal fixation.

In the Gillies approach (Figs. 36.11A and B), the incision is made in the temporal area, about 2 cm posterior to the anterior hairline. Dissection continues until the temporalis muscle is reached. A large curved clamp-like Rowe elevator is tunneled downward just deep to the deep temporal fascia and fractured zygoma and upward traction applied taking care not to fulcrum off the squamous portion of the temporal bone, as this is a weak bone and prone to fracture. It is critical to achieve the reduction in one attempt otherwise the bony fragment will become loose and uneducable. Should this happen some packing or inflated Foley catheter can be placed on the medial aspect of the arch to support it for 5–7 days so that it can start healing in the correct position. Alternatively, an external splint like a wooden or metal spatula may be applied to the zygomatic area and the unstable zygomatic arch fragment stabilized in the reduced position by transcutaneous sutures that span the fracture fragment and splint.

In the keen intraoral approach, an upper gingival buccal mucosa incision is made with a monopolar cautery near the inferior part of ZM buttress. A zygoma elevator is then placed medial to the zygomatic arch and used to elevate it into its proper position.

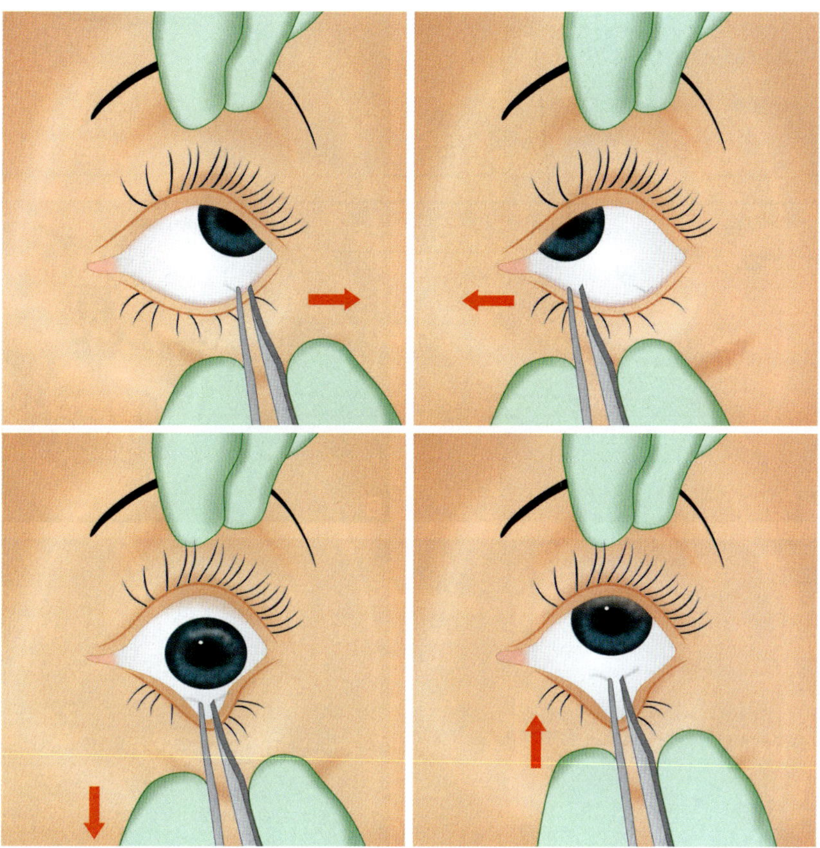

Fig. 36.7: Forced duction test is performed by grasping the conjunctiva inferior or lateral to the cornea and moving the globe medially, laterally, superiorly, and inferiorly. Any restriction to smooth movement of globe is a sign of extraocular muscle entrapment.

High-energy fractures will require access to FZ, ZM, and IO sites, which may require multiple approaches. Loss of lateral projection usually means that there has been comminution at the ZM and IO areas, allowing the zygomatic complex to be displaced medially. Loss of AP projection is associated with comminution of the zygomatic arch. Proper reduction in these fractures will re-establish lateral and AP projections. After reduction of comminuted fractures, it is not uncommon to find missing bone at the orbital floor, ZM area, or zygomatic arch. For this reason, the surgeon should be prepared to perform bone grafting in high-energy fractures, especially if they are associated with severe displacement. Although it is imperative to protect the frontal branch of facial nerve during this approach, the nerve has usually been injured from trauma leading to injury.

Failure to obtain appropriate reduction or delay in treatment can result in post-traumatic deformity including enophthalmos, hypophthalmos, or lack of malar eminence projection. Correction of these deformities can be challenging and often requires osteotomies and bone grafts.

Maxillary Fractures

The first step in treatment consists of maxillomandibular fixation. This requires nasotracheal intubation, after skull base fractures have been ruled out, or a tracheostomy. Some surgeons, especially oral surgeons, prefer submandibular intubation. Patients with mandible fractures will require reduction and fixation of those fractures before or during maxillomandibular fixation. Sometimes the maxilla will be impacted posteriorly and require mobilization using the Rowe disimpaction forceps (Figs. 36.12A to C).

After maxillomandibular fixation, the maxillary fracture is reduced and plated with 1.5 mm titanium plates at the NM and ZM buttresses. This will require an intraoral approach for Le Fort I, associated with IO approach for Le Fort II and upper lid blepharoplasty/lateral eyebrow approach for Le Fort III fractures. Also, a coronal approach may be used for a Le Fort III fracture. If there are other associated fractures, the authors prefer to work from a solid base (mandible inferiorly, frontal bone superiorly). Similarly, reduction is carried out from lateral to medial

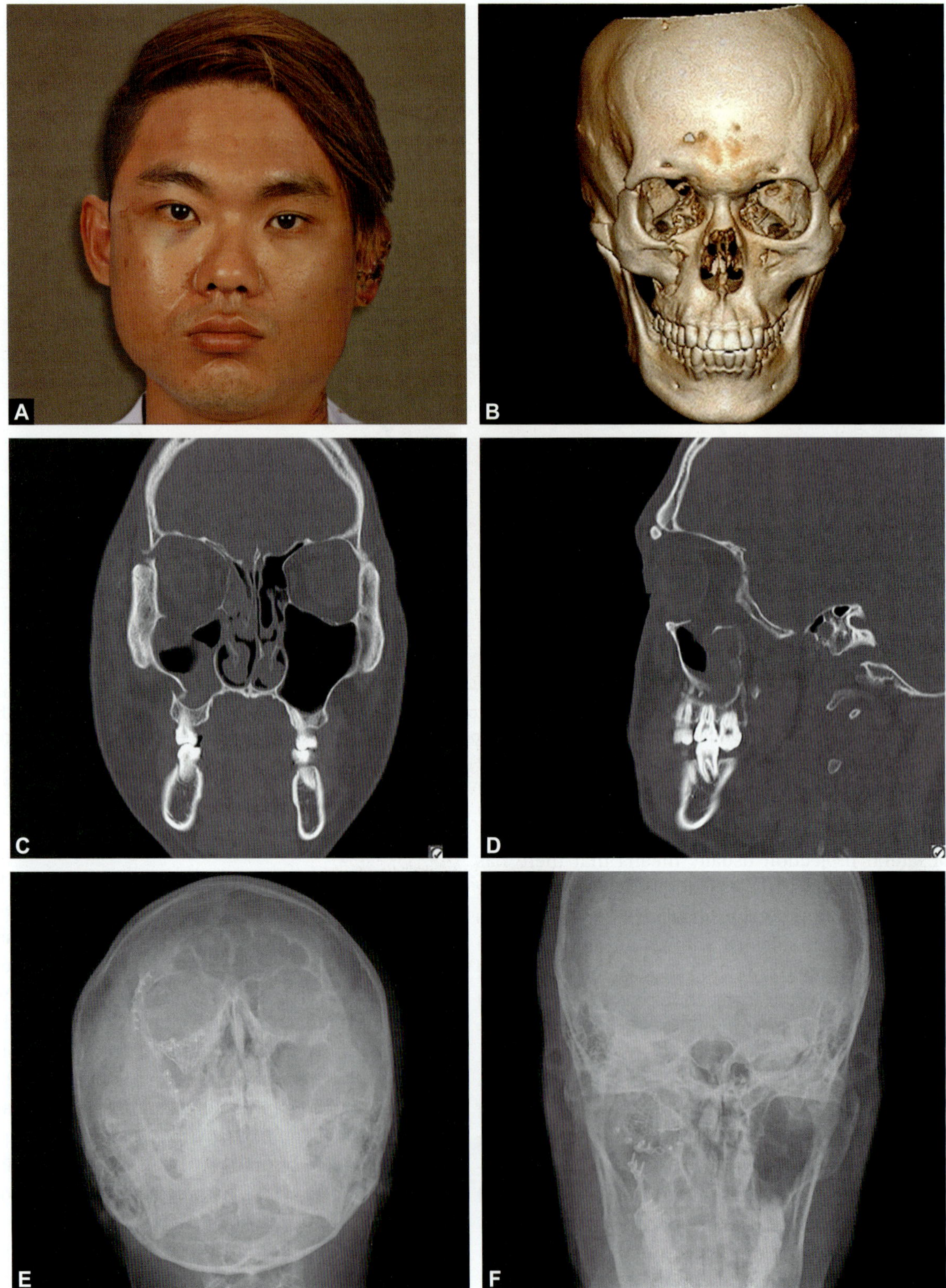

Figs. 36.8A to F: (A) Patient with malposition of the right globe due to an internally rotated tripod fracture. (B) Three-dimensional reconstruction computerized tomography scan showing the tripod fracture. (C and D) Right orbital floor fracture. (E and F) Postoperative radiographs showing three-point fixation using miniplates and orbital floor reconstruction using titanium mesh plate.

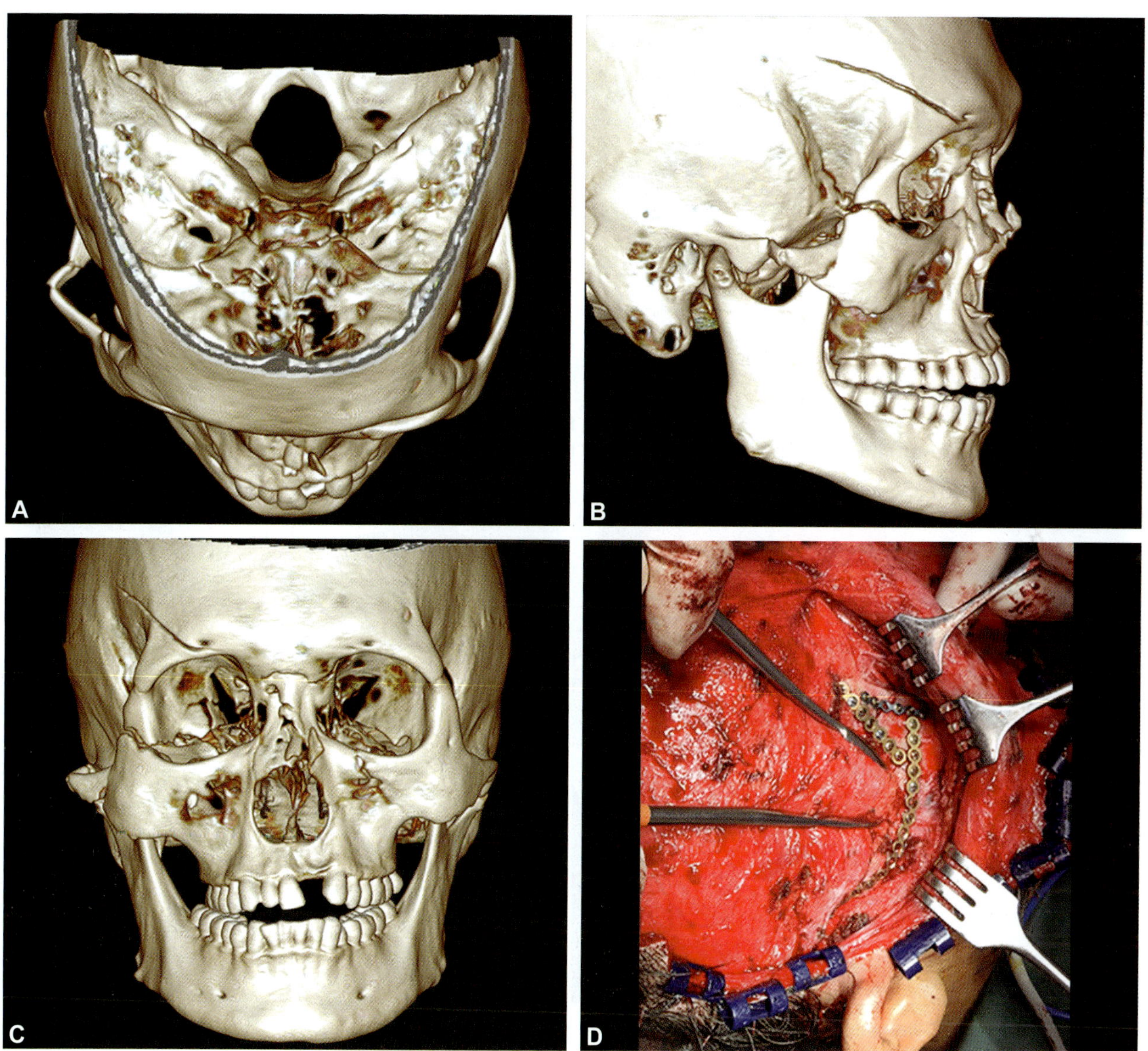

Figs. 36.9A to D: (A to C) Three-dimensional reconstruction computerized tomography scans of a patient with depressed right zygomatic arch and lateral orbital wall fracture. (D) Coronal approach was used for open reduction and internal fixation of the fractures.

(zygomatic fractures first and NOE fractures last). Like any other place in the facial skeleton, fractures associated with severe comminution will need bone graft repair.

The other challenge is the treatment of patients with poor dentition. In this case, maxillomandibular fixation may not be possible. Palatal splints and gunning splints can be used to achieve a better maxillomandibular relationship.

36.5 TREATMENT OUTCOME(S)

Treatment outcomes will depend on the severity of the fractures, patient's overall health status, and experience of the surgeon. The most common complications are malocclusion, orbital and facial deformity, paresthesia, infection, and malunion. Malocclusion is commonly seen when maxillary fractures are associated with comminution and/or mandibular fractures.

Orbital complications are common and have been reported in up to 20% of patients (O'Sullivan, et al., 1999). One of the most feared but rare complications is blindness. In the postoperative setting, blindness can be caused by retrobulbar hemorrhage/hematoma, retinal artery spasm, or optic nerve compression by a bone fragment. Enophthalmos and hypophthalmos can be caused by failure to reconstruct the orbital walls properly or by bone resorption.

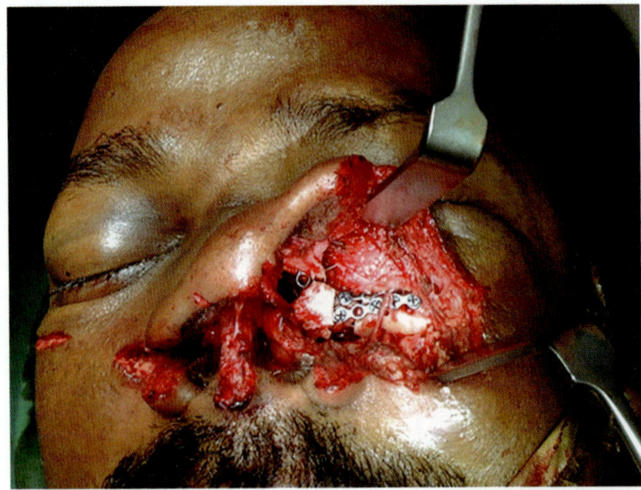

Fig. 36.10: Anterior maxillary wall and orbital floor fractures being treated through a facial laceration.

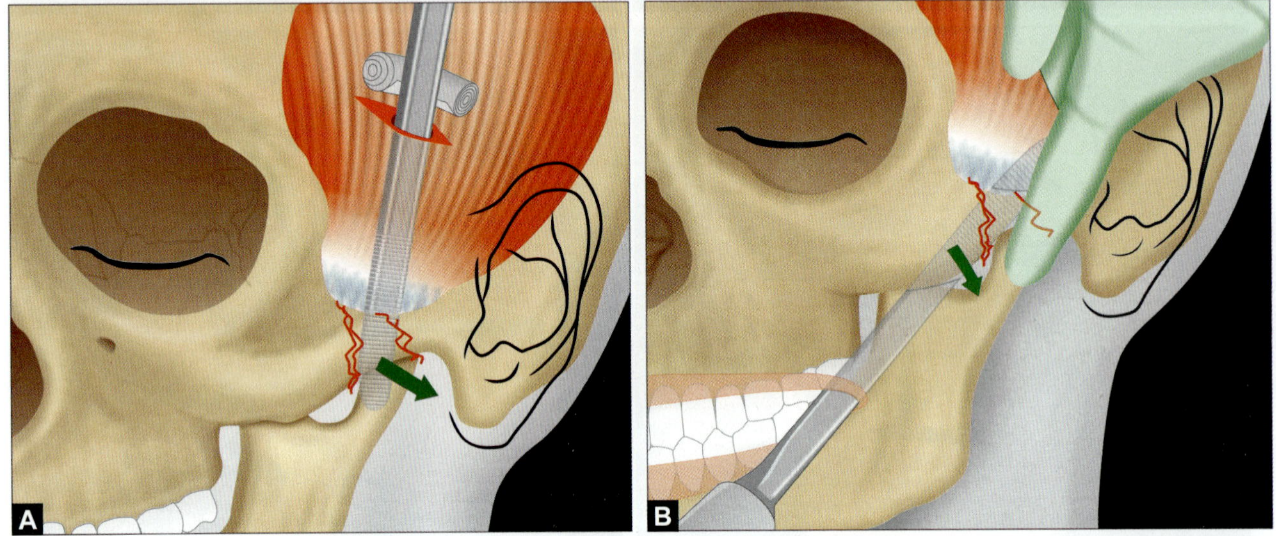

Figs. 36.11A and B: (A) Gilles and (B) Keen approaches to open reduction in depressed zygomatic arch fractures.

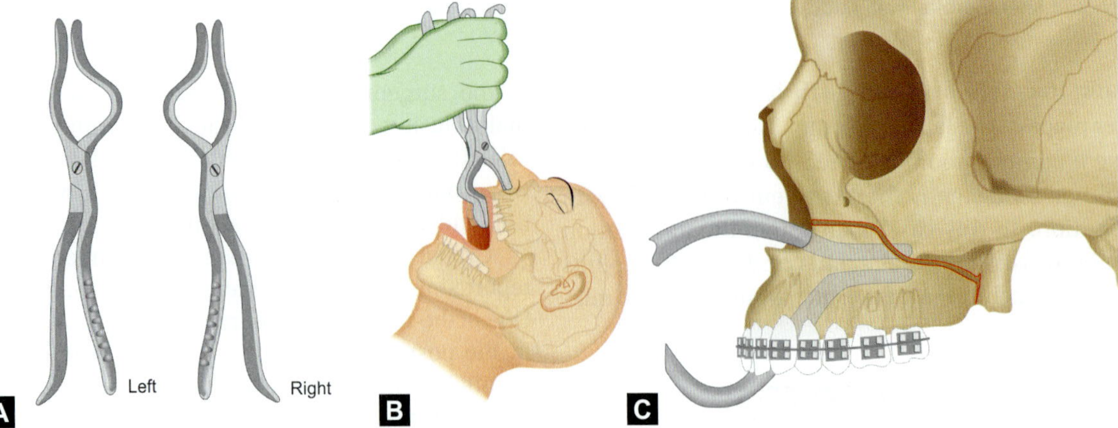

Figs. 36.12A to C: (A) Illustrations showing left and right Rowe disimpaction forceps. (B and C) The forceps are being used to mobilize an impacted Le Fort I fracture.

Malunion and infection are usually associated with technical problems that result in loose screws and lack of stability. Bone fragment mobility precludes ossification and can cause pseudoarthrosis and subsequent infection.

REFERENCES

Gassner, R., Tuli, T., Hachl, O., Rudisch, A. and Ulmer, H., 2003. Cranio-maxillofacial trauma: a 10-year review of 9,543 cases with 21,067 injuries. *Journal of Craniomaxillofacial Surgery,* 31, pp. 51-61.

Kim, S.T., Go, D.H., Jung, J.H., Cha, H.E., Woo, J.H. and Kang, I.G., 2011. Comparison of 1-point fixation with 2-point fixation in treating tripod fractures of the zygoma. *Journal of Oral and Maxillofacial Surgery,* 69, pp. 2848-52.

Manson, P.N., Markowitz, B., Mirvis, S., Dunham, M. and Yaremchuk, M., 1990. Toward CT-based facial fracture treatment. *Plastic and Reconstructive Surgery,* 85, pp. 202-12; discussion 213-4.

Markowitz, B.L., Manson, P.N., Sargent, L., Vander Kolk, C.A., Yaremchuk, M., Glassman, D. and Crawley, W.A., 1991. Management of the medial canthal tendon in nasoethmoid orbital fractures: the importance of the central fragment in classification and treatment. *Plastic and Reconstructive Surgery,* 87, pp. 843-53.

McGovern, M.K., Murphy, R.X., Jr., Okunski, W.J. and Wasser, T.E., 2000. The influence of air bags and restraining devices on extremity injuries in motor vehicle collisions. *Annals of Plastic Surgery,* 44, pp. 481-5.

O'Sullivan, S.T., Snyder, B.J., Moore, M.H. and David, D.J., 1999. Outcome measurement of the treatment of maxillary fractures: a prospective analysis of 100 consecutive cases. *British Journal of Plastic Surgery,* 52, pp. 519-23.

APPENDIX 36.1: FACIAL TRAUMA ANALYSIS

History

Mode of trauma	
Time of trauma	
Loss of consciousness	Yes/No
Headache	Yes/No
Vomiting	Yes/No
Vision	Decreased right/Decreased left/Decreased both/Not affected
Difficulty breathing	Yes/No
Hoarseness	Yes/No
Hearing	Decreased right/Decreased left/Decreased both/Not affected
Facial sensation	• Not affected/Decreased right upper face/Decreased left upper face/Decreased upper face on both sides • Decreased right midface/Decreased left midface/Decreased midface on both sides • Decreased right lower face/Decreased left lower face/Decreased lower face on both sides
Change in occlusion	Yes/No
Last meal/drink	

Past Medical History

TMJ disease	
Malocclusion	Yes/No
Dental treatment	Yes/No
Diabetes	No/Well controlled/Poorly controlled
Epilepsy	Yes/No
Other medical problems	

Examination

Airway	
Denture	Present/Missing/Cannot be assessed/Not applicable
Teeth fragments	Present/Missing/Cannot be assessed/Not applicable
Foreign body	Yes/No/Cannot be assessed/Not applicable
Circulation	Blood pressure: mmHg, Heart rate: beats/min, O_2 saturation: %
C-spine tenderness, deformity, etc.	Yes/No/Cannot be assessed/Not applicable
GCS	EVM

Inspection

Right side of face	No abnormality detected	**Left side of face**	No abnormality detected
Swelling	Yes/No	Swelling	Yes/No
Bruising	Yes/No	Bruising	Yes/No
Laceration	Yes/No	Laceration	Yes/No

Avulsion	Yes/No	Avulsion	Yes/No
Tattooing from debris	Yes/No	Tattooing from debris	Yes/No
Foreign body	Yes/No	Foreign body	Yes/No
Deformity	Yes/No	Deformity	Yes/No
Others		Others	

Right eye	No abnormality detected	**Left eye**	No abnormality detected
Laceration	Yes/No	Laceration	Yes/No
Periorbital ecchymosis	Yes/No	Periorbital ecchymosis	Yes/No
Subconjunctival hemorrhage	Yes/No	Subconjunctival hemorrhage	Yes/No
Epiphora	Yes/No	Epiphora	Yes/No
Lacrimal system injury	Yes/No	Lacrimal system injury	Yes/No
Direct light reflex	Yes/No	Direct light reflex	Yes/No
Consensual light reflex	Yes/No	Consensual light reflex	Yes/No
Visual acuity	Normal/Abnormal/Cannot be assessed	Visual acuity	Normal/Abnormal/Cannot be assessed
Visual field defect	Yes/No	Visual field defect	Yes/No
Diplopia	Yes/No	Diplopia	Yes/No
Ophthalmoplegia	Up/Down/Lateral/Medial	Ophthalmoplegia	Up/Down/Lateral/Medial
Eye protrusion	Exophthalmos/Enophthalmos	Eye protrusion	Exophthalmos/Enophthalmos

Nose, right side	No abnormality detected	**Nose, left side**	No abnormality detected
Laceration	Yes/No	Laceration	Yes/No
Deviation	Yes/No	Deviation	Yes/No
Saddle nose	Yes/No	Saddle nose	Yes/No
Swelling	Yes/No	Swelling	Yes/No
Telecanthus	Yes/No	Telecanthus	Yes/No
Increased nostril show	Yes/No	Increased nostril show	Yes/No
Deviated nasal septum	Yes/No	Deviated nasal septum	Yes/No
Septal hematoma	Yes/No	Septal hematoma	Yes/No

Right ear	No abnormality detected	**Left ear**	No abnormality detected
Auricle hematoma	Yes/No	Auricle hematoma	Yes/No
Auricle laceration	Yes/No	Auricle laceration	Yes/No
Battle sign	Yes/No	Battle sign	Yes/No
Bleeding	Yes/No	Bleeding	Yes/No
CSF leak	Yes/No	CSF leak	Yes/No
External auditory canal narrowing	Yes/No	External auditory canal narrowing	Yes/No

Tympanic membrane perforation	Yes/No	Tympanic membrane perforation	Yes/No
Hemotympanum	Yes/No	Hemotympanum	Yes/No
Others		Others	

Oral cavity, right side	No abnormality detected	**Oral cavity, left side**	No abnormality detected
Dentures	Normal/Missing/Cannot be assessed	Dentures	Normal/Missing/Cannot be assessed
Trismus	Yes/No/Cannot be assessed	Trismus	Yes/No/Cannot be assessed
Laceration (lip/mucosal/palatal)	Yes/No/Cannot be assessed	Laceration (lip/mucosal/palatal)	Yes/No/Cannot be assessed
Alveolar fracture	Yes/No/Cannot be assessed	Alveolar fracture	Yes/No/Cannot be assessed
Hard palate fracture	Yes/No/Cannot be assessed	Hard palate fracture	Yes/No/Cannot be assessed
Avulsed teeth	Yes/No/Cannot be assessed	Avulsed teeth	Yes/No/Cannot be assessed
Floor of mouth hematoma	Yes/No/Cannot be assessed	Floor of mouth hematoma	Yes/No/Cannot be assessed
Malocclusion	Yes/No/Cannot be assessed	Malocclusion	Yes/No/Cannot be assessed
Cross bite deformity	Yes/No/Cannot be assessed	Cross bite deformity	Yes/No/Cannot be assessed
Open bite deformity	Anterior/Lateral/Posterior/No	Open bite deformity	Anterior/Lateral/Posterior/No

Palpation

Right eye	No abnormality detected	**Left eye**	No abnormality detected
Supraorbital rim	Normal/Abnormal	Supraorbital rim	Normal/Abnormal
Infraorbital rim	Normal/Abnormal	Infraorbital rim	Normal/Abnormal
Lateral wall	Normal/Abnormal	Lateral wall	Normal/Abnormal
Medial wall	Normal/Abnormal	Medial wall	Normal/Abnormal
Forced duction test	Normal/Abnormal	Forced duction test	Normal/Abnormal
Intercanthal distance (if telecanthus)		Intercanthal distance (if telecanthus)	

Right side of face	No abnormality detected	**Left side of face**	No abnormality detected
Frontal bone	Normal/Abnormal	Frontal bone	Normal/Abnormal
Maxilla	Normal/Abnormal	Maxilla	Normal/Abnormal
Zygomatic arch	Normal/Abnormal	Zygomatic arch	Normal/Abnormal
Teeth and alveolus	Normal/Abnormal	Teeth and alveolus	Normal/Abnormal

Right side of nose	No abnormality detected	**Left side of nose**	No abnormality detected
Nasal bone	Normal/Crepitus	Nasal bone	Normal/Crepitus

Right side of mandible	No abnormality detected	**Left side of mandible**	No abnormality detected
TMJ	Normal/Abnormal/ Cannot be assessed	TMJ	Normal/Abnormal/ Cannot be assessed

Mandible	Normal/Abnormal/ Cannot be assessed	Mandible	Normal/Abnormal/ Cannot be assessed
Range of motion	Normal/Abnormal/ Cannot be assessed	Range of motion	Normal/Abnormal/ Cannot be assessed
Interincisal distance	0–8 cm	Interincisal distance	0–8 cm
Lateral excursion	Normal/Abnormal/ Cannot be assessed	Lateral excursion	Normal/Abnormal/ Cannot be assessed
Protrusion	Normal/Abnormal/ Cannot be assessed	Protrusion	Normal/Abnormal/ Cannot be assessed

Right side of larynx	No abnormality detected	**Left side of larynx**	No abnormality detected
Surgical emphysema neck	Yes/No	Surgical emphysema neck	Yes/No

Right facial sensation	No abnormality detected	**Left facial sensation**	No abnormality detected
Supraorbital/ Supratrochlear nerves	Normal/Decreased sensation/ Cannot be assessed	Supraorbital/ Supratrochlear nerves	Normal/Decreased sensation/ Cannot be assessed
Infraorbital nerve	Normal/Decreased sensation/ Cannot be assessed	Infraorbital nerve	Normal/Decreased sensation/ Cannot be assessed
Mental nerve	Normal/Decreased sensation/ Cannot be assessed	Mental nerve	Normal/Decreased sensation/ Cannot be assessed

Right facial nerve	No abnormality detected	**Left facial nerve**	No abnormality detected
Temporal branch	House Brackmann grades 1–6	Temporal branch	House Brackmann grades 1–6
Zygomatic branch	House Brackmann grades 1–6	Zygomatic branch	House Brackmann grades 1–6
Buccal branch	House Brackmann grades 1–6	Buccal branch	House Brackmann grades 1–6
Marginal mandibular branch	House Brackmann grades 1–6	Marginal mandibular branch	House Brackmann grades 1–6
Cervical branch	House Brackmann grades 1–6	Cervical branch	House Brackmann grades 1–6

Nasal endoscopy	No abnormality detected
Septal hematoma	Yes/No/Cannot be assessed
Epistaxis	Yes/No
Larynx	Edema/Hematoma/Avulsed vocal cords/Dislocated arytenoids

(TMJ: Temporomandibular joint; O_2: Oxygen; C-spine, cervical spine; GCS: Glasgow coma scale; E: Eye; V: Voice; M: Movement; CSF: Cerebrospinal fluid).

37 Orbital Floor Fracture

Yip Chee Chew

Chapter Overview

Pearls and Pitfalls

Pearls

- Orbital pain and proptosis may indicate a developing orbital hematoma.
- Surgical repair of orbital floor fractures may be delayed till resolution of the soft tissue swelling except in fractures with muscle entrapment.
- Indications for surgery include severe enophthalmos and muscle entrapment.
- White-eyed blowout fracture requires urgent and immediate surgical intervention.
- Computed tomography (CT) scan of orbits is the radiological investigation of choice in patients with suspected orbital wall fractures.
- Transconjunctival approach is preferred over conventional subciliary approach.
- The implant used for repair of orbital floor fracture should be stable and supported by the adjacent intact orbital bone beyond the edges of the fracture.

Pitfalls

- Placing the implant too far posteriorly can likely damage the orbital apex structures.
- Failure to close the conjunctiva and lower lid retractors meticulously may lead to complications.
- It is important to detect abnormalities of pupil size and relative afferent papillary defect early to identify any developing compressive optic neuropathy.

37.1 INTRODUCTION

Orbital floor fractures are not uncommonly encountered in the injuries involving the periorbital region. They are often associated with blunt trauma to the orbit. The assessment and treatment of these injuries present unique challenges that will be discussed in this chapter.

37.2 EPIDEMIOLOGY OF ORBITAL FLOOR FRACTURES

Orbital floor fractures may occur in isolation in about one-fifth of cases presenting to trauma centers (Antoun and Lee, 2008; Hwang, You and Sohn, 2009) or associated with fractures of the adjacent bones such as the orbital medial wall, roof, and lateral wall. In more severe cases, the zygomaticomaxillary complex and/or mandible may also be involved.

37.3 ANATOMY OF THE ORBITAL FLOOR

- The orbit is pyramidal in shape with four walls: a roof, lateral wall, floor, and medial wall.
- The bony pyramid base is the orbital entrance (4 cm wide and 3.5 cm high), which is rotated laterally. The lateral walls of the right and left orbits are at right angles to each other.
- The orbital floor is comprised of three bones: orbital plate of the maxilla anteromedially, zygoma anterolaterally, and the palatine bone posteriorly. The orbital floor separates the orbit from the maxillary sinus. It is triangular in shape and slopes gradually upward to merge with the medial wall at the maxilloethmoidal suture. The orientation of the floor implant should respect this anatomical configuration to restore the orbital cavity volume.
- Near the middle of the posterior part of the orbital surface of the maxilla is the infraorbital groove, for the passage of the infraorbital vessels and nerve. The groove leads to the infraorbital canal, which transmits the infraorbital nerve and artery, both of which exit the anterior face of the maxilla through the infraorbital foramina. Medial to the infraorbital nerve, the orbital floor is relatively thin and fractures easily. Orbital floor fracture may involve the infraorbital nerve to cause hypoesthesia of the V2 distribution such as the ipsilateral cheek, upper gums, and teeth.
- Its posterolateral two thirds is separated from the lateral wall by the inferior orbital fissure through which it transmits the zygomatic nerve, a branch of the maxillary division of the trigeminal nerve (V2), the ascending branches from the pterygopalatine ganglion, and the infraorbital vessels.
- The volume of the orbit is about 30 cm^3 and that of the globe about 7 cm^3. The length of the medial orbital wall from the anterior lacrimal crest is 44–50 mm, whereas the distance along the lateral wall from the rim to the superior orbital fissure measures 40 mm. The optic nerve, ophthalmic artery, and sympathetic fibers from the carotid plexus pass through the optic foramen. The lateral part of the superior orbital fissure transmits the lacrimal and frontal nerve branches of V1, trochlear nerve, meningeal branch of lacrimal artery, and anastomotic branch of middle meningeal artery. The middle part transmits the upper and lower divisions of the oculomotor nerve, the nasociliary nerve (V1), and abducent nerve. The medial part transmits the superior ophthalmic vein and sympathetic nerves. These structures along with those passing through the inferior orbital fissure can get stretched or compressed in orbital wall fractures to affect vision, ocular motility, and facial sensation.

37.4 PATHOPHYSIOLOGY OF ORBITAL FLOOR FRACTURES

Orbital floor fractures may occur due to direct impact on the inferior orbital rim or indirectly as in a blowout fracture. The two mechanisms postulated to explain the latter are as follows:

- *Hydraulic theory*: According to this theory (Rhee, et al., 2002), the orbital floor fractures from an increase in intraorbital pressure. This is generally due to the impact of an object of greater size than the orbital entrance exerting a diffuse force to the orbital contents to cause the weaker orbital floor to give way.
- *Buckling theory*: The orbital floor buckles and breaks due to a high-compressive force applied to the inferior orbital rim (Warwar, et al., 2000).

In a blowout fracture, entrapment and/or herniation of the periorbital and orbital contents into the maxillary antrum results in limitation of extraocular movements. Expansion of the orbital volume also causes globe retroplacement and enophthalmos.

In the pediatric age group, due to the "elastic" nature of the orbital bones, the orbital floor fracture site may impose a trapdoor-like effect to impinge upon the herniated extraocular muscles. In this population, entrapment may occur without obvious eye signs (white eye syndrome) and represents a surgical emergency (Jordan, et al., 1998) to avoid ischemia and fibrosis of the entrapped extraocular muscle.

37.5 ASSESSMENT OF PATIENT WITH ORBITAL FLOOR FRACTURE

Clinical History

- The surgeon should ascertain the mechanism of injury, whether it is blunt or sharps-related trauma. Sometimes, the patient may have sustained a combination of both types of injury, as in a motor vehicle accident.

- A history of sharps-related trauma may be associated with intraocular or orbital foreign body; this needs to be excluded.
- A history of binocular diplopia may suggest extraocular muscle involvement.
- Numbness of the lower eyelid, cheek, gums, and/or teeth may suggest infraorbital nerve injury.
- Epistasis may occur due to the involvement of the paranasal sinuses, especially the ethmoidal sinus, in concomitant orbital floor and medial wall fractures.
- A compliant of blurred vision may indicate the need for referral to an ophthalmologist for an eye evaluation to exclude ocular or optic nerve injuries.
- The presence of painful eye movements, nausea, vomiting, and syncopy may suggest acute extraocular muscle entrapment, as in white-eyed blowout fracture in children (Jordan, et al., 1998).

Clinical Examination

The patient presents with one or more of the following (Fig. 37.1):

- Periorbital ecchymosis and edema.
- Subconjunctival hemorrhage due to damage to the superficial conjunctival vessels.
- In pediatric orbital floor fractures, the external signs may be minimal with an uncongested eye. However, these white-eyed blowout fractures are commonly associated with acute and severe entrapment of the extraocular muscles. The patient may also present with a history of syncope due to oculocardiac reflex (*Aschner phenomenon*) being triggered by attempted eye movements. This reflex is mediated by the neural connections between the ophthalmic branch of the fifth cranial nerve via the ciliary ganglion and the vagus nerve (parasympathetic).
- Limitation in up-gaze and rarely down-gaze (due to inferior rectus injury) with vertical diplopia.
- Forced duction test may be positive on an entrapped extraocular muscle. The test is used to check for restrictive myopathy by moving the affected muscle (at its insertion) with a nontoothed forceps away from its field of action under topical anesthesia. However, the author feels that it is much more comfortable for the patient if a cotton-tipped applicator is used in replacement of the forceps.
- Subcutaneous emphysema in the periorbital region.
- Hypoesthesia over the distribution of the infraorbital nerve.
- Step over the inferior orbital rim (with orbital rim fracture) on palpation.
- Exophthalmometry is mandatory to measure the globe position and assess the severity of enophthalmos.
- Enophthalmos may not be apparent in the acute stage due to orbital soft tissue swelling. Rarely, proptosis may occur due to orbital hemorrhage.

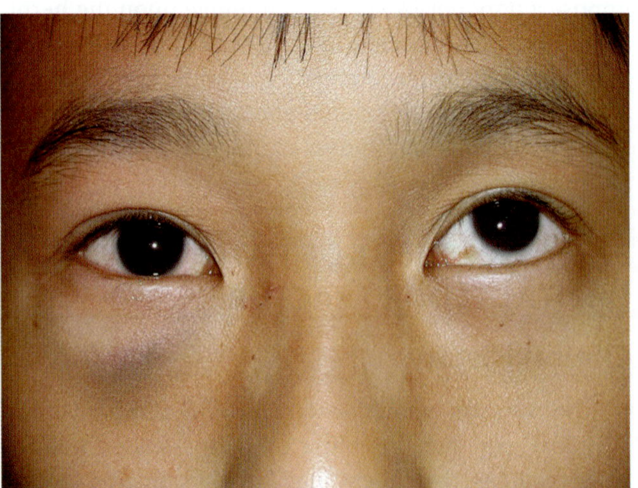

Fig. 37.1: Patient presenting with right-sided blowout fracture showing periorbital bruising and limitation in up-gaze.

In the clinical evaluation of the orbital trauma patient, traumatic optic neuropathy, intraocular foreign body, and globe injuries should be excluded and managed promptly, if present. A careful pupil examination is mandatory to exclude optic nerve injury and severe ocular damage.

37.6 INVESTIGATIONS

- Clinical photography to document the relevant clinical signs is important.
- Binocular single vision chart (Fig. 37.2) is indicated (if available) to quantify the degree of gaze beyond which diplopia occurs.
- Hess chart (Fig. 37.3) is the gold standard in documenting the range of extraocular movements in all nine positions of gaze.
- Computed tomography of the orbit (Fig. 37.4) should be done to determine the location and extent of orbital fracture(s), the severity of orbital soft tissue herniation into the maxillary antrum, and to exclude intraocular or orbital foreign body. The conventional orbital radiograph has generally been replaced by CT orbit, given the imaging superiority of the latter.

37.7 TREATMENT

Indications for Surgery

- Acute entrapment of the extraocular muscle as in white-eyed blowout fracture requires urgent and immediate surgical intervention as soon as the operating facility is available (Burnstine, 2002).
- Large orbital fracture involving more than half of the orbital floor should be repaired in view of the significant enophthalmos that may ensue.
- Severe enophthalmos (> 2 mm).

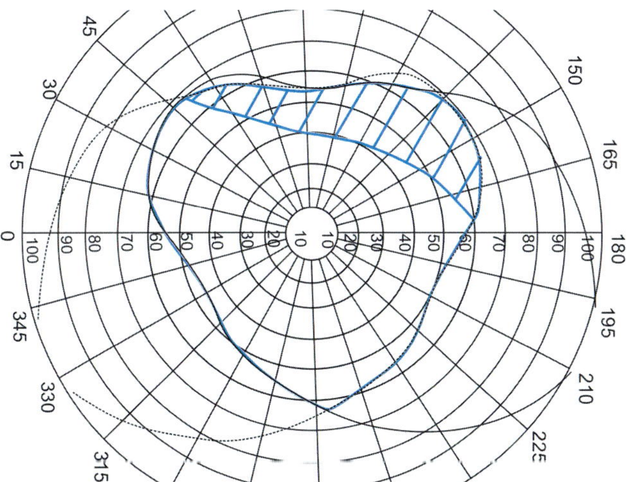

Fig. 37.2: Binocular single vision chart of a patient showing the extent of diplopia (shaded area). Diplopia is present from 30° of up-gaze onward.

- Combined orbital floor and medial wall fractures are often associated with significant enophthalmos that requires correction.

Surgical Repair of Orbital Floor Fracture

- Surgical repair may be done electively under general anesthesia after resolution of the soft tissue swelling except in fractures with muscle entrapment.
- A short course (about 1 week) of oral steroids with broad-spectrum antibiotic coverage before surgery is useful to reduce soft tissue inflammation and edema.
- Transconjunctival approach is preferred over conventional transcutaneous (subciliary) approach. The former avoids the problems of scarring, eyelid retraction, and ectropion. The orbital floor may be reached via a pre- or post-septal plane after incising into the conjunctiva and lower eyelid retractors.
- In the preseptal approach, after incising the conjunctiva and lower eyelid retractors below the inferior tarsal border, the orbicularis oculi is dissected bluntly with a Steven's scissors or cotton-tipped applicators from the orbital septum down to the level of the inferior orbital rim. The dissection is aided by anterosuperior countertraction on the anterior lamella (skin and orbicularis oculi) with a lacrimal rake or Desmarres retractor. In the postseptal approach, the incision is made in the inferior fornix and the dissection is carried through the orbital fat to the inferior orbital rim.

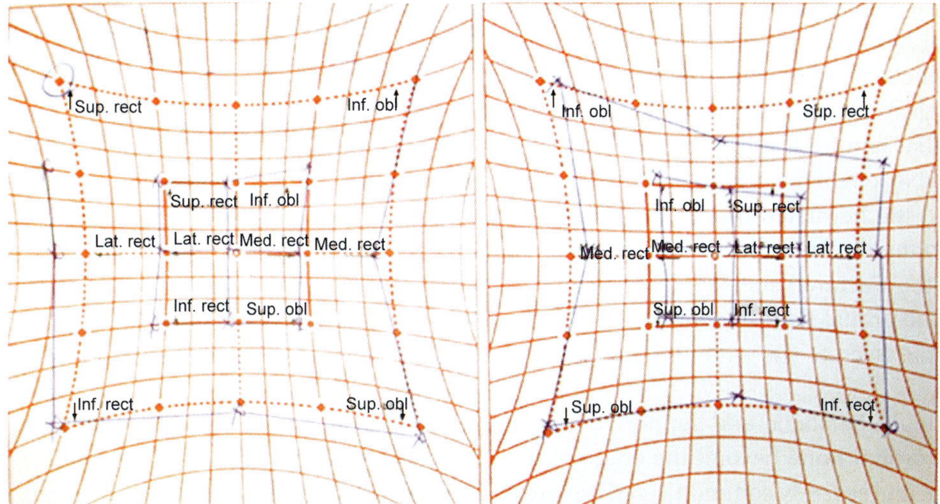

Fig. 37.3: Hess charts in a patient with right-sided blowout fracture showing limitation in movement of right eye (right chart) on up-gaze (due to entrapped inferior rectus) and corresponding overaction of the left superior rectus (left chart).

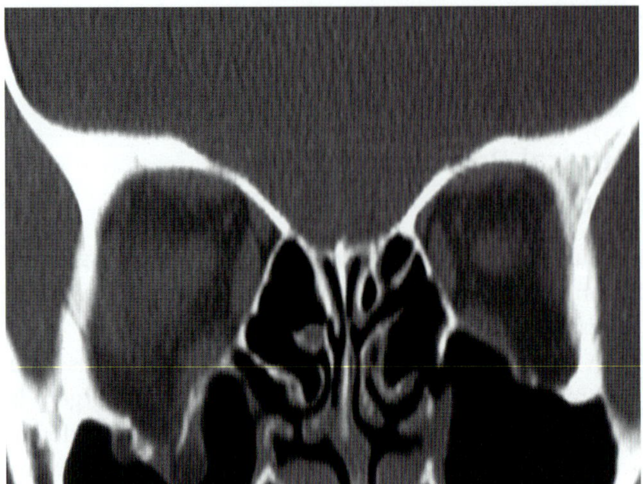

Fig. 37.4: Coronal computed tomography scan of orbit showing right orbital floor and lateral wall fractures with herniation of the orbital soft tissue into the maxillary antrum.

- The preseptal plane avoids the problem of orbital fat prolapsing into the surgical field. However, dissection in this surgical plane may be difficult for the novice surgeon and carries the risk of full-thickness penetration through the skin. In comparison, the postseptal approach may be an easier dissection plane that is favored by some.
- The orbital periosteum is incised at the arcus marginalis widely with a No. 15 blade and then reflected off the orbital floor with a periosteal elevator to expose the fractured site.
- Further surgical exposure may be improved with a lateral canthotomy and inferior cantholysis. However, proper reconstruction of the lateral canthus is required to avoid canthal dystopia and eyelid malpositioning.
- The transconjunctival approach may be combined with a transgingival approach in the presence of maxillary fractures that require fixation.
- The location and extent of the orbital floor fracture are determined and the herniated orbital contents repositioned back to their normal anatomical position. All the borders of the fractured site should be identified to ensure that the orbital floor implant covers the full dimensions of the fracture site with no herniated soft tissues.
- The implant should be stable and supported by the adjacent intact orbital bone beyond the edges of the fracture. In large and severely communicated fractures without stable or sufficient margins to support one or more sides of the implant, special implants designed for orbital rim fixation may be needed. The fracture site can be repaired with a nonabsorbable material, e.g. Supramid, titanium plates, or the newer bioabsorbable material such as Osteopore. The choice of implant material depends on cost consideration and the surgeon's training, preference, and experience. It is crucial to ensure that the entire fracture site is visualized and covered by the implant. However, care should be exercised not to place the implant too far posteriorly as this is likely to damage the orbital apex structures.
- Closure of the incised orbital periosteum is advisable to prevent migration of the implant.
- A meticulous closure of the conjunctiva and lower eyelid retractor is necessary to avoid complications.

37.8 POSTOPERATIVE CARE

- The patient is advised to avoid blowing the nose, and to sneeze with the mouth open and nose unobstructed. This helps reduce the risk of developing orbital surgical emphysema. Avoidance of strenuous physical activity for a few weeks is also advisable.
- Regular monitoring of the pupil size and the presence of relative afferent papillary defect are important to detect any early signs of compressive optic neuropathy due to orbital hemorrhage. The surgeon should also be alert to orbital pain and proptosis, which may indicate a developing orbital hematoma.
- Cold compresses are advised to reduce surgical edema and soft tissue swelling.
- Topical steroid eye drops are helpful to reduce ocular surface inflammation.
- A short course (1–2 weeks) of oral steroid with broad-spectrum antibiotic coverage is prescribed.

37.9 POSTOPERATIVE COMPLICATIONS

The patient should be informed of following potential complications (Gosau, et al., 2011) following repair of orbital floor fracture.

- Over- or undercorrection of enophthalmos may occur and require further surgery.
- Lower eyelid retraction and ectropion may occur but are less likely with the transconjunctival approach.
- Infraorbital nerve damage may lead to numbness over the cheek area. This may be temporary if the nerve has been stretched at the time of surgery, or permanent if the nerve has been transected due to the initial injury or because of iatrogenic injury.

- Inferior oblique injury may lead to diplopia.
- Orbicularis oculi paresis or paralysis may manifest as ectropion and impaired blinking.
- Symblepharon may follow the transconjunctival approach and may lead to cicatricial entropion.
- Infection.
- Implant extrusion or migration.
- Persistent eyelid edema or chemosis due to lymphedema.
- Optic nerve damage and blindness.

REFERENCES

Antoun, J.S. and Lee, K.H., 2008. Sports-related maxillofacial fractures over an 11-year period. *Journal of Oral and Maxillofacial Surgery*, 66(3), pp. 504-8.

Burnstine, M.A., 2002. Clinical recommendations for repair of isolated orbital floor fractures: an evidence-based analysis. *Ophthalmology*, 109(7), pp. 1207-10.

Gosau, M., Schöneich, M., Draenert, F.G., Ettl, T., Driemel, O. and Reichert, T.E., 2011. Retrospective analysis of orbital floor fractures—complications, outcome, and review of literature. *Clinical Oral Investigations*, 15(3), pp. 305-13.

Hwang, K., You, S.H. and Sohn, I.A., 2009. Analysis of orbital bone fractures: a 12-year study of 391 patients. *Journal of Craniofacial Surgery*, 20(4), pp. 1218-23.

Jordan, D.R., Allen, L.H., White, J., Harvey, J., Pashby, R. and Esmaeli, B., 1998. Intervention within days for some orbital floor fractures: the white-eyed blowout. *Ophthalmic Plastic and Reconstructive Surgery*, 14(6), pp. 379-90.

Rhee, J.S., Kilde, J., Yoganadan, N. and Pintar, F., 2002. Orbital blowout fractures: experimental evidence for the pure hydraulic theory. *Archives of Facial Plastic Surgery*, 4(2), pp. 98-101.

Warwar, R.E., Bullock, J.D., Ballal, D.R. and Ballal, R.D., 2000. Mechanisms of orbital floor fractures: a clinical, experimental, and theoretical study. *Ophthalmic Plastic and Reconstructive Surgery*, 16(3), pp. 188-200.

Mandible Fracture 38

Lai Juen Bin

Chapter Overview

Pearls and Pitfalls

Pearls

- Achieving form and function (occlusion) is the main objective in the management of mandibular fractures.
- The surgeon should utilize his/her knowledge of ideal lines of osteosynthesis and principles of load-bearing and load-sharing osteosynthesis to treat each individual fracture.
- Sublingual hematoma is pathognomonic of mandibular body fractures and should alert one to its presence.

Pitfalls

- Relying only on mandibular radiographs without carrying out a detailed physical examination of a patient with a suspected mandibular fracture may lead to mismanagement of mandibular fractures.
- Ignoring dental occlusion during reduction in mandibular fractures will lead to postoperative malocclusion that may require extensive revision surgery.
- Prescribing closed reduction is not suitable for all mandibular condylar fractures.

38.1 ETIOLOGY

Mandibular fractures are the second most common facial fractures in facial trauma due to the position and prominence of the mandible (Ogundare, Bonnick and Bayley, 2003; Thaller, 1994). Common causes include road traffic accidents 43%, assault 34%, sport injuries 4%, and falls 7% (Hagan and Huelke, 1961). Mandibular fractures are less common in children due to greater elasticity of the bone.

38.2 ANATOMY OF THE MANDIBLE AND ITS RELATED STRUCTURES

It is important to understand the mandible osteology, dental occlusion, and structures related to the mandible to manage mandibular fractures adequately.

Mandible Osteology

The mandible is a U-shaped bone that supports the lower dentition and makes up the lower facial skeleton. It has no bony attachments to the skull. It is suspended below the maxilla by muscles, ligaments, and other soft tissues, which provide the mobility necessary to function with the maxilla.

The superior aspect of the mandible consists of the alveolar process and the teeth. The anterior part of the mandible between the lower canines is the symphysis that transits the parasymphysis around the lower canine and first premolar region. The mandibular bone curves backward to form the body. The body of the mandible extends posteroinferiorly to form the mandibular angle and posterosuperiorly to form the ascending ramus. The ascending ramus of the mandible is formed by a vertical plate of bone that extends upward as two processes. The anterior process is the coronoid process where the temporalis muscle inserts. The posterior process is the condyle that articulates with the temporal cranial base to form the temporomandibular joint (TMJ).

The TMJ provides both hinging movement around the inferior joint compartment and gliding movement around the superior joint compartment when the mouth opens widely. It is therefore considered as a ginglymoarthrodial joint.

Nerve

Inferior alveolar nerve (IAN) is a branch of the mandibular division of the trigeminal nerve. It enters the mandibular foramen that lies in the medial surface of the ramus of the mandible and runs intraosseously until the mandibular body. It exits the mandible below the lower premolars' root region from the mental foramen to supply sensation of the lower lip and chin. Anatomical knowledge is important especially during placement of osteosynthesis plates and screws to avoid damage to the nerve.

The lingual nerve is also a branch of the mandibular division of the trigeminal nerve. It lies anterior to the IAN and first descends deep to the lateral pterygoid muscle and superficial to the medial pterygoid muscle. It lies close to the lingual cortex of the mandible over the retromolar trigone and lower third molar region. This makes it susceptible to damage during open reduction and internal fixation of osteosynthesis plates and screws over the fractured mandibular angle region.

Facial Nerve

The marginal mandibular branch of the facial nerve is at risk of injury in transfacial approaches to the ramus and angle aspect of the mandible.

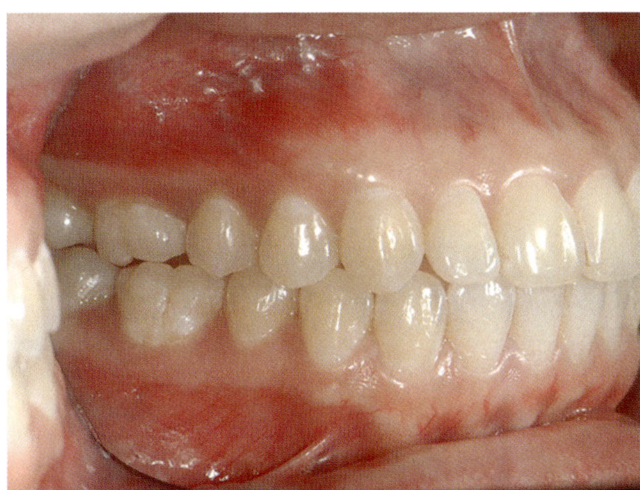

Fig. 38.1: Class I occlusion. The relative mesiodistal position of the dental arches is normal with permanent first molars usually in normal occlusion.

The frontotemporal branches of the facial nerve are at risk in preauricular approach to mandibular condyle.

Facial Vessels

The facial vessels cross the inferior border of the mandible around the body region. These vessels are responsible for hemorrhage if they are accidentally damaged during open reduction and internal fixation of mandibular fractures.

Dental Occlusion

Understanding dental occlusion is important in the management of mandibular fractures in order to restore patient back to preinjury occlusion and function.

There are three variations in occlusion in the general population as defined by Angle's classification of malocclusion: Class I (Fig. 38.1), Class II (Fig. 38.2), and Class III (Fig. 38.3) occlusions. The classification is based on the relationship of the mesiobuccal cusp of the maxillary first molar and the buccal groove of the mandibular first molar. If this molar relationship exists, then the teeth can align into normal occlusion. The prevalence of Class I, II, and III occlusions varies from ethnic racial groups to geographic locations. The relative distribution of various types of occlusions in Singapore is: Class I occlusion (48.1%), Class II occlusion (29.5%), and Class III occlusion (22.4%), with Indians having a higher incidence of Class II occlusion (Soh, Sandham and Chan, 2005).

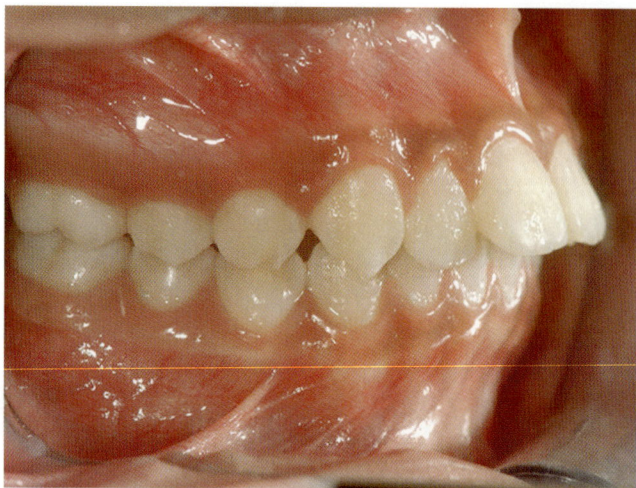

Fig. 38.2: Class II occlusion. The relative mesiodistal relations of the dental arch are abnormal with all the lower teeth occluding distal to normal, producing a disharmony in the incisor region and facial lines.

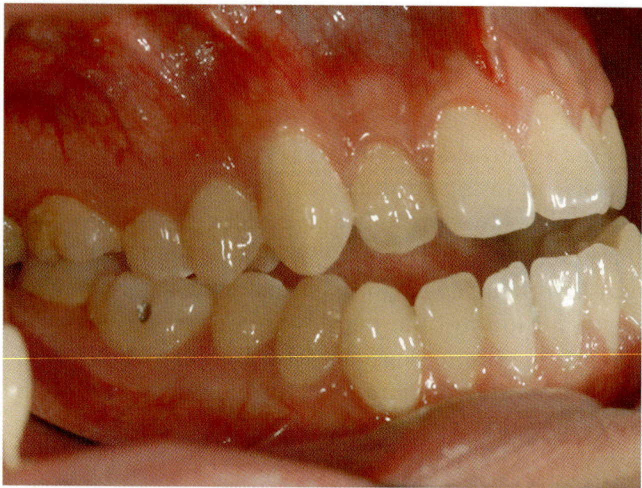

Fig. 38.3: Class III occlusion. The relative mesiodistal relations of the arches are abnormal with all the lower teeth occluding mesial to normal, producing a disharmony in the incisor region and facial lines.

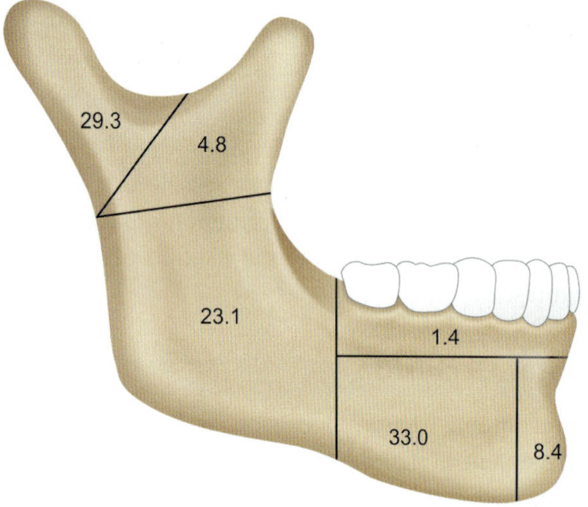

Fig. 38.4: The percentage distribution of mandibular fracture sites. *Source*: Luyk, N.H., 1992. Principles of management of fractures of the mandible. In: Peterson, L.J., et al., eds. *Principles of oral and maxillofacial surgery*. Philadelphia, PA: Lippincott-Raven; pp. 381-434.

38.3 CLASSIFICATION OF MANDIBULAR FRACTURES

There are two main classifications of mandibular fractures. The common classifications are by the anatomic location affected and the other by the fracture patterns. Classification of mandibular fractures by anatomic location affected is as follows (Fig. 38.4):

- Condyle—condylar head, condylar neck, and subcondylar
- Angle
- Body
- Symphyseal and parasymphyseal
- Dentoalveolar
- Ramus
- Coronoid process

Classification of mandibular fractures by the type of fracture is as follows:

- *Greenstick fracture*: This means it is not a through and through fracture, the fracture either involves buccal or lingual cortex or does not extend to the lower border of the mandible.
- *Simple fracture*: The fracture does not extend to tooth-bearing area of the mandible and does not communicate with the periodontal ligament space of the dentoalveolar segment.
- *Compound fracture*: The fracture extends to tooth-bearing area of the mandible and communicates with the periodontal ligament space of the dentoalveolar segment.
- *Comminuted fracture*: The fracture consists of multiple fracture lines and segments.
- *Favorable versus unfavorable fractures:* These depend on the fracture patterns with respect to the displacing forces by the masticatory muscles. In unfavorable fractures, the fractured fragments are pulled apart by the action of muscles, whereas in favorable fractures the pull exerted by the muscles helps keep the fractured fragments aligned (Figs. 38.5 and 38.6).

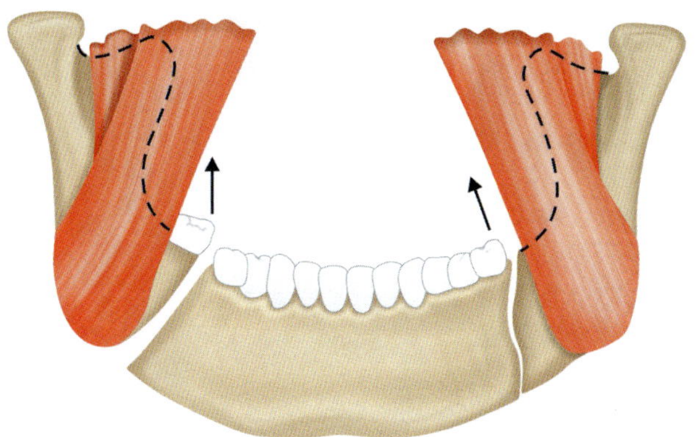

Fig. 38.5: Diagram of horizontally unfavorable (left) and favorable (right) fracture lines. Arrows indicate displacing forces from the masseter and medial pterygoid muscles.
Source: Luyk, N.H., 1992. Principles of management of fractures of the mandible. In: Peterson, L.J., et al., eds. *Principles of oral and maxillofacial surgery*. Philadelphia, PA: Lippincott-Raven; pp. 381-434.

38.4 SIGNS AND SYMPTOMS OF MANDIBULAR FRACTURES

- Patients may complain of intraoral bleeding, pain, and tenderness over the lower border of the mandible, chin area, and temporomandibular region.
- Malocclusion that develops acutely after a traumatic impact to the mandible is the most common sign. Patients will invariably complain that their bite is different. Acute facial asymmetry may develop with deviation of the chin point from the central facial midline.
- Patients may complain about difficulty in mouth opening and trismus. Examination may identify limited mandibular range of movements. There may also be deviation of lower jaw on mouth opening.
- Palpation of the mandible may indicate step-off deformity as well as tenderness at the fracture site. Mandibular stress test is useful to identify subtle fractures. The test is performed by pushing the lingual surfaces of the body of mandible outward with the volar pads of the examiner's thumbs. The location of pain experienced by the patient helps localize the site of the fracture. Skin laceration under the chin should also alert the clinician to possible condylar and/or symphysis fractures. Intraoral mucosal and gum laceration may also suggest underlying fractures.
- Sublingual hematoma due to tear in the lingual periosteum of the mandible may be observed. It is pathognomonic of mandibular body fractures.
- When fractures transverse the mental foramen and the IAN, patient can develop numbness of the lower lip and chin. It is important to ask the patient about the lower lip and chin sensation whenever mandibular fractures are suspected.

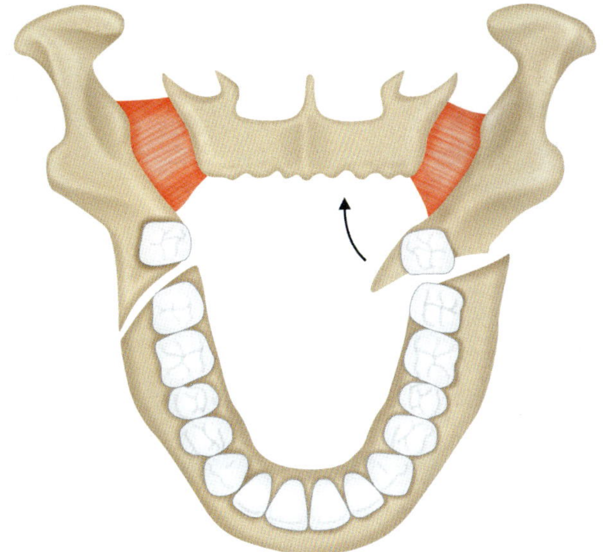

Fig. 38.6: Diagram of vertically favorable (right) and unfavorable (left) fracture lines. Arrow indicates displacing force from the medial pterygoid muscle.
Source: Luyk, N.H., 1992. Principles of management of fractures of the mandible. In: Peterson, L.J., et al., eds. *Principles of oral and maxillofacial surgery*. Philadelphia, PA: Lippincott-Raven; pp. 381-434.

38.5 RADIOGRAPHIC INVESTIGATIONS FOR MANDIBULAR FRACTURES

- There are various radiographs that can be performed to screen for mandibular fractures. Orthopantomogram (OPG) and intraoral radiographs are commonly ordered to investigate for mandibular fractures. For OPG, the patients need to be able to stand upright and this may not be possible in polytrauma and unconscious patients. However, OPG is able to identify 92% of mandibular fractures compared with standard radiographs (Chayra, et al., 1986). It should be born in mind that the symphyseal region is not clearly visualized due to overlapping images used to generate an OPG and fractures around the area may be missed.
- The most common radiographs are the mandible X-ray series that include posteroanterior , right and left oblique views, and reverse Towne's to screen for condylar fractures. These can be performed in a patient who is unable to stand erect and can detect 66% of fractures of the mandible (Chayra, et al., 1986).

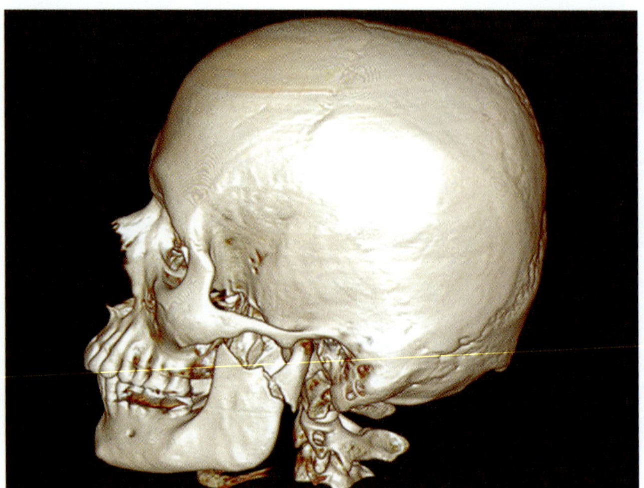

Fig. 38.7: Three-dimensional reconstruction computed tomography scan of a patient with medially displaced left subcondylar fracture.
Image courtesy: Dr Sandeep Uppal.

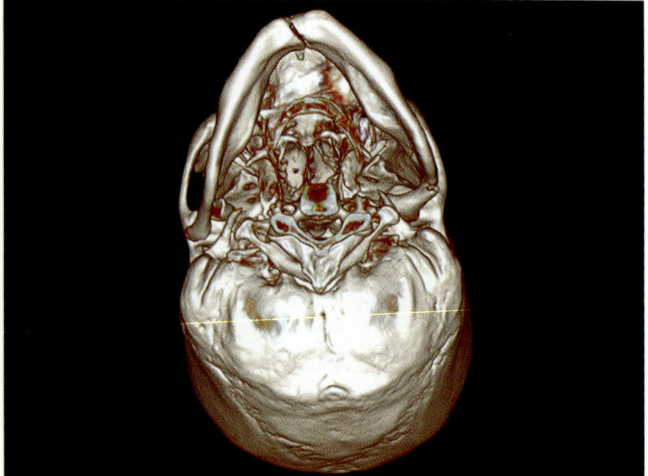

Fig. 38.8: Three-dimensional reconstruction computed tomography scan of the same patient as in Figure 38.7 showing medially displaced left subcondylar fracture, medially displaced right head of condyle fracture, and right symphyseal fracture. Three-dimensional reconstruction images help familiarize the surgeon with the orientation of the fractured condylar fragments and inform surgical planning.
Image courtesy: Dr Sandeep Uppal.

- Cone beam computed tomography (CT) and conventional CT scan can render three-dimensional images of the mandible and the associated fractures. Although costlier than mandible X-ray series and OPG, this gold standard investigation can prove very useful in surgical planning especially in displaced condylar, subcondylar, and comminuted fractures (Figs. 38.7 and 38.8).

38.6 TREATMENT PRINCIPLES

- In any trauma patient, the appropriate sequence of management includes primary survey (**A**irway and cervical spine control, **B**reathing and ventilation, **C**irculation and hemorrhage control, **D**isability, and **E**xposure and environment) with concurrent resuscitation; regular assessment of ABCDE; secondary survey, and then definitive care. Following these principles, mandibular fractures are only managed once the patient has been comprehensively assessed to rule out other life-threatening injuries and stabilized adequately.
- The aim of mandible fracture management is anatomical reduction and stabilization of the fracture fragments until bony union is established. Preinjury dental occlusion should be established and complications like infection should be prevented by timely use of antibiotics in patients with open fractures.
- Dentoalveolar injuries can also be present at the same time as mandibular fractures. These injuries must be identified and treated appropriately. The management of mandibular fracture and teeth in the line of fracture is controversial. The surgeon must consider whether to remove the offending tooth or leave the tooth in place if it is thought not to compromise the fracture management. In general, the tooth in line of fracture is often left in situ if it does not interfere with reduction and fixation of the fracture, otherwise removal of the tooth may cause loss of bone that makes placement of plates and screws difficult.

38.7 BIOMECHANICS OF THE MANDIBLE

The mandible is subjected to masticatory forces during function. Zones of compression and tension (Fig. 38.9) are formed in the mandible depending on where the bite force is located in the mandibular arch. The tension zone is formed at the superior portion of the mandible and the compression zone is formed at the inferior portion of the mandible. Champy described the ideal lines of osteosynthesis (Fig. 38.10) that are utilized for fracture fixation.

Principle of Fracture Reduction

The fracture fragments need to be stabilized at least along the zone of tension as there is a tendency for the fragments to splay away from each other in this area due to

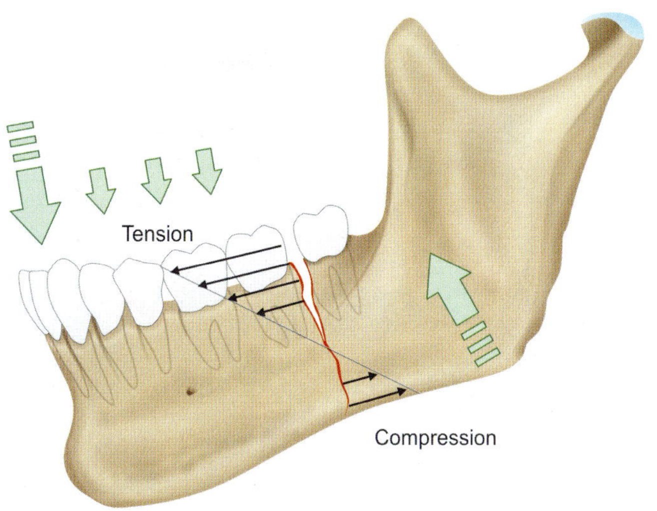

Fig. 38.9: The zones of compression and tension formed in the mandible due to forces of mastication. The superior border of the mandible is the tension zone and the inferior border is the compression zone.
Source: AO Surgery Reference (https://www.aofoundation. org/wps/portal/surgery).

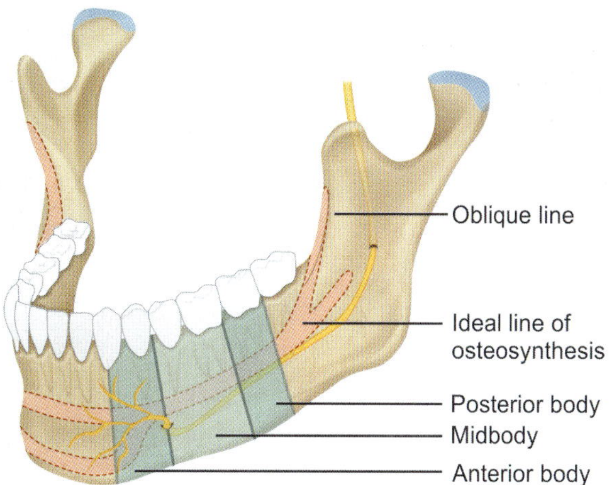

Fig. 38.10: Champy's ideal lines of osteosynthesis (shown in pink). *Source*: AO Surgery Reference (https://www.aofoundation. org/wps/portal/surgery).

the forces of mastication. There is debate in the literature regarding the need for fixation along the zone of compression since the fragments tend to be naturally compressed together along this zone due to masticatory forces. Surgeons have differing philosophies regarding utilizing one or two plate technique for fracture fixation depending on the configuration and location of the fracture, but the common denominator is that fracture needs to be stabilized along the zone of tension either with a plate or by using an arch bar.

Single-Plate Fixation

The single miniplate technique along Champy's line may be employed in the management of simple isolated mandibular angle fractures or when the other mandibular fractures can be treated with rigid fixation. For angle fractures, this will involve using a single monocortical plate along the oblique line. A simple fracture involving the anterior mandible (symphysis and parasymphysis) requires fixation along the zones of tension and compression. These fractures can be treated using the combination of a stable arch bar along the zone of tension and one plate just above the inferior border of mandible (zone of compression). This is particularly useful when it is physically not possible to place two plates, e.g. in situations where the vertical dimension of the mandible is reduced and the apices of teeth are in danger of being damaged, or in edentulous patients. In condylar fractures, if the fracture morphology is unfavorable and the available bone stock is limited, a single strong plate placed along the long axis of the condylar process may be used for reconstruction.

Two-Plate Fixation

In angle fractures, two monocortical miniplates, one along Champy's line along the superior part of the mandible and the other along the inferior part of the lateral cortex below the IAN, are used when other mandibular fractures cannot be stabilized with rigid fixation, e.g. contralateral condylar fracture being treated by closed reduction, bilateral angle fractures (one side should be treated with two miniplates), and associated maxillary fractures when it is important to have an intact and stable mandible from condyle-to-condyle for proper reduction in maxillary fractures to achieve preinjury occlusion. One plate each along Champy's lines is also employed in complex anterior fractures of the mandible (Figs. 38.11 and 38.12). One reconstruction plate along the inferior border of the mandible and miniplate higher up on the mandible just below the apices of the teeth is used in patients with communited fractures of the anterior part, body, or angle of mandible (Fig. 38.13). In other patients, reconstruction plate may be used with arch bar fixation. In condylar fractures, fixation using two miniplates is preferred, with one plate inferior to the sigmoid notch and the other along the posterior border, if the fracture configuration allows it.

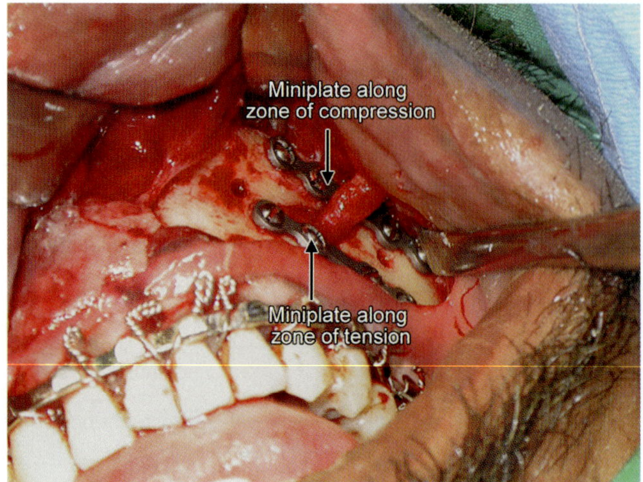

Fig. 38.11: Intraoperative photograph showing open reduction and internal fixation with one miniplate each along the zone of compression and tension to repair a fracture of right mandibular body.

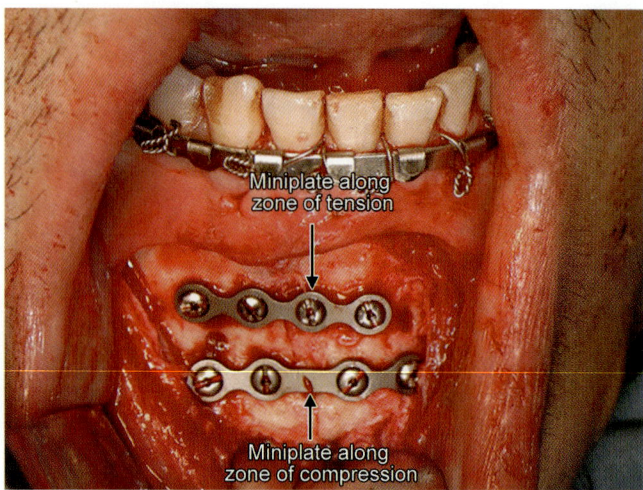

Fig. 38.12: Intraoperative photograph showing open reduction and internal fixation with one miniplate each along the zone of compression and tension to repair a symphyseal fracture.

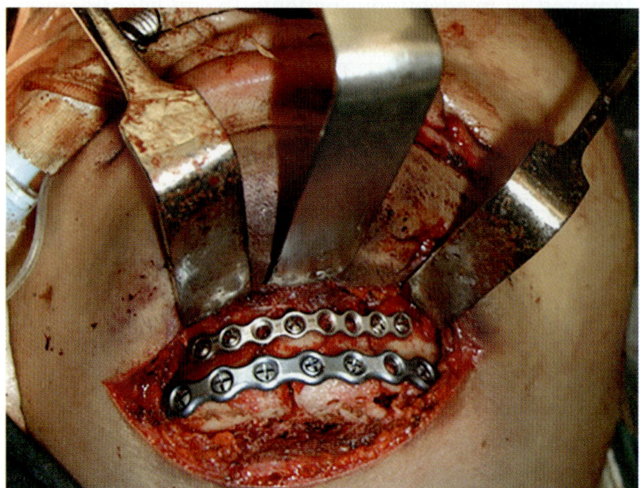

Fig. 38.13: Intraoperative photograph showing open reduction and internal fixation of symphyseal and left parasymphyseal fracture with a universal reconstruction plate along the inferior border of mandible and miniplate along the zone of tension.

38.8 TREATMENT OPTIONS FOR MANDIBULAR FRACTURES

Closed Reduction with Intermaxillary Fixation

For minimally displaced mandibular fractures, closed reduction with intermaxillary fixation (semirigid fixation) can be prescribed. This involves application of upper and lower arch bars on dentate patients along with elastics to close the jaws together in preinjury occlusion. For edentulous patients, intermaxillary fixation can be applied using patients' existing dentures (after laboratory modifications) or gunning splints. Other options for intermaxillary fixation include ivy loops and four screw intermaxillary fixation.

Open Reduction and Internal Fixation (Load Sharing versus Load-Bearing Osteosynthesis)

For displaced mandibular fractures and unfavorable fractures, open reduction and internal fixation are required to achieve mandibular form and function to preinjury state. There are various techniques of internal fixation using lag screws, miniplates, locking miniplates, dynamic compression plates or universal fracture plates and screws, and reconstruction plates or locking reconstruction plates (thicker and stronger) and screws.

There are two techniques available depending on the amount of comminution of mandibular fractures. They are either load-bearing osteosynthesis or load-sharing osteosynthesis. The load-sharing technique is indicated for simple mandibular fractures where the load is "shared" between the miniplates, monocortical screws, and the bone. The load-bearing technique is for comminuted mandibular fractures, fractures with defect, and atrophic mandibles where the load is "borne" by the thicker reconstruction plates and bicortical screws.

38.9 SOFT TISSUE APPROACHES TO MANDIBULAR FRACTURES

There are various approaches to the mandible depending on the site of fractures:

- *Existing lacerations*: Sometimes the existing lacerations over the lower border of the mandible can be used to access the underlying fracture sites.
- *Intraoral approach*: Intraoral vestibular approach is the usual method to access fractures located in the symphysis, parasymphysis, body, and angle. However, as the fractures are located more posteriorly, intraoral approach may need to be supplemented with the transbuccal approach.
- *Submental approach*: This approach can be used to reach mandibular symphysis and anterior body. This approach allows the surgeon to check the alignment of reduced fracture fragments along the lingual cortex.
- *Submandibular approach*: This approach allows exposure of the mandibular body and angle region when intraoral approach is not suitable.
- *Retromandibular approach*: This approach allows access from the ramus all the way up to the condylar neck region.
- *Preauricular approach*: This approach allows access to the condylar head and neck region. Sometimes, this approach is combined with retromandibular approach.
- *Facelift (rhytidectomy) approach*: This approach provides similar exposure to the preauricular and retromandibular approach combined. The incision is placed in a more cosmetically acceptable location.

38.10 CONDYLAR FRACTURES

Mandibular condylar fractures account for 29.3% of mandibular fractures, and form the second most common site of mandibular fractures. The condylar fractures deserve separate discussion due to the controversies surrounding their management.

The classification of condylar fracture is based on three features: anatomical fracture level, the fractured condyle relative to the mandible, and the fractured condyle relative to the glenoid fossa (Lindahl, 1977).

Classification based on anatomical fracture level:

- Intracapsular condylar head fracture
- Condylar neck fracture
- Subcondylar fracture

Classification based on fractured condyle relative to the mandible:

- Undisplaced
- Displaced
- Deviated
- No bony contact

Classification based on fractured condyle relative to the glenoid fossa:

- Undisplaced
- Displaced (condylar head still in the fossa)
- Dislocated (condylar head is out of the fossa)

There are many controversies surrounding the management of condylar fractures in regard to closed treatment versus open reduction and internal fixation. This is because closed treatment gives "satisfactory" results in majority of the cases. There is no large case series reported in the literature where patients have been followed up after surgical treatment because the management of condylar fractures has been historically closed treatment. In addition, surgery to condylar fractures is difficult because of the anatomical hazards such as injury to the facial nerve. However, with improved surgical techniques and instrument armamentarium in the recent years, open reduction and internal fixation have become popular. In a prospective multicentered comparison study in 2006, open treatment fared significantly better than closed treatment in terms of jaw movements, temporomandibular dysfunction, pain, and malocclusions (Eckelt, et al., 2006).

There are absolute and relative indications for open reduction in condylar fractures (Zide and Kent, 1983).

Absolute indications for open reduction in condylar fractures are as follows:

- Displacement into the middle cranial fossa
- Inability to obtain adequate occlusion with closed reduction
- Lateral extracapsular displacement of the condyle
- Invasion of foreign body, e.g. gunshot wound.

Relative indications for open reduction in condylar fractures are as follows:

- Bilateral condylar fractures in edentulous patient when splints are unavailable or impossible
- Unilateral or bilateral condylar fractures when splinting is not recommended for medical reasons or where adequate physiotherapy is impossible
- Bilateral condylar fractures associated with comminuted midfacial fractures
- Bilateral condylar fractures and associated gnathologic problems (e.g. lack of posterior teeth and unstable occlusion due to orthodontics).

38.11 COMPLICATIONS

Complications following treatment of mandibular fractures are uncommon.

The most common complication is infection or osteomyelitis. The incidence varies between 5% and 10%. Preoperative oral sepsis with grossly carious and periodontally involved teeth in the fracture line contributes to the problem. Inadequate immobilization of fracture segments and prolonged delay in treatment contribute to infection as well.

Malunion with malocclusion is also a possible complication in the treatment of mandibular fractures. Lack of knowledge in occlusion or failure to apply intraoperative intermaxillary fixation during open reduction and internal fixation of mandibular fractures may lead to malunion and malocclusion.

Ankylosis of the TMJs is a rare complication in mandibular condyle fractures in particular intracapsular condylar head fractures. This has some genetic predisposition. Prolonged splinting of the jaws and lack of aggressive postoperative jaw physiotherapy can contribute to TMJ ankylosis resulting in trismus.

Facial widening can occur if the plates are not correctly bent and placed. The type of mandibular fracture that is most prone to this complication is symphyseal fracture. This is particularly so when it is associated with condylar fractures and poor dentition where correct occlusion is not present to aid in accurate reduction. The muscle pull from the tongue and suprahyoid muscles causes lateral flaring of the mandibular angles and lingual tipping of the buccal segments. The buccal fracture line at the symphysis remains deceivingly intact while the lingual cortex gets separated.

REFERENCES

Chayra, G.A., Meador, L.R. and Laskin, D.M., 1986. Comparsion of panoramic and standard radiographs for the diagnosis of mandibular fractures. *Journal of Oral and Maxillofacial Surgery*, 44(9), pp. 677-9.

Eckelt, U., Schneider, M., Erasmus, F., Gerlach, K.L., Kuhlisch, E., Loukota, R., Rasse, M., Schubert, J. and Terheyden, H., 2006. Open versus closed treatment of fractures of the mandibular condylar process—a prospective randomized multi-centre study. *Journal of Craniomaxillofacial Surgery*, 34(5), pp. 306-14.

Hagan, E.H. and Huelke, D.F., 1961. Analyses of 319 case reports of mandibular fractures. *Journal of Oral Surgery*, 19, pp. 93.

Lindahl, L., 1977. Condylar fractures of the mandible. I. Classification and relation to age, occlusion, and concomitant injuries of teeth and teeth-supporting structures, and fractures of the mandibular body. *International Journal of Oral Surgery*, 6(1), pp. 12-21.

Luyk, N.H., 1992. Principles of management of fractures of the mandible. In: Peterson, L.J., et al., eds. *Principles of oral and maxillofacial surgery*. Philadelphia, PA: Lippincott-Raven, pp. 381-434.

Ogundare, B.O., Bonnick, A. and Bayley, N., 2003. Pattern of mandible fractures in an urban major trauma center. *Journal of Oral and Maxillofacial Surgery*, 61, pp. 713-8.

Soh, J., Sandham, A. and Chan, Y.H., 2005. Occlusal status in Asian male adults: prevalence and ethnic variation. *Angle Orthodontist*, 75(5), pp. 814-20.

Thaller, S.R., 1994. Management of mandibular fractures. *Archives of Otolaryngology—Head and Neck Surgery*, 120, pp. 44-7.

Zide, M.F. and Kent, J.N., 1983. Indications for open reduction of mandibular condyle fractures. *Journal of Oral and Maxillofacial Surgery*, 41(2), pp. 89-98

39 Cleft Lip and Palate

Mahdi Shkoukani

Chapter Overview

Pearls and Pitfalls

Pearls

- Microform cleft lip may go unnoticed for months. Pediatricians need to be familiar with such mild deformity.
- The three signs of submucosal cleft palate: bifid uvula, notched hard palate, and zona pellucida.
- The care of such patients requires a multidisciplinary approach. Educating the parents and family early on about the condition and the stages of treatment is critical to have cooperative and compliant parents.
- The cleft lip and palate should be repaired in a timeline as mentioned in Table 39.1, patient's health permitting; otherwise, the repair should be delayed.
- In bilateral cleft lip repair, the best cosmetic outcome is achieved by utilizing the muscle from bilateral–lateral segment to re-establish the muscular sphincter. The midportion of prolabium skin is utilized to reconstruct the philtral segment of the upper lip.
- Nasal deformity should be addressed initially at the time of cleft lip repair.
- The author recommends repairing the cleft palate as early as 6 months if the following conditions are met: medical health permits; palate tissue is bulky enough to withstand repair; and the patient is tolerating spoon-feeding.
- The author recommends using two-flap palatoplasty for complete cleft palates, Von Langenbeck for secondary palate clefts, and intravelar veloplasty for soft palate clefts. Double opposing Z-plasty may be considered for revision cases. Some surgeons may incorporate this technique with the two-flap palatoplasty and Von Langenbeck palatoplasties.

Pitfalls

- Failure to do a thorough work up especially to patients with cleft palate alone may result in missing associated syndromic symptoms as such features may reach as high as 50% among this population.
- Failure to release orbicularis Oris attachment to anterior nasal spine and alar base will result in tethering of muscle and failure to re-establish the muscular sphincter.

39.1 EPIDEMIOLOGY AND PATHOGENESIS

- *Cleft lip* and palate is the most common *craniofacial anomaly* (Marazita and Mooney, 2004).
- There is no universal classification for cleft lip and/or palate. However, they are usually divided into cleft lip with or without *cleft palate* (CL±P) or cleft palate alone based on embryological development.
- The upper lip usually develops between 4th and 8th week of gestation. *Primary palate* (anterior to incisive foramen) develops around the same time as the lip (6–9th weeks; Bender, 2000). On the contrary, *secondary palate* (posterior to the incisive foramen) develops

between 8th and 12th week of gestation (Sykes and Tollefson, 2005). In 1942, Fogh-Anderson (1942) found that the risk of CL±P was not increased in relatives of patients with isolated cleft palate. Similarly, the risk of isolated cleft palate was not increased in relatives of patients with CL±P.

- Unilateral and bilateral cleft lips are further divided into complete and incomplete. In the complete case, there is no communication between the orbicularis oris muscle fibers at the medial and lateral segments of the cleft. Incomplete cleft lips can range from minimal muscle diastasis in the upper lip with slight dermal changes to a tiny bridge of tissue between the lateral and medial segments that is called "*Simonart's band*." Microform cleft lip is a very mild case of incomplete cleft lip where there is a mild asymmetry of philtral columns. Nasal asymmetry might be seen in microform cleft lip as well (Figs. 39.1 and 39.2).
- Unilateral and bilateral cleft palates are divided into complete and incomplete. Complete cleft palate includes soft palate, hard palate, and alveolar ridge. Veau (1931) classified cleft palates on the basis of site involvement: I—soft palate; II—secondary palate; III—soft palate, hard palate, and alveolar ridge (complete unilateral); IV—bilateral complete cleft palates (Figs. 39.3A to D).
- The prevalence of cleft lip with or without cleft palate is 14 per 10,000 live births. The prevalence of cleft palate alone is about 4 per 10,000 live births (Thigpen and Kenner, 2003).
- The percentage of having other syndromic features in patients with cleft lip and palate, cleft lip without cleft palate, and cleft palate alone is 10%, 30%, and 50%, respectively.
- A review of over 100 references by Karsten and Gundlach in 2006 showed that clefts are more likely to affect the left side (52%; Karsten and Gundlach, 2006). In the same study, both bilateral and right-sided clefts had the same prevalence at 24%.
- The etiology of cleft lip and palate is considered multifactorial and possibly dependent on a mixture of demographic characteristics, genetic disorders, and environmental factors (Merritt, 2005).
- Genetic factors form a significant component of risk factors. Clefts are seen in about 40–50% of monozygotic

Table 39.1: Recommended timing of surgery in patients with orofacial clefting.

Time	*Procedure*
0–3 months	Taping and/or presurgical orthopedics
3 months	Repair of cleft lip, primary rhinoplasty
9 months	Repair of cleft palate, possible myringotomy with tube placement
3–4 years	Repair of VPI if speech therapy fails
School-age years	Revision lip/nasal deformity as needed
6–9 years	Secondary alveolar bone graft
12–16 years	Orthodontics
15–17 years (females) 18–21 years (males)	Orthognathic surgery, final rhinoplasty

(VPI: Velopharyngeal insufficiency).

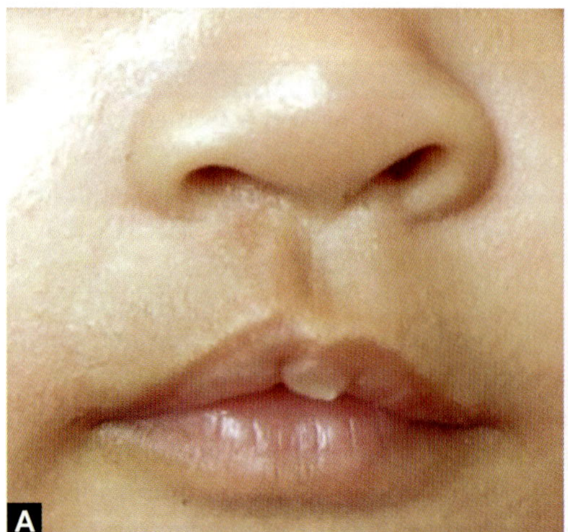

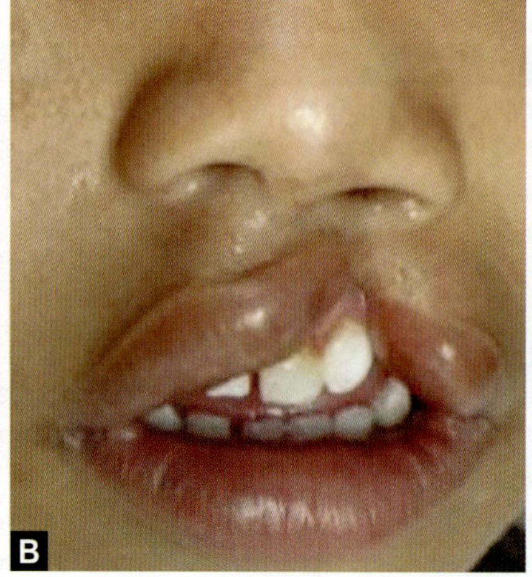

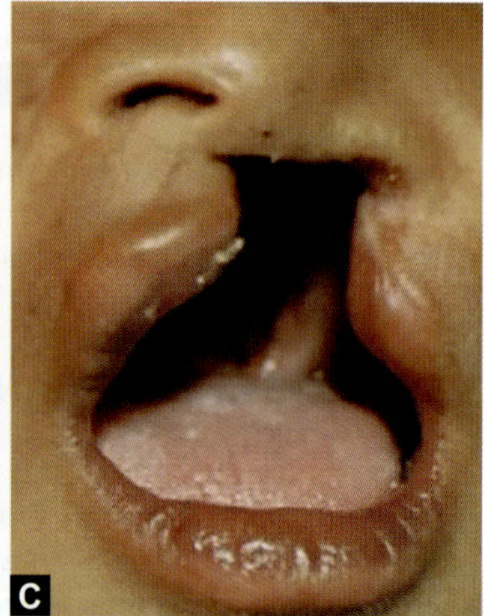

Figs. 39.1A to C: Unilateral cleft lip classification. (A) Microform cleft type. (B) Incomplete cleft type. (C) Complete cleft type.

twins concurrently whereas this percentage drops down to 5% in dizygotic twins (Murray, 2002). The risk associated with general population without any family history of clefts is 0.04–0.10%. Having one parent with a cleft increases the risk to 3–5% (Bender, 2000). Having a nephew/niece with a cleft carries a risk of about 1%. The risk goes down to 0.5% when the affected relative is a first cousin (Bender, 2000). Having a positive history in one sibling and one parent increases this risk to around 15% (Curtis, Fraser and Warburton, 1961).

- Although the genes responsible for some of the syndromes associated with clefts have been identified, no single universal gene has been found to cause cleft syndrome (Kerrigan, et al., 2000). Pierre Robin sequence and various syndromes associated with cleft lip and/or palate include, but are not limited to, van der Woude syndrome, Apert syndrome, Crouzon syndrome, Treacher Collins syndrome, Stickler syndrome, and hemifacial microsomia.
- Prevalence of clefts among Mongolians, American-Indians, and Far East Asians is considered the highest and may reach over 30 per 10,000 live births in some populations. Caucasians have a moderate prevalence rate. African-Americans have the least documented rates (2.1–4.6 per 10,000 live births). There are limited studies from the continent of Africa (Karsten and Gundlach, 2006).
- Cleft lip with or without cleft palate is more common among men, whereas cleft palate (CP) is more common among women (Fogh-Anderson, 1942).
- Teratogenic and environmental factors play a major role particularly in nonsyndromic cases. Medications taken in the first trimester such as anticonvulsants (i.e. phenytoin), cortisone, ethanol, diazepam, hypoxia, ionizing radiation, and others have been shown to increase the risk for clefting in animal models (Houdayer and Bahuau, 1998). Mothers who take anticonvulsants regularly are recommended to take folate supplements months before initiating pregnancy. Rubella and toxoplasmosis infection during first pregnancy has been reported to lead to clefting of the newborn child (Georgiade, 1992). Smoking and alcohol are considered serious risk factors as well.

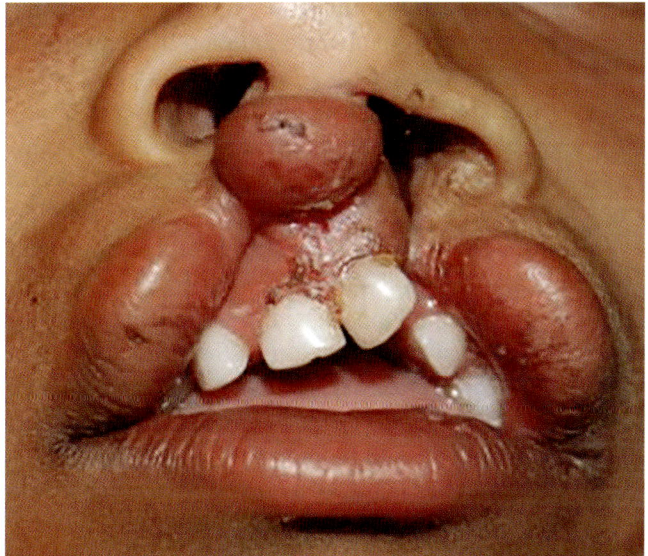

Fig. 39.2: Bilateral cleft lip: this case represent a right incomplete and left complete type.

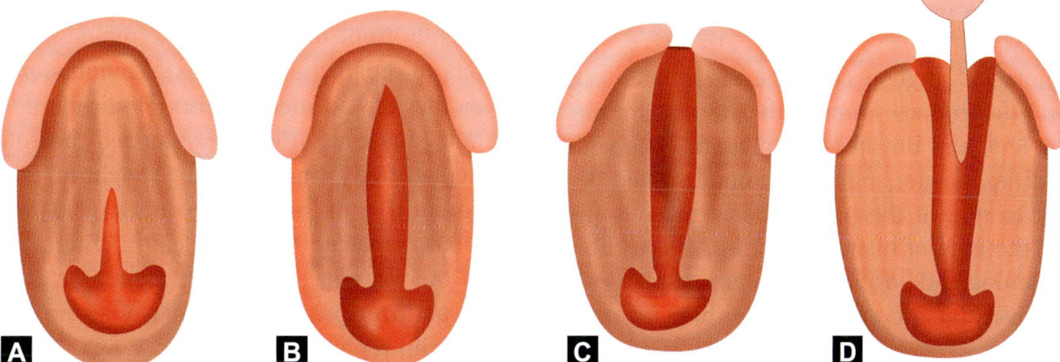

Figs. 39.3A to D: Veau classification for cleft palates. (A) Type I: involves soft palate only. (B) Type II: involves secondary palate soft and hard palate up to the incisive foramen. (C) Type III: Complete unilateral cleft palate involves soft palate, hard palate and alveolar ridge. (D) Type IV: Bilateral complete cleft palates.

39.2 CLINICAL FEATURES

Features in Clinical History

- A craniofacial surgeon is usually consulted after the examination of newborns by the pediatrician. A fissured lip and/or palate would be noted. However, a microform cleft lip may go unnoticed till the infants follow up with the pediatrician in the outpatient setting. Occasionally, if the cleft lip is noted on ultrasound during pregnancy, the surgeon may get consulted prenatally.
- A complete pre/peri/postnatal history should be obtained. It should be focused on exposure to any of the risk factors mentioned above. History of infections or any other complications in the antenatal period should be obtained. Family history for any congenital abnormalities including clefting should be obtained.
- Nursing the newborn child with a cleft palate is a major concern for the mother. Breast-feeding is not an option especially in moderate/severe clefting. Standard bottles may not be appropriate for cleft children. It is important to make sure that by the time the patient and his/her mother are discharged from the hospital, they have been trained using assisted delivery bottles (i.e. Haberman or Mead Johnson) or nonassisted delivery bottles such as the Pigeon bottle. Assisted delivery bottles help the parents to feed milk to the child by squeezing the part of the bottles. Others may benefit from a standard bottle with a large bore nipple.

39.3 TYPICAL FINDINGS ON EXAMINATION

- A complete head-and-neck examination with extra attention to the upper lip, alveolus, palate, and nose is performed.
- The craniofacial surgeon classifies the cleft lip and palate and determines whether the cleft is complete or incomplete, and unilateral or bilateral. The width of the cleft lip, palate, and/or alveolus is noted. It is important to note if the premaxilla is severely protruded in the case of bilateral cleft lip. The width of alveolus clefting and position of premaxilla may influence the decision for presurgical orthopedic treatment.
- In a unilateral cleft lip, the philtral column on the ipsilateral side is shorter as a result of the Cupid's bow being asymmetrically rotated upwardly toward the cleft side. Also, there is loss of volume of the philtral tubercle. The columella is shorter; the domes are asymmetric with the ipsilateral dome being less prominent. The caudal septum is deviated to the contralateral side. Alar cartilage is flattened on the cleft side due to its lateral, posterior, and inferiorly displacement. The ala on the cleft side is displaced posteriorly, laterally, and superiorly due to maxillary hypoplasia.
  - The majority of cases in bilateral cleft lip are symmetrical (bilateral complete or bilateral incomplete). However, about 25% of cases are asymmetrical (Yuzuriha, Oh and Mulliken, 2008). In patients with complete cleft lip, there is no orbicularis muscle in the prolabium. The premaxilla protrusion varies from one patient to another. In symmetrical cases, the Cupid's bow is symmetrical and parallel to the horizontal plane. The nasal tip is broad, columella short, and ala flat and broad bilaterally. Asymmetric bilateral cleft lips should be viewed as two different unilateral cleft lips. Each side has unique features that need to be recognized and managed accordingly.
  - Cleft palate patients may have submucosal, incomplete or complete clefting. The three signs of submucosal cleft palate are bifid uvula, notched posterior edge of hard palate, and zona pellucida.
- Cleft children should be managed in the setting of a multidisciplinary team, which includes a geneticist to perform a genetics evaluation and family counseling. This becomes particularly important when the case involves syndromic features.

39.4 PREFERRED TREATMENT

- Timing of repair is critical (Table 39.1). It may vary slightly from one center to another. The author prefers to repair the cleft lip at 3 months of age as long as there is no medical contraindication. Wilhelmsen and Musgrave (1966) popularized the rule of 10s to be satisfied prior to repair: weight of 10 lbs, hemoglobin 10 g/dL, and white count <10,000/mm^3. Millard (1957) replaced the white count criteria with the age of the patient, at least 10 weeks. The author prefers to perform primary rhinoplasty at the same time of cleft lip repair.
- In regard to the cleft palate, it is usually repaired between 6 and 12 months of age. The author has performed cleft palate repair involving the soft palate

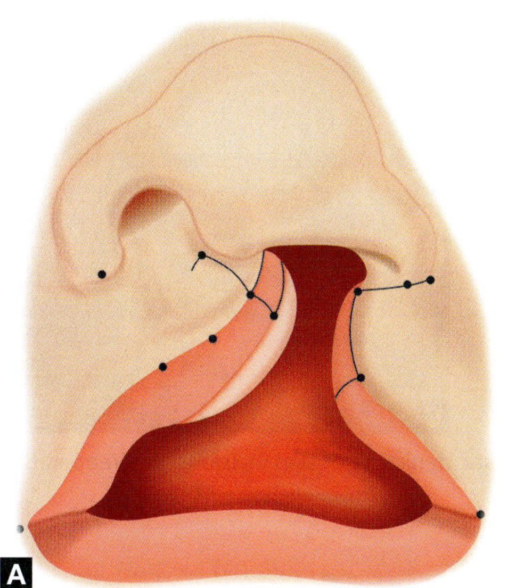

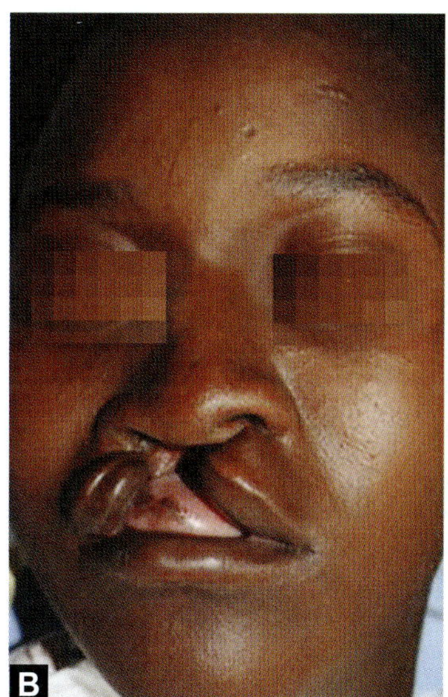

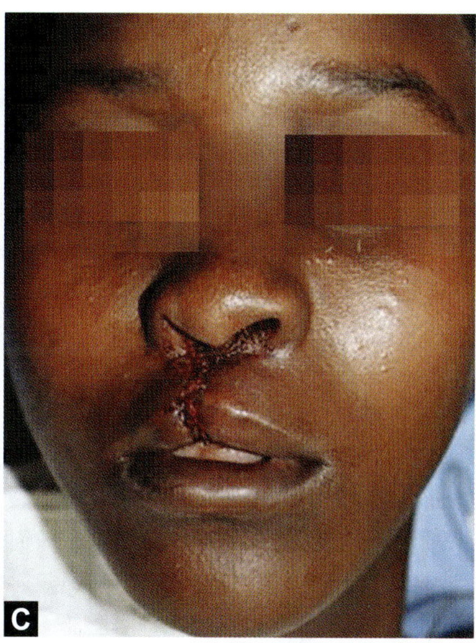

Figs. 39.4A to C: Advancement-rotation flap technique for unilateral cleft lip repair. (A) Diagrammatic depiction of skin incisions. (B) Preoperative view. (C) Postoperative view.

alone as early as 6 months. If cleft palate involves more than just the soft palate, repair is performed around 9 months of age. Our goal is to repair the palate as early as possible, so that it will have minimal effect on speech. However, the palate needs to be repaired at a point when there is enough tissue to mobilize to allow closure. It is recommended that these patients are able to be spoon fed at the time of repair so that bottle-feeding can be stopped for about 2 weeks.

- *Lip taping, lip adhesion,* and presurgical orthopedics are options available prior to lip repair to help the surgeon in approximating the alveolar ridges. This helps the surgeon to narrow the width of the cleft and allows for better cosmetic closure. *Presurgical orthopedics* is divided into active and passive types. Active appliances such as Latham appliance approximate the alveolar ridges using a direct and controlled force. It has to be applied in the operating room. On the other hand, passive appliances do not deliver a force but rather help in molding the alveolar ridges to the desired position. Nasoalveolar molding is one of the most recent developments in passive presurgical orthopedics. The appliance has a piece that helps the surgeon to mold the nasal structures and also to elongate the collumella, thus giving the nose a more symmetrical appearance.
- Unilateral cleft lip is commonly repaired with advancement-rotation flaps popularized by Millard (Figs. 39.4A to C). The medial side of the cleft is downwardly rotated to lengthen the philtral column on the cleft side. The lateral segment is advanced medially to bulk up the soft tissue deficiency in the cleft area. The mucosal edges of the cleft can be used to bulk up the newly reconstructed upper lip and recreate the nasal floor. The lateral crus of alar cartilage has to be released from its abnormal attachment at the level of the pyriform aperture and resecured more medially, superiorly, and anteriorly. The cupid bow is reconstructed and the scar mainly falls in the philtral column. This technique usually requires experience and is not recommended for a beginner surgeon.
- Another useful technique to address unilateral cleft lips is triangular-flap technique. The principle of such technique is to interdigitate triangular flaps arising from the lateral segment to be inserted into the medial segment to increase the height of philtral column (Figs. 39.5A to C). It is a recommended technique for inexperienced surgeons and for cases where wide clefts are encountered. Minimal tissue is discarded using this technique.
- The straight-line closure is usually reserved for microform cleft lip closure and rarely used to close an incomplete or complete cleft lip. It may also be used for lip adhesion prior to definite repair to minimize tension and help narrow a wide alveolar cleft. It does sacrifice normal tissue during repair and the scar contracture tends to cause lip notching (Figs. 39.6A and B).

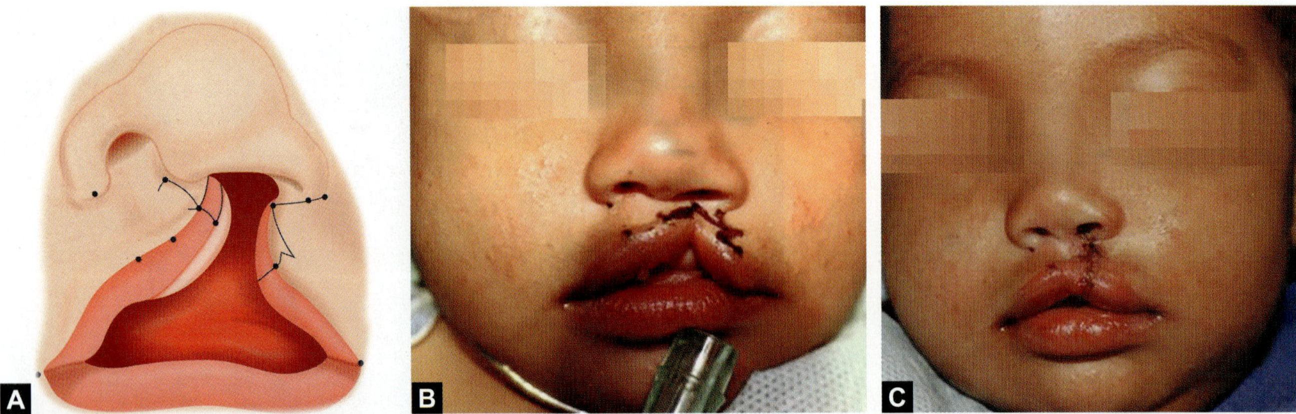

Figs. 39.5A to C: Triangular flap technique for unilateral cleft lip repair. (A) Diagrammatic depiction of skin incisions. (B) Preoperative view with skin marking. (C) Postoperative view.

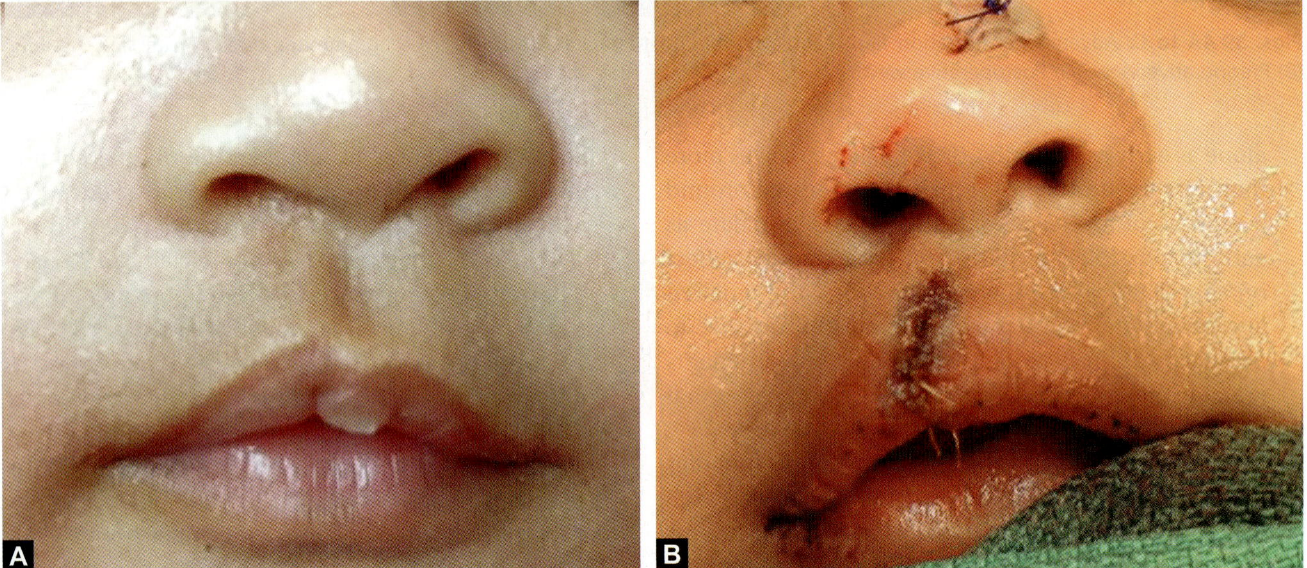

Figs. 39.6A and B: Straight line closure for unilateral microform cleft lip repair. (A) Preoperative view. (B) Postoperative view.

- Bilateral cleft lip repair follows the same principles followed in unilateral cleft repair. Besides the involvement of both sides, what complicates such repairs is that the prolabium carries no muscle fibers and has deficiency in volume to replace a natural bulky median tubercle. The author uses a revised version of Mulliken technique (Mulliken, 2004). A superiorly based central philtral flap is raised. The skin on either side of this flap is de-epithelialized. The rest of mucosa on the prolabium is sutured at the anterior nasal spine to recreate the gingival side of the gingivolabial sulcus mesially. The lateral labial segments are bilaterally released from the alar bases. The orbicularis oris is undermined on the mucosal and cutaneous sides to help mobilize the muscle. Using the incisions medially and laterally, the alar cartilage is undermined to release it from the overlying skin. The mucosa is approximated first and sutured to recreate the labial side of the gingivolabial sulcus anteriorly. Then the muscle is sutured to meet in the midline. This move brings in mucosa from the lateral segment to create a more natural-looking bulky median tubercle. The skin from the lateral segments is sutured to the central philtral flap. It is critical to narrow the alar base width by securing the deep alar soft tissue to the anterior nasal spine area. Depending on the case, the author suspends the lower lateral cartilage to the contralateral upper lateral cartilages via a suture.

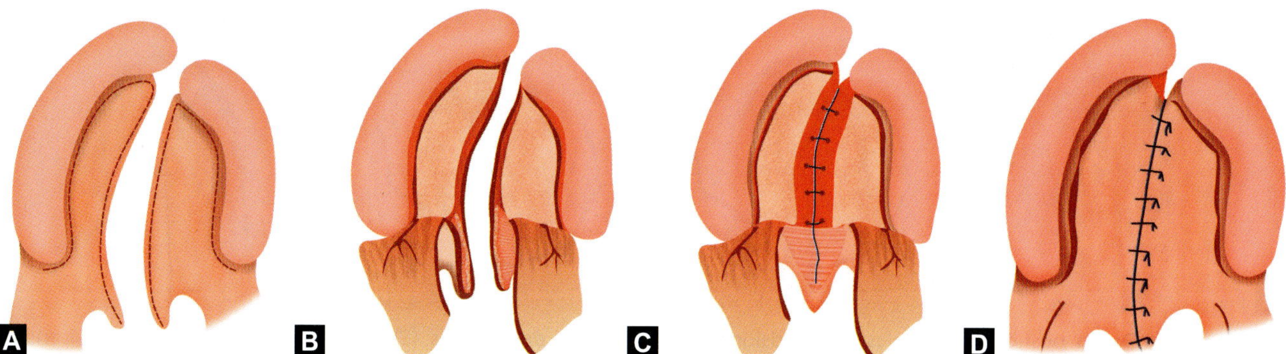

Figs. 39.7A to D: Two-flap palatoplasy. (A) Incision are marked with dotted lines. (B) Oral mucoperiosteal flap is raised and greater palatine vascular pedicle is well preserved. (C) Nasal mucoperiosteum is elevated and sutured in tension-free closure. (D) Oral mucosa is sutured.

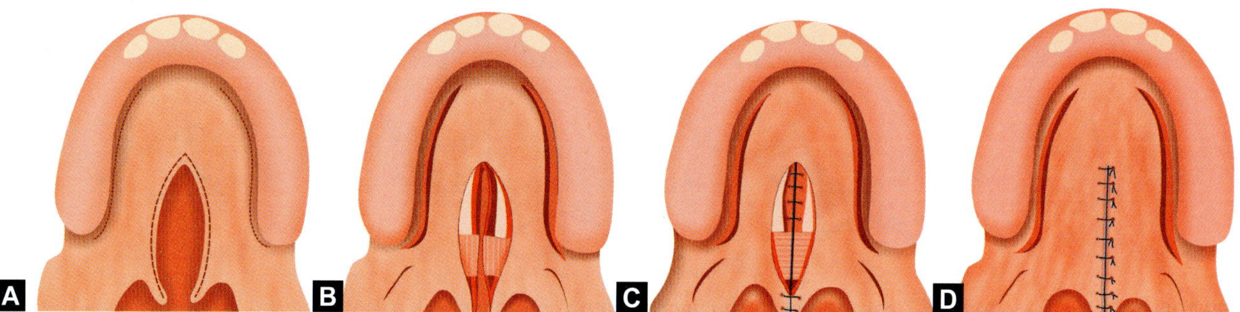

Figs. 39.8A to D: Von Langenbeck technique. (A) Incisions are marked with dotted lines. (B) Oral and nasal mucoperiosteal flaps are raised. During this step, greater palatine vascular pedicle is identified and protected throughout the case. (C) Palatal muscles are released from posterior edge of hard palate and closed in transverse direction. nasal mucoperiosteum is closed. (D) Oral mucosa is sutured.

- In cleft palate repair, the goal is to have a multilayer closure. At the level of soft palate, the nasal mucosa, muscle, and oral mucosa are closed in a tension-free matter. The author has performed intravelar veloplasty to reconstruct the levator sling. At the level of hard palate, the oral and nasal mucosa should be closed in a tension-free matter. The oral mucosa is sutured in a vertical mattress fashion to reduce the dead space between tissue layers and to secure the layers together.
- In symptomatic submucosal cleft palate, intravelar veloplasty should be adequate in most cases. A midline incision is made in the soft palate. The oral and nasal mucosa on both sides are elevated. The muscle is dissected on both sides and sutured together to form the levator sling after closing the nasal mucosa. Finally, the oral mucosa is closed in a vertical mattress fashion.
- *Two-flap palatoplasty* (Bardach and Salyer, 1987; Figs. 39.7A to D) is the technique of choice for complete cleft palates. The entire oral mucoperiosteum is elevated off the bone. The vascular pedicle is dissected to help mobilize the oral mucosa. The author occasionally osteotomizes the posterior end of the greater palatine foramen to completely release the vascular pedicle. The nasal mucoperiosteum is elevated completely using a periosteal elevator. The muscle is dissected off the posterior edge of hard palate to perform intravelar veloplasty at the time of closure. The nasal and oral mucosal layers are elevated off velar muscle. Next, the three layers are closed in a tension-free matter.
- There are two common techniques for secondary palate cleft. In these cases, the author prefers the *Von Langenbeck technique* (Trier and Dreyer, 1984; Figs. 39.8A to D). The medial edge of the cleft is incised, and both oral and nasal mucosa are elevated. The muscle should be dissected off the posterior edge of the hard palate to reorient it in a transverse rather than longitudinal direction. Finally, release incisions are made laterally on the hard palate extending form the palatine–maxillary suture line anteriorly to just

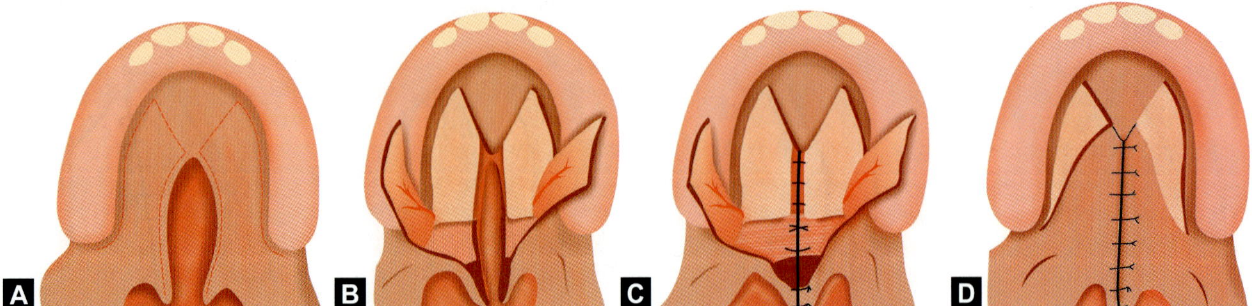

Figs. 39.9A to D: V–Y pushback palatoplasty. (A) Incisions are marked with dotted lines. (B) Oral mucoperiosteal flaps are raised and greater palatine vascular pedicle is well preserved. (C) Palatal muscles are released from posterior edge of hard palate and closed in transverse direction. Nasal mucoperiosteum is elevated and sutured in tension-free closure. (D) Oral mucosa is sutured by pushing the oral flaps posteriorly.

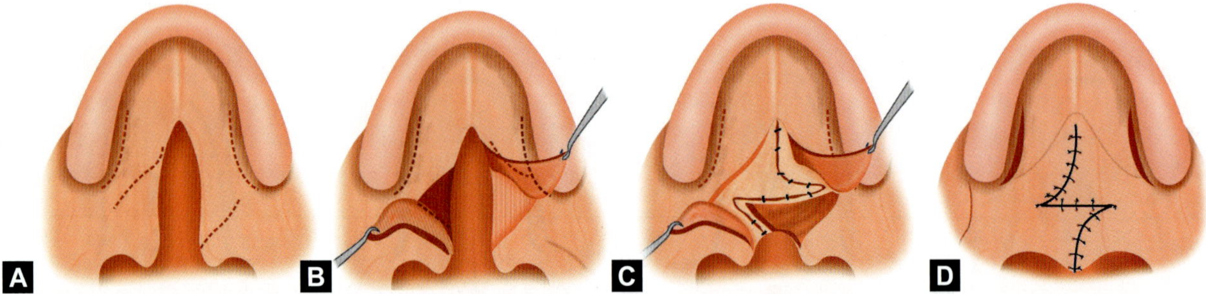

Figs. 39.10A to D: Double opposing Z-palatoplasty in conjunction with Von Langenbeck palatoplasty. (A) Incisions are marked with dotted lines. (B) Oral mucoperiosteal flaps are raised and opposing Z-plasty cuts are marked on the nasal mucosa with dotted lines. Flaps that are transposed anteriorly carry mucosa only. Flaps that are transposed posteriorly carry palatal muscles. (C) Nasal flaps are sutured. (D) Oral flaps are sutured.

lateral to the hammulus abutting and marching posterior to the maxillary tuberosity. At this point, mucoperitosteum is elevated and care should be taken to protect the greater palatine pedicle. In many cases, vascular pedicle should be dissected to cut down the tension upon oral mucosal closure. The three layers are closed as mentioned above. The other technique is Veau-Wardill-Kilner *V-Y pushback palatoplasty* (Krause, Tharp and Morris, 1976; Figs. 39.9A to D). It is similar to the Von Langenbeck technique, but in this case the lateral and medial incisions are connected via an oblique incision extending from the palatine-maxillary suture laterally to the midline at the anterior point of the medial incisions. Upon closure, the oral mucosa is pushed posteriorly to close it in a V-Y fashion. Consequently, a part of the hard palate is left uncovered with mucosa. A few studies have shown that this technique suffers from the possible drawback of stunting the maxillary growth secondary to keeping the hard palate exposed (Pigott, et al., 2002; Semb and Shaw, 1998).

- Soft palate cleft may get closed in a direct fashion by incising both sides of the cleft and then perform an intravelar veloplasty as mentioned above. Others may perform a double opposing Z-plasty (*Furlow palatoplasty*; Furlow, 1986) repair in these cases (Figs. 39.10A to D). An opposing Z-plasty is performed on the oral and nasal mucosa, so incisions on both sides do not overlap. The muscle is kept attached to one of the two triangles created by the Z-plasty. The muscle is kept on the triangle that will be transposed posteriorly to strengthen the muscle sling posteriorly, and prevent velopharyngeal insufficiency (VPI).

39.5 COMPLICATIONS

- Having a cleft lip and/or palate increases the risk of developing several complications. Cleft lip results in poor cosmetic appearance at the level of nose and upper lip. If the cleft lip extends to the alveolus, then these patients develop problems with incisor eruption and issues with occlusion. Having a cleft palate results in problems with speech and swallowing. Most patients suffer from hypernasal speech and VPI. Cleft palate patients may also suffer from recurrent otitis media requiring tympanostomy with tube placement.

- There are many complications of surgical repair of cleft lip. Infection and bleeding are possible but uncommon. Scarring is unavoidable but correct surgical techniques and experience help the surgeon to make surgical scars more favorable. Scar contracture may lead to notching of the lip. Inadequate volume restoration of vermillion and scar contracture may lead to *whistle deformity*. Surgery may result in asymmetry of the lip and/or nose. This is usually secondary to inadequate dissection, inappropriate technique, and inexperience.
- Complications of cleft palate include infection and bleeding. If bleeding is noted, then the wound may need to be re-examined in the operating room. Oronasal fistula, persistent VPI, and persistent otitis media with effusions are other complications. The most common site for oronasal fistula is the junction of hard and soft palates where wound tension is highest. Although uncommon, postoperative airway compromise is a dreaded complication. This may be due to blood collection around the endotracheal tube during surgery, or secondary to postoperative swelling in the oral cavity or oropharynx. It is highly recommended that hypopharyngeal packing be placed prior to starting surgery to prevent aspiration of blood. For this reason, we observe these patients for at least one postoperative day in the pediatric intensive care unit.

REFERENCES

Bardach, J. and Salyer, K., 1987. *Surgical techniques in cleft lip and palate.* Chicago: Year Book Medical Publishers.

Bender, P.L., 2000. Genetics of cleft lip and palate. *Journal of Pediatric Nursing,* 15, pp. 242-9.

Curtis, E.J., Fraser, F.C. and Warburton, D., 1961. Congenital cleft lip and palate. *American Journal of Diseases of Children,* 102, pp. 853-7.

Fogh-anderson, P., 1942. *Inheritance of harelip and cleft palate.* Copenhagen, NYT: Nordisk Forlog.

Furlow, L.T., Jr., 1986. Cleft palate repair by double opposing Z-plasty. *Plastic and Reconstructive Surgery,* 78, pp. 724-38.

Georgiade, G.S., 1992. *Textbook of plastic, maxillofacial, and reconstructive surgery.* 2nd Ed. Philadelphia: Lippincott Williams and Wilkins and Wilkins, pp. 299-306.

Houdayer, C. and Bahuau, M., 1998. Orofacial cleft defects: inference from nature and nurture. *Annales de Genetique,* 41, pp. 89-117.

Karsten, K.H. and Gundlach, M.C., 2006. Epidemiological studies on the frequency of clefts in Europe and world-wide. *Journal of Maxillofacial Surgery,* 34(Suppl. S2), pp. 1-2.

Kerrigan, J.J., Mansell, J.P., Sengupta, A., Brown, N. and Sandy, J. R., 2000. Palatogenesis and potential mechanisms for clefting. *Journal of the Royal College of Surgeons of Edinburgh,* 45, pp. 351-8.

Krause, C.J., Tharp, R.F. and Morris, H.L., 1976. A comparative study of results of the von Langenbeck and the V-Y pushback palatoplasties. *The Cleft Palate Journal,* 13, pp. 11-9.

Marazita, M.L. and Mooney, M.P., 2004. Current concepts in the embryology and genetics of cleft lip and cleft palate. *Clinics in Plastic Surgery,* 31, pp. 125-40.

Merritt, L., 2005. Part 1. Understanding the embryology and genetics of cleft lip and palate. *Advances in Neonatal Care,* 5, pp. 64-71.

Millard, R.T., 1957. The role of cineradiography with image amplification for evaluation of post operative cleft palate cases. *Acta Oto-rino-laringologica Ibero-americana,* 8, pp. 225-7.

Mulliken, J.B., 2004. Bilateral cleft lip. *Clinics in Plastic Surgery,* 31, pp. 209-20.

Murray, J.C., 2002. Gene/environment causes of cleft lip and/or palate. *Clinical Genetics,* 61, pp. 248-56.

Pigott, R.W., Albery, E.H., Hathorn, I.S., Atack, N.E., Williams, A., Harland, K., Orlando, A., Falder, S. and Coghlan, B., 2002. A comparison of three methods of repairing the hard palate. *The Cleft Palate-craniofacial Journal,* 39, pp. 383-91.

Semb, G. and Shaw, W.C., 1998. Facial growth after different methods of surgical intervention in patients with cleft lip and palate. *Acta Odontologica Scandinavica,* 56, pp. 352-5.

Sykes, J.M. and Tollefson, T.T., 2005. Management of the cleft lip deformity. *Facial Plastic Surgery Clinics of North America,* 13, pp. 157-67.

Thigpen, J. and Kenner, C., 2003. *Assessment and management of the gastrointestinal system.* Philadelphia, PA: WB Saunders.

Trier, W.C. and Dreyer, T.M., 1984. Primary von Langenbeck palatoplasty with levator reconstruction: rationale and technique. *The Cleft Palate Journal,* 21, pp. 254-62.

Veau, V., 1931. *La division palatine.* Paris: Masson.

Wilhelmsen, H.R. and Musgrave, R.H., 1966. Complications of cleft lip surgery. *The Cleft Palate Journal,* 3, pp. 223-31.

Yuzuriha, S., Oh, A.K. and Mulliken, J.B., 2008. Asymmetrical bilateral cleft lip: complete or incomplete and contralateral lesser defect (minor-form, microform, or mini-microform). *Plastic and Reconstructive Surgery,* 122, pp. 1494-504.

40 Craniosynostosis

Mahdi Shkoukani

Chapter Overview

Pearls and Pitfalls

Pearls

- Sagittal craniosynostosis is the most common, and lambdoid craniosynostosis is the least common.
- Early diagnosis is critical so intervention can be planned within the first year of age.
- Surgeon has to be vigilant in differentiating deformational plagiocephaly from unilateral lambdoid craniosynostosis or unilateral coronal craniosynostosis. Mostly, a thorough physical examination and computerized tomogram (CT) scan can accomplish such differentiation.
- Development of intracranial hypertension is an indication for abrupt surgical intervention. Ophthalmology need to be consulted as untreated intracranial pressures may lead to papilledema and eventually to blindness.
- Goal of surgery is to correct the fused sutures and repair accompanying craniofacial deformity to maximize success.
- During surgical repair, surgeon might leave up to 1.5-cm bony defect without any concern as long as the patient is <2 years old.
- Strip craniectomy is reserved for mild cases where vault remodeling is indicated for moderate to severe deformities.

Pitfalls

- Not recognizing premature closure of sutures and associated increased intracranial pressure can lead to papilledema, optic nerve injury, and blindness.
- Failure to repair craniosynostosis in a timely manner might lead to restricted brain growth and cognitive impairment. Abnormal facial growth also develops secondary to cranial deformity.

40.1 EPIDEMIOLOGY AND PATHOGENESIS

- Cranial sutures add malleability to the head during transvaginal delivery and provide a growth center for the growing calvarium.
- The sutures allow the calvarium to expand during the first 2 years of life when the brain is growing rapidly.
- There are eight main sutures (Fig. 40.1): one metopic suture (between frontal bones), two coronal sutures (between frontal and parietal bones), one sagittal suture (between parietal bones), two lambdoid sutures (between parietal and occipital bones), and two squamosal sutures (between parietal and temporal bones).
- Normally, these sutures start closing at variable dates in early infancy. Metopic suture is the first one to close

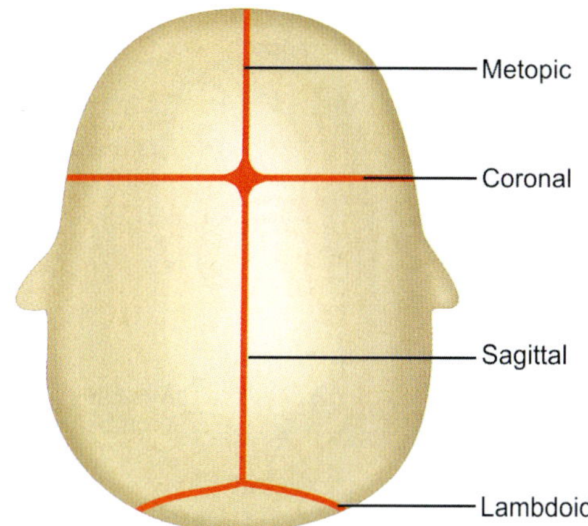

Fig. 40.1: Normocephaly.

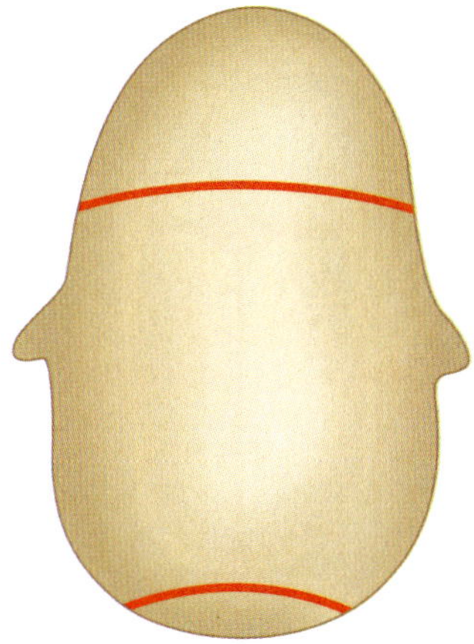

Fig. 40.2: Synostotic scaphocephaly (Sagittal).

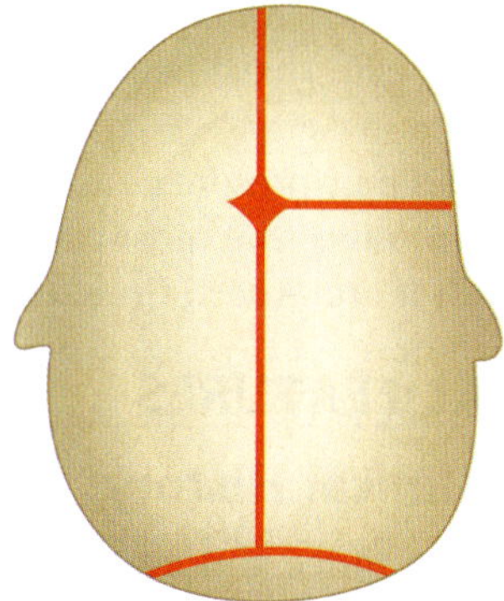

Fig. 40.3: Synostotic anterior plagiocephaly (Unicoronal).

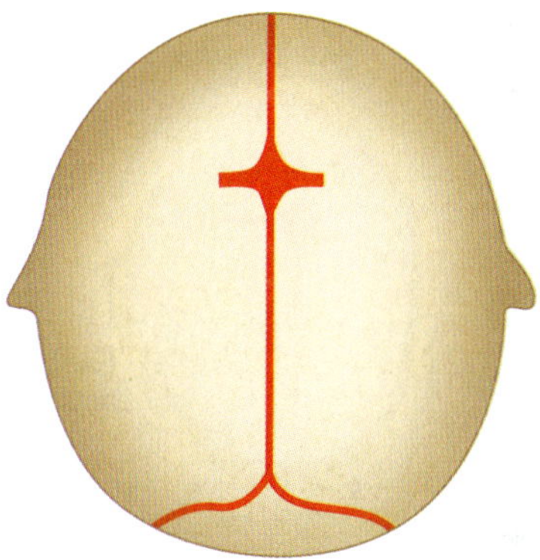

Fig. 40.4: Synostotic brachycephaly (Bicoronal).

at 2 months of age followed by sagittal, coronal, and lambdoid that start closing at 22, 24, and 26 months of age, respectively.

- Premature suture fusion permits growth parallel to that suture but restricts growth perpendicular to it. For example, a premature closure of a coronal suture would permit the skull growth in the mediolateral direction but would limit the ventrodorsal direction.
- A sagittal craniosynostosis gives a scaphocephaly skull where the calvarium gets elongated in the anteroposterior dimension. It may present as a complete or partial fusion (Fig. 40.2).
- A unicoronal craniosynostosis gives a frontal plagiocephaly skull. In these patients, the ipsilateral skull appears to be short in the ventrodorsal dimension, but the contralateral side continues to grow out normally (Fig. 40.3).
- A bicoronal craniosynostosis gives a brachycephaly skull. These patients will have a skull with a short axis in the ventrodorsal direction and long axis in the mediolateral direction. In severe cases, exorbitism may develop (Fig. 40.4).
- A metopic craniosynostosis gives a trigonocephaly skull where the forehead is pointed with a prominent and pointed ridge in the midline (Fig. 40.5).
- A lambdoid craniosynostosis leads to an occipital plagiocephaly where the occiput is flat on the involved side and more rounded on the contralateral side (Fig. 40.6).
- Deformational plagiocephaly (Fig. 40.7), where the occiput is flat, is not due to craniosynostosis, but rather it is caused by having the baby lay down supine. This can be confused with lambdoid craniosynostosis.
- The craniofacial skeleton grows as one unit. Asymmetry in the cranium will lead to asymmetry in facial skeleton, with the orbit being the most common site affected.
- Premature closure of sutures may result in increased intracranial pressure, in particular when more than one suture is involved. Hydrocephalus has been reported

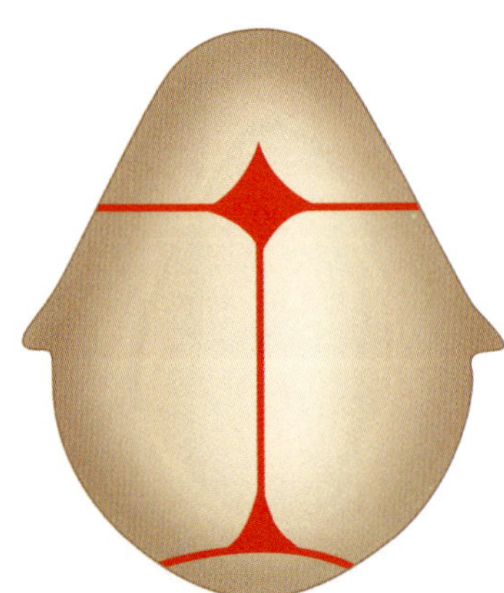

Fig. 40.5: Synostotic trigonocephaly (Metopic).

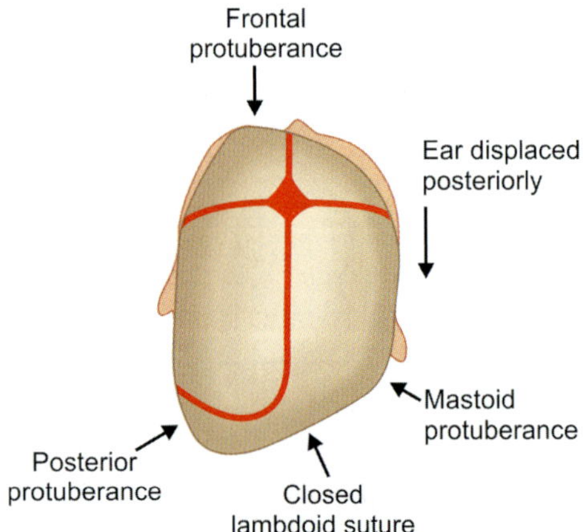

Fig. 40.6: Lambdoid synostosis.

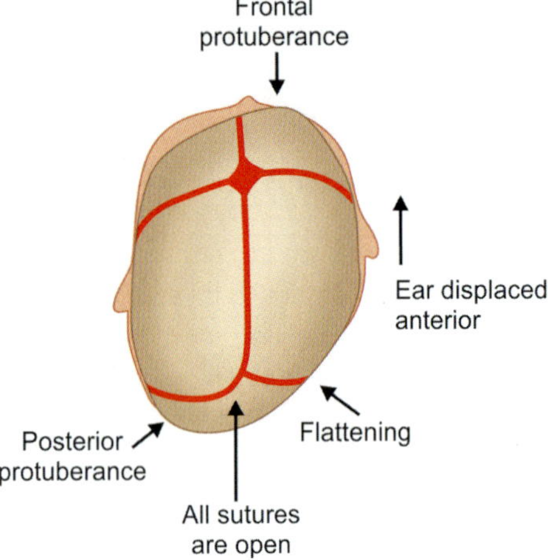

Fig. 40.7: Positional molding.

in patients with multiple craniosynostosis. Prolonged elevated pressures can lead to papilledema and optic nerve injury, which may ultimately result in blindness.

- Most studies show that the sagittal synostosis is the most common, and the lambdoid synostosis is the least common (Pattisapu, et al., 2010).
- Worldwide and the US studies have shown that the prevalence of craniosynostosis is nearly 3–5 per 10,000 live births (Lajeunie, et al., 1995; Lenton, et al., 2005; Boulet, Rasmussen and Honein, 2008).
- Mutations in the fibroblast growth factor receptor family and the transcription factors TWIST and MSX2 (Lajeunie, et al., 1995; Wilkie, 1997; Lenton, et al., 2005; Boulet, Rasmussen and Honein, 2008) are present in most syndromic craniosynostosis patients.
- It is more prevalent among Caucasian males (Boulet, Rasmussen and Honein, 2008). Prenatal smoke exposure (Kallen, 1999) and anticonvulsant therapy (Kallen and Robert-Gnansia, 2005) have been documented as risk factors.
- Craniosynostosis may present as an isolated finding or as part of a syndrome. The most common syndromes associated with it are: Apert, Crouzon, and Pfeiffer.

40.2 CLINICAL FEATURES

Features in Clinical History

- The parents may notice abnormally shaped head that is worsening with time, and it has been present since birth. Deformational plagiocephaly is usually noted few months after birth, and the parents may report a more symmetrical head in the first two months after birth. Parents should be asked if the patient sleeps in one position all the time.
- A complete pre/peri/postnatal history should be obtained. It should be focused on exposure to any of the risk factors mentioned earlier, infections, or any other complications in the perinatal period.
- If craniosynostosis is part of a syndrome, then midfacial and limb abnormalities may be noted.
- If premature suture fusion goes untreated, intracranial hypertension may develop. Symptoms include poor feeding, sleep disturbances, decreased cognitive function, behavioral changes, and vomiting.
- Family history of any congenital abnormalities should be obtained.

Typical Findings on Examination

- Evaluate the head shape and symmetry. Look for flat forehead or occiput. Does the head appear elongated, broad, or triangular in shape? Also, measure the head circumference.

- On examination, it is very difficult to differentiate deformational plagiocephaly from either unilateral coronal craniosynostosis or unilateral lambdoid craniosynostosis. In deformational plagiocephaly, the head has a parallelogram shape, has no ipsilateral occipitomastoid bossing. On the contrary, patients with unilateral lambdoid craniosynostosis will have a head that has a trapezoidal shape; there will be prominence of ipsilateral occipitomastoid bossing and the ipsilateral ear is displaced posteriorly. In cases of unilateral coronal craniosynostosis, a step off might be appreciated at the occipitoparietal junction and the ipsilateral ear is displaced anteriorly.
- Evaluate for increased intracranial pressure.
- Evaluate for physical findings other than premature suture fusion when syndromic cases are suspected. In Apert syndrome, patients usually develop midfacial hypoplasia, exorbitism (ocular proptosis), hypertelorism, high-arched cleft palate, low-set ears, and syndactyly. In Crouzon syndrome, patients differ from Apert syndrome patients by having normal hands and feet, normal intelligence, and no cleft palate. Also, it is critical to rule out any cervical spine abnormalities in Crouzon patients prior to any surgical intervention. In Pfeiffer syndrome, patients have a midfacial hypoplasia, partial syndactyly, broad fingers/toes, hydrocephalus, and imperforate anus.
- These patients require a complete examination by an ophthalmologist to assess for proptosis (exorbitism) secondary to decreased bony orbital volume as seen in coronal suture synostosis. These patients may develop ocular trauma due to prolonged corneal exposure. Hypertelorism is not uncommon and may coincide with strabismus. Most importantly, it is critical to assess the retina and optic disk and check for papilledema and/or atrophy of the optic nerve, which are all signs of increased intracranial pressure. Eventually, if this goes untreated, complete blindness may pursue.

Investigations

- *Plain radiographs (skull series)*: It is a simple but inaccurate investigation. If there is any further suspicion, then a CT scan should be obtained.
- *CT scan*: It is more accurate than plain radiographs in evaluating the sutures. Also, it gives more detailed information in regard to brain abnormalities, hydrocephalus, orbital anatomy, skull base shape, and three-dimensional shape of the skull. This investigative test is more helpful in cases of multiple craniosynostosis or single synostosis involving the lambdoid suture. The CT scan helps to differentiate between lambdoid craniosynostosis and deformational plagiocephaly.
- Failure to repair craniosynostosis in a timely manner might lead to restricted brain growth, in particular when fontanels close down. Sequelae such as increased intracranial pressure and hydrocephalus may develop. Uncorrected craniosynostosis might result in abnormal facial growth secondary to cranial deformity.

40.3 PREFERRED TREATMENT

- The goal of surgery is to release the fused sutures and repair accompanying craniofacial deformities (Ghali, Sinn and Tantipasawasin, 2002; Panchal and Uttchin, 2003; Warren, et al., 2012). Timing is critical, and it is highly recommended to perform the primary surgery before the patient turns 1 year of age. Some surgeons advocate early surgery (3–6 months) to prevent sequelae associated with craniosynostosis. However, the bone is softer at this early age, which makes it more difficult to perform internal fixation. Moreover, there is a higher chance of refusion. On the contrary, others prefer to perform the primary surgery between 9 and 12 months of age when the bone is firmer, and it is easier to perform internal fixation.
- Depending on the case and surgeon's preference, the surgery may range from simple suture strip craniectomy (Fig. 40.8) to complete vault reshaping (Fig. 40.9). Releasing the fused suture alone will not reshape the malformed cranium. However, in mild cases, wearing a helmet postoperatively may help in molding the calvarium. During remodeling surgery, as long as the patient is <2 years of age, the surgeon may leave a complete bony defect up to 1.5-cm-wide without a need for a bone graft or bone substitute. It is believed that at this age, dura and pericranium carry an osteogenic potential and lead to new bone formation.
- Revision cases and correction of midface deformities are addressed between 4 and 8 years of age.
- *Sagittal craniosynostosis*
    - Initially, removal of fused suture (strip craniectomy) was utilized as a surgical option. This is usually performed between 3 and 6 months of age. A major drawback of this simpler technique is higher risk of refusion of the suture. Recently, endoscopic

strip craniectomy has been described followed by molding helmet therapy for 1 year (Jimenez and Barone, 2010).
    - Cranial vault remodeling is a more extensive procedure with higher blood loss and longer hospital stay. However, studies have shown that this extensive approach has a better success rate than strip craniectomy (Francel, 1995). It involves excising and reshaping the frontal, parietal, and occipital bones.
- *Unicoronal craniosynostosis*
    - The goal of surgery is to advance the ipsilateral supraorbital rim ventrally so that it is 2 to 3 mm ventral to the corneal line, widen the ipsilateral superior orbital rim, and narrow the contralateral superior orbital rim. When the fronto-orbital bar is released, osteotomies are made vertically to advance the ipsilateral side ventrally. Also, the bone graft that is removed on the contralateral side is inserted on the ipsilateral side to accommodate

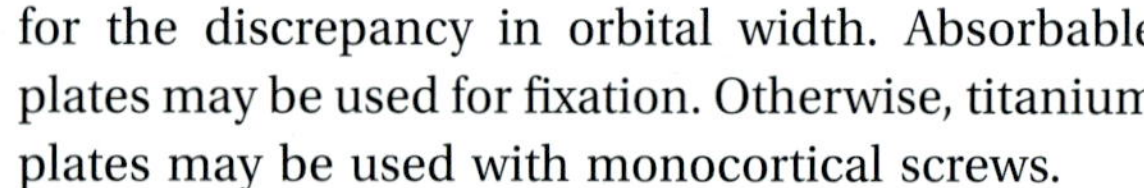

for the discrepancy in orbital width. Absorbable plates may be used for fixation. Otherwise, titanium plates may be used with monocortical screws.
- *Bicoronal craniosynostosis*
    - The goal of surgery is to advance the frontoparietal bones including the fronto-orbital bar to address the short anteroposterior dimension of the skull. Ideally, the supraorbital rims have to be around 2 to 3 mm ventral to the corneal line.
- *Metopic craniosynostosis*
    - The goal of surgery is to advance the fronto-orbital bar. Also, it is critical to remodel the frontal bone to increase the volume of the anterior cranial fossa.
- *Unilateral lambdoid craniosynostosis*
    - As we have mentioned this is a rare presentation and there is no agreement among surgeons regarding the best approach to manage these patients. A group of surgeons advocate the simpler suture strip craniectomy, whereas others argue that open cranial vault approach with reshaping is the way to address such synostosis.

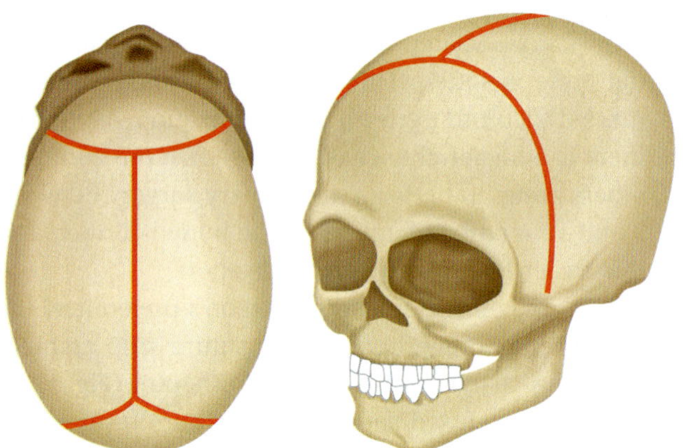

Fig. 40.8: Simple suture strip craniectomy.

40.4 POSTOPERATIVE CARE

- Postoperatively, the patient is usually extubated and sent to the pediatric intensive care unit for a day or two. Periorbital edema is expected, and cold compresses may help. If Helmet usage is indicated as in endoscopic repair, it may get started immediately postoperatively. The patient is prescribed ceftriaxone for up to 5 days while in the hospital. Most centers may obtain a CT scan within the first week to assess the craniofacial skeleton. Sutures are removed 10 to 14 days postoperatively. Regular follow-up is needed to assess craniofacial growth and neurologic development.

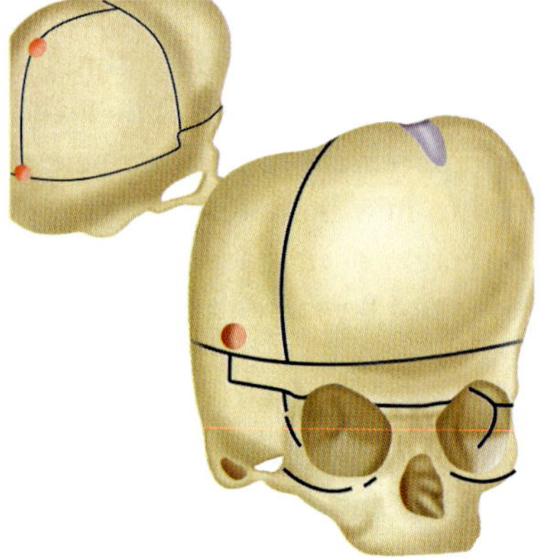

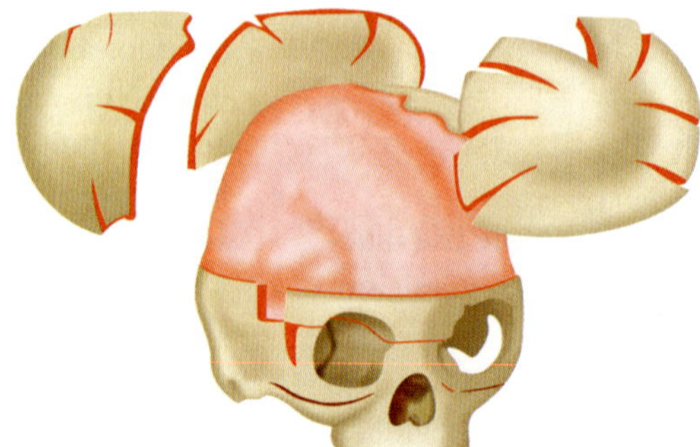

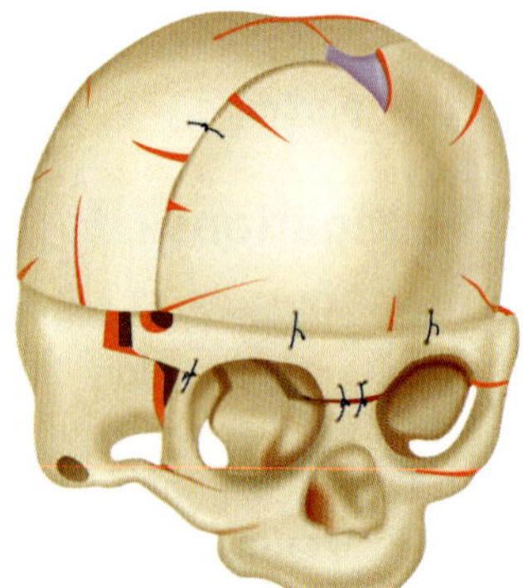

Fig. 40.9: Complete vault reshaping.

40.5 COMPLICATIONS OF TREATMENT

- Possible complications from surgery include but are not limited to: death due to high volume blood loss, wound infection, cerebrospinal fluid (CSF) leak, and persistent asymmetry. Hemostasis during the procedure is critical to minimize blood loss. It is important that the neurosurgeon perform a tight dural closure to prevent postoperative CSF leak. Mild asymmetry may get addressed by applying hydroxyapatite paste, whereas major asymmetry may require revision osteotomies.

REFERENCES

Boulet, S.L., Rasmussen, S.A. and Honein, M.A., 2008. A population-based study of craniosynostosis in metropolitan Atlanta, 1989-2003. *American Journal of Medical Genetics Part A,* 146A, pp. 984-91.

Francel, P.C., 1995. *Evolution of the treatment for sagittal synostosis: a personal record.* New York: Thieme Medical Publisher.

Ghali, G.E., Sinn, D.P. and Tantipasawasin, S., 2002. Management of nonsyndromic craniosynostosis. *Atlas of the Oral and Maxillofacial Surgery Clinics of North America,* 10, pp. 1-41.

Jimenez, D.F. and Barone, C.M., 2010. Endoscopic techniques for craniosynostosis. *Atlas of the Oral and Maxillofacial Surgery Clinics of North America,* 18, pp. 93-107.

Kallen, B. and Robert-Gnansia, E., 2005. Maternal drug use, fertility problems, and infant craniostenosis. *The Cleft Palate-Craniofacial Journal,* 42, pp. 589-93.

Kallen, K., 1999. Maternal smoking and craniosynostosis. *Teratology,* 60, pp. 146-50.

Lajeunie, E., Le Merrer, M., Bonaiti-pellie, C., Marchac, D. and Renier, D., 1995. Genetic study of nonsyndromic coronal craniosynostosis. *American Journal of Medical Genetics,* 55, pp. 500-504.

Lenton, K.A., Nacamuli, R.P., Wan, D.C., Helms, J.A. and Longaker, M.T., 2005. Cranial suture biology. *Current Topics in Developmental Biology,* 66, pp. 287-328.

Panchal, J. and Uttchin, V., 2003. Management of craniosynostosis. *Plastic and Reconstructive Surgery,* 111, pp. 2032-48; quiz 2049.

Pattisapu, J.V., Gegg, C.A., Olavarria, G., Johnson, K.K., Ruiz, R.L. and Costello, B.J., 2010. Craniosynostosis: diagnosis and surgical management. *Atlas of the Oral and Maxillofacial Surgery Clinics of North America,* 18, pp. 77-91.

Warren, S.M., Proctor, M.R., Bartlett, S.P., Blount, J.P., Buchman, S.R., Burnett, W., Fearon, J.A., Keating, R., Muraszko, K.M., Rogers, G.F., Rubin, M.S. and Mccarthy, J.G., 2012. Parameters of care for craniosynostosis: craniofacial and neurologic surgery perspectives. *Plastic and Reconstructive Surgery,* 129, pp. 731-7.

Wilkie, A.O., 1997. Craniosynostosis: genes and mechanisms. *Human Molecular Genetics,* 6, pp. 1647-56.

Index

Note: Page numbers followed by f refer to figure, fc refer to flowchart and t refer to table.

D

E

N

O

P

Q

R

S